Hematopoietic Stem Cell Transplantation

A Manual for Nursing Practice

Edited by
Susan Ezzone, MS, RN, CNP

Authors
Joyce J. Adams, RN, MN
Debra Adornetto, RN, MS
Lowell Anderson-Reitz, RN, MS, ANP, AOCN®
Beth E. Mechling Baumert, RN, MS, CNS, AOCN®
Shelley Burcat, RN, MSN
Mary Reilly Burgunder, RN, BSN, MS, OCN®
Kathleen Clifford, RN, MSN, FNP, CS, AOCN®
Kathleen M. Duffy, RN, MSN, CRNP, BC
Wendy Holmes, RN, PhD
Gail B. Johnson, MSN, RN, AOCN®
Claire A. Keller, RN, MN, OCN®
Frances Walker McAdams, RN, MSN, AOCN®
Sandra A. Mitchell, CRNP, MScN, AOCN®
Joyce L. Neumann, RN, MS, AOCN®
Dawn Niess, MS, RN, CNP
Kimberly Quiett, RN, MSN, AOCN®
Kim Schmit-Pokorny, RN, MSN, OCN®
Sheryl P. Shannon, RN, MSN, OCN®, APRN
Michelle M. Stevens, RN, BS, OCN®
Elizabeth (Beth) Warnick, RN, MSN, CRNP, BC
Lori Williams, RN, MSN, OCN®, AOCN®

Field Reviewers
Linda Z. Abramovitz, RN, MSN
Rosemary C. Ford, RN, BSN, OCN®
Stephanie Jardine, BSN, RN, OCN®
Cathleen Poliquin, MS, APN-BC, AOCN®
Teresa J. Wikle-Shapiro, RN, MSN, CRNP

Oncology Nursing Society
Pittsburgh, PA

ONS Publishing Division
Publisher: Leonard Mafrica, MBA, CAE
Director, Commercial Publishing: Barbara Sigler, RN, MNEd
Production Manager: Lisa M. George, BA
Technical Publications Editor: Dorothy Mayernik, RN, MSN
Staff Editor: Lori Wilson, BA
Graphic Designer: Dany Sjoen

Hematopoietic Stem Cell Transplantation: A Manual for Nursing Practice

Library of Congress Control Number: 2004104799

ISBN 1-890504-41-6

Publisher's Note

This book is published by the Oncology Nursing Society (ONS). ONS neither represents nor guarantees that the practices described herein will, if followed, ensure safe and effective patient care. The recommendations contained in this book reflect ONS's judgment regarding the state of general knowledge and practice in the field as of the date of publication. The recommendations may not be appropriate for use in all circumstances. Those who use this book should make their own determinations regarding specific safe and appropriate patient-care practices, taking into account the personnel, equipment, and practices available at the hospital or other facility at which they are located. The editors and publisher cannot be held responsible for any liability incurred as a consequence from the use or application of any of the contents of this book. Figures and tables are used as examples only. They are not meant to be all-inclusive, nor do they represent endorsement of any particular institution by ONS. Mention of specific products and opinions related to those products do not indicate or imply endorsement by ONS.

ONS publications are originally published in English. Permission has been granted by the ONS Board of Directors for foreign translation. (Individual tables and figures that are reprinted or adapted require additional permission from the original source.) However, because translations from English may not always be accurate or precise, ONS disclaims any responsibility for inaccuracies in words or meaning that may occur as a result of the translation. Readers relying on precise information should check the original English version.

Printed in the United States of America

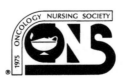

Oncology Nursing Society
Integrity • Innovation • Stewardship • Advocacy • Excellence • Inclusiveness

Contributors

Editor

Susan Ezzone, MS, RN, CNP
Nurse Practitioner, Blood & Marrow Stem Cell Transplant
Arthur G. James Cancer Hospital and Solove Research Institute
The Ohio State University Medical Center
Columbus, Ohio

Authors

Joyce J. Adams, RN, MN
Supervisor of Medical Operations
Case Management
Wellpoint Health Networks
Thousand Oaks, California
Chapter 5: Considerations in Hematopoietic Stem Cell Transplant Program Development and Sites of Care Delivery

Debra Adornetto, RN, MS
Clinical Administrative Director
University of Texas M.D. Anderson Cancer Center
Houston, Texas
Chapter 5: Considerations in Hematopoietic Stem Cell Transplant Program Development and Sites of Care Delivery

Lowell Anderson-Reitz, RN, MS, ANP, AOCN®
Blood & Marrow Transplant Nurse Practitioner
Blood and Marrow Transplant Program
Baylor-Charles A. Sammons Cancer Center
Dallas, Texas
Chapter 9: Hepatorenal Complications of Hematopoietic Stem Cell Transplant

Beth E. Mechling Baumert, RN, MS, CNS, AOCN®
Program Manager
Rocky Mountain Cancer Center
Denver, Colorado
Chapter 9: Hepatorenal Complications of Hematopoietic Stem Cell Transplant

Shelley Burcat, RN, MSN
Clinical Nurse Specialist
Blood and Marrow Transplant Unit
Thomas Jefferson University Hospital
Philadelphia, Pennsylvania
Chapter 16: Current Research and Future Directions in Hematopoietic Stem Cell Transplantation

Mary Reilly Burgunder, RN, BSN, MS, OCN®
Infusion/Oncology Specialty Clinician
University of Pittsburgh Medical Center South Hills Health System Home Health, LP
Formerly Hematopoietic Stem Cell Transplant Program Leader
University of Pittsburgh Medical Center
Pittsburgh, Pennsylvania
Chapter 4: Transplant Course

Kathleen Clifford, RN, MSN, FNP, CS, AOCN®
Nurse Practitioner, Blood and Marrow Transplant Coordinator
St. Luke's Mountain State Tumor Institute
Boise, Idaho
Chapter 5: Considerations in Hematopoietic Stem Cell Transplant Program Development and Sites of Care Delivery

Kathleen M. Duffy, RN, MSN, CRNP, BC
Oncology Clinical Coordinator
Genentech, Inc.
South San Francisco, California
Chapter 2: Basic Concepts of Transplantation

Wendy Holmes, RN, PhD
Clinical Nurse Specialist
Bone Marrow Transplant
University of Massachusetts Medical Center
Worcester, Massachusetts
Chapter 15: Quality-of-Life Issues in Hematopoietic Stem Cell Transplantation

Gail B. Johnson, MSN, RN, AOCN®
Nurse Clinician
Blood and Marrow Transplant Program
Jewish Hospital
Cincinnati, Ohio
Chapter 7: Hematologic Effects

Claire A. Keller, RN, MN, OCN®
BMT Clinical Nurse Specialist
Fairview University Medical Center
Minneapolis, Minnesota
Chapter 10: Cardiopulmonary Effects

Frances Walker McAdams, RN, MSN, AOCN®
Clinical Director for Oncology Services
Temple University Hospital
Philadelphia, Pennsylvania
Chapter 4: Transplant Course

Sandra A. Mitchell, CRNP, MScN, AOCN®
Oncology Nurse Practitioner, National Institutes of Health
Bethesda, Maryland
Faculty Associate, School of Nursing
University of Maryland
Baltimore, Maryland
Chapter 6: Graft Versus Host Disease

Joyce L. Neumann, RN, MS, AOCN®
Program Director, BMT
University of Texas M.D. Anderson Cancer Center
Houston, Texas
Chapter 14: Ethical Considerations in Hematopoietic Stem Cell Transplantation Nursing

Dawn Niess, MS, RN, CNP
Certified Nurse Practitioner and Stem Cell Coordinator
Children's Hospitals and Clinics
St. Paul, Minnesota
Chapter 2: Basic Concepts of Transplantation

Kimberly Quiett, RN, MSN, AOCN®
Assistant Professor of Nursing
University of Mobile
Mobile, Alabama
Chapter 7: Hematologic Effects

Kim Schmit-Pokorny, RN, MSN, OCN®
Manager/PSCT Case Manager
Blood and Marrow Stem Cell Transplantation Program
University of Nebraska Medical Center
Omaha, Nebraska
Chapter 3: Stem Cell Collection

Sheryl P. Shannon, RN, MSN, OCN®, APRN
Nurse Practitioner
Oncology Hematology West, PC
Omaha, Nebraska
Chapter 12: Relapse and Secondary Malignancies Following Hematopoietic Stem Cell Transplantation

Michelle M. Stevens, RN, BS, OCN®
Leukemia/Bone Marrow Transplant Coordinator
Stony Brook University Hospital
Stony Brook, New York
Chapter 8: Gastrointestinal Complications of Hematopoietic Stem Cell Transplantation

Elizabeth (Beth) Warnick, RN, MSN, CRNP, BC
Nurse Practitioner, Stem Cell Transplant Program
Department of Medicine, Division of Hematology-Oncology
University of Pittsburgh Hillman Cancer Center
Pittsburgh, Pennsylvania
Chapter 11: Neurologic Complications

Lori Williams, RN, MSN, OCN®, AOCN®
Graduate Student Research Assistant and Project Manager
University of Texas Health Science Center
School of Nursing at Houston
Houston, Texas
Chapter 1: Comprehensive Review of Hematopoiesis and Immunology
Chapter 13: Post-Transplant Follow-Up

Field Reviewers

Linda Z. Abramovitz, RN, MSN
Clinical Nurse Specialist
Pediatric Bone Marrow Transplant
Children's Hospital at University of California San Francisco Medical Center
San Francisco, California

Rosemary C. Ford, RN, BSN, OCN®
Nurse Manager, Transplant Clinic
Seattle Cancer Care Alliance
Seattle, Washington

Stephanie Jardine, BSN, RN, OCN®
Clinical Research Coordinator
University of Pittsburgh Medical Center
Pittsburgh, Pennsylvania

Cathleen Poliquin, MS, APN-BC, AOCN®
Nurse Practitioner
Massachusetts General Hospital
Boston, Massachusetts

Teresa J. Wikle-Shapiro, RN, MSN, CRNP
Nurse Practitioner, Bone Marrow Transplant Program
University Physicians – University of Arizona
Tucson, Arizona

The Oncology Nursing Society (ONS) would like to thank the editors, authors, and reviewers of the original editions that preceded this new manual:

Manual for Bone Marrow Transplant Nursing: Recommendations for Practice and Education

Editors
Susan Ezzone, RN, MS, OCN®
Dawn Camp-Sorrell, RN, MSN, OCN®

Writers
Joyce Adams, RN, MS
Diane Bell, CRNP, MSN, OCN®
Deborah Brisch-Cramer, RN, OCN®
Mary Burgunder, RN, BSN, OCN®
Mary Callaghan, RN, MS
Deborah Davison, CRNP, MSN
Susan Ezzone, RN, MS, OCN®
Sarah Griffin, RN, BAN
Joanne Howard, RN
Cheryl Lindsay, RN, BSN, OCN®
Teri Nobbs, RN, BAN, OCN®
Margaret Rosenzweig, RN, MS, CRNP, OCN®
Barbara Rutecki, RN, MSN, CRNP
Patricia Schaefer, RN, MDiv, OCN®
Teresa Wickle Shapiro, RN, BA, BSN
Shirley Sutliff, RN, BSN, OCN®

Reviewers
1992–1993 ONS Clinical Practice Committee:
Kim Rumsey, RN, MSN, OCN®, Chair
Cindy Horrell, RN, MSN, OCN®
Mary Mrozek-Orlowski, RN, MSN
Lorrie Powel Schwager, RN, MSN, OCN®
Karen Stanley, RN, MSN, OCN®

Field Reviewers
Tess Artig, RN, BSN
Patricia C. Buchsel, RN, MSN
Mary Ann Crouch, RN, MSN
Rosemary Ford, RN, BA, BS
Ruth Ford, RN, MSN, OCN®

Debra McCorkindale, RN, MS, OCN®
Paula McCue, RN, MA
Jean Nelson, RN, BS, OCN®
Nancy Ohanian, RN, MS, OCN®
Cathleen Poliquin, RN, OCN®
Mary Beth Riley, RN, MSN, OCN®
Marie Whedon, RN, MSN, OCN®

ONS Staff
Bridget Culhane, RN, MN, OCN®
Linda Worrall, RN, BSN, OCN®

Peripheral Blood Stem Cell Transplantation: Recommendations for Nursing Education and Practice

Editor
Susan Ezzone, MS, RN, ANP

Writers
Wendy Holmes, RN, MSN
Pamela M. Kapustay, RN, MSN
Frances Walker, RN, MSN, AOCN®
Lori Williams, RN, MSN, OCN®

Field Reviewers
Patricia C. Buchsel, RN, MSN
Elaine Demeyer, RN, MSN, OCN®
Patricia F. Jassak, MS, RN, OCN®
Cynthia R. King, RN, NP, MSN, PhD(c)
Susan A. O'Connell, MSN, RN, OCN®
Deborah M. Rust, MSN, CRNP, OCN®
Kim Schmit-Pokorny, RN, MSN, OCN®

ONS Staff
Michele R. McCorkle, RN, MSN, OCN®
Barbara A. Sigler, RN, MNEd

Table of Contents

CHAPTER 16. CURRENT RESEARCH AND FUTURE DIRECTIONS IN HEMATOPOIETIC STEM CELL TRANSPLANTATION **249**

Preface

Over the past five decades or more, the use of hematopoietic stem cell transplantation (HSCT) has continued to evolve as a specialty for the treatment of hematologic malignancies, nonmalignant hematologic diseases, and select solid tumors. Each year, new, more advanced, treatment methods and strategies for use of HSCT as a treatment option emerge.

Traditionally, stems cells were collected from the bone marrow, which led to the treatment name *bone marrow transplantation*. Since the mid-80s, the use of stem cells collected from the peripheral blood have become the source used most often with stem cells. Peripheral blood stem cells can be collected and used for autologous, allogeneic, and nonmyeloablative transplant. The umbilical cord also has been identified as a third source of stem cells and is a readily available source of stem cells. Because of the expanded sources for stem cell collection, HSCT usually will be referred to in the book to describe the transplant process.

The Oncology Nursing Society (ONS) and ONS Publishing Division were leaders in publishing two guideline books on transplantation for nurses: *Manual for Bone Marrow Transplant Nursing: Recommendations for Practice and Education* (1994) and *Peripheral Blood Stem Cell Transplantation: Recommendations for Nursing Education and Practice* (1997). As the specialty of HSCT has continued to grow and change, it is now appropriate to combine these two publications into one reference book. This book is intended to provide basic and advanced concepts as well as the most current trends related to the specialty of HSCT.

Acknowledgments

A Note of Thanks

Many individuals have been involved in the development of this resource book for nurses on hematopoietic stem cell transplantation (HSCT). First, thanks to the ONS Publishing Division and ONS Board for their willingness to combine the previous transplant publications into an up-to-date book on HSCT. Thanks for their helpful persistence and patience as each step of the completion of this book was undertaken. Thanks to all the authors who through their expertise in HSCT have developed content that will be an invaluable tool for nurses. Nursing experts in HSCT also served as field reviewers for the book. Thanks to them for sharing their expertise through helpful comments for improvement. Lastly, thanks to my family—husband Jay and children Nathan and Sara—for their understanding, patience, and encouragement during the completion of this project.

Susan Ezzone, MS, RN, CNP
Editor

Comprehensive Review of Hematopoiesis and Immunology: Implications for Hematopoietic Stem Cell Transplant Recipients

Introduction

Hematopoiesis and immunology provide part of the scientific basis for hematopoietic stem cell transplant (HSCT). Hematopoiesis describes the process of blood cell development from pluripotent stem cell to mature blood cell. Immunology is the study of the immune system's response to foreign substances. Because the specialized cells of the immune system develop from hematopoietic stem cells, immune function is partially dependent on hematopoiesis.

Hematopoiesis

Hematopoiesis is the process of growth, division, and differentiation of blood cells. The end products of hematopoiesis are mature red blood cells (RBCs), white blood cells (WBCs), and platelets. RBCs provide all other cells in the body with oxygen necessary for cell respiration and remove from them the cellular waste product, carbon dioxide. WBCs, the foundation of the immune system, defend the body from a variety of foreign invaders that may cause harm. Platelets are vital to hemostasis and the control of bleeding (Lowell, 1997).

CD34+ Cells

Hematopoiesis begins with the most basic and primitive blood cell, the pluripotent hematopoietic stem cell (PHSC). Most PHSCs are found in the bone marrow, although some also circulate in the peripheral blood. Under normal conditions, PHSCs represent no more than 0.01% of the cells in the bone marrow. Morphologically, PHSCs are small cells with round nuclei and little cytoplasm that are similar to some other types of cells in the bone marrow. PHSCs are identified by CD34, a characteristic protein produced on the surface of the cells (Baum, 1994).

CD is an abbreviation for cluster of differentiation. CD is a nomenclature developed to identify proteins or protein complexes that occur on the surface of cells (Wujcik, 1997). The biologic function of a CD protein is usually unknown when it is identified, but it can be differentiated from other proteins by its physical properties. Each identifiable protein or protein complex is given the designation CD followed by a unique number. CD proteins may not be related to each other either structurally or functionally. CD proteins occur most often on the surface of hematopoietic cells. Other immature human hematopoietic cells besides PHSCs express CD34. PHSCs are further identified by the fact that they do not produce the CD38 protein, which is produced by cells more differentiated than PHSCs that express CD34. PHSCs are cells that are CD34+CD38– (Lowell, 1997).

PHSCs are capable of either dividing and producing other PHSCs or developing into committed hematopoietic progenitor cells (HPCs) that become mature blood cells. The capacity to produce other PHSCs is called self-renewal. This ability prevents the depletion of the pool of PHSCs. Rather than self-renewing, PHSCs often become committed to one of several differentiation pathways. These pathways eventually lead to the production of mature blood cells (Ratajczak & Gewirtz, 1995). A typical pathway includes multiple (five or more) cell divisions before a mature blood cell is produced. With each division, cells acquire more of the characteristics of the mature blood cells they will become. Because these pathways progress with cell division, greater numbers of more mature cells are produced, as demonstrated in Figure 1-1. As cells differentiate, their capacity to replicate and self-renew declines. Hematopoietic cells lose the ability to replicate when they are fully mature and are said to be terminally differentiated. Less differentiated cells in a pathway are less common, but they replicate actively. More differen-

Figure 1-1. Hematopoietic Cell Division

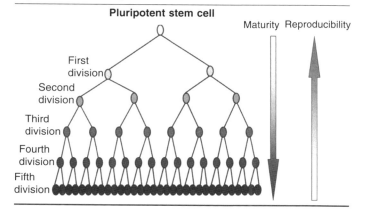

tiated cells are more numerous but reproduce less frequently (Baum, 1994).

It has traditionally been thought that PHSCs and stem cells of other tissues are pluripotent only for their tissue of origin. Embryonic stem cells were known to be totipotent—that is, able to differentiate into cells from all types of tissues (Abkowitz, 2002). However, recent evidence from allogeneic HSCT recipients suggests that PHSCs may be able to differentiate and mature into cells of other tissues. Donor-derived epithelial cells and hepatocytes have been found in biopsy specimens of the skin, gastrointestinal tract, and liver of patients following allogeneic peripheral blood stem cell transplant (PBSCT) and bone marrow transplant (BMT). These cells were found as early as two weeks and as late as one year post-transplant (Korbling et al., 2002). This finding raises the intriguing possibility that tissue-specific stem cells, such as PHSCs, might be stimulated to differentiate into cells of other types of tissues (Abkowitz). Cell replacement therapy with PHSCs for a variety of damaged tissues might be possible in the future (Muller et al., 2002).

Bone Marrow Microenvironment

HPCs and PHSCs cannot reproduce and differentiate alone. They are tightly packed in the marrow space with other cells and substances, which are collectively referred to as the bone marrow microenvironment. The bone marrow microenvironment is critical to the process of hematopoiesis (Sutherland, 2000). Without it, the HPCs and PHSCs would not be able to produce mature blood cells.

The bone marrow microenvironment, also called the bone marrow stroma, is composed of mesenchymal cells, which include fibroblasts, osteoblasts, and endothelial cells, and a three-dimensional extracellular matrix (ECM). In addition, monocytes, basophils, megakaryocytes, and mature cells of lymphoid lineage, including T cells, B cells, and natural killer (NK) cells, move freely in and out of the marrow and are part of the microenvironment. HPCs, PHSCs, and the microenvironment are continuously bathed in a large volume of rapidly circulating RBCs and plasma. The RBCs and plasma continually supply the marrow constituents with large amounts of oxygen and nutrients necessary for hematopoiesis and remove toxic waste products of cellular metabolism (Emerson, Adams, & Taichman, 2000).

The bone marrow microenvironment supports hematopoiesis by secreting cytokines and producing adhesion molecules. Cytokines regulate hematopoiesis. Adhesion molecules hold onto HPCs and PHSCs so that they are exposed to high concentrations of cytokines and experience direct contact with the ECM and with other cells like themselves (Lowell, 1997). Proliferation and maturation of PHSCs and HPCs is facilitated by contact with other cells of the same type and with substances in the ECM. Production of colonies of mature cells by the same type of HPCs tends to occur in close proximity. This causes the bone marrow to appear as discrete areas of the same type of cell rather than as a mixture of all types of cells (Lowell).

Cytokines

Cytokines are a group of polypeptide hormones that control hematopoiesis. Blood cells and bone marrow stromal cells secrete cytokines. They have unique effects on the proliferation, differentiation, and other functions of blood cells. Cytokines may either upregulate or downregulate cell activities, and therefore may be stimulatory or inhibitory at different times or to different cells. The cytokines that have the most influence on hematopoiesis are known as colony-stimulating factors (CSFs) and interleukins (ILs) (Broudy, Kaushansky, Harlan, & Adamson, 1987). The main cytokines that influence PHSC proliferation are interleukin-3 (IL-3), granulocyte macrophage–colony-stimulating factor (GM-CSF), and stem cell factor (SCF) (Lowell, 1997).

During hematopoiesis, cytokines function primarily to promote the growth and survival of lineage-specific cells. The actions of many cytokines overlap or interact (Emerson, Yang, Clark, & Long, 1988). Cytokine control of hematopoiesis should be viewed as a matrix rather than a series of separate actions. Although HPCs deprived of the group of cytokines specific to their lineage often will undergo apoptosis and die, the absence of a single cytokine has much more of an effect on the functioning of mature cells than it has on hematopoiesis (Leary et al., 1988).

All blood cells possess cytokine receptors. Cytokine receptors are made up of three parts: an extracellular portion on the surface of the cell membrane that binds to the cytokine, a transmembrane portion, and an intracellular portion called a cytoplasmic tail. When a cytokine binds to the external portion of the cytokine receptor, a signal is sent to the interior of the cell to initiate a specific cell response by a process called signal transduction. The extracellular portion of cytokine receptors consists of an α-chain, a β-chain, and, in some cases, a γ-chain. The α-chain determines the specificity of the receptor, whereas the β-chain ensures maximal binding. The γ-chain, when it is present, increases the binding ability of the α- and β-chains. Many cytokine receptors share a common chain. This accounts for the overlap in action of cytokines (Lowell, 1997).

The cytoplasmic tail of cytokine receptors contains the enzyme protein tyrosine kinase (PTK). When the cytokine receptor is bound, PTK begins to phosphorylate tyrosine residues in the cytoplasm of the cell. This initiates signal transduction. Most signals are transmitted to the nucleus of the cell by one of two common pathways, the Ras-dependent signaling pathway or the Jak-Stat pathway, and the cytokine-specific cellular response is induced (Lowell, 1997).

Cytokine activity is regulated by several feedback mechanisms. In response to specific stimuli, cells will begin producing a cytokine and will continue to produce it until the stimulus is removed. However, the ability of the cytokine to act can be modulated by substances produced by the cells that the cytokine affects. In response to various cues related to the activity of the cytokine, other cells in the microenvironment also may produce substances to regulate the cytokine activity. Many cytokines have soluble receptors, produced by the cells that they affect. Soluble receptors function to downregulate the action of the cytokine. As more and more cytokine is produced in response to a stimulus, cells acted on by the cytokine begin to produce receptors that break off from the surface of the cell and circulate in the microenvironment with the cytokine. A cytokine that forms a complex with its soluble receptor is not available to bind with receptors on the surface of the cell and stimulate the cell. Cytokine receptor antagonists also exist. These proteins bind with cytokine receptors on the surface of cells and prevent cytokines from binding and stimulating the cell (Oppenheim & Ruscetti, 1994).

Based on studies in animal models, PHSC proliferation appears to occur by processes called clonal succession and quantal mitosis. Clonal succession means that, at any given time, a small number of PHSCs are stimulated to proliferate. This small group of PHSCs replicates through multiple cell divisions, as is seen in Figure 1-1, eventually producing a large number of completely mature blood cells of all types (Reincke, Rosenblatt, & Hellman, 1984). At the same time, by quantal mitosis, only a limited number of pluripotent stem cells are produced in multiple cell divisions (Holtzer et al., 1983). As these PHSCs are completing proliferation, other small groups of PHSCs are being stimulated by cytokines to begin the proliferative process. When a PHSC divides and produces HPCs, each HPC is capable of producing a cluster or colony of mature cells. For this reason, HPCs are sometimes called colony-forming units (CFUs). The type of mature cells produced by the HPC is dependent on the lineage that the HPC is committed to and on the cytokine stimulation it receives (Messner & McCulloch, 1994).

Adhesion Molecules

Large molecules, called adhesion molecules, are found on the surface of HPCs. These molecules are essential to hematopoiesis and allow different types of hematopoietic cells to bind securely to each other or to the bone marrow microenvironment. Adhesion molecules include integrins and selectins (Simmons, Zannettino, Gronthos, & Leavesley, 1994).

Integrins are proteins with an α-chain and a β-chain. There are 15 different α-chains and 7 different β-chains that can combine in various ways to produce adhesion molecules with distinct properties. Integrins may bind with ECM proteins or with proteins on bone marrow stromal cells. They are responsible for the sequestration of HPCs in various areas of the bone marrow. Binding of integrins also may send a signal to proliferate, differentiate, or perform other functions to the HPC expressing the integrin (Lowell, 1997).

Selectins bind to residues of mucin glycoproteins expressed on cell surfaces. CD34, found on PHSCs, is a mucin that binds L-selectin, found on the surface of mature WBCs. HPCs and bone marrow stromal cells produce a variety of selectins and mucins that govern interactions between these types of cells. These cell-to-cell interactions have a profound effect on the process of hematopoiesis (Lowell, 1997).

Cell Proliferation Control and Apoptosis

Cytokines, ECM proteins, and intercellular interactions control the rate at which hematopoietic cells proliferate by cell division. The cell cycle is a sequence of events during which cell division occurs. The four phases of the cell cycle are G_1, S (synthesis of DNA), G_2, and M (mitosis). Certain tasks must be completed before a cell can progress from one phase of the cell cycle to the next and cell division take place. Regulation of cell proliferation occurs mainly at the transition points between phases of the cell cycle. Three types of proteins are directly involved in regulating the passage of cells through the transition points in the cell cycle: cyclins, cyclin-dependent kinases (CDKs), and CDK inhibitors (CDKIs). Cytokines, ECM proteins, and other products of hematopoietic cell interactions stimulate expression of cyclins, CDKs, and CDKIs in different hematopoietic cell lineages at various times (Nussbaum, McInnes, & Williard, 2001). Based on the type of stimulation received, hematopoietic cells will progress through the cell cycle and proliferate or remain in one phase of the cell cycle and not complete cell division (Miyasaki, n.d.).

Apoptosis, or programmed cell death, is critical for rapidly dividing cell populations, such as hematopoietic cells, to maintain appropriate numbers of each type of blood cell. The changes in cells that occur during apoptosis seem to be consistent across most types of cells. The intracellular proteins that appear to control apoptosis are related to the oncoprotein Bcl2. Certain cytokines regulate apoptosis by stimulating or inhibiting expression of Bcl2 proteins. As new cells are produced, other cells of the same type are stimulated to die so that the total number of each type of cell present in the body remains in the correct range (Snustad & Simmons, 2000).

Hematopoietic Cell Lineages

Initially, HPCs belong to one of two main differentiation pathways, also called lineages, the myeloid and the lymphoid. As cell division and maturation occur, the cells of the myeloid lineage divide into both the myeloid and erythroid lineages. The earliest forms of each cell lineage cannot be identified by structure and appearance, but biologic assays allow inference of their existence. Cells of myeloid lineage comprise 60% of marrow cells; erythroid lineage cells account for 25% of marrow cells; and lymphoid lineage cells make up the remaining 15% of marrow cells (Lowell, 1997). Mature cells of the myeloid lineage include neutrophils, monocytes, mast cells, eosinophils, NK cells, dendritic cells, and megakaryocytes.

Large numbers of blood cells are continually produced by the PHSCs in the bone marrow. In general, as cells proceed down the pathway to full maturity, they are released into the blood stream. However, under normal conditions, 10%–20% of marrow cells will be mature neutrophils, stored in the marrow and available for rapid mobilization if needed to defend against foreign invaders. Both processes of blood cell production and release into the blood stream are carefully controlled in response to physiologic needs (Emerson et al., 2000). This control is exerted by the interaction of PHSCs and HPCs with other cells and soluble factors in the tissues where hematopoietic cells reside.

PHSCs are stimulated to proliferate and differentiate by a variety of cytokines. To induce proliferation and differentiation into the myeloid lineage, PHSCs are stimulated primarily by IL-1, IL-3, IL-6, SCF, and granulocyte–colony-stimulating factor (G-CSF). IL-1, IL-6, SCF, and *fms*-like tyrosine kinase-3 ligand (FLT-3L) induce proliferation and differentiation into the lymphoid lineage (Kripps, 2001).

Red Blood Cells

The average number of red cells in the circulation of normal adult males is 4.6–6.2 x 10^6/μl, and normal adult females is 4.1–5.4 x 10^6/μl (Wujcik, 1997). RBCs are released into the blood stream from the bone marrow in a slightly immature form, called a reticulocyte. A reticulocyte still contains a few remnants of intracellular structures. Final maturation of reticulocytes occurs in the circulation over one to two days. When fully mature, RBCs no longer contain any intracellular structures. The larger the percentage of reticulocytes in the peripheral circulation, the more actively the bone marrow is producing new cells. RBCs have the longest life span of any blood cell and may remain in circulation for up to four months. RBC production is stimulated primarily by erythropoietin, a cytokine produced by the kidney. IL-3 and GM-CSF play minor roles in erythropoiesis (Kripps, 2001).

Platelets

Platelets, responsible for clotting and hemostasis, are not actually cells themselves. Rather, they are small fragments of cytoplasm from megakaryocytes. Although megakaryocytes are a mature cell of the myeloid lineage, they do not circulate in the blood stream. Rather, they remain in the bone marrow and release platelets. The average number of platelets circulating in a normal adult is 150,000–350,000/μl (Wujcik, 1997). Platelets possess the ability to secrete both microbicidal and clotting substances. This allows platelets to take an active role in the immediate defense against microbial invaders at the site of an injury (Miyasaki, n.d.). Platelets remain in circulation for four to seven days. Megakaryocyte production is controlled by the cytokines IL-3 and IL-11 (Kripps, 2001).

White Blood Cells

Two lineages of hematopoietic cells produce different kinds of WBCs. The primary function of all WBCs, regardless of lineage, is to protect the body from foreign invaders that may be harmful. Mature WBCs from the myeloid lineage include neutrophils, eosinophils, basophils, monocytes, dendritic cells, and mast cells. Neutrophils are the most common type of myeloid WBC. Out of a total of 5,000–11,000/μl WBCs, the average adult under normal conditions will have approximately 3,000–6,000/μl circulating neutrophils. The other WBCs of myeloid lineage combined make up less than 15% of the total number of WBCs. The remaining circulating WBCs come from the lymphoid lineage. They include T lymphocytes, B lymphocytes, and NK cells (Wujcik, 1997).

WBC production is primarily stimulated by inflammation or infection (Miyasaki, n.d.). The cytokines IL-3 and GM-CSF provide stimulus for myeloid WBC production throughout the entire proliferation and differentiation process, whereas G-CSF plays an important role in the later stages of neutrophil maturation (Kripps, 2001). Macrophage colony-stimulating factor, IL-4, and IL-5 stimulate later maturation of monocytes, basophils, and eosinophils, respectively. Lymphoid WBC production is stimulated in the B cell lineage primarily by IL-1, IL-2, IL-4, IL-5, and IL-6. In the T cell lineage, lymphoid WBC production is stimulated primarily by IL-2 and IL-4 (Kripps).

Age-Dependent Hematopoiesis

Hematopoiesis varies across the life span. During fetal development, most hematopoiesis occurs in the liver and is devoted to red cell development. Platelet production does not begin until the third month of gestation, and WBCs are not produced until the fifth month of gestation. As bones form prior to birth, the marrow cavities are produced with a network of epithelial cells called bone marrow stroma. Shortly before birth, PHSCs fully populate the marrow cavities. During childhood, much hematopoiesis occurs in the long bones. By adulthood, hematopoiesis occurs almost exclusively in the axial skeleton, pelvis, vertebrae, ribs, sternum, and skull. However, if the bone marrow is injured at any age, hematopoiesis can resume in the liver and spleen. This is referred to as extramedullary hematopoiesis (Nussbaum et al., 2001).

Immunology

The immune system is a complex network of cells, tissues, and organs with an intricate communication structure that protects the body from invasion by foreign organisms. The immune system initially attempts to protect the body by preventing entry by foreign organisms. When organisms overcome the immune system and gain entry, the body's defenses go into action to seek and destroy the invaders. The immune system displays both diversity and specificity to control and eliminate all possible threats. The elaborate communication network activates and regulates the functioning of the various components of the immune system to effectively control an invasion .

Antigens are substances capable of being recognized by the immune system and triggering immune system responses. Epitopes protrude from the surface of antigens and allow the immune system to recognize antigens as foreign substances. This recognition leads to the initiation of an immune response. Epitopes may be more or less effective in initiating an immune response, depending on how foreign and threatening they appear to the immune system (Schlinder, Kerrigan, & Kelly, 2003).

Organs of the Immune System

Organs of the immune system are involved with production, maturation, and activity of immune cells. Bone marrow produces WBCs, which are the basic cells of the immune system. The thymus, a butterfly-shaped organ located behind the sternum, is involved in the maturation of certain WBCs. The lymphatic vessels and blood vessels provide immune transportation systems (Parslow, 1997; Parslow & Bainton, 1997).

There are multiple organs in which WBCs meet and interact with each other and with antigens. They are strategically located to intercept invaders and allow immune cells to efficiently eliminate the invaders. Lymph nodes are encapsulated organs located along the lymphatic vessels. The spleen is also an encapsulated lymphoid organ located in the abdomen. It screens the blood for foreign substances. Nonencapsulated lymphoid organs include the tonsils and adenoids in the upper respiratory tract and Peyers patches and the appendix in the abdomen (Schlinder et al., 2003).

Cells of the Immune System

WBCs are the primary cells of the immune system. WBCs include lymphocytes, phagocytes, and dendritic cells.

Lymphocytes

An adult has about 1×10^{12} lymphocytes. There are two basic types of lymphocytes: B cells and T cells. B cells are produced and mature in the bone marrow and are responsible for humoral immunity that is mediated by antibodies. B cells have two primary functions, to present antigens to T cells and to produce antibodies. When a B cell is stimulated to produce its antibody, it may develop into a plasma cell, which is a large cell that produces large amounts of a particular antibody (Snustad & Simmons, 2000).

Antibodies, also called immunoglobulins, are specific soluble proteins that bind to specific antigens. Antibodies can defend the body against antigens in several different ways.

- Direct inactivation of toxins (This type of antibody is called an antitoxin.)
- Blockage of viruses from entering host cells
- Release of complement, a group of lethal serum enzymes, by antigen-antibody complexes
- Coating (opsinizing) invaders to make them more attractive to scavenger cells
- Coating invaders to increase vulnerability to attack by killer WBCs (antibody-dependent cell-mediated cytotoxicity) (Schlinder et al., 2003)

Antibodies are Y-shaped structures that contain two light chains and two heavy chains. The molecular configuration of the upper part of the Y varies to match a specific antigen. The molecular configuration of the tail of the Y is constant based on the class of the immunoglobulin. It matches the immune system components to which it relates. There are five known classes of immunoglobulins: IgG, IgA, IgM, IgE, and IgD. The primary actions of the classes of antibodies are listed in Table 1-1 (Schlinder et al., 2003; Snustad & Simmons, 2000).

Table 1-1. Action of Immunoglobulins

Immunoglobulin	Number of Kinds	Action
IgG	4	Coat invaders to speed uptake by other immune cells in the blood
IgA	2	Concentrate in body fluids to protect guard entrances to body
IgM	1	Link together in blood stream to kill invaders
IgE	1	Participate in allergic reactions
IgD	1	Regulate cell activation on B cell membranes

T cells are produced in the bone marrow and then travel to the thymus to complete maturation. They are responsible for cell-mediated immunity. There are three main types of T cells: regulatory, cytotoxic, and NK cells. Regulatory T cells are vital to the proper function of the immune system. There are two primary types of regulatory T cells: helper/inducer cells and suppressor cells. Helper/inducer T cells also are called T4 cells and carry the CD4 antigen on the surfaces of their cell membranes (Snustad & Simmons, 2000). T4 cells initiate an immune response by activating B cells, other T cells, NK cells, and macrophages. Equally as important are suppressor cells that can stop an immune response when it is no longer needed. Suppressor cells are called T8 cells and carry the CD8 antigen on their cell surfaces. These cells produce substances called lymphokines that signal activated immune cells to become inactive or stop responding to activation signals (Snustad & Simmons).

Cytotoxic T cells also have the CD8 antigen on their cell surfaces. They are programmed to recognize a specific antigen. These antigens may identify cells that have been infected with a virus, malignant cells, or cells from foreign tissues and organs. When a cytotoxic T cell recognizes an antigen on a cell, it kills the cell on contact (Snustad & Simmons, 2000).

The final type of T cell is the NK cell. Unlike cytotoxic T cells, NK cells do not need to come to contact with a specific antigen before acting. Once stimulated in act, they will directly destroy any foreign cell, including tumor cells and microorganisms. NK cells also secrete large amounts of lymphokines that regulate immune system function (Schlinder et al., 2003).

Lymphokines

Lymphokines are cytokines that are secreted by lymphocytes or that act on lymphocytes. They are very important to immune system communication and function. Table 1-2 lists some of the more common lymphokines, the primary secretory cell, the target cell, and the action of the lymphokine.

Phagocytes

There are two main types of phagocyte WBCs: monocyte/macrophages and granulocytes. Monocytes are scavenger cells in the blood stream, and macrophages are scavenger

Table 1-2. Common Lymphokines, Secretory Cells, Target Cells, and Actions

Lymphokine	Primary Secretory Cells	Primary Target Cells	Action
Interferon-alpha	T cells, macrophages	Macrophages	Activates macrophages and inflammatory responses
Lymphotoxin	Lymphocytes	Tumor cells	Kills tumor cells
Tumor necrosis factor	Macrophages, T cells	B cells, T cells	Kills tumor cells, inhibits parasites and viruses, activates cells, induces inflammatory response
IL-1	Macrophages, B cells	B cells, T cells	Activates cells, induces inflammatory response, stimulates cell proliferation
IL-2	T cells, natural killer cells	B cells, T cells	Stimulates clonal expansion and cell maturation
IL-3	T cells	Immature precursor cells	Stimulates cell proliferation
IL-4	T cells	B cells, T cells, macrophages	Stimulates proliferation and differentiation, induces major histocompatibility complex class II expression, inhibits proinflammatory cytokine production
IL-5	T cells	Eosinophils	Stimulates cell proliferation and activation
IL-6	B cells, T cells	B cells	Stimulates cell differentiation
IL-7	Thymic and bone marrow stromal cells	T cells, macrophages	Stimulates cell proliferation and activation
IL-8	Macrophages	B cells, T cells, neutrophils	Enhances cell migration into tissues and chemotaxis
IL-9	T cells	T4 cells	Inhibits apoptosis
IL-10	B cells, T cells, macrophages	B cells, macrophages	Inhibits antigen presentation, inflammatory cytokine production, and cell activation
IL-11	Bone marrow stromal cells	Hematopoietic progenitor cells	Stimulates hematopoiesis and thrombopoiesis
IL-12	B cells, macrophages	Macrophages, natural killer cells	Stimulates cell-mediated immunity (Gazzinelli, Hieny, Wynn, Wolf, & Sher, 1993; Scott, 1993)
IL-13	T cells	B cells	Stimulates cell differentiation
IL-14	B cells, T cells	B cells	Stimulates cell proliferation
IL-15	Monocytes	B cells, T cells	Stimulates clonal expansion and cell maturation
IL-16	T cells	T4 cells	Attracts cells and stimulates cell differentiation
IL-18	Monocytes, macrophages	T4 cells	Stimulates interferon-alpha production

Note. Based on information from Oppenheim & Ruscetti, 1994; Roitt, Brostoff, & Male, 1996.

cells in the tissues (Parslow & Bainton, 1997). Monocyte/macrophages also present antigen to T cells, secrete monokines that stimulate and regulate immune system function, and have numerous lymphokine receptors to permit them to respond to signals from other WBCs (Snustad & Simmons, 2000). Granulocytes include neutrophils, basophils, and eosinophils, which circulate in the blood stream, and mast cells, which are found in tissues. Granulocytes digest any invader that they encounter. Neutrophils primarily attack microorganisms, especially bacteria and fungi, whereas basophils respond to environmental antigens and eosinophils defend against parasites (Parslow & Bainton).

Dendritic Cells

The final type of WBC is a dendritic cell. Dendritic cells have no capacity to destroy invaders directly but are extremely efficient at presenting antigens to other immune system cells so that an immune response can be initiated and the invaders destroyed (Schlinder et al., 2003).

Immune System Activity

Immune responses can be nonspecific or specific. Nonspecific responses are carried out by cells that respond to an invader without regard to the characteristics of the antigens that the invader carries. Nonspecific responses provide the diversity of the immune system and usually are the first action by the immune system against an invasion. Granulocytes and NK cells are primarily responsible for nonspecific immune responses (Snustad & Simmons, 2000).

Specific immune responses can be cell-mediated or humoral. In these responses, immune system cells must recognize a specific antigen before they react. Specific responses give the immune system a high degree of specificity. This specificity causes them to take longer to initiate than nonspecific responses but allows a more sustained assault on an invader without exhausting the rest of the body and causing excessive harm to normal tissues and organs. In a cell-mediated immune response, a macrophage initially recognizes an antigen and digests it. The macrophage then presents to T cells the antigen attached to a glycoprotein molecule produced by genes of the major histocompatibility complex (MHC) (Snustad & Simmons, 2000). If the antigen is attached to a class I MHC molecule, it will be recognized by and activate cytotoxic T8 cells. The activated T8 cells will kill invaders expressing the antigen and cells infected with the invader on contact. If the antigen is attached to a class II MHC molecule, it will be recognized by and activate T4 cells. When activated by the antigen presented with a class II MHC molecule, the T4 cells will secrete lymphokines that stimulate T cell growth, attract other immune cells to the area, and regulate the immune response to the invader (Nussbaum et al., 2001). Once the invasion has been controlled, suppressor T8 cells will be activated by lymphokines from the T4 cells to turn off the immune response (Snustad & Simmons).

B cells initiate a humoral immune response when they recognize a specific antigen that matches receptors on their cell surface. The B cells will take in the antigen, process it, and present the antigen with a class II MCH molecule to T4 cells. When the B cells enlist the help of the T4 cells, the T4 cells secrete lymphokines that cause clonal expansion of the B cells, which produce antibodies to the specific antigen. As the B cells produce and release antibody, antigen-antibody complexes are formed that initiate the complement cascade. Complement is a group of powerful blood proteins that will destroy bacteria, produce inflammation, and regulate the immune reaction. Antigen attached to antibody in an antigen-antibody complex is removed in the liver or spleen (Snustad & Simmons, 2000).

Genetic Basis of Immunity

Mapping of the human genome has greatly increased the knowledge of the human immune system while uncovering increased complexity that is not yet fully understood (Nussbaum et al., 2001). Genes responsible for human immunity in the MHC were some of the earliest genes identified (Bach & Amos, 1967). They provided understanding of the great variations, called polymorphisms, which are present in some human genes. These polymorphisms allow the immune system to display great diversity over relatively few chromosomal loci (Nussbaum et al.).

The MHC is located on the short arm of chromosome 6 (Roitt, Brostoff, & Male, 1996). Some of the MHC genes en-code glycoproteins called human leukocyte antigens (HLAs). Because HLAs are unique to the individual, they permit identification of self from nonself. This is how the body is able to identify invaders that do not belong in the body. Invaders can be substances that come from outside of the body, but they can also be cells from the body, called somatic cells, that have undergone a malignant transformation. The main function of HLAs is to present portions of foreign antigens to immune cells to facilitate the destruction of the invaders (Roitt et al.). The MHC genes that produce HLAs often are referred to as the HLA genes. HLA genes are clinically important to BMT because of their critical role in immunocompetence and because of their involvement in transplant rejection, graft verses host disease (GVHD), and the development of self-tolerance (Nussbaum et al., 2001).

Determination of the HLA alleles of an individual is called HLA typing. It is done to uniquely identify individuals and to facilitate and predict outcomes of cell, tissue, and organ transplantation. HLA typing traditionally has been performed by serologically identifying HLA protein expression on WBCs. This testing is accomplished by mixing sera-containing antibodies to specific HLAs (Nussbaum et al., 2001). Production of antigen-antibody complexes is evidence that the specific HLA is produced by WBCs. This type of testing identifies the phenotype of the individual but not the genotype. However, advances in molecular biology now permit routine molecular identification of HLA alleles. Molecular identification permits more precise identification of the individual's HLA type. Some HLA alleles will appear serologically identical when they are not molecularly identical. Although some of these molecular variations in HLA alleles are not clinically significant, others can have important implications for outcomes in BMT and solid organ transplantation, such as graft rejection and GVHD (Petersdorf et al., 2001). This technology also allows the use of cells that can be obtained noninvasively, such as cheek or hair cells, for HLA typing.

MHC genes have been divided into three classes based on structural and functional similarities and differences. The class I and II genes are the HLA genes (Nussbaum et al., 2001). There are three major class I HLA genes, identified as HLA-A, -B, and -C, which can be found at the A, B, and C loci in the MHC. Class I HLA genes are very polymorphic and are expressed on virtually all nucleated cells in the body. There are three major class II HLA genes, identified as HLA-DR, -DP, and –DQ, which are found at the DR, DP, and DQ loci in the MHC. The DR locus is divided into 10 subregions, DRA and DRB1 to DRB9. The DQ locus is divided into two subregions, DQA1 and DQB1. The DP locus is divided into two subregions, DPA1 and DPB1. Class II HLAs are expressed on only a select set of antigen-presenting immune system cells, such as B cells, macrophages, and activated T cells. HLA-A, -B, and -DR have been found to be especially important in predicting the success and complications of allogeneic BMT (Nussbaum et al.). In addition to the major class I and class II HLAs, minor histocompatibility antigens may have a significant effect on HSCT outcomes. The exact nature and function of these antigens is less well understood than that of the major antigens (Morishima et al., 2002). The class III MHC genes are very diverse. They are not involved with histocompatibility, although some of the proteins they encode, such as complement, are involved in immunity (Snustad & Simmons, 2000).

As more has been understood about HLA allele polymorphism, the naming of HLA alleles has become more complex. When HLA alleles were identified serologically, they were designated by the letter of their gene and the number of the allele, such as HLA-A1 or HLA-B37. When HLA alleles are identified molecularly, the name consists of
- HLA, for the HLA region
- The name of the HLA gene or locus
- Two digits for the group number of alleles that encode a particular antigen
- Two digits for the number of the specific allele.

An example of this designation is HLA-A*0103. This identifies the third HLA-A allele in the 01 group. Some alleles will have an N added to their designation, for example HLA-B*1307N. This indicates that the allele is a null allele with a mutation that makes it incapable of producing an antigen. Some alleles will have a fifth digit in their designation. This number indicates that there are synonymous mutations in the allele (Marsh, 2003). A synonymous mutation is one that has a point mutation in a single nucleotide that does not change the amino acid that is coded for by the codon of which the nucleotide is a member. This is possible because more than one codon triplet can code for a single amino acid. An example of synonymous mutation designations are HLA-DRB1*03011 and HLA-DRB1*03012. Finally, an allele may have a sixth and seventh digit that indicates that the allele contains a mutation outside of the coding region of the gene. This mutation may have no effect on the protein expression of the gene, or it may affect the part of the gene that regulates protein expression (Marsh). An example of these designations are HLA-B*4006101 and HLA-B*4006102.

The number of currently recognized HLA alleles for each major HLA gene and loci , as of October 2003, are in Table 1-3. Recognized HLA alleles are updated frequently. Internet resources for information on HLA typing and listings of currently recognized HLA alleles are in Table 1-4.

Some HLA alleles are very common in all populations, and others are very rare. Some HLA alleles are also common in certain ethnic populations and rare in others. Ethnic tendencies in HLA inheritance can make HLA matching with an unrelated transplant donor difficult among members of ethnic minorities or people with mixed ethnic heritage (Nussbaum et al., 2001). The HLA loci are very close together on chromosome 6. There is a strong tendency for HLA genes to be inherited together as a haplotype rather than as single genes. Crossovers occur occasionally, especially between class I and II genes. HLA genes also exhibit linkage disequilibria, with certain combinations of genes tending to occur much more frequently than would be expected by chance. HLA genes are co-dominant, with each gene normally encoding a functional protein (Nussbaum et al.).

Table 1-3. Major Recognized Human Leukocyte Antigen Alleles

HLA Gene or Locus	Number of Recognized Alleles
A	290
B	553
C	140
DRA	3
DRB1	354
DRB2	1
DRB3	39
DRB4	12
DRB5	17
DRB6	3
DRB7	2
DRB8	1
DRB9	1
DQA1	25
DQB1	56
DPA1	20
DPB1	106

Note. Based on information from Marsh, 2003.

Each nucleated human cell has two HLA haplotypes, one inherited from the mother and the other inherited from the father. Aside from monozygotic twins, who share exactly the same HLA haplotype, full siblings are most likely to share the same HLA haplotypes because they come from the same gene pool. As can be seen in Figure 1-2, there is a one in four chance of full siblings having the same haplotype. Except in cases of coincidence or consanguinity, children and parents will only share single haplotypes (Nussbaum et al., 2001).

The Immune System and Hematopoietic Stem Cell Transplantation

Immune Reconstitution Post-Transplant

Recovery of the immune system following PBSCT or BMT is slow. WBC engraftment occurs fairly promptly, usually within the first three weeks after transplant for PBSCT and the first four weeks for BMT. The average time to engraftment for umbilical cord blood cells is three to four weeks (Lewis, 2002). However, recovery of humoral and cell-mediated immunity with full lymphocyte function takes much longer. This accounts for patient susceptibility to viral and opportunistic infections for several months after autologous transplant and for many months to years after allogeneic transplant. A decrease in the CD4/CD8 lymphocyte ratio occurs very quickly after transplant. For autologous transplant, this decrease starts one week post-transplant, nadirs at approxi-

Table 1-4. Internet Resources for Information on HLA Typing and Currently Recognized Alleles

Resource	URL
American Society for Histocompatibility and Immunogenetics	www.ashi-hla.org
Bone Marrow Donors Worldwide	www.bmdw.org
International Immunogenetics Project	www.ebi.ac.uk/imgt/hla
Anthony Nolan Trust	www.anthonynolan.org.uk/HIG/index.html
National Marrow Donor Program	www.nmdpresearch.org/index.html
Online Mendelian Inheritance in Man (OMIM)	www.ncbi.nlm.nih.gov/entrez/query.fcgi?db=OMIM

mately three weeks post-transplant, and starts to recover two months post-transplant. However, the ratio remains abnormally low for approximately one year post-transplant (Steingrimsdottir, Gruber, Bjorkholm, Svensson, & Hansson, 2000). Patients who receive CD34+ selected autologous PBSCTs experience more immune dysfunction post-transplant than patients receiving unselected autologous PBSCTs (Sica et al., 2001). For allogeneic transplant, the decrease starts slightly later, at about two weeks post-transplant, does not nadir until two months post-transplant, and does not begin to show recovery until more than three months post-transplant (Marin et al., 1999). NK cells are elevated post-transplant. In autologous transplant, they are increased by the first week post-transplant. They continue to rise and peak at approximately two months post-transplant. Although not back to normal, they are beginning to decline at three months post-transplant. In allogeneic transplantation, NK cells begin to increase approximately three weeks post-transplant. They usually peak about two months post-transplant, but they do not begin to decline until well after three months post-transplant (Marin et al.). B cells are severely depressed following both autologous and allogeneic transplant and do not start to recover until more than three months after transplant regardless of the stem cell source. T cell depletion to prevent GVHD, HLA mismatch between the donor and recipient, immunosuppressive therapy, and GVHD all contribute to the length of time and severity of immune dysfunction post-allogeneic transplantation. The type of cells used for transplantation (e.g., peripheral blood stem cells, bone marrow) do not seem to influence immune system dysfunction or recovery post-transplant (Marin et al.).

Human Leukoctye Antigen Matching and HSCT

Prior to establishment of donor hematopoiesis, recognition of donor stem cells by immunocompetent host T cells can cause failed, delayed, or inadequate engraftment of donor hematopoietic stem cells. Eradication of the host immune system and immunologic similarity between the pa-

tient and donor is important to ensure strong donor engraftment (Janeway, Travers, Walport, & Shlomchik, 2001).

Once donor hematopoietic stem cell engraftment has occurred, immunocompetent donor T cells may recognize host cells as foreign and may attempt to destroy them. This process begins prior to the HSCT with the administration of a high-dose conditioning regimen for the transplant. This regimen causes extensive damage to host cells with the release of a cascade of inflammatory cytokines and increased expression of MHC antigens in the recipient (Krenger, Hill, & Ferrara, 1997). When donor T cells become established in the host, they are stimulated by recognition of foreign host antigens and become activated and proliferate (Goker, Haznedaroglu, & Chao, 2001). It is important that the patient and donor be as immunologically similar as possible to prevent this potentially fatal complication, referred to as GVHD (Morishima et al., 2002).

Immunocompetent donor T cells can induce immune-mediated antimalignancy effects, if the donor cells can recognize the tumor cells as foreign. This effect, referred to as graft versus tumor (GVT) effect, has been clinically established in certain hematologic malignancies and in some solid tumors amenable to immunologic interventions (Childs, 2002). It is the most potent form of cancer immunotherapy currently available and is potentially curative. The power of the GVT effect to control or eliminate malignant cells is currently being tested in nonmyeloablative HSCTs (Champlin et al., 2000).

Mismatches of HLA alleles between patient and donor in allogeneic HSCT, which lead to disparities of major and minor histocompatibility antigens, are responsible for transplant outcomes such as GVHD, engraftment failure, or GVT effects (Morishima et al., 2002). Traditionally, candidates and potential donors for allogeneic HSCT have been matched at HLA-A, -B, and -DR (Nussbaum et al., 2001). The

Figure 1-2. Possible HLA Haplotype Inheritance Combinations Without Occurrence of Crossovers

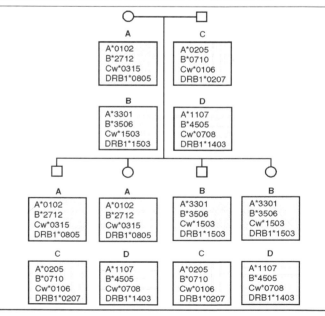

HLA typing for allogeneic HSCT has been performed serologically for HLA-A and -B and serologically or molecularly for HLA-DR (Morishima et al.). Genomic sequencing was performed retrospectively for HLA-A, -B, -C, -DRB1, and -DQB1 on 1,298 recipient-donor pairs after allogeneic HSCT, which was based on serological HLA-A, -B, and -DR typing. HLA-A, -B, -C, and DRB1 molecular disparities were found to be independent and significant factors for the development of severe acute GVHD. Although mismatching at HLA-C had less effect alone on the development of severe acute GVHD than mismatching of HLA-A or HLA-B, it was synergistic with other mismatches in the development of severe acute GVHD. Severe acute GVHD in patients with a single HLA-C molecular mismatch was more responsive to treatment than severe acute GVHD associated with other mismatches (Morishima et al.). Chronic GVHD, a syndrome of immune dysfunction that results in immunodeficiency and autoimmunity, appears to be closely related to class I HLA genes. Mismatching at HLA-A and -B was significantly correlated with the development of chronic GVHD, whereas mismatching at HLA-C showed a nonsignificant tendency to an increased incidence of chronic GVHD. The incidence of graft failure was very low among these patients. No single allele mismatch was significantly correlated with graft failure, but molecular mismatches in general increased the risk of graft failure. HLA-A and -B molecular mismatches resulted in significantly poorer overall survival (Morishima et al.). In patients with leukemia, HLA-C molecular mismatches have been found to reduce leukemic relapse (Sasazuki et al., 1998). Patients with single HLA-C molecular mismatches did not have poorer overall survival than patients with no mismatches. The increased incidence of severe acute GVHD related to the mismatch was offset by the reduced rate of relapse and the responsiveness to treatment of the acute GVHD. Multiple HLA molecular mismatches that included HLA-C mismatches also had significantly poorer overall survival (Morishima et al.). Molecular mismatches at both class I and II antigens have not been found to be synergistic for the development of severe acute GVHD, but they do result in poorer overall survival than mismatches in a single class of antigens (Petersdorf et al., 1998).

Other Immunologic Factors Associated With GVHD

Recently genetic predispositions, unrelated to the closeness of the HLA match, have been postulated to influence the occurrence of GVHD. The initial phase of GVHD is stimulated by proinflammatory lymphokines, including tumor necrosis factor (TNF). A polymorphism in the gene of the HSCT recipient that encodes TNF and results in increased levels of TNF in response to tissue damage, such as that caused by preparative regimens, has been associated with increased acute GVHD (Middleton, Taylor, Jackson, Proctor, & Dickinson, 1998). In addition, a second polymorphism has been identified in the gene that encodes IL-10, which downregulates the affects of TNF. This polymorphism in genes in both recipients and donors that results in decreased levels of IL-10 also has been associated with increased severe acute GVHD (Middleton et al.; Socie et al., 2001) and early mortality following allogeneic HSCT (Cavet et al., 1999). A polymorphism in a recipient gene that encodes for the inflammatory lymphokine IL-6 and causes increased levels of IL-6 is associated with increased risk for the development of chronic GVHD (Socie et al.). Cell surface receptors to IL-2 and IL-6 are increased on peripheral blood mononuclear cells in patients with acute GVHD and graft failure following allogeneic HSCT (Tanaka et al., 1995). Polymorphisms in these and other genes that encode lymphokines and their receptors may help to explain some of the differences in the occurrence of acute GVHD that cannot be explained by disparities in HLA matching.

Approximately 10 years ago, a major shift occurred in the source of cells for HSCT from bone marrow to peripheral blood. The shift initially began in autologous transplantation because of a concern for increased acute GVHD in allogeneic transplants (Tayebi, Kuttler, et al., 2001). Peripheral blood stem cells are almost always collected following mobilization with a CSF. The total number of mononuclear cells as well as T cells is increased approximately 10-fold in a peripheral blood stem cell product for transplant. The increase in T cells infused during the transplant led to concern for an increased risk of GVHD. Experience has shown no increased incidence of acute GVHD following allogeneic PBSCT; however, the incidence of chronic GVHD is higher (Blaise et al., 2000). It is now known that both quantitative and qualitative differences exist in the lymphocytes infused in a BMT versus a PBSCT. Approximately 10 times as many suppressor T cells are present in BMT as compared to PBSCT. The sheer volume of these cells may be enough to suppress the inflammatory reactions associated with severe acute GVHD (Tayebi, Kuttler, et al.). Mobilization with G-CSF also decreases the number of activated T cells that are infused with peripheral blood compared with the number infused with bone marrow (Tayebi, Tiberghien, et al., 2001). Suppressor T cells have a longer life span than activated T cells, which would help to explain no increased incidence of acute GVHD but an increased incidence of chronic GVHD (Tayebi, Kuttler, et al.).

Recently, attempts have been made to take advantage of GVT effects while decreasing the toxicity of extremely high-dose myeloablative preparative regimens. Preparative regimens that are highly immunosuppressive but nonmyeloablative will allow engraftment of donor hematopoietic stem cells. This therapy has potential usefulness for patients of advanced age or in poor physical condition who are unable to withstand the toxicity of extremely high-dose myeloablative preparative regimens used for standard allogeneic HSCTs. However, this therapy is not practical or effective for malignant disease with a large tumor burden (Champlin et al., 2000).

Strong antitumor responses have been observed following nonmyeloablative stem cell transplant (NST) in some hematologic malignancies. For reasons that are not completely understood, some malignant diseases are more amenable to this immunologic approach than others. Research is ongoing in hematologic malignancies and some solid tumors that are known to be responsive to immunologic interventions (Baron & Beguin, 2002). GVT effects have been observed between one and nine months post-NST in patients with metastatic renal cell carcinoma (Childs et al., 2000). One complete response has lasted for four-and-a-half years (Childs, 2002). Acute GVHD is positively associated with a GVT effect. However, it is not required for GVT to occur. This indicates that distinct populations of T cells that are able to recognize and respond to tumor-specific antigens are involved in GVT (Childs).

When a myeloablative preparative regimen is not used, there may be some degree of autologous hematopoietic recovery. This situation of mixed chimerism, in which both donor and recipient hematopoietic stem cells are present in the bone marrow, increases the immunologic tolerance between host and donor cells and decreases the risk of GVHD. However, a mix of donor and recipient cells may increase donor tolerance of tumor cells and decrease GVT effects. In addition, a mix of donor and recipient cells may delay full donor immune engraftment, especially in recipients with solid tumors and intact immune systems. If a mix of donor and recipient cells develops, methods to convert patients to only donor cells may be necessary, including rapid removal of immunosuppressive therapy and donor lymphocyte infusions (Champlin et al., 2000).

Conclusion

Basic understandings of hematopoiesis and immunology provide the foundation for the therapy of HSCT. Recent dramatic advances in the field of genomics because of the Human Genome Project are quickly increasing knowledge in these two areas. The field of HSCT is changing rapidly, with therapies becoming more effective and less toxic because of these advances. Nurses and other healthcare professionals are being challenged to remain knowledgeable about these advances and to develop methods to effectively educate patients and families about the effect of these advances on therapy options, treatments, and outcomes.

References

Abkowitz, J.L. (2002). Can human hematopoietic stem cells become skin, gut, or liver cells? *New England Journal of Medicine, 346,* 770–772.

Bach, F.H., & Amos, D.B. (1967). Hu-1: Major histocompatibility locus in man. *Science, 156,* 1506–1508.

Baron, F., & Beguin, Y. (2002). Nonmyeloablative allogeneic hematopoietic stem cell transplantation. *Journal of Hematotherapy and Stem Cell Research, 11,* 243–263.

Baum, C.M. (1994). Isolation and characterization of hematopoietic progenitor and stem cells. In S.J. Forman, K.G. Blume, & E.D. Thomas (Eds.), *Bone marrow transplantation* (pp. 53–71). Boston: Blackwell Scientific.

Blaise, D., Kuentz, M., Fortanier, C., Bourhis, J.H., Milpied, N., Sutton, L., et al. (2000). Randomized trial of bone marrow versus lenograstim-primed blood cell allogeneic transplantation in patients with early-stage leukemia: A report from the Societe Francaise de Greffe de Moelle. *Journal of Clinical Oncology, 18,* 537–546.

Broudy, V.C., Kaushansky, K., Harlan, J.M., & Adamson, J.W. (1987). Interleukin 1 stimulates human endothelial cells to produce granulocyte-macrophage colony-stimulating factor and granulocyte colony-stimulating factor. *Journal of Immunology, 139,* 464–468.

Cavet, J., Middleton, P.G., Segall, M., Noreen, H., Davies, S.M., & Dickinson, A.M. (1999). Recipient tumor necrosis factor-alpha and interleukin-10 gene polymorphisms associate with early mortality and acute graft-versus-host disease severity in HLA-matched sibling bone marrow transplants. *Blood, 94,* 3941–3946.

Champlin, R., Khouri, I., Shimoni, A., Gajewski, J., Kornblau, S., Molldrem, J., et al. (2000). Harnessing graft-versus-malignancy: Non-myeloablative preparative regimens for allogeneic haematopoietic transplantation, an evolving strategy for adoptive immunotherapy. *British Journal of Haematology, 111,* 18–29.

Childs, R.W. (2002). Immunotherapy of solid tumors: Nonmyeloablative allogeneic stem cell transplantation. *Medscape Hematology-Oncology eJournal, 5*(3). Retrieved July 2, 2002, from http://www.medscape.com/viewarticle/436456

Childs, R.W., Chernoff, A., Contentin, N., Bahceci, E., Schrump, D., Leitman, S., et al. (2000). Regression of metastatic renal-cell carcinoma after nonmyeloablative allogeneic peripheral-blood stem-cell transplantation. *New England Journal of Medicine, 343,* 750–758.

Emerson, S.G., Adams, S., & Taichman, R. (2000). The hematopoietic microenvironment. In J.O. Armitage & K.H. Antman (Eds.), *High-dose cancer therapy: Pharmacology, hematopoietins, stem cells* (3rd ed., pp. 185–192). Philadelphia: Lippincott Williams and Wilkins.

Emerson, S.G., Yang, Y.C., Clark, S.C., & Long, M.W. (1988). Human recombinant granulocyte-macrophage colony stimulating factor and interleukin 3 have overlapping but distinct hematopoietic activities. *Journal of Clinical Investigation, 82,* 1282–1287.

Gazzinelli, R.T., Hieny, S., Wynn, T.A., Wolf, S., & Sher, A. (1993). Interleukin 12 is required for the T-lymphocyte-independent induction of interferon gamma by an intracellular parasite and induces resistance in T-cell-deficient hosts. *Proceedings of the National Academy of Science USA, 90,* 6115–6119.

Goker, H., Haznedaroglu, I.C., & Chao, N.J. (2001). Acute graft-vs-host disease: Pathobiology and management. *Experimental Hematology, 29,* 259–277.

Holtzer, H., Biehl, J., Antin, P., Tokunaka, S., Sasse, J., Pacifici, M., et al. (1983). Quantal and proliferative cell cycles: How lineages generate cell diversity and maintain fidelity. *Progress in Clinical and Biological Research, 134,* 213–227.

Janeway, C.A., Jr., Travers, P., Walport, M., & Shlomchik, M. (2001). *Immunobiology* (5th ed.). New York: Garland Publishing.

Korbling, M., Katz, R.L., Khanna, A., Ruifrok, A.C., Rondon, G., Albitar, M., et al. (2002). Hepatocytes and epithelial cells of donor origin in recipients of peripheral-blood stem cells. *New England Journal of Medicine, 346,* 738–746.

Krenger, W., Hill, G.R., & Ferrara, J.L. (1997). Cytokine cascades in acute graft-versus-host disease. *Transplantation, 64,* 553–558.

Kripps, T. (2001). *UCSD School of Medicine SOM 214 course syllabus fall 2001 I. Cytokines.* Retrieved October 5, 2001, from http://medschool.ucsd.edu/curricular_resources/HEM/syllabus/supplement/i/index.html

Leary, A.G., Ikebuchi, K., Hirai, Y., Wong, G.G., Yang, Y.C., Clark, S.C., et al. (1988). Synergism between interleukin-6 and interleukin-3 in supporting proliferation of human hematopoietic stem cells: Comparison with interleukin-1 alpha. *Blood, 71,* 1759–1763.

Lewis, I.D. (2002). Clinical and experimental uses of umbilical cord blood. *Internal Medicine Journal, 32*, 601–609.

Lowell, C. (1997). Fundamentals of blood cell biology. In D.P. Stites, A.I. Terr, & T.G. Parslow (Eds.), *Medical immunology* (9th ed., pp. 9–24). Stamford, CT: Appleton and Lange.

Marin, G.H., Mendez, M.C., Menna, M.E., Malacalza, J., Bergna, M.I., Klein, G., et al. (1999). Immune recovery after bone marrow and peripheral blood stem cells transplantation. *Transplantation Proceedings, 31*, 2582–2584.

Marsh, S.G.E. (2003, October 13). *HLA Informatics Group. Anthony Nolan Trust.* Retrieved November 17, 2003, from http://www.anthonynolan.org.uk/HIG/index.html

Messner, H.A., & McCulloch, E.A. (1994). Mechanisms of human hematopoiesis. In S.J. Forman, K.G. Blume, & E.D. Thomas (Eds.), *Bone marrow transplantation* (pp. 41–52). Boston: Blackwell Scientific.

Middleton, P.G., Taylor, P.R., Jackson, G., Proctor, S.J., & Dickinson, A.M. (1998). Cytokine gene polymorphisms associating with severe acute graft-versus-host disease in HLA-identical sibling transplants. *Blood, 92*, 3943–3948.

Miyasaki, K. (n.d.). *UCLA School of Dentistry basic immunology course materials. Chapter I. Overview of the immune system.* Retrieved July 17, 2003, from http://www.dent.ucla.edu/sod/courses/OB471b/Ch01.pdf

Morishima, Y., Sasazuki, T., Inoko, H., Juji, T., Akaza, T., Yamamoto, K., et al. (2002). The clinical significance of human leukocyte antigen (HLA) allele compatibility in patients receiving a marrow transplant from serologically HLA-A, HLA-B, and HLA-DR matched unrelated donors. *Blood, 99*, 4200–4206.

Muller, P., Pfeiffer, P., Koglin, J., Schafers, H.J., Seeland, U., Janzen, I., et al. (2002). Cardiomyocytes of noncardiac origin in myocardial biopsies of human transplanted hearts. *Circulation, 106*, 31–35.

Nussbaum, R.L., McInnes, R.R., & Williard, H.F. (2001). *Thompson and Thompson genetics in medicine* (6th ed.). Philadelphia: W.B. Saunders.

Oppenheim, J.J., & Ruscetti, F.W. (1994). Cytokines. In D.P. Stites, A.I. Terr, & T.G. Parslow (Eds.), *Medical immunology* (9th ed., pp. 146–168). Stamford, CT: Appleton and Lange.

Parslow, T.G. (1997). Lymphocytes and lymphoid tissues. In D.P. Stites, A.I. Terr, & T.G. Parslow (Eds.), *Medical immunology* (9th ed., pp. 43–62). Stamford, CT: Appleton and Lange.

Parslow, T.G., & Bainton, D.F. (1997). Innate immunity. In D.P. Stites, A.I. Terr, & T.G. Parslow (Eds.), *Medical immunology* (9th ed., pp. 25–42). Stamford, CT: Appleton and Lange.

Petersdorf, E., Anasetti, C., Martin, P.J., Woolfrey, A., Smith, A., Mickelson, E., et al. (2001). Genomics of unrelated-donor hematopoietic cell transplantation. *Current Opinion in Immunology, 13*, 582–589.

Petersdorf, E.W., Gooley, T.A., Anasetti, C., Martin, P.J., Smith, A.G., Mickelson, E.M., et al. (1998). Optimizing outcome after unrelated marrow transplantation by comprehensive matching of HLA class I and II alleles in the donor and recipient. *Blood, 92*, 3515–3520.

Ratajczak, M.Z., & Gewirtz, A.M. (1995). The biology of hematopoietic stem cells. *Seminars in Oncology, 22*, 210–217.

Reincke, U., Rosenblatt, M., & Hellman, S. (1984). An in vitro clonal assay of adherent stem cells (ASC) in mouse marrow. *Journal of Cell Physiology, 121*, 275–283.

Roitt, I., Brostoff, J., & Male, D. (Eds.). (1996). *Immunology* (4th ed.). London: Mosby.

Sasazuki, T., Juji, T., Morishima, Y., Kinukawa, N., Kashiwabara, H., Inoko, H., et al. (1998). Effect of matching of class I HLA alleles on clinical outcome after transplantation of hematopoietic stem cells from an unrelated donor. Japan Marrow Donor Program. *New England Journal of Medicine, 339*, 1177–1185.

Schlinder, L., Kerrigan, D., & Kelly, J. (2003, January [update]). *Understanding the immune system. National Cancer Institute.* Retrieved July 17, 2003, from http://newscenter.cancer.gov/sciencebehind/immune/immune00.htm

Scott, P. (1993). IL-12: Initiation cytokine for cell-mediated immunity. *Science, 260*, 496–497.

Sica, S., Laurenti, L., Sora, F., Menichella, G., Rumi, C., Leone, G., et al. (2001). Immune reconstitution following transplantation of autologous peripheral CD34+ cells. *Acta Haematologica, 105*, 179–187.

Simmons, P.J., Zannettino, A., Gronthos, S., & Leavesley, D. (1994). Potential adhesion mechanisms for localisation of haemopoietic progenitors to bone marrow stroma. *Leukemia and Lymphoma, 12*, 353–363.

Snustad, D.P., & Simmons, M.J. (2000). *Principles of genetics* (2nd ed.). New York: John Wiley and Sons.

Socie, G., Loiseau, P., Tamouza, R., Janin, A., Busson, M., Gluckman, E., et al. (2001). Both genetic and clinical factors predict the development of graft-versus-host disease after allogeneic hematopoietic stem cell transplantation. *Transplantation, 72*, 699–706.

Steingrimsdottir, H., Gruber, A., Bjorkholm, M., Svensson, A., & Hansson, M. (2000). Immune reconstitution after autologous hematopoietic stem cell transplantation in relation to underlying disease, type of high-dose therapy and infectious complications. *Haematologica, 85*, 832–838.

Sutherland, C.W. (2000). The immunology of peripheral stem cell transplantation. In P.C. Buchsel & P.M. Kapustay (Eds.), *Stem cell transplantation: A clinical textbook* (pp. 2.1–2.24). Pittsburgh, PA: Oncology Nursing Society.

Tanaka, J., Imamura, M., Kasai, M., Zhu, X., Kobayashi, S., Hashino, S., et al. (1995). Cytokine receptor gene expression in peripheral blood mononuclear cells during graft-versus-host disease after allogeneic bone marrow transplantation. *Leukemia and Lymphoma, 19*(3–4), 281–287.

Tayebi, H., Kuttler, F., Saas, P., Lienard, A., Petracca, B., Lapierre, V., et al. (2001). Effect of granulocyte colony-stimulating factor mobilization on phenotypical and functional properties of immune cells. *Experimental Hematology, 29*, 458–470.

Tayebi, H., Tiberghien, P., Ferrand, C., Lienard, A., Duperrier, A., Cahn, J.Y., et al. (2001). Allogeneic peripheral blood stem cell transplantation results in less alteration of early T cell compartment homeostasis than bone marrow transplantation. *Bone Marrow Transplantation, 27*, 167–175.

Wujcik, D. (1997). Hematopoiesis. In M.B. Whedon & D. Wujcik (Eds.), *Blood and marrow stem cell transplantation: Principles, practice, and nursing insights* (2nd ed., pp. 25–42). Sudbury, MA: Jones and Bartlett.

Dawn Niess, MS, RN, CNP
Kathleen M. Duffy, RN, MSN, CRNP, BC

CHAPTER 2

Basic Concepts of Transplantation

History of Transplantation

The area of hematopoietic stem cell transplantation (HSCT) has grown immensely in the past several years. The roots of bone marrow transplant (BMT) can be traced back to 1949 when Leon Jacobson and his colleagues performed mouse experiments and discovered that mice could recover from lethal irradiation if their spleen was shielded (Appelbaum, 1996). Lorenz, Uphoff, Reid, and Shelton (1951) demonstrated in 1951 that irradiation protection could be provided with the infusion of syngeneic marrow. In 1955, Main and Prehn showed that mice protected with an allogeneic marrow infusion could permanently accept a skin graft from a marrow donor. By the mid-1950s, several laboratories had shown by cytogenetic markers that the radioprotective effect of BMT was the result of the replacement of the damaged hematopoietic system of the host with healthy cells from a donor (Appelbaum). In 1959, Dr. E. Donnall Thomas initiated the first attempts to treat leukemia using high-dose chemotherapy followed by syngeneic (identical twin) marrow transplantation (Appelbaum). In early trials, transplantation using donors other than identical twins proved unsuccessful because of a lack of understanding of human leukocyte antigens (HLAs) and their importance to histocompatibility (Thomas, 1995). "By the mid-1960s, it had been discovered, in dogs, that matching at the major histocompatibility complex allowed for successful allogeneic marrow transplantation" (Appelbaum, p. 152).

The first successful allogeneic transplant for leukemia occurred in the late 1960s, at the University of Minnesota. The donor was a matched sibling, and the recipient was an infant with an immune deficiency disease (Appelbaum, 1996). Autologous marrow transplantation was first used successfully in patients with lymphoma in the late 1970s and became more widespread throughout the 1980s (Appelbaum). Currently, HSCT is used in a wide variety of malignant, nonmalignant, and genetically determined diseases. Transplantation may be referred to by a number of different terms, including BMT, HSCT, or peripheral blood stem cell transplant (PBSCT).

HSCT is the transplantation of hematopoietic progenitor cells that have the ability to proliferate and repopulate the marrow spaces. Historically, hematopoietic stem cells (HSCs) were collected from the bone marrow. More recently, it has been well documented that these cells may be mobilized out of the bone marrow and collected from the peripheral blood, via apheresis, or harvested from umbilical cord blood (UCB) following delivery of a baby (Blume & Thomas, 2000). The first successful PBSCTs were performed in the 1980s (Duncombe, 1997). Transplantation of UCB was successfully performed for the first time in 1988 to treat a child with Fanconi's anemia. The patient received cord blood from a sibling who was a perfect HLA match (Gluckman, 2001). Since then, much has been learned about UCB and the role it can play in transplant. Multiple cord-blood banks have been established in the United States and Europe. With these and other advances, cord blood transplantation is now a viable option for adult HSCT (Laughlin, 2001).

The use of HSCT has increased for several reasons. First, it allows administration of dose-intensive systemic chemotherapy and radiotherapy that would be lethal without transplantation. In addition, HSCT from an allogeneic donor has an additional antitumor effect (Sullivan et al., 1989). There are also several characteristics of HSCs that make transplant possible. The first is the ability of the stem cells to regenerate in the marrow. A small number of stem cells can replicate to repopulate a patient's entire hematopoietic system. The second characteristic is the ability of the cells to find their way to the marrow following intravenous infusion, a process that is not yet clearly understood (Appelbaum, 1996). The final characteristic of HSCs is that they can be cryopreserved with little or no damage, allowing storage for future use (Appelbaum).

Types of Hematopoietic Stem Cell Transplant

HSCT can be divided into categories based on the origin of the cell source. These include autologous, allogeneic, and syngeneic (see Table 2-1). Autologous HSCT refers to the use of stem cells collected from a patient, or "self," to be reinfused, or "transplanted," at a later date following myeloablative or high-dose chemotherapy. Stem cells are collected and cryopreserved and may be stored indefinitely

Table 2-1. Types of Allogeneic Hematopoietic Stem Cell Transplantation

Type of Transplant	Cell Source	Advantages	Disadvantages
Syngeneic	Identical twin	No need for immunosuppression	No graft versus tumor effect
Matched sibling/related	Human leukocyte antigen (HLA) identical relative	No potential for stem cell contamination Access to cells since donor related	Only 25% of population has a sibling match Risk of graft versus host disease (GVHD)
Mismatched related	HLA nonidentical relative	No potential stem cell contamination Increased number of potential donors	Increased risk of GVHD Increased risk of graft failure related to HLA disparity
Matched unrelated	HLA identical unrelated donor	No potential stem cell contamination	Increased risk of GVHD Limited numbers of non-Caucasian donors Waiting period to identify donor
Mismatched unrelated	HLA nonidentical unrelated donor	No potential stem cell contamination	Increased risk of GVHD High treatment-related mortality
Cord blood	Umbilical cord unit	Easy access to cell source	Limited number of cells Delayed time to engraftment Increased infection rates

until needed for reinfusion at the time of stem cell rescue. Autologous transplantation following myelosuppressive therapy is utilized in a variety of diseases and disease states. For some diseases, it is considered part of the initial treatment plan; for others, it is reserved for relapse or persistent disease states. Diseases treated with this modality include multiple myeloma, non-Hodgkin's lymphoma, Hodgkin's disease, germ cell tumors, and neuroblastoma. Autologous transplant also has been used as a treatment option for patients with acute myeloid and acute lymphoid leukemias. Clinical trials continually evaluate the effectiveness of this treatment for other solid tumors, severe autoimmune disease, and some rheumatologic disorders (Fassas, Anagnostopoulos, & Kazis, 1997) (see Table 2-2). Advantages to this type of transplant include easier access to the stem cells, decreased incidence and severity of side effects, earlier engraftment, and no risk of graft versus host disease (GVHD) (Forte & Norville, 1998). However, the risk of potential tumor contamination in the infused cell product and the lack of the immunologic graft versus tumor (GVT) effect may contribute to relapse (Blume & Thomas, 2000). The International Bone Marrow Transplant Registry (IBMTR) and the Autologous Blood and Marrow Transplant Registry (ABMTR) comprehensive HSCT databases report a less than 10% treatment-related mortality, attributed primarily to organ toxicity from high-dose chemotherapy for patients undergoing this type of transplantation (IBMTR/ABMTR, 2002).

Allogeneic HSCT uses a related or unrelated donor as the source of stem cells. It is the treatment of choice for patients with diseased or damaged bone marrow or patients with genetic diseases (Dix & Yee, 1997; O'Connell & Schmit-Pokorny, 1997) (see Table 2-2). Standard allogeneic transplantation uses myeloablative chemotherapy followed by infusion of stem cells from a compatible donor. Appropriate donors are identified through HLA typing. HLA compatibility is a key factor in predicting transplant-related morbidity and mortality. Because the antigens are genetically acquired, siblings are more likely to have similar HLA-matched stem cells. However, because of the pairing and various combinations of HLA antigens in a family, only 25% of the population will have an HLA-matched sibling. If an HLA compatible match is not found in the family, unrelated donors may be sought through bone marrow donor registries or placental cord blood registries, the largest of which is the National Marrow Donor Program (NMDP). Advantages to allogeneic HSCT include not only replacement of diseased or damaged stem cells with healthy ones but also the addition of a powerful immune reaction in which the newly transplanted immune cells may react against any residual disease. This is known as the graft versus leukemia or GVT effect (Sullivan et al., 1989).

In addition, as a result of the immune modulation, patients are at risk for GVHD, a powerful immune reaction in which the immunocompetent donor cells recognize and attack healthy tissues in the recipient or host (Porter, Roth, McGarigle, Ferrara, & Antin, 1994). Patients undergoing allogeneic HSCT are at higher risk for organ toxicity, infection, and bleeding because of myeloablative chemotherapy and radiation. As a result of these potential complications, the treatment-related mortality for these transplants as reported by IBMTR/ABMTR in 2002 approaches 50% in some cases, with a range of approximately 10%–50% (IBMTR/ABMTR, 2002).

The term *syngeneic transplant* refers to an allogeneic transplant in which stem cells are collected from one identical twin and infused into the other twin following high-dose chemotherapy. Because identical twins are genetically the same, this syngeneic transplant is similar to an autologous transplant in terms of morbidity and mortality (Forte & Norville, 1998). The disadvantage of this type of transplant is the lack of GVT effect. Collection of stem cells from UCB has been gaining interest in recent years (Forte & Norville). UCB is a rich source of stem cells collected at the time of childbirth. The UCB stem cells could be frozen and stored or saved through a cord blood bank to be used in the unrelated registry.

Nonmyeloablative Hematopoietic Stem Cell Transplant

Because of the potential dangers of allogeneic HSCT, this treatment has been traditionally reserved for patients younger than age 60 without comorbidities. Evidence suggests that the dose-intensive chemotherapy previously thought to be the curative agent in allogeneic HSCT may not be solely responsible for patients' durable remissions. Rather, the powerful GVT effect may be concurrently responsible for remissions (Porter et al., 1994). It is upon this principle that newer, potentially safer, ways to perform these transplants have been developed. Nonmyeloablative allogeneic HSCT, a treatment using standard doses of chemotherapy followed by infusions of donor stem cells, has been developed in an effort to take advantage of the GVT effect while providing an effective yet less toxic modality for performing allogeneic HSCT. Results of published studies demonstrate that allogeneic HSCT following nonmyeloablative conditioning has significant activity for a heterogenous group of patients, including patients with non-Hodgkin's lymphomas, Hodgkin's disease, multiple myeloma, and chronic lymphocytic leukemia (Bhatia & Porter, 2001). Complete response rates for various hematologic malignancies have varied. There is evidence to suggest activity in solid tumors, including renal cell carcinoma, although only small numbers of patients have been treated (Childs et al., 2000). Nonmyeloablative therapy is under investigation as a method of consolidating remissions in high-risk patients (e.g., poor-risk acute myelogenous leukemia), treating patients who are ineligible for standard allogeneic HSCT, and salvaging patients after relapse from previous autologous HSCT.

Table 2-2. Common Diseases Treated With Hematopoietic Stem Cell Transplant

Type of Disease	Autologous HSCT	Allogeneic HSCT
Malignant		
Hematologic malignancies	Hodgkin's disease Non-Hodgkin's lymphoma Multiple myeloma	Acute lymphocytic leukemia Acute myelogenous leukemia Chronic myelogenous leukemia Myelodysplastic syndrome Non-Hodgkin's lymphoma
Solid tumors	Neuroblastoma Sarcoma Germ cell tumor	
Nonmalignant		
Hematologic		Severe aplastic anemia Fanconi's anemia Thalassemia Sickle cell disease Diamond Blackfan anemia Chédiak-Higashi syndrome Chronic granulomatous disease Congenital neutropenia
Immunodeficiency		Severe combined immunodeficiency disease Wiskott-Aldrich syndrome Functional T cell deficiency
Genetic		Adrenoleukodystrophy Metachromatic leukodystrophy Hurler's syndrome Hunter's disease Gaucher's syndrome
Miscellaneous		
		Osteoporosis Langerhan's cell histiocytosis Glycogen storage diseases

Sources of Stem Cells

Stem cells may be collected from bone marrow, peripheral blood, or UCB. There are several advantages and disadvantages to each of these sources.

Traditionally, bone marrow was used exclusively as the source of stem cells. When cells are collected or harbored from the bone marrow, the donor is placed under general or epidural anesthesia in an operating room. Stem cells are obtained by performing multiple needle aspirations of marrow from the posterior or anterior iliac crests. The cells are mixed with anticoagulant and filtered to remove bone chips, fat cells, and blood clots. If the donor and recipient are ABO incompatible, further processing also will be conducted (Forte & Norville, 1998).

Advantages to bone marrow collection are that the collection can be completed in several hours and is generally well tolerated; therefore, it may be performed as an outpatient or require only a one night stay. Maybe more significant is the finding that the use of bone marrow may result in a decreased risk of chronic GVHD, which may have a profound impact on the patient's long-term outcome and quality of life (Morton, Hutchins, & Durrant, 2001). Disadvantages include the need for general anesthesia or epidural anesthesia along with the risk of infection, bleeding, and bone damage (Forte & Norville, 1998).

During the past 10–15 years, the use of peripheral blood stem cells (PBSCs) as a rescue following myeloablative therapy has increased significantly (Blume & Thomas, 2000). Initially, PBSCs were only used for autologous transplants; however, in recent years, the collection of PBSCs from allogeneic donors has grown. Research in this area continues to expand. Stem cells are "mobilized" or moved out of the bone marrow into the peripheral blood with the use of granulocyte–colony-stimulating factor (G-CSF) or granulocyte macrophage–colony-stimulating factor (GM-CSF). Once the cells are mobilized into the blood stream, they can then be collected from the peripheral blood by a process called apheresis. Apheresis uses centrifugation to remove the stem cells from the blood with the remaining components of the blood being returned to the donor. In autologous transplants, the donor may receive mobilization chemotherapy followed by G-CSF or GM-CSF. Once the stem cells are obtained, they then are mixed with an anticoagulant and a preservative followed by cryopreservation (Buchsel, Leum, & Randolph, 1997). In the allogeneic setting, where fresh stem cells are used, the cells usually are not cryopreserved. Instead, the stem cells are infused "fresh" into the transplant recipient.

One advantage of collecting PBSCs is that it can be performed as an outpatient procedure with no need for anesthesia, and generally donors of all ages tolerate this procedure well. Another important advantage to the use of PBSCs is that cells obtained from the blood engraft earlier than cells obtained from bone marrow (Bensinger et al., 1996). This quicker hematologic recovery time has many advantages, including decreased length of neutropenia, fewer infections, decreased antibiotic use, decreased length of thrombocytopenia, decreased risk for episodes of bleeding, decreased use of blood products, and decreased organ toxicity. All of these lead to decreased lengths of hospital stays and decreased costs.

An important consideration in the collection of PBSCs is to determine how the stem cells will be collected. Tunneled multiple-lumen apheresis catheters are inserted into autologous patients for stem cell collection, which may stay in throughout treatment. Peripheral IV access is usually used for allogeneic donors if good venous access is available and the patient can tolerate this for the duration of the apheresis procedure (Buschel & Kapustay, 1997). Patients and donors need education that the apheresis procedure may last four to six hours per day and may take multiple days.

UCB stem cell collections also have occurred more frequently in recent years. Harvesting cord blood units involves collecting stem cells from an umbilical cord and placenta immediately following birth. The cord blood is HLA typed, cryopreserved, and stored in one of various cord blood banks throughout the world. Advantages include easy access to the cord blood units and a simple collection procedure with no risk to the mother or child (Forte & Norville, 1998). Another advantage over unrelated BMT is that cord blood transplants have a lower risk of GVHD (Hegland, 1997). Disadvantages include the potential of passing genetic diseases to the recipient and a limited and finite number of cells (Laughlin, 2001). There also may be additional costs to patients because of storage costs of cord blood stem cells (Hegland).

National Marrow Donor Program

For patients who do not have an HLA-compatible related donor, registries including the NMDP provide potential unrelated donor options. The NMDP was founded in 1986 and is the world's largest single database of unrelated marrow and stem cell donors. It contains more than four million committed volunteer donors. Through NMDP, approximately 130 transplants are performed per month. Up to 40% of the facilitated transplants involve an international recipient or donor. With a mission to facilitate unrelated marrow transplantation and PBSCT, NMDP offers a single point of access to finding unrelated marrow, blood stem cells, and cord blood units. Since its inception, NMDP has facilitated approximately 12,000 unrelated donor transplants for patients with blood disorders (e.g., leukemia, aplastic anemia), as well as certain genetic and immune system disorders. At any point in time, approximately 3,000 patients are actively being searched in the registry.

NMDP is associated with a network of both domestic and international facilities, including apheresis and collection centers. There are also cord blood banks, donor centers, laboratories, transplant centers, recruitment groups, and repositories. In addition to facilitating transplants, NMDP initiatives include research (comprehensive database), patient empowerment (Office of Patient Advocacy), educating medical professionals, and reducing search and time to transplant intervals.

Donor recruitment is a priority. Although Caucasians are well represented on the registries, powerful initiatives are under way for targeted minority recruitment. Efforts are focused on African Americans, American Indians/Alaska Natives, Asian/Pacific Islanders, and Hispanics/Latinos. Approximately 34,000 new donors per month are added to the registry.

The median time from initiation of a formal search to transplant is four months. The initial step is to obtain the patient's HLA typing using the recommended molecular (DNA) testing methods. A preliminary search can then be performed. The preliminary search is a "single snapshot" of potential donors on the registry. It is a computerized search of all stem cell donor and cord blood unit information contained in the registry the day the search is performed. The preliminary search is free, and results are usually available within 24 hours of submission of the search request. The search can be performed for any physician by the NMDP or by an NMDP-approved transplant center. After the preliminary search is run for the first time, patients and physicians receive information about unrelated donor transplantation from the NMDP's Office of Patient Advocacy.

If a physician and patient decide to proceed with the transplant process, the patient must be referred to the NMDP transplant center. A formal search then can be initiated. Formal searches include further laboratory testing performed at the NMDP transplant center. This testing is done to confirm initial HLA results as well as potential matches. Once a donor is identified and the typing is confirmed to be an appropriate match with the patient, the transplant center may proceed with the next step. At this time, the transplant center's physicians may request a donor to proceed to the workup phase. The volunteer donor will be contacted and educated about the donation process for the stem cell product that has been requested (bone marrow versus PBSC). If he or she agrees, the patient will undergo a comprehensive physical examination, including blood work and any additional medical testing deemed necessary for safe procurement of the blood cell product.

Preparative Regimens

There are many combinations of preparative regimens consisting of chemotherapy, immunotherapy, and/or radiation therapy given pretransplant. The agents used in preparative regimens vary depending on the type of transplant (allogeneic versus autologous), disease treated, and desired effects. The goals of the preparative regimens in traditional (myeloablative) allogeneic transplants include eradicating any malignant disease, suppressing the immune system to prevent graft rejection, and ablating the host's bone marrow to make room for growth of donor stem cells (Dix & Yee, 1997). In autologous transplants, immunosuppression is not necessary because the host is the source of the new stem cell. Thus, the main goals are to eradicate disease and to ablate the bone marrow. The use of HSCT for treatment of nonmalignant diseases is to provide immunosuppression and bone marrow ablation (Dix & Yee).

Preparative regimens have evolved over time as more is learned about various diseases and their responses to different drugs. Early BMTs used total body irradiation (TBI) alone for conditioning. TBI is the exposure of the entire body to gamma radiation. It is delivered in varying doses and may be given as a single dose or in fractionated doses (Dreifke & DeMeyer, 1992). Although TBI can produce immunosuppression, ablation, and some antitumor effects, it is not entirely effective in eradicating diseased marrow; therefore, chemotherapy is added to optimize the conditioning regimen (Dix & Yee, 1997). Preparative regimens vary depending on the disease, stem cell source, type of transplant, and goals of conditioning. Some common myeloablative preparative regimens for transplants are listed in Table 2-3 (Dix & Yee).

Choice of a preparative or conditioning regimen is largely based on the disease being treated and the goal of therapy. For hematologic and immunodeficiency diseases, high doses of chemotherapy will eradicate stem cells in the bone marrow to make space for engraftment of healthy allogeneic cells. The new donor cells will produce normal white blood cells, red blood cells, and platelets (O'Connell & Schmit-Pokorny, 1997). The goal of HSCT for treatment of lymphomas or solid tumors is to administer high-dose chemotherapy to aggressively treat the disease, followed by the reinfusion of stem cells to rescue the patient from the side effect of myeloablation. In genetic and metabolic disorders, chemotherapy is given to destroy the abnormal cells in the bone marrow. Donor cells are infused and upon engraftment produce ad-

Table 2-3. Common Myeloablative Preparative Regimens

Preparative Regimen	Diseases Treated
Busulfan + Cyclophosphamide	AML/CML (allogeneic/auto)
Cyclophosphamide + TBI	AML/CML/AA/NHL (allo/auto)
Carmustine + Cisplatin + Cyclophosphamide	NHL/HD (allo/auto)
Carmustine + Cyclophosphamide + Etoposide	NHL/HD (auto)
Carmustine + Etoposide + Cytarabine + Melphalan	NHL/HD (auto)
Etoposide + TBI	ALL (allo/auto)
Melphalan	MM (auto)
Busulfan + Melphalan	AML/CML, solid tumors (auto/allo)
Thiotepa + Cyclophosphamide + Etoposide	Solid tumors (auto)
Thiotepa + Cyclophosphamide + Carboplatin	Breast (auto)
Busulfan + Cyclophosphamide + Etoposide	NHL/HD/MM (allo/auto)

AA—aplastic anemia; AML—acute myelogenous leukemia; CML—chronic myelogenous leukemia; HD—Hodgkin's disease; MM—multiple myeloma; NHL—non-Hodgkin's lymphoma; TBI—total body irradiation

Note. Based on information from Dix & Yee, 1997.

equate amounts of deficient enzymes, thus curing the underlying disorder (O'Connell & Schmit-Pokorny).

The preparative regimen for nonmyeloablative allogeneic HSCT is different than that of traditional allogeneic HSCT because although the process is similar, the goals are different. Patients are conditioned with chemotherapy and/or radiation. The goal of this preparative regimen is not to eradicate the malignancy; rather, the intent is to provide adequate immune suppression to achieve mixed chimera initially and, ultimately, full donor chimera engraftment of an allogeneic blood cell graft. The optimal conditioning regimen is yet to be determined. Regimens typically consist of highly immunosuppressive chemotherapeutic agents, such as purine analogs (e.g., fludarabine) or alkylating agents (e.g., busulfan, cyclophosphamide) in nonmyeloablative doses alone or in combination with immunosuppressive agents (e.g., antithymocyte globulin), monoclonal antibodies (Campath-1H®, ILEX Pharmaceuticals, San Antonio, TX), or low-dose total nodal irradiation or TBI (200 cGy). The combination of chemo/radio/immunotherapy is intended to suppress the immune system of the host and allow engraftment of donor cells as well as induce a GVT response in which the donor's immune cells attack the host malignancy.

Clinical Evaluation

Because many life-threatening complications are associated with HSCT, the decision to use this treatment is based on a thorough evaluation of the patient. Some variation may exist among transplant centers in terms of eligibility requirements, diseases treated, and the components of the pretransplant clinical evaluation. In an effort to standardize as well as promote quality medical practices, the Foundation for the Accreditation of Cellular Therapy (FACT) was developed (FACT, 1997). FACT is a national voluntary inspection and accreditation program that encompasses all phases of hematopoietic collection, processing, and the actual transplant. It was developed to oversee and encourage standardization of quality practices in transplant centers. Centers that meet rigorous standards of quality medical care and laboratory practice are recognized with certificates of accreditation. FACT requirements for patient evaluation are indicated in Figure 2-1.

General considerations for eligibility include determining that patients have chemotherapy-sensitive disease, adequate organ function, and no life-threatening viral exposures or comorbidities. Additionally, the patient's age, performance status, and ability to comply with treatment are considered (Secola, 1997). A clinical evaluation, including a complete health history documenting the history of present illness, should be obtained. Information should include disease and treatment course from diagnosis to the time of transplant. A general health history, including past medical and surgical history and family, social, and travel history, should be obtained as well as documentation of allergies, medications, and female gynecologic history. A psychosocial assessment and various diagnostic tests to evaluate the

patient's general health and disease status also should be performed. A complete physical examination, including laboratory studies and diagnostics assessing vital organ function and infectious disease testing, should be performed.

In addition to the clinical assessment, a psychological assessment of the patient and family should be performed (Secola, 1997). The patient should be evaluated for his or her comprehension of the procedure, potential risks, side effects, and complications and the ability to comply with therapy. Psychosocial evaluation should include social and spiritual issues, psychological well-being, financial issues, and family concerns. Children should have neuropsychological testing performed to have a baseline for further assessments. Finally, consent must be obtained prior to HSCT. If the patient is a minor, a parent or guardian must consent. Children younger than 18 years of age may sign an assent form.

Allogeneic transplant donors also must undergo a thorough clinical evaluation and a psychosocial assessment. The donor should have a complete medical history and physical examination to rule out genetic or infectious diseases and significant health problems that may pose a risk to either the patient or donor during the collection of stem cells (see Figure 2-1). The stem cell donor evaluation is described in detail in Chapter 3. Psychological intervention also may allow the donor to express fears he or she may have regarding stem cell donation and discuss ways to cope with those fears. Intervention should be provided to assist donors in processing feelings of guilt or anxiety related to the transplant recipient's outcome. The identity of an unrelated donor is kept confidential for at least one year following HSCT, at which time the donor and recipient may be introduced. Informed consent for the collection of peripheral blood or bone marrow stem cells is obtained prior to donation.

Patient/Family Education

Nurses have an excellent opportunity to provide education to patients and families undergoing HSCT. Transplantation is a very intense and complicated process that requires educational efforts throughout all phases of treatment. These should include patients, donors, and families/support people at each transplant phase.

Donors should be instructed about the diagnostic studies and laboratory tests required to evaluate their health status prior to donation of stem cells. Donors should have a thorough understanding of the collection process, the potential risks and complications, and the potential outcomes that they may experience, along with the potential outcomes for the recipient of their donated cells. Donors also should know how to seek medical attention if they develop complications or questions following collection. The donor must sign informed consent papers prior to the collection being performed.

Pre-HSCT education for patients and families should be individualized and ongoing, with continued evaluation of their comprehension and understanding of this process.

Figure 2-1. Clinical Evaluation Requirements for Transplant

Laboratory Evaluation
- CBC with differential
- Chemistry profile
- Electrolytes, LFTs, BUN/Cr, PT/PTT, INR
- Hep B surface Ag*+
- Hep C AB*+
- HIV Ab*+
- HIV1/2Ab*+
- HTLV 1*+
- RPR*+
- CMV IgG, IgM*+
- HSV IgG
- ABO/Rh*+
- HLA typing for allogeneic transplants+
- Toxoplasmosis Ab
- Cpcco serologies
- VZV IgG
- GFR/creatinine clearance
- Pregnancy test*+

Organ Function Testing
- MUGA/echocardiogram
- Pulmonary function test
- 12 lead ECG
- Dental examination

Disease Evaluation
- Bone marrow aspirates and biopsies
- Lumbar puncture
- CT scans
- MRI
- Bone scan
- Gallium scan
- PET scan
- Tumor markers
- 24-hour urine protein electrophoresis
- Immunoglobulins
- Urine catecholamines (VMA/HVA)

* = FACT requirement; + = donor requirement also

Many patients have received other therapies prior to HSCT and may have previous experience with chemotherapy or radiation therapy and hospitalization. Assessment of a patient's prior experience with side effects may guide the nurse in providing appropriate pretransplant education. The nurse should discuss the route of administration, dosage, side effects, and administration of all medications, such as chemotherapeutic agents, anti-infectives, immunosuppressives, antiemetics, immunomodulators, analgesics, and growth factors. Information should be provided regarding the actual reinfusion and potential side effects and complications occurring during aplasia, including organ toxicity, infection, and bleeding. For patients undergoing allogeneic HSCT, education should include risks, clinical presentation, and treatments for GVHD. Additionally, the potential side effects of immunosuppressive medications, such as high risk of infection, hepatotoxicity, and nephrotoxicity, should be discussed.

Because of the level of caregiver burden for families and support people of patients undergoing HSCT, family structure and function should be assessed early on in the transplant process (DeMeyer, Whedon, & Ferrell, 1997). Efforts should include educating families in both the physical and psychosocial elements of this process. Helping families identify key support people and teaching them to delegate activities to maximize available resources is a key element in managing caregiver burden. Family members should be encouraged to express their fears and concerns regarding the possibility of the death of a loved one and their expectations and hope for a positive outcome (Wochna, 1997). Nurses, social workers, and psychosocial staff should address these issues and acknowledge changing roles within the family and the impact they may have on the HSCT process (DeMeyer et al.). Whenever possible, families and support people should be encouraged to participate in groups and use other available support networks.

The education of the child requires special attention. Many pediatric transplant centers employ child life specialists who can assist with developing appropriate education. Educational efforts should be directed toward the child's developmental stage (Secola, 1997). Although children may not understand everything, an attempt should be made to help them understand why they are in the hospital, what is going to happen, how they may feel, and what they can do during the transplant process. Teaching should be conducted at appropriate times, and children should always be told what to expect prior to procedures or administering medications. Children should be given the opportunity to ask questions and to share their concerns. Parents may need help in addressing their children's questions or needs. Child life specialists, nurses, and other staff should be available to assist with education of children and families.

Much of the basics of PBSCT and BMT can be applied to both adults and children. However, there are special considerations for children. Pediatric patients have special and unique growth and developmental needs. The child's ability to cope will be dependent upon his or her developmental level along with the trust and support he or she feels from the family and the transplant staff (Secola, 1997). Children should have opportunities to have their emotional needs met along with developmental needs. This could include such things as providing the ability to continue schoolwork, activities, play, and exercise, if possible. Peer interaction should be continued via computers, videophones, and letters, if age appropriate. Social interaction with family, friends, and staff also will be very important (Secola). Staff familiar with pediatric patients and their needs should be involved in the care of these patients when at all possible. Family involvement is crucial when a child is undergoing the transplant experience, and the entire family will need to be cared for and included.

Finally, discharge education is very important and should be initiated early to optimize planning and resources. Because of the high level of anxiety of patients and their caregivers, information should be presented clearly and reinforced frequently during the hospital stay. Discharge instructions should be explained verbally by the nurse and reinforced by providing printed materials to take home, and should be realistic regarding life after transplant (Boyle et al., 2000). Information provided should include risk of infection, practices to prevent infection, physical activity expectations and restrictions, and medication administration. To combat fatigue, the patient and caregiver need information on how to meet daily nutritional requirements. The possibility of GVHD and long-term complications of each organ system should be addressed. A follow-up plan also should be outlined for the patient and family.

Discharge teaching should include family members and support people. It is notable that the family roles may change throughout the transplant process, as the patient requires changing levels of support. Family members should be instructed in ways to cope with the stress associated with this dynamic process (Wochna, 1997). It is anticipated that every day family life may be disrupted with frequent follow-up office visits, in addition to the long-term effects of treatment (e.g., fatigue, GVHD). The family also may be dealing with financial issues, uncertainty about the future, fear of relapse, and fear of death (Rivera, 1997). Recurrence anxiety is a predominant theme rarely addressed by the professional team because the assessment of symptoms and recovery from transplant take priority (Boyle et al., 2000). The family should be provided with a time to discuss all of these issues and express any concerns prior to the patient's discharge from the hospital so that a follow-up plan can be cooperatively developed.

HSCT is a very complex process that continues to grow and develop. It is essential for nurses to maintain current knowledge of the basics so that they can continually improve the quality of care provided to patients and families. Treatment advances are occurring rapidly, and nurses have a wonderful opportunity to prepare and assist patients throughout the transplant process.

References

Appelbaum, F. (1996). The use of bone marrow and peripheral blood stem cell transplantation in the treatment of cancer. *CA: A Cancer Journal for Clinicians, 46*(3), 143–164.

Bensinger, W.I., Clift, R., Martin, P., Applebaum, F.R., Demirer, T., Gooley, T., et al. (1996). Allogeneic peripheral blood stem cell transplantation in patients with advanced hematologic malignancies: A retrospective comparison with marrow transplantation. *Blood, 88,* 2794–2800.

Bhatia, V., & Porter D.L. (2001). Novel approaches to allogeneic stem cell therapy. *Expert Opinion in Biologic Therapy, 1*(1), 3–15.

Blume, K.G., & Thomas, E.D. (2000). A review of autologous hematopoietic cell transplantation. *Biology of Blood and Marrow Transplantation, 6,* 1–12.

Boyle, D., Blodgett, L., Gnesdiloff, S., White, J., Bamford, A., Sheridan, M., et al. (2000). Caregiver quality of life after autolo-

gous bone marrow transplantation. *Cancer Nursing, 23,* 193–203.

Buchsel, P., & Kapustay, P. (1997). Models of ambulatory care for blood cell and bone marrow transplantation. In M.B. Whedon & D. Wujcik (Eds.), *Blood and marrow stem cell transplantation: Principles, practice, and nursing insights* (pp. 43–45). Sudbury, MA: Jones and Bartlett.

Buchsel, P., Leum, E., & Randolph, S. (1997). Nursing care of the blood cell transplant recipient. *Seminars in Oncology Nursing, 13,* 172–183.

Childs, R., Chernoff, A., Contentin, N., Bahceci, E., Schrump, D., Leitman, S., et al. (2000). Regression of metastatic renal cell after non-myeloablative allogeneic peripheral blood stem cell transplantation. *New England Journal of Medicine, 343,* 750–758.

DeMeyer, E., Whedon, M.B., & Ferrell, B.R. (1997). Quality of life after transplantation. In M.B. Whedon & D. Wujcik (Eds.), *Blood and marrow stem cell transplantation: Principles, practice, and nursing insights* (pp. 400–428). Sudbury, MA: Jones and Bartlett.

Dix, S., & Yee, G. (1997). Pharmacologic and biologic agents. In M.B. Whedon & D. Wujcik (Eds.), *Blood and marrow stem cell transplantation: Principles, practice, and nursing insights* (pp. 100–150). Sudbury, MA: Jones and Bartlett.

Dreifke, L., & DeMeyer, E. (1992). Information guide for patients receiving total body irradiation before bone marrow transplantation. *Cancer Nursing, 15,* 206–210.

Duncombe, A. (1997). Bone marrow and stem cell transplantation. *BMJ, 314,* 1179–1182.

Fassas, A., Anagnostopoulos, A., & Kazis, A. (1997). Peripheral blood stem cell transplantation in the treatment of progressive multiple sclerosis: First results of a pilot study. *Bone Marrow Transplantation, 20,* 631–638.

Forte, K., & Norville, R. (1998). Hematopoietic stem cell transplantation. In M. Hockenberry-Eaton (Ed.), *Essentials of pediatric oncology nursing: A core curriculum* (pp. 100–110). Glenview, IL: Association of Pediatric Oncology Nurses.

Foundation for the Accreditation of Cellular Therapy. (1997). *Hematopoietic progenitor cell collection, processing, and transplantation accreditation manual.* Omaha, NE: Author.

Gluckman, E. (2001). Hematopoietic stem-cell transplants using umbilical cord blood. *New England Journal of Medicine, 344,* 1860–1861.

Hegland, J. (1997). Transplant immunology: HLA and issues of stem cell donation. In M.B. Whedon & D. Wujcik (Eds.), *Blood and marrow stem cell transplantation: Principles, practice, and nursing insights* (pp. 43–45). Sudbury: MA: Jones and Bartlett.

International Bone Marrow Transplant Directory/Autologous Blood and Marrow Transplant Directory. (2002). Report on state of the art in blood and marrow transplantation. *IBMTR/ABMTR Newsletter, 9,* 4–11.

Laughlin, M.J. (2001). Umbilical cord blood for allogeneic transplantation in children and adults [Review]. *Bone Marrow Transplantation, 27,* 1–6.

Lorenz, E., Uphoff, D., Reid, T.R., & Shelton, E. (1951). Modification of irradiation injury in mice and guinea pigs by bone marrow injections. *Journal of the National Cancer Institute, 12,* 197–201.

Main, J.M., & Prehn, R.T. (1955). Successful skin homografts after the administration of high dose x radiation and homologous bone marrow. *Journal of the National Cancer Institute, 15,* 1023–1029.

Morton, J., Hutchins, C., & Durrant, S. (2001). Granulocyte-colony-stimulating factor (G-CSF)-primed allogeneic bone marrow: Significantly less graft-versus-host disease and comparable engraftment to G-CSF-mobilized peripheral blood stem cells. *Blood, 98,* 3186–3191.

O'Connell, S., & Schmit-Pokorny, K. (1997). Blood and marrow stem cell transplantation: Indications, procedure, process. In M.B. Whedon & D. Wujcik (Eds.), *Blood and marrow stem cell transplan-*

tation: Principles, practice, and nursing insights (pp. 66–99). Sudbury, MA: Jones and Bartlett.

Porter, D.L., Roth, M., McGarigle, C., Ferrara, J., & Antin, J. (1994). Induction of graft-versus-host disease as immunotherapy for relapsed chronic myelogenous leukemia. *New England Journal of Medicine, 330*, 251–266.

Rivera, L. (1997). Blood cell transplantation: Its impact on one family. *Seminars in Oncology Nursing, 13*, 194–199.

Secola, R. (1997). Pediatric blood cell transplantation. *Seminars in Oncology Nursing, 13*, 184–193.

Sullivan, K., Weiden, P., Storb, R., Witherspoon, R., Fefer, A., Fisher, L., et al. (1989). Influence of acute and chronic graft versus host disease on relapse and survival after bone marrow transplantation from HLA-identical siblings as treatment of acute and chronic leukemia. *Blood, 73*, 1720–1728.

Thomas, E. (1995). Transplantation of hematopoietic progenitor cells with emphasis on the results in children. *Turkish Journal of Pediatrics, 37*, 31–43.

Wochna, V. (1997). Anxiety, needs and coping in family members of the bone marrow transplant patient. *Cancer Nursing, 20*, 244–250.

Stem Cell Collection

Introduction

Stem cells may be collected for transplantation from bone marrow (BM), blood, and umbilical cord blood (UCB). In the previous chapter, advantages and disadvantages to each method were discussed. In summary, collecting stem cells from the blood has demonstrated several major advantages in comparison to surgically harvesting stem cells from BM. Patients who receive stem cells from the blood may experience a more rapid hematopoietic recovery, receive a stem cell product that has a lower risk of contamination by tumor cells in comparison to stem cells harvested from BM, and experience a better overall outcome. Smith et al. (1997) also described significant cost savings for patients who are transplanted with blood stem cells (BSC). Savings are achieved through lower collection costs, shorter hospital stays, and less supportive care. However, Smith et al. indicated that cost savings would vary depending on individual practice patterns. In addition, BSC collections may be performed in an outpatient setting, without general anesthesia. Patients who have tumors in the marrow or have had pelvic irradiation that caused BM fibrosis also may have stem cells collected from the blood. Advantages that UCB transplants may have are that UCB products contain many immature progenitor cells and may have the lowest incidence of graft versus host disease (GVHD).

Evaluation of Autologous and Allogeneic Donors for Collection

Prior to BM harvest or BSC collection, the transplant recipient must be evaluated to determine eligibility for transplant (as discussed in Chapter 2). The recipient, if autologous stem cells are to be harvested, or the allogeneic donor also must be evaluated in terms of undergoing the harvest or collection procedure. The evaluation specific to harvest or collection involves a history and physical, blood tests, and possibly radiological tests. A thorough explanation of the marrow harvest or BSC collection procedure must be provided. The Foundation for the Accreditation of Cellular Therapy (FACT) outlined specific standards to protect the safety of the patient and the product. Figure 3-1 lists the evalu-

ation tests required for an allogeneic donor or a patient who is undergoing autologous transplant prior to BM harvesting or BSC collection. In addition, written informed consent from the donor must be obtained. FACT (1996) also requires the recipient's physician to write an order to collect and process the stem cells that includes recipient and donor information, treatment plan, collection protocol, processing and cryopreservation method, and any assays to be performed on the stem cell product. Figure 3-2 is an example of an order sheet that may be used for BSC collection. Buckner, Petersen, and Bolonesi (1994) described the necessity of including a psychological and social evaluation during the physical evaluation of the allogeneic donor. Legal and ethical aspects also should be considered, especially when using minors as donors.

Bone Marrow Harvest

BM, which contains more stem cells than peripheral blood, is harvested from the posterior iliac crests via multiple large-bore needle aspirations. Occasionally, the anterior iliac crest or the sternum may be used to obtain enough cells for transplant. Usually, the procedure is performed in an operating room under general or spinal anesthesia. Typically the procedure lasts one to two hours, following which the patient may be admitted to the hospital. The patient lies on the operating table, and BM is collected from both posterior iliac crests by multiple needle aspirations. The number of nucleated cells that is attempted to be harvested ranges from $1–2.5 \times 10^8$/kg. The total fluid volume obtained is usually 500–1,000 ml. Following the marrow stem cell harvest, the BM is filtered though progressively smaller filter screens to remove fat and bone particles, and then it is processed. If the recipient and the donor have a major ABO incompatibility, the product will be red cell or plasma depleted. The marrow may be frozen if the cells are from a donor, or on the day of transplant, the cells will be infused.

Side effects donors may experience following the harvest include bleeding, infection, pain, hypovolemia, hypotension, hematoma, electrolyte imbalances, and side effects from general anesthesia. The nurse should assess the harvest sites frequently for bleeding, drainage, or development of a he-

Figure 3-1. Evaluation of the Donor for Bone Marrow Harvest or Blood Stem Cell Collection

Autologous Donor
- Complete blood count (CBC), differential (diff), platelet (plt)—a CBC, diff, plt must be obtained within a 72-hour period prior to the first blood stem cell (BSC) collection and within 24 hours before each subsequent BSC collection (Foundation for the Accreditation of Cellular Therapy [FACT], 1996)
- Chemistries (liver and kidney function)
- Prothrombin time (PT)/partial thromboplastin time (PTT)/international ratio (INR)
- Blood grouping and Rh typing (ABO and Rh)
- Infectious disease tests (hepatitis B surface antigen, hepatitis B core antigen, hepatitis C antibody, human immunodeficiency virus (HIV)-1 antibody, HIV-2 antibody, HIV antigen, human T cell lymphotropic viruses (HTLV), syphilis, and cytomegalovirus) performed within 30 days prior to collection or on the day of the first collection (FACT)
- Electrocardiogram (bone marrow [BM] donors only)
- Chest x-ray (BM donors only)
- Pregnancy assessment (FACT) within 72 hours prior to the start of growth factor (American Association of Blood Banks, 2000)
- History and physical (FACT)

The following must be documented:
- Suitability of donor to undergo stem cell collection
- Abnormal findings and rationale for proceeding
- Counseling of patient regarding abnormal findings
- Patient informed of tests performed to protect the health of the patient
- Patient informed of right to review test results

Allogeneic Donor
- HLA-A, B, DR typing
- Recipient evaluation to prove eligibility for transplant
- CBC, diff, plt—a CBC, diff, plt must be obtained within a 72-hour period prior to the first BSC collection and within 24 hours before each subsequent BSC collection (FACT)
- Chemistries (liver and kidney function)
- PT/PTT/INR
- ABO group and Rh type, blood bank—bone marrow transplant evaluation (type and irregular antibody screen, red cell phenotype, red blood cell crossmatch between donor and recipient, anti-A, anti-B titers as appropriate)
- Infectious disease tests (hepatitis B surface antigen, hepatitis B core antigen, hepatitis C antibody, HIV-1 antibody, HIV-2 antibody, HIV antigen, HTLV, syphilis, and cytomegalovirus) performed within 30 days prior to collection
- Electrocardiogram (BM donors only)
- Chest x-ray (BM donors only)
- Pregnancy assessment (FACT) within 72 hours prior to the start of growth factor (American Association of Blood Banks)
- Screening questions for infectious disease and high-risk behavior
- History and physical (FACT)

The following must be documented:
- Suitability of donor to undergo stem cell collection
- Vaccination history
- Recent blood transfusion history
- Abnormal findings and rationale for proceeding
- Counseling of patient regarding abnormal findings
- Determine if recipient may be informed of abnormal findings and document.
- Inform recipient and document in recipient's chart.
- Patient informed of tests performed to protect the health of the patient
- Patient informed of right to review test results

---

matoma. Mild analgesics may be prescribed for pain. Following BM harvest, donors may become anemic and require a blood transfusion. The allogeneic donor should consider storing autologous red blood cells prior to the procedure, which may need to be infused at the time of the harvest. Autologous donors may need additional intravenous (IV) fluids or a transfusion of irradiated packed red blood cells. Typically, the BM cells that were removed from the donor will regenerate within a few weeks. The nurse should instruct the donor or family member to assess the harvest sites daily for signs of bleeding or infection following the harvest, avoid tub baths for several days (a shower within 24 hours may be permitted at some centers), and avoid heavy lifting.

Buckner et al. (1994) reviewed 1,549 marrow donations for complications following the harvest. The most common complications were postaspiration hypotension (27%), bleeding and need for transfusions (14%), excess pain (8%), and fever (5%). Life-threatening complications (e.g., severe hypotension, cardiac arrest, severe hypoxemia, septicemia, osteomyelitis), usually experienced in the operating room, were encountered by 0.4% of the marrow donors, some of whom had preexisting medical problems (Buckner et al.).

Even though BM harvesting has been performed on a large number of autologous and allogeneic donors, complications are possible, and the donors should be followed.

Pain at the harvest site is a common complaint following BM harvest. Some donors have described the pain similar to a fall on ice. Chern, McCarthy, Hutchins, and Durrant (1999) assessed the duration and severity of pain following BM harvest. They evaluated the effectiveness of a local analgesic, bupivacaine, which was infiltrated into one of the harvest sites, by having donors record the level of pain at each of the harvest sites. BM donors reported a significant reduction in pain at the harvest site that was injected with the analgesic; thus, the authors recommended that bupivacaine be infiltrated into the harvest site routinely following harvest (Chern et al.).

Allogeneic donors may not only experience physical side effects from the BM harvest but also may experience psychological stress. Christopher (2000) conducted an exploratory, descriptive, and qualitative study to describe the experience of donating BM to a relative. Twelve BM donors were interviewed using semistructured questions. Findings of the study indicated that allogeneic donors were not reluctant to donate, would repeat the experience, and felt great personal

Figure 3-2. Peripheral Blood Progenitor Cell Physicians Order Form

PERIPHERAL BLOOD PROGENITOR CELL PHYSICIANS ORDER FORM

RECIPIENT INFORMATION: AUTOLOGOUS ☐ ALLOGENEIC ☐ DONOR LEUKOCYTE INFUSION ☐ OTHER

NAME:		MEDICAL RECORDS #:
HOME ADDRESS: ☐		

DATE OF BIRTH: / /	SOCIAL SECURITY NUMBER - -	WT _____ KG	ABO/Rh	DIAGNOSIS

DONOR INFORMATION:
DONOR NAME: **MEDICAL RECORDS #**

DATE OF BIRTH: / /	SOCIAL SECURITY NUMBER - -	WT _____ KG	ABO/Rh

COLLECTION INFORMATION:

COLLECTION PROTOCOL:_____VOLUME OF BLOOD TO PROCESS EACH DAY:_____liters

MINIMUM NUMBER OF COLLECTIONS: ___ 1 ___ 2 ___ 3 ___ 4 ___OTHER   ANTICIPATED DATE OF FIRST COLLECTION / /

MOBILIZING CYTOKINE:_____

CHEMOTHERAPY MOBILIZED: ____ Yes _____No   DATE_____/_____/_____

DESIRED CELL DOSE FOR TRANSPLANT (#MNC/kg or CD34/kg) _____ x 10^8 MNC/ kg OR _____ x 10^6 CD34+/ kg OR _____OTHER

PROCESSING AND CRYOPRESERVATION: (All collections will be processed by the same method unless otherwise noted)

_____5% DMSO, 6% HES _Investigational; must have documented informed consent on file and plan to store < 2 year_	_____10% DMSO; Controlled Rate Freezing (Standard Method)	_____ OTHER

ASSAYS:

_____ CD34+ CELL ENUMERATION BY FLOW CYTOMETERY (daily on fresh collections)	_____ CFU-GM FRESH DAILY ASSAY	___ CFU-GM FROZEN POOLED ASSAY	_____OTHER

ANTICIPATED DATE OF INFUSION / / _____ UNKNOWN

PHYSICIAN
NAME:_____PHONE_____FAX_____

PHYSICIANS SIGNATURE: _____ DATE_____

TRANSPLANT FACILITY

ADDITIONAL INFORMATION

SUBMIT THE COMPLETED FORM BEFORE THE FIRST COLLECTION TO:

AMERICAN RED CROSS
MIDWEST REGION BLOOD SERVICES
APHERESIS DEPARTMENT
3838 DEWEY AVENUE
OMAHA, NE 68105
or FAX to (402) 341-8107

ARC TO SEND COPY TO:
CELL PROCESSING LABORATORY COORDINATOR
NHS-UNIVERSITY OF NEBRASKA MEDICAL CENTER
600 SO. 42ND STREET
OMAHA, NE 68198-1180
FAX to (402) 559-8838

Version 07/2001

(Continued on next page)

Peripheral Progenitor Cell Physician's Order Form Completion Instructions

Recipient Information:
1. Mark the appropriate box for the type of collection procedure requested, either autologous or allogeneic.
2. Enter the name and medical records number of the recipient.
3. Enter the address, including street address, city, state, and zip code, if known.
4. Enter the date of birth, the social security number, weight in kilograms, ABO/Rh and diagnosis.
5. For allogeneic donors, enter the name and medical records number, the date of birth, social security number, weight, and ABO/Rh of the donor.

Collection Information:
1. Enter the collection protocol, if known, and the volume of blood to process each day in liters.
2. Enter the minimum number of collections and anticipated date of first collection.
3. Enter the mobilizing cytokine, if known.
4. Mark the appropriate blank for chemotherapy mobilized and date, if known.
5. Enter the desired transplant dose for both/or either CD34 or MNC/kg or other.

Processing and Cryopreservation:
1. Mark the appropriate processing and cryopreservation method.

Assays:
1. Mark the appropriate blanks for type of assays requested.

Remaining Information:
1. Enter the anticipated date of infusion, or mark the blank for unknown.
2. The physician name, phone numbers, signature, and date are to be recorded in appropriate blanks.
3. Document the name of the transplant facility.
4. Record any additional information, if applicable.

Note. Figure copyright 2001 by the American Red Cross Midwest Region. Used with permission.

satisfaction following the donation. Issues that created stress in the donor were pain following the harvest, negative patient outcomes, and the donor's relationship with the patient's family. Christopher concluded that adequate education should be provided to the donors and an assessment of their coping should be conducted throughout the transplant course. She suggested that formal donor support programs might be necessary.

Autologous and allogeneic bone marrow stem cell (BMSC) harvesting has been mostly replaced by BSC collections; however, there may be the occasion where it is still appropriate (i.e., inadequate BSC collections or specific study protocols). Currently, unrelated BMSC harvesting is more common than unrelated BSC collection, but this may soon change.

Blood Stem Cell Collection

The use of stem cells collected from the peripheral blood for both autologous and allogeneic transplantation has grown during the last 15 years. In 1986, six independent transplant centers reported successful autologous blood cell transplants (BCTs) (Bell, Figes, Oscier, & Hamblin, 1986; Castaigne et al., 1986; Kessinger, Armitage, Landmark, & Weisenburger, 1986; Korbling et al., 1986; Reiffers et al., 1986; Tilly et al., 1986). Kessinger et al. (1989) reported the first related allogeneic BCT in 1989.

According to the International Bone Marrow Transplant Registry (IBMTR)/Autologous Blood and Marrow Transplant Registry (ABMTR), the number of autologous BCTs has surpassed the number of BMTs per year (see Figure 3-3). The number of allogeneic BCTs also has increased in the last few years (see Figure 3-4) (IBMTR/ABMTR, 2002).

Collecting stem cells from the blood as compared to harvesting stem cells from BM has shown to be more advantageous to the transplant recipient in several aspects. Primarily, BSCs result in more rapid hematopoietic recovery. Following the Second International Meeting on Blood Stem Cell Transplants, Gale, Henon, and Juttner (1992) summarized that this result only occurs when BSCs are mobilized with chemotherapy and/or growth factors. They suggested that the difference is due to the increased number of mature granulocyte progenitors in the stem cell product. Other variables that may affect the rate of hematopoietic recovery include dose of cells given, the intensity of the preparative regimen, and the amount of prior BM damage. They stated that although a minimum number of cells may be required for transplant, there are many factors (e.g., infections, antibiotics) that impact and obscure correlations between cell dose and hematopoietic recovery (Gale et al.). The rapid hematopoietic recovery that patients receiving BCTs experience results in a decrease in infections, transfusions, hospital days, and overall cost as compared to bone marrow transplant (BMT) (To et al., 1992).

A second advantage (discussed later in this chapter) for patients who receive BSCs in comparison with stem cells harvested from BM is the BSC product may have a lower risk of contamination by tumor cells (Gale et al., 1992; Sharp et al.,

Figure 3-3. Autologous Stem Cell Sources by Age, 1996–2001

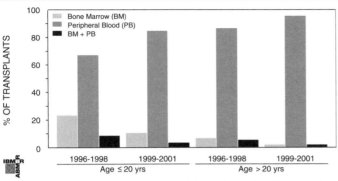

More than 95% of autotransplants in adults and 80% in children and adolescents use hematopoietic progenitor cells collected from blood. The remainder use bone marrow alone or in combination with cells collected from blood.

Note. From *2002 IBMTR/ABMTR Summary Slides: State-of-the-Art in Blood and Marrow Transplantation,* by the International Bone Marrow Transplant Directory and Autologous Blood and Marrow Transplant Directory, 2002, retrieved May 22, 2003, from http://instruct.mcw.edu/ IBMTR/BWebServer/summarysldset/summset_files/v3_document.htm. Copyright 2002 by IBMTR/ABMTR. Reprinted with permission.

1992). An advantage noted by many authors is that BSC collections may be performed in an outpatient setting, without general anesthesia. Also, patients who have tumor in the marrow or have had pelvic irradiation that caused BM fibrosis may undergo successful BSC collection.

Mobilization of Stem Cells

The number of circulating stem cells in the blood is low as compared with the number of stem cells in BM. Stem cells may be collected from the blood, whereas BM is in a steady state, and the patient has to have recovered from all chemotherapy or radiation. This method of collecting will result in an adequate product but may require multiple apheresis procedures. Mobilization of stem cells refers to methods of stimulating the stem cell that originates in BM to move into the peripheral blood.

Two methods have been used to increase the number of circulating stem cells. These include chemotherapy and, more recently, growth factors. Gianni et al. (1990) mobilized stem cells in patients with a combination of chemotherapy and growth factors. Because no growth factors were administered to the patients post-transplant, the accelerated hematopoietic recoveries that were observed were attributable solely to the infusion of mobilized stem cells.

Chemotherapy

Following standard chemotherapy, there is a transient increase, or "overshoot," in the number of circulating stem cells (Richman, Weiner, & Yankee, 1976). As the white blood cells (WBCs) start to recover, the stem cells also recover and may be harvested during this transient increase in number. In one of the earliest reports, To et al. (1990) reported the use of cy-

clophosphamide at a dose of 4 g/m^2 to mobilize stem cells in 30 patients with lymphoma, myeloma, breast carcinoma, ovarian carcinoma, and sarcomas. They found that at approximately 16 days following the chemotherapy, there was approximately a 14-fold increase above baseline in the number of circulating granulocyte macrophage–colony-forming units (CFU-GM), which lasts for approximately four to five days. Following this report, cyclophosphamide or chemotherapy regimens used for the treatment of the patient's malignancy became one of the most common mobilization methods. Bishop (1994) indicated that the administration of chemotherapy for mobilization should be started when the patient has recovered from prior chemotherapy or radiation. Patients should be closely monitored, and apheresis should begin when the patient starts to recover from his or her neutrophil nadir, approximately 10–14 days postchemotherapy (Bishop).

Chemotherapy for mobilization may result in more rapid hematopoietic recovery following transplant but may have several disadvantages. To et al. (1990) reported that several patients who received myelosuppressive chemotherapy for mobilization developed neutropenic sepsis and required antibiotic therapy. To et al. (1990) also reported on one patient who died while neutropenic from the chemotherapy mobilization. The patient developed streptococcal septicemia and died of a probable cardiac arrhythmia. Other disadvantages to using chemotherapy for mobilization are that patients who have received multiple courses of chemotherapy or patients with tumor in their BM may fail to mobilize (To et al., 1990). Using chemotherapy for mobilization also may be time consuming. The patient must receive chemotherapy, wait approximately 10–16 days for the optimal time to collect, collect over several days, and then com-

Figure 3-4. Allogeneic Stem Cell Sources by Age, 1996–2001

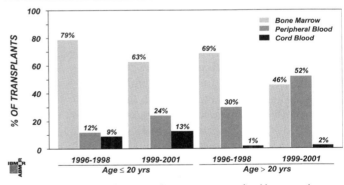

Most allogeneic transplants use bone marrow grafts. However, in 1998–2000 there was a steady increase in use of peripheral blood stem cells, especially in older recipients. There also was an increase in use of umbilical cord blood stem cells in recipients aged ≤ 20 years but very few cord blood transplants in older recipients.

Note. From *2002 IBMTR/ABMTR Summary Slides: State-of-the-Art in Blood and Marrow Transplantation,* by the International Bone Marrow Transplant Directory and Autologous Blood and Marrow Transplant Directory, 2002, retrieved May 22, 2003, from http://instruct.mcw.edu/ IBMTR/BWebServer/summarysldset/summset_files/v3_document.htm. Copyright 2002 by IBMTR/ABMTR. Reprinted with permission.

pletely recover from the toxicities of chemotherapy. If an insufficient number of stem cells are collected, the process must be repeated (Kessinger, 1993).

Chemotherapy mobilization side effects are similar to side effects encountered with standard doses of chemotherapy, including pancytopenia, infection, hair loss, mucositis, nausea, vomiting, or other side effects associated with the specific chemotherapy agent. Patients should be closely monitored for side effects of the chemotherapy.

Hematopoietic Growth Factors

Another method to mobilize stem cells is the use of hematopoietic growth factors to stimulate the number of stem cells in the blood. Socinski et al. (1988) conducted a three-phase study in which patients with sarcoma received granulocyte macrophage–colony-stimulating factor (GM-CSF). The study found that GM-CSF alone increased the number of circulating progenitor cells by approximately 18-fold. In patients who received GM-CSF and chemotherapy, the number of circulating progenitor cells increased by approximately 60-fold. This initial study concluded that the utilization of GM-CSF might expedite collecting stem cells from the blood for transplantation.

Haas et al. (1990) reported the use of GM-CSF used to mobilize 12 patients with hematologic malignancies. GM-CSF was given as a continuous IV infusion. In these patients, a 8.5-fold increase was noted in progenitor cells. Haas et al. also noted a decrease in the platelet count (median 21%, range 7%–67%) during GM-CSF administration but prior to the start of the apheresis collection procedures.

In a sequential study (Bishop et al., 1994) involving hard-to-mobilize patients (i.e., extensive prior chemotherapy and/ or BM deficiencies, presence or history of morphologic tumor contamination and/or hypocellularity), GM-CSF mobilization demonstrated that adequate numbers of stem cells could be collected. This study also noted that transplantation with GM-CSF–mobilized stem cells resulted in significantly earlier recovery for granulocytes and shorter time to platelet and red blood cell transfusion independence. Bishop et al. (1994) reported that following BCT, the rate of engraftment between the nonmobilized and mobilized groups of patients was not affected by growth factors.

Currently, the most commonly used dose of GM-CSF is 125–250 mcg/m^2/day, and the most commonly used dose of granulocyte–colony-stimulating factor (G-CSF) is 5–10 mcg/kg/day. Typically, the growth factors are given as a subcutaneous injection, although initially there were many reports of continuous IV infusion (Gianni et al., 1990; Haas et al., 1990; Socinski et al., 1988). Although growth factors usually are given in a once-daily injection, Lee et al. (2000) gave G-CSF 5 mcg/kg twice daily to mobilize stem cells in healthy donors and pediatric patients for autologous backup before receiving an allogeneic stem cell transplant. This group of patients was compared to historical controls who had received G-CSF 10 mcg/kg daily. The conclusion of the study was that the twice-daily dose of G-CSF was more efficient in mobilizing stem cells (Lee et al.).

Many current mobilization protocols include chemotherapy and hematopoietic growth factors. The growth factors not only help to reduce cytopenia following chemotherapy but also dramatically increase the number of circulating progenitor cells (Gianni, Siena, et al., 1989). This combination method of mobilization may produce the most stem cells possible, but patients may experience significant side effects from the chemotherapy.

The most common side effects associated with growth factors used for mobilization include bone pain, fever, and malaise. Other less common symptoms are chills, headache, nausea, vomiting, diarrhea, edema, rash, irritation at injection site, dyspnea, pleural or pericardial effusion, and nasal congestion. Most symptoms are minimal and easily treated and resolve upon the discontinuation of the growth factor. Daily nursing assessments should include a discussion of symptoms and an evaluation of temperature, pulse, respirations, blood pressure, and weight. Patients may be instructed to take acetaminophen for the bone pain or headache. Occasionally, a patient will request a stronger pain reliever, such as acetaminophen with codeine. Other side effects should be assessed and treated symptomatically. More serious side effects (e.g., pleural or pericardial effusions) may necessitate stopping the growth factors.

Other types of growth factors that have been used for mobilization of stem cells are included in a study by Vose et al. (1992), who examined the effect of interleukin- (IL-) 3 on the stem cell product. The conclusion of this study was that even though there was an increase in the progenitor cell content, use of the cells for autologous transplantation did not result in quicker hematopoietic recovery.

Another study by Bishop et al. (1996) reported that the use of PIXY321 (Immunex Corp., Seattle, WA), a fusion protein that consists of GM-CSF and IL-3, successfully mobilized progenitors into the peripheral blood, and hematopoietic recovery was rapid following transplantation. Bishop et al. (1996) concluded that PIXY321, if combined with other mobilization methods, might improve the quality of the stem cell product.

Recombinant human stem cell factor (SCF), usually in combination with G-CSF, is another growth factor that has been studied (Glaspy et al., 1997). SCF is active on early progenitor cells and also on the erythroid and myeloid cell lines. SCF is able to synergize with other growth factors (Shpall, 1999). Shpall reported the use of SCF with G-CSF or G-CSF alone to mobilize patients with breast cancer. Hard-to-mobilize patients who were mobilized with SCF plus G-CSF were able to reach the target CD34+ cell number and had a more sustained increase in the number of CD34+ cells, resulting in a lesser number of apheresis collections (Shpall).

Kessinger and Sharp (1996) reported on the administration of recombinant human erythropoietin (epoetin alfa) during BSC collections for 12 patients. Patients received epoetin alfa 200 units/day until an adequate product was obtained. In the 11 assessable patients, the peak mobilization effect was noted on the fourth day of the growth factor. Nine of the patients received high-dose therapy and were transplanted with these BSCs. Engraftment was comparable to patients who had received autologous BMT. Kessinger and Sharp concluded that the administration of epoetin alfa increases the number of circulating progenitor cells, even from nonerythropoietic lineages. However, because of the need for more clinical trials, the clinical significance of epoetin alfa as a mobilizing agent still needs to be determined.

Other growth factors that have been used in studies include recombinant Mpl ligands and the flt-3 ligand. The use of both chemotherapy and growth factors for mobilization appears to result in the quickest collection time and the quickest recovery time following transplant.

Tumor Cell Mobilization

Circulating tumor cells have been detected in stem cell products from patients with lymphoma and metastatic breast cancer (Sharp et al., 1992). Sharp et al. found that detection of tumor cells in the BSC product was significantly less than in BM products. They also found that patients with non-Hodgkin's lymphoma who received BSC products, even though they had tumor in their BM, had a better survival outcome than patients who received BM. Brugger et al. (1994) demonstrated that patients who had circulating tumor cells prior to mobilization showed an increase in the number of tumor cells present following mobilization. In patients who did not demonstrate any circulating tumor cells premobilization, 21% (9 of 42) were found to have circulating tumor cells following mobilization, especially in patients who had stage IV breast cancer or extensive-disease small-cell lung cancer (Brugger et al., 1994). The significance of harvesting tumor cells in the stem cell product is not verified, but infusing a product containing tumor cells might contribute to relapse.

In patients with stage IV breast cancer, Kahn et al. (1997) showed that as the number of apheresis procedures increases, the amount of tumor cell contamination in the product also increases. They noted that the incidence of tumor contamination from the first apheresis (5.4%) increased dramatically in the second apheresis (15.4%). Kahn et al. concluded that decreasing the number of apheresis collections would decrease the amount of tumor contamination for patients with stage IV breast cancer.

Mobilization Failure

Patients who have received multiple courses of chemotherapy or who have BM metastases may not achieve an increased number of circulating stem cells with mobilization and may not be able to collect enough stem cells for transplant. Stiff (1999) listed several chemotherapeutic agents (melphalan, nitrosoureas, procarbazine, nitrogen mustard, alkylating agents, and platinum compounds) that appear to be more toxic to the patient and may cause difficulties in collecting stem cells. Other risk factors that also may make it difficult to mobilize and collect adequate stem cells are type of malignancy (breast cancer, Hodgkin's disease, non-Hodgkin's lymphoma, and ovarian cancer), an age older than 60, and prior radiation to marrow-producing sites (Stiff). He reviewed four strategies to obtain adequate stem cells: (a) BM harvesting, (b) remobilization, (c) mobilization with growth factors plus chemotherapy, and (d) dose escalation of growth factors.

Addition of Bone Marrow to Blood Stem Cells

Studies have reported the addition of BSCs to BM harvests in efforts to achieve quicker engraftment or to augment a below-minimum BM stem cell harvest. Lobo et al. (1991) randomized 35 patients with various malignancies to receiving BCT in combination with BM or BM alone. No manipulations were performed on the BSC products. BSCs were collected with four-hour leukapheresis procedures on three consecutive days. Lobo et al. found that the addition of nonmobilized BSCs to autologous marrow did not accelerate marrow recovery.

However, another team (Gianni, Bregni, et al., 1989) treated 19 patients with high-dose melphalan and total body irradiation (TBI). Six patients received BSCs harvested with chemotherapy-induced mobilization in addition to BM. Patients receiving BSCs had an earlier recovery of granulocytes, received fewer platelets and red blood cell transfusions, and had a shorter hospitalization period than those who received BM alone.

In a report by Watts et al. (1998), back-up BM was harvested in patients who had a poor BSC collection. In their conclusion, harvesting and infusing back-up BM does not improve engraftment, possibly suggesting that patients who have poor BSC mobilization may have poor marrow function. Stiff (1999) concluded that, overall, the addition of BM stem cells to BSC products offers little value to the patient.

Remobilization

Patients who are not able to collect enough cells for transplant may be able to repeat the mobilization procedure. Weaver et al. (1998) retrospectively reviewed the results of 119 patients who underwent a second mobilization and collection attempt. These patients had failed to collect $\geq 2.5 \times 10^6$ CD34+ cells/kg after mobilization with chemotherapy and/or G-CSF. Weaver et al. (1998) found that 48% of the patients were able to obtain an adequate number of stem cells after the second mobilization attempt, which usually yielded more CD34+ cells per apheresis than the first, suggesting a priming effect of the first mobilization efforts. Also, during the second attempt at mobilization, no difference was found between the number of CD34+ cells harvested in either mobilization method, growth factor alone, or chemotherapy plus growth factor. This is distinctly different from CD34+ cell numbers from the first mobilization attempt, in which more CD34+ cells were harvested following chemotherapy plus G-CSF (Weaver et al., 1998).

Stiff (1999) concluded that remobilizing patients who initially mobilize poorly with chemotherapy and growth factors may yield an adequate stem cell product. However, Stiff cautioned that the costs involved in the remobilization and the additional side effects must be considered.

Mobilization With Growth Factors and Chemotherapy

Stiff (1999) reviewed the data from several centers using chemotherapy and growth factors initially for mobilization. He concluded that the data suggested that this method of mobilization may be advantageous for the patient, but comparative trials consisting of hard-to-mobilize patients using a variety of mobilization techniques have not been conducted.

Dose-Escalation of Growth Factors

Several studies have compared the use of varying doses of growth factors on the stem cell product (Bishop et al., 1994; Stiff, 1999). These studies indicated that higher doses of growth factors resulted in a lesser number of apheresis procedures for those patients. Stiff noted that the cost associated with higher doses of growth factors may be offset by the cost of the additional apheresis procedures and platelet and red cell transfusions required by the lower-dose group.

Stiff (1999) suggested trying to target groups of patients at risk for poor mobilization instead of targeting individual patients. The options presented above need more research, including randomized trials to determine their usefulness in patients who are hard-to-mobilize or fail mobilization.

Apheresis Issues

Peripheral Venous Access Versus Central Venous Catheters

Antecubital veins may be used to harvest BSCs, but patients who have received multiple courses of chemotherapy may not have adequate venous access. Most centers use a thick-walled, large lumen (10–18.5 French) apheresis or hemodialysis catheter, which allows flow rates up to 250 ml/hour or greater, to withdraw blood during apheresis (Camp-Sorrell, 2004). Apheresis catheters are usually inserted into the subclavian vein and may be tunneled to provide long-term access. However, other venous access sites that have been used are the jugular vein (Bishop et al., 1997; Camp-Sorrell), the inferior vena cava (Haire et al., 1990), and the femoral vein (Camp-Sorrell). Pediatric patients may require a smaller catheter (7–8 French) (Secola, 1997). Antecubital veins are most commonly used in allogeneic donors. However, if peripheral venous access cannot be obtained or maintained in allogeneic donors, Bishop et al. (1997) described the use of a 13.5 French right atrial double-lumen apheresis catheter that is placed temporarily in the jugular vein. Ultimately, the transplant team must consider the size and type of catheter, along with patient or donor comfort, that will yield the highest flow rate during apheresis. Often the catheter used for apheresis also may be used for venous access during the high-dose therapy, reinfusion of stem cells, and recovery phases.

Buchsel, Leum, and Randolph (1997) noted several adverse events that may occur during the placement of a catheter, including perforation of the vein, pneumothorax, or hemothorax. In addition, the authors also described other complications associated with the catheter such as infection, occlusion, thrombus, catheter rupture, and phlebitis. Table 3-1 describes symptoms and management of these complications.

Care of the apheresis catheter varies widely from institution to institution. Camp-Sorrell (2004) described a common maintenance procedure for tunneled and nontunneled catheters using a transparent dressing, changed every 5–7 days, or gauze, changed every day. Dressings should be changed more frequently if they become soiled or wet. The catheter should be flushed daily with heparin or saline. Stephens et al. (1997) compared the incidence of thrombotic occlusions in catheters in 78 patients undergoing apheresis in which heparin or saline was used for routine flushing. Stephens et al. (1997) concluded that there was no significant difference in clotting problems between the two groups of patients, suggesting saline may be as effective as heparin in maintaining catheter patency.

Timing and Initiation of Apheresis

Initiation of collection of stem cells following chemotherapy mobilization can be difficult to determine but usually begins when the WBC count reaches 1.0^9/liter. Assessing the number of CD34+ cells in the peripheral blood may indicate the best time to start the collection, but this assay is expensive. Usually, once the WBC count starts to rise following nadir, the number of stem cells also start to increase. Stem cell collection following growth factor mobilization usually begins when the WBC count reaches 10.0^9/liter or greater, or approximately 4–5 days following the start of the growth factor. If both chemotherapy and growth factors are used to mobilize stem cells, collection of stem cells also begins during the recovery of WBCs, approximately when the WBC count reaches 1.0^9/liter.

Type of Apheresis Device

Following mobilization, the BSCs from the patient or donor are collected via a process called apheresis. The apheresis process involves using a commercial cell separator to centrifuge the blood and separate the components by density into various layers. The white cell and platelet layer is located between the red cell and plasma layers. Located in the white cell layer are the mononuclear cells and stem cells. Several apheresis machines are available that may be programmed to harvest stem cells. They include the COBE® Spectra™ (COBE BCT, Lakewood, CO), Haemonetics® V-50™ (Haemonetics, Braintree, MA), and the Fenwall CS-3000™ (Baxter Healthcare, Deerfield, IL). (See picture of patient collecting stem cells, Figure 3-5.) The patient's blood is withdrawn through the central venous catheter into the apheresis machine and centrifuged. As the blood is drawn into the apheresis machine, an anticoagulant, citrate dextrose solution (ACD-A), is added to prevent clotting. The ratio of ACD-A to blood is usually 1:12. The apheresis machine centrifuges the blood, transfers the stem cells into a collection bag, and returns the remaining blood to the patient via the central venous catheter.

Table 3-1. Complications of Central Venous Catheters

Complications	Time of Onset	Symptoms	Cause	Clinical Management	Nursing Management
Exit site bleeding/ hematoma	Insertion	Oozing or frank bleeding from exit site; discoloration or bruising	Introducer sheath larger than catheter left in place or traumatic insertion. Patient may have coagulopathies or thrombocytopenia or be on anticoagulants	Additional sutures may be necessary, possible removal of catheter	Apply local pressure, change dressings as needed.
Pneumothorax or hemothorax	Insertion	Chest pain, tachypnea, dyspnea, decreased breath sounds	Air or blood in the pleural cavity because of pleura, vein, or thoracic duct injury	Chest x-ray, oxygen, needle aspirations, and chest tube drainage	Administration of oxygen, care of chest tube
Exit site infection	Duration of catheter placement	Fever, skin breakdown, local erythema, pain, tenderness at catheter insertion site, possible purulent drainage, sepsis	Neutropenia secondary to chemo-mobilization, poor catheter management techniques, commonly gram-positive organisms	Antibiotics	Blood and exit site cultures, administration of antibiotics if indicated. Teach aseptic technique in dressing changes and catheter flushing, signs and symptoms of infection, and emergency instructions.
Tunnel infection	Duration of catheter placement	Erythema, induration, tenderness along subcutaneous track of catheter, possible purulent exudate	Neutropenia secondary to chemomobilization, poor catheter management techniques, commonly gram-positive organisms	Antibiotics, possible catheter removal	Blood cultures, culture exudate if present, administration of appropriate antibiotics
Line infections	Duration of catheter placement	Cellulitis	Neutropenia secondary to chemomobilization, poor catheter management techniques, commonly gram-positive organisms, colonization of infecting organism (i.e., *Staphylococcus epidermis, Staphylococcus aureus*)	Antibiotics, possible catheter removal	Blood cultures, culture exudate if present, administration of appropriate antibiotics
Catheter occlusion	Duration of catheter placement, particularly during apheresis procedure	Inability to aspirate from or flush catheter, arm swelling, pain may be asymptomatic	G-CSF, GM-CSF, thrombus, technical or mechanical problems, blood clotting, drug precipitate	Venogram, Doppler study, dye study, chest x-ray, alteplase (2 mg)	Gentle catheter flushing with heparin, reposition patient, possible catheter removal. Instill alteplase (2 mg) into lumen of catheter and let stand for 30 minutes. Attempt to aspirate, may repeat.
Catheter-related venous thrombus	Duration of catheter placement, particularly during mobilization and stem cell collection	Arm swelling, pain may be asymptomatic. Venous congestion in neck on side of catheter	Venous collateral circulation	Venogram, Doppler study, dye study, chest x-ray, alteplase (2 mg)	Reposition patient, gentle catheter flushing, possible catheter removal, monitor daily prothrombin time/partial thromboplastin time
Catheter rupture	Duration of catheter placement, particularly during mobilization and stem cell collection	Pain, shortness of breath, air and blood emboli, leakage from catheter, inability to aspirate catheter	Frequent catheter manipulation, forceful flushing against resistance	Replace catheter	Turn patient on left side and call physician; clean and secure catheter; repair or exchange if possible; possible catheter removal

Note. From "Nursing Care of the Blood Cell Transplant Recipient," by P.C. Buchsel, E. Leum, and S.R. Randolph, 1997, *Seminars in Oncology Nursing, 13,* pp. 174–175. Copyright 1997 by W.B. Saunders; and *Access Device Guidelines: Recommendations for Nursing Practice and Education* (2nd ed., pp. 14–15), by D. Camp-Sorrell (Ed.), 2004, Pittsburgh, PA: Oncology Nursing Society. Copyright 2004 by the Oncology Nursing Society. Adapted with permission.

Figure 3-5. Patient Collecting Stem Cells

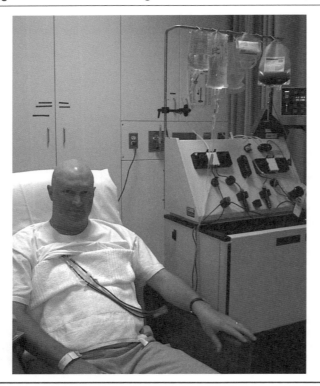

Kessinger, Schmit-Pokorny, Smith, and Armitage (1990) reported that stem cell products that contain larger volumes of red cells resulted in a higher frequency of reinfusion toxicities. One hundred consecutive autologous BCT patients were evaluated for the type and frequency of side effects during BSC infusion. Side effects that were associated with a larger volume of red cells were hypertension, chills, nausea, and fever. Side effects that were associated with a larger volume of red cells and larger overall volume were tachypnea, elevated serum bilirubin, and elevated serum creatinine (Kessinger et al., 1990). Implementing methods during apheresis or processing to completely remove red cells from the stem cell product is possible; however, Kessinger et al. (1990) reported that while there were fewer side effects during reinfusion, it resulted in slower engraftment.

Amount of Blood to Process

In adults, approximately 12–15 liters of blood, at a flow rate between 50 and 100 ml/minute, are commonly processed from a patient each day. Each apheresis procedure takes two to four hours, and an adequate number of cells may be achieved in one collection. The average number of collections is four; however, patients may need to undergo collection many days. Apheresis procedures that process large volumes of blood in a single collection result in the collection of large numbers of BSCs. In a report by Pettengell et al. (1993), 45 patients mobilized using chemotherapy and G-CSF underwent a single apheresis collection procedure, processing a median of 14 liters of blood (range, 5.6–23 liters). The me-

dian number of CD34+ cells harvested was 10.6×10^6/kg (range 1.9–398). Forty patients underwent high-dose therapy and BSC transplantation. All patients achieved rapid hematopoietic engraftment. Pettengell et al. concluded that a single apheresis collection could result in adequate engraftment. In another study, Feremans et al. (1996) reported using large-volume apheresis in one collection to harvest stem cells. In 26 patients who were mobilized with chemotherapy plus G-CSF or G-CSF alone, 24 were able to harvest adequate numbers of stem cells for transplant in one large-volume (median volume 20 liters, range 10–22 liters) apheresis. Kapustay and Buchsel (2000) described large-volume apheresis in which 40 liters of blood are processed in one six- to seven-hour apheresis session. They indicated that increased citrate toxicity occurs during large volume apheresis collections. Oral calcium given prophylactically and administration of 1 gram of IV calcium gluconate every hour may be necessary to manage the toxicities associated with the large amount of citrate. Collecting adequate BSCs in one collection enables BCT to be a cost-effective option for patients; however, some patients may not be able to tolerate the lengthy procedure or side effects. Also, reducing the number of collections results in a decrease in the amount of dimethyl sulfoxide (DMSO) necessary to preserve the product, thus potentially minimizing side effects during infusion of the stem cells.

Stem Cell Collection

The amount of stem cells collected is related to the rate of engraftment. Higher amounts of stem cells collected usually result in quicker engraftment, although complications associated with the high-dose therapy play a role (Pecora, 1999). A variety of methods have been used to determine an adequate number of stem cells to collect for transplant. Initially, the number of mononuclear cells present in the product was used to determine an adequate product. Mononuclear cells are easy to measure, but these mature cells may not be the most efficient method to determine the number of stem cells present. The colony assay, which detects committed progenitors, specifically CFU-GMs, became the more common method to determine the number of cells required for transplant. To et al. (1992) reported that BCT recipients who received a higher dose of CFU-GM in comparison to autologous and allogeneic BMT recipients recovered from neutropenia and thrombocytopenia significantly faster. Also, in comparison, the BCT recipients required less supportive care. A disadvantage of using CFU-GM assays for determining adequate stem cell dosage are that the assays must incubate for approximately two weeks following each collection. After two weeks have passed, it may be determined that the product is inadequate, and the mobilization and collection process must be repeated. A second disadvantage to using the CFU-GM assay is the different techniques used between laboratories and the lack of a consistent method, resulting in an inability to compare outcomes between centers (Bender, Bik, Williams, & Schwartzberg, 1992).

Currently, the most commonly used method to determine an adequate dose of stem cells for transplant is the use of flow cytometric analysis to measure the number of cells expressing the CD34 antigen in the product. The CD34 antigen is present on committed hematopoietic progenitor cells and pluripotent stem cells (Golde, 1991). As BSCs mature, the expression of the CD34 antigen decreases, and these cells are no longer identified as CD34 positive (Vescio et al., 1994). An advantage of flow cytometric analysis over colony assays is that the results are available in less than three hours after collection.

Siena et al. (1991) reported that the number of CD34+ cells correlates well with the number of circulating CFU-GM colonies in chemotherapy and growth factor–mobilized patients. Unfortunately, the laboratory method of conducting the CD34+ assay may vary from center to center, again making it difficult to compare CD34+ numbers between centers. The dose of CD34+ cells infused also varies widely from center to center. Several studies indicate that a dose of $\geq$ 5 x 10^6 CD34+ cells/kg ensures rapid engraftment, whereas doses < 1 x 10^6 CD34+ cells/kg may result in delayed engraftment (Bensinger, Appelbaum, et al., 1995; Bensinger, Weaver, et al., 1995; Weaver et al., 1995).

Another method that may be able to predict the number of stem cells collected is using the number of morphologically identified blast cells in the stem cell product as a marker of stem cell content. Mijovic, Fishlock, Pagliuca, and Mufti (1998) found that the number of blast cells reported in the stem cell product correlated with the number of CD34+ cells, CFU-GM colonies, and engraftment following autologous transplantation. They found that if the number of reported blasts in the product was above 1.3 x 10^6/kg, hematopoietic recovery would most likely be rapid.

Side Effects of Collection

Common side effects encountered during the apheresis procedure are hypocalcemia, hypovolemia, thrombocytopenia, anemia, chilling, and headache. Usually these side effects are minimal and well tolerated. Table 3-2 describes potential complications of stem cell collections. Another complication frequently encountered during the apheresis is catheter occlusion. Occlusion may result from the catheter resting against the wall of the vein, a kink in the catheter, or a clot or fibrin sheath around the end of the catheter. Stephens, Haire, Schmit-Pokorny, Kessinger, and Kotulak (1993) compared patients who did not receive growth factors for mobilization with patients who were mobilized with continuous-infusion GM-CSF. Even though all patients received aspirin 325 mg daily as a prophylaxis, the GM-CSF-mobilized patients had a significantly higher rate of catheter occlusions. Although the exact mechanism for the formation of the clot is unknown, the authors suggested that contributing factors may include proliferation of "sticky" neutrophils, which aggregate at the catheter tip, the method of administration of the GM-CSF, or changes in the coagulation and fibrinolytic systems caused by the GM-CSF (Stephens et al., 1993). Flushing the catheter with normal saline or repositioning the patient may correct the obstruction. A fibrinolytic agent, Activase® (alteplase, recombinant) (Genentech,

South San Francisco, CA) may be necessary to lyse or dissolve the clot. Occasionally, a cathetergram or dye injected into the catheter may be necessary to determine the exact cause of the obstruction. If a clot is noted at the end of the catheter, additional injections of alteplase may be necessary to dissolve the clot. Occasionally, a catheter may need to be repositioned or replaced if the clot cannot be corrected.

During the apheresis procedure, the platelet count or hemoglobin may decrease because of removal of the cells into the product collection bag. Patients may need to receive irradiated packed red blood cells or platelets to replenish the cells removed. Patients who have received chemotherapy for mobilization may need to receive blood products prior to the apheresis to ensure a safe procedure. Transfusions should be considered for patients with a hemoglobin count < 9 g/dl and a platelet count < 80,000/mm^3.

Allogeneic Blood Stem Cell Collections

The first reported related allogeneic BCT was in an 18-year-old male diagnosed with acute lymphocytic leukemia (Kessinger et al., 1989). Stem cells were collected from his 21-year-old human leukocyte antigen- (HLA-) identical sibling because he was unwilling to undergo general anesthesia and marrow harvesting. Ten apheresis collections were performed, and the product was T lymphocyte depleted. A BM biopsy and cytogenetic studies on day +27 showed trilineage engraftment with donor cells. Unfortunately, the patient died from a fungal infection on day +32, and long-term engraftment could not be evaluated. Advantages of an allogeneic BCT include more rapid hematopoietic and immune recovery, avoidance of general anesthesia, and avoidance of the side effects associated with BM harvest (Goldman, 1995; Russell & Hunter, 1994). Disadvantages may include the theoretical concern of an increased risk of GVHD (Henon et al., 1992; Roberts et al., 1993; Weaver, Longin, Buckner, & Bensinger, 1994). Several more recent reports indicated a decrease in acute GVHD, decreased initial hospital stay, and decreased overall morbidity as compared with BMT (Bensinger, Weaver, et al. 1995; Korbling et al., 1995; Schmitz et al., 1995), whereas other authors have reported increased chronic GVHD (Shea, 1999; Storek et al., 1997). Shea suggested that the large number of T cells in the peripheral blood is responsible for the possible increase in chronic GVHD.

Allogeneic donors usually are mobilized using G-CSF 5–10 mcg/kg, similar to autologous patients. Bishop et al. (1997) mobilized 41 donors with G-CSF 5 mcg/kg and gathered a minimum of three collections per donor. Toxicities were evaluated daily by the clinical nurse coordinator and the apheresis nurse. Each donor also maintained a diary to record any adverse effect of G-CSF administration and apheresis procedures. The most common side effects were arthralgias/myalgias (83%), headache (44%), fever (27%), and chills (22%). Other side effects noted were nausea/emesis, paresthesias, chest pain, cough, diarrhea, sore throat, and hypertension. Except for one, all recorded side effects

Table 3-2. Potential Complications During Stem Cell Collection

Potential Complications	Etiology	Assessment	Interventions
Hypocalcemia	Sodium citrate used to prevent blood from clotting in the apheresis machine binds ionized calcium.	• Baseline serum calcium • Hourly ionized calcium* • Patient age • Assess for paresthesias of the extremities or circumoral area during the procedure.	• Notify physician if calcium is low. • Slow flow rate and offer oral calcium, liquid or tablets. • Increase calcium-containing foods. • Advise patient to take oral calcium supplements. • Administer IV calcium gluconate (for severe symptoms).

Hypovolemia	Extracorporeal volume greater than patient tolerance	• Baseline pulse, blood pressure, hemoglobin/hematocrit, and health history
		• Brief physical assessment and vital signs every five minutes initially, gradually decreasing frequency as patient's tolerance is established
		• Assess for
		  - Hypotension
		  - Tachycardia
		  - Light-headedness
		  - Diaphoresis
		  - Dysrhythmias
			• Notify physician of abnormal or unexpected findings before proceeding.
			• Interrupt the procedure until the patient is stable, then resume at a slower flow rate and minimal extracorporeal volume.
			• Monitor physical status and vital signs closely. Notify physician if symptoms persist or progress.
			• Administer blood products.
			• Administer fluid.

Thrombocytopenia	Collection of platelets into product	• Baseline platelet count • Ascertain whether platelet-rich plasma will be returned at the procedure's completion.	• Notify physician if count is less than 50,000/mm³. • Monitor for signs of post-procedure bleeding. • Administer platelet products.
Miscellaneous effects Chilling	• Cooling of blood while circulating in the apheresis machine	• Observe for chilling.	• Provide warmth (e.g., blankets, heating pad).
Severe headache	• Growth factor side effect • Intracranial metastases unique to patient with cancer	• Pain relievers • CT or MRI of the brain in patients prone to intracranial metastases prior to beginning apheresis	• Administer analgesics.
Prolonged cytopenia	• Previous chemotherapy regimens • Pediatric patients with less developed hematopoietic progenitor pool*	• Observe for headache. • Observe daily complete blood count, platelets, and differential.	• Transfusion support

*Applies to pediatric patients

Note. From "Peripheral Blood Stem Cell Transplantation," by P.J. Hooper and E.J. Santos, 1993, *Oncology Nursing Forum, 20,* p. 1218. Copyright 1993 by the Oncology Nursing Society. Adapted with permission.

were grade 1, according to the Common Toxicity Criteria of the National Cancer Institute (1999). One patient experienced hypertension, grade 3, and was treated with nifedipine. Bishop et al. (1997) concluded that low doses of G-CSF can effectively and safely be used for mobilization.

Wiesneth et al. (1998) reported the use of G-CSF 10–12 mcg/kg to mobilize 96 related donors. BSC harvest was started on day four of the growth factor, and donors collected in an average of two days (range 1–4). Wiesneth et al. found that the peak level of CD34+ cells occurred between days four and six of the G-CSF administration. They also found that female and older donors tended to have a decreased response to the G-CSF; however, this was not

statistically significant. Retransfusion of platelets collected during the apheresis procedure was necessary in 16% of the donors because of a platelet count < 80,000/mm³ post-apheresis (Wiesneth et al.).

A report of a serious adverse event in an allogeneic donor possibly related to the mobilization technique was splenic rupture and pneumothorax that occurred with a 22-year-old male (Becker et al., 1997). The donor received six days of G-CSF prior to apheresis. Four days following the completion of apheresis, the donor presented with left-sided abdominal pain, dyspnea, hypotension, and tachycardia. A CT scan revealed a ruptured spleen, and emergency surgery was required. Becker et al. concluded that even though growth factors have proved to be advantageous for recipients, potentially serious adverse effects are possible. In most circumstances, growth factor–mobilized stem cells can be safely collected from donors; however, because serious side effects may occur, donors should be thoroughly educated about potential complications.

Pediatric Blood Stem Cell Collections

Special consideration must be given to pediatric patients during the collection of BSCs. The volume of blood processed during the apheresis procedure must be based on the child's size. Commonly, 200–250 ml of blood per kilogram of body weight may be processed, dependent on the patient's tolerance of the procedure. Schmit-Pokorny and Nuss (2000) reported large volume apheresis procedures, processing up to 450 ml of blood per kilogram of body weight (up to 15 liters total). In an effort to decrease the amount of blood lost during priming of the apheresis machine, a pediatric-sized centrifuge bowl may be used with small children. Also, the apheresis machine and tubing may need to be preprimed with irradiated red blood cells if more than 10%–15% of the child's total blood volume (a child weighing 20 kg or less) is needed for priming the apheresis machine (Chan & Bond, 1994). Another method to decrease the amount of blood loss from the child is to dilute the red cells with albumin to approximate the same value as the patient's hematocrit, or slightly higher, prior to priming the apheresis machine. Calcium gluconate may be administered to prevent hypocalcemia. Kanold et al. (1998) reported using 0.5 g per 10 kg body weight of oral calcium gluconate at 12 hours and 1 hour prior to apheresis. During apheresis, the child is given calcium gluconate every 60 minutes either orally or IV bolus.

Pediatric allogeneic donors undergo mobilization and collection similar to the adult allogeneic donor. Controversy remains about whether it is appropriate to give growth factors for mobilization to minor donors, as the long-term effects of growth factors are still unknown. Many centers mobilize and collect peripheral stem cells from sibling donors older than 13; however, few harvest cells from donors younger than 13. Pahys et al. (2000) reported the collection of stem cells from a 6.1 kg, seven-month-old female donor who received G-CSF 10 mcg/kg/day and was apheresed for approximately six hours. The apheresis machine was primed with irradiated paternal whole blood. A slow flow rate of blood was anticipated and, because of the possibility of platelet clumping, 80 mg of aspirin was given to the child the evening prior to collection. During the procedure, ionized calcium levels and coagulation parameters were assessed, and the donor received a bolus of calcium gluconate. An adequate product was achieved in one collection. The donor's catheter site was oozing following the procedure, and the platelet count was 65,000/mm³. Single donor platelets were administered. The investigators (Pahys et al.) concluded that even though peripheral stem cell collections may be less painful than a BM harvest, they are

unable to determine that donor safety is improved for small children.

Unrelated Blood Stem Cell Collections

Until very recently, the use of BSCs was limited to related allogeneic and autologous transplants. One reason for the reluctance to use BSCs from unrelated donors was because of the lack of knowledge about the long-term side effects of growth factors. In one study (Cavallaro et al., 2000), 95 related donors (age range 12–65 years) were contacted three to six years following stem cell donation. Donors had received G-CSF for mobilization for 3–15 days. Donors who had prior medical problems (cancer, Grave's disease, hypertension, sinusitis, or hepatitis C) experienced no progression or worsening of their medical problem. Cavallaro et al. concluded that health changes (chest pain, enlarged lymph nodes, cancer, Parkinson's disease, and diabetes) that occurred after the growth factor mobilization were unrelated to the mobilization and collection.

The National Marrow Donor Program (NMDP), established in 1986, has facilitated nearly 13,000 unrelated transplants. Initially, all unrelated transplant patients received bone marrow transplants. In 1999, the NMDP began to facilitate BSC and UCB transplants. Currently, more than four million donors are listed on the NMDP registry. The NMDP protocol for harvesting stem cells from an unrelated donor involves mobilizing and collecting the donor cells similar to the process with related donors. Donors receive G-CSF for four or five consecutive days and then undergo apheresis to collect stem cells. Following stem cell collection, NMDP continues to follow the donors on an annual basis.

Ringden et al. (1999) transplanted 45 patients with unrelated BSCs and compared the outcome to 45 BMT recipients. Their conclusion was that in comparing BSCs harvested from unrelated compatible donors with BMT controls, the BCT can result in quicker engraftment and is a safe alternative to a BMT. Although their follow-up is only two years, there is no difference in survival, relapse, and relapse-free survival. Advantages for the donor that the authors noted include ability to collect the cells on an outpatient basis, and no general anesthesia or blood transfusions were necessary. The only disadvantage cited by the authors was the potential risk of receiving G-CSF.

Mismatched Donors

Many patients who are candidates for high-dose therapy do not have an HLA-matched related allogeneic sibling or are unable to locate an HLA-matched unrelated donor through national registries. In these cases, a partially mismatched related donor could be considered. Henslee-Downey et al. (1997) reported the use of partially mismatched related donors for 72 patients. The patients received TBI and high-dose chemotherapy followed by transplantation of T lymphocyte-depleted BM. The authors concluded that a partially mismatched related donor transplant can be performed with acceptable rates of graft failure and GVHD; however, more studies are needed.

Cord Blood Stem Cell Transplantation

Another option for obtaining stem cells is the use of UCB and placental blood. UCB may be collected, cryopreserved, and stored for the donor (autologous) or a family member (related allogeneic) or donated to a UCB registry bank for an unrelated recipient (unrelated allogeneic transplant). The first report of a successful UCB transplant was provided in 1989 by Gluckman et al. (1989), in which a five-year old boy with Fanconi's anemia was transplanted with his sibling's cord blood. Since that time, many UCB transplants have been reported, and determining the proper use of these stem cells has generated substantial research. Advantages for harvesting UCB seem to outweigh any disadvantages (see Figure 3-6). The potential for a low incidence of GVHD may be one of the most important advantages for using UCB. Because of the decreased effectiveness of the lymphocytes, UCB transplants result in significantly less incidence and severity of GVHD, as compared to matched or mismatched transplants (Kline & Bertolone, 1998). Unfortunately, this also may result in less graft versus tumor effect.

Identifying a suitable cord blood match is much quicker than identifying an unrelated BM or BSC donor (Kline & Bertolone, 1998). The cord blood has already undergone viral testing; samples for confirmatory testing are already available; and the UCB, once identified, is already stored. For ethnic or minority populations, there is the potential for increased participation in donating to the UCB bank. There also may be a lower risk of viral contamination (specifically

cytomegalovirus and Epstein-Barr), because few infants are infected with these viruses (Kline & Bertolone).

Initially, there were concerns that insufficient progenitor cells would be available for larger patients, and recipients were limited to 40 kg. Rubinstein et al. (1998) reported on 562 patients who had received unrelated UCB transplants, of which 185 recipients weighed more than 40 kg. They noted that the heaviest patient (116 kg) received the lowest number of cells and achieved successful engraftment.

Another significant disadvantage for using UCB is the possible transfer of undiagnosed genetic diseases. Currently, cord blood donors are not followed past birth to determine if a congenital disease developed. However, extensive individual and family questionnaires are completed prior to birth to try to sort out potential problems.

Other possible disadvantages include microbial or maternal T lymphocyte contamination of the UCB product. Also, as discussed by Kline and Bertolone (1998), the amount of time a UCB product may be stored and still maintain its viability is unknown.

Collection of stem cells from the umbilical cord usually is accomplished by one of two methods. The main goal is not to disrupt the normal labor, delivery, and postpartum period.

The most common method of collection is to remove the placenta to a site outside the delivery room and puncture the umbilical vein with a 16-gauge needle (Rubinstein, Rosenfield, Adamson, & Stevens, 1993). The blood then is drained by gravity into a blood bag or withdrawn into a 60 ml syringe containing anticoagulant. This method takes approximately 5–10 minutes and may be accomplished in a sterile fashion. Another option is to collect blood from the placenta while it is still in utero, after the baby has been delivered but prior to delivery of the placenta. Uterine contractions are used to force blood out of the placenta. Delay in delivery of the placenta may not be possible, and contamination with either maternal blood or infectious organisms is highly possible.

A number of UCB banks have been established, with the largest in the United States at the New York Blood Center, established in 1992 (American Association of Blood Banks, 2000). The NMDP began facilitating UCB transplants in 1999. NMDP has developed a central registry of UCB units that are available at a number of UCB banks (see Figure 3-7).

Many ethical issues surround the use of UCB transplantation. First is the issue of for-profit companies that store UCB for potential future use by the donor or a family member versus donation of UCB to registries with the intention of an unrelated UCB transplant. A number of facilities that offer cryopreservation and storage for a fee are available around the country. Kline and Bertolone (1998) and Sugarman et al. (1997) questioned the ethics in marketing this service to new parents when the probability of actually using the cord blood is highly unlikely.

Another issue involves informed consent. Consent is obtained from the mother for UCB banking; however, the question of "whose" stem cells these really are may arise. If the cells have not been used by the time the child reaches maturity, the question arises as to whether the cells belong to the

---

Figure 3-6. Umbilical Cord Blood

Advantages
- Abundant source, usually discarded
- Ease and safety of collection
- May be stored for unrelated patients
- Potential for increased ethnic or minority participation
- Low incidence of graft versus host disease
- Low risk of viral contamination (e.g., cytomegalovirus, Epstein-Barr)

Disadvantages
- Possible slightly lowered hemoglobin for neonate, if the umbilical cord is clamped less than 30 seconds after delivery
- Potential maternal T lymphocyte contamination
- Possible microbial contamination
- Limited number of stem cells harvested (may not be adequate for transplant)
- Potential for decreased graft versus tumor effect
- Possible delayed engraftment
- Potential for graft failure
- Impossible to obtain additional cells from unrelated donor
- Transmission of undiagnosed genetic diseases
- Transmission of infectious disease
- Ethical issues

Note. Based on information from Bertolini et al., 1995; Forte, 1997; Rubinstein et al., 1993.

American Red Cross North Central Blood Services
Cord Blood Program
100 South Robert Street
St. Paul, MN 55107
651-290-8633

American Red Cross Western Area Community Cord Blood Bank Portland
3131 North Vancouver Avenue
Portland, OR 97227
877-783-3560

Ashley Ross Cord Blood Program of the San Diego Blood Bank
440 Upas Street
San Diego, CA 92103-4900
619-296-6393 ext. 161

Bonfils Cord Blood Services Belle Bonfils Memorial Blood Center
717 Yosemite Circle
Denver, CO 80230
800-421-9529 ext. 2350
www.bonfils.org/bonfils.php?section=donor&page=donor

Children's Hospital of Orange County Cord Blood Bank
455 South Main Street
Orange, CA 92868
714-516-4335
www.choc.com/services/blood_bank.lasso

ITxM Cord Blood Services
ITxM Clinical Services
1205 Milwaukee Avenue
Glenview, IL 60025
800-486-0680

J.P. McCarthy Cord Stem Cell Bank
110 E. Warren Avenue
Detroit, MI 48102

LifeCord
1221 Northwest 13th Street
Gainesville, FL 32601
352-334-1000
http://crbs.org/lifecord/lifecord.htm

New Jersey Cord Blood Bank at the Coriell Institute for Medical Research
403 Haddon Avenue
Camden, NJ 08103
856-757-9752
http://njcbb.umdnj.edu

Puget Sound Blood Center
Northwest Tissue Center
921 Terry Avenue
Seattle, WA 98104
206-292-1896
www.psbc.org

St. Louis Cord Blood Bank
3662 Park Avenue
St. Louis, MO 63110
888-453-2673
www.slcbb.org

StemCyte, Inc.
400 Rolyn Place
Arcadia, CA 91007
866-STEMCYTE
www.stemcyte.com

Note. Based on information from National Marrow Donor Program, National Headquarters, Minneapolis, MN, www.marrow.org. Current as of 12/1/03.

child. Parents of a sick child may choose to become pregnant with the hopes of creating a compatible donor. There is also the potential for liability issues arising from undiagnosed genetic diseases that may be transferred to the recipient. UCB transplantation will continue to be studied to determine its place in stem cell transplantation.

Stem Cell Processing

Once the stem cells from the BM, blood, or umbilical cord are collected, they are further processed, usually cryopreserved, and stored between –80°C and –196°C in a freezer. Autologous stem cell products usually are frozen until after the patient has received high-dose therapy and is ready for reinfusion or transplant. Allogeneic stem cell products may be infused immediately following collection and processing, stored in a refrigerator at 4°C, infused the day following collection, or frozen. Unrelated allogeneic stem cell products are collected at an NMDP-approved collection center and shipped via courier to the transplant center. At the transplant center, they will undergo appropriate processing and then are transplanted.

All stem cell products require additional processing prior to freezing. The stem cells are tested for sterility and infec-

tious diseases, and blood typing is completed to ensure a safe product. Usually the overall volume of each product is reduced to decrease the amount of cryoprotectant required. Letheby, Jackson, and Warkentin (2000) indicated that increased volumes of cryoprotectant and cell lysis are associated with increased clinical toxicities during the reinfusion or transplant. Kessinger et al. (1990) reported that stem cell products that contain larger volumes of overall infusate and DMSO result in a higher frequency of reinfusion toxicities. Larger volumes of infusate were associated with a higher incidence of headache following transplant. As discussed earlier, a larger infused volume and larger infused red cell volume were associated with tachypnea, elevated serum bilirubin, and elevated serum creatinine. According to Letheby et al., BSC products are concentrated to 2×10^8 nucleated cells/ml, maintaining at least a 50 ml volume. BM products are concentrated to 1×10^8 nucleated cells per ml. Allogeneic, related or unrelated, products may be red cell- or plasma-depleted prior to infusion or freezing if there is an ABO incompatibility between the recipient and the donor.

Following processing, the stem cells are cryopreserved. During this phase, a cryoprotectant is added to the cells to prevent cell damage during either freezing or thawing. Without some form of cryopreservation, ice crystals form in cells during the freezing or thawing process. This results in ruptured cell membranes. The most common current method of cryopreservation is using 5% DMSO, an intracellular cryoprotectant, and 6% hydroxyethyl starch (HES), an extracellular cryoprotectant, followed by placement of the product in a –80°C freezer for 24 hours (Stiff, Koester, Weidner, Dvorak, & Fisher, 1987). The stem cell product then may be placed in a long-term storage freezer, in the vapor phase of liquid nitrogen. According to Letheby et al. (2000), two disadvantages in using HES are that it is not available commercially and its use as a cryoprotectant requires Investigational New Drug approval from the U.S. Food and Drug Administration. Another cryopreservation method involves using 10% DMSO followed by controlled-rate freezing and then placement of the product into a long-term storage freezer in liquid nitrogen or, more commonly, the vapor phase of liquid nitrogen (Gorin, 1992). Disadvantages, noted by Letheby et al., include the necessity of strictly controlled freezing rates and granulocytes are not preserved.

Sugrue et al. (1998) reported on the effect of overnight storage of BSC products. Prospectively, they stored BSC products from 12 patients overnight on ice. The product was combined with the next day's stem cell product and frozen. Cell counts, viability, bacterial cultures, and colony assays were assessed before and after storage. Median viability following storage was reported to be between 95% and 100% recovery, and there was no detected clotting or bacterial contamination. All patients engrafted quickly. A retrospective analysis of an additional 124 patients' BSC products demonstrated that all engrafted successfully. Sugrue et al. concluded that it is not only safe and cost effective to allow overnight storage and combination of two BSC products, but it also allows for a greater efficiency in laboratory staffing.

Stem Cell Purging

Prior to cryopreservation, autologous stem cells may be purged to remove tumor contamination. There are two main methods of purging: negative cell selection and positive cell selection. Negative cell selection involves attempts to remove tumor cells from the stem cell product. Blume and Thomas (2000) described a variety of methods, including the use of physical separation, chemotherapy, monoclonal antibodies, toxins, magnetic beads, and radionuclides. Blume and Thomas stated that immunologic purging did not affect engraftment following transplant; however, chemotherapy purging often delayed engraftment. They concluded that even though clinical trials of purging using negative cell selection showed promising results, prospective randomized trials were needed to confirm that purged products were preferable over nonpurged stem cell products (Blume & Thomas).

Positive stem cell selection involves removing the stem cells from the product that are needed for the transplant. Sorting devices, such as columns containing antibody-coated beads or magnetic cells, target antigens (e.g., CD34 antigens) on the surface of the cell (Blume & Thomas, 2000). These enriched products have a decrease in tumor cell contamination and have successfully engrafted following transplant (Blume & Thomas). One type of semiautomated selection system used to choose CD34+ cells from the leukapheresis product is the Nexell Isolex 300 or 300i Cell Selection System® (Nexell Therapeutics, Irvine, CA). The BSC leukapheresis product may be processed daily on the selection system, or two consecutive collections may be pooled and then processed without harming viability (Dyson et al., 2000). Stem cell selection or purging is more labor intensive than standard processing methods and is more costly. The cost for purging one product on the Nexell Selection System is approximately $7,000. The clinical efficacy of stem cell selection systems must be studied and reported before purging becomes the standard processing method (Bensinger, 1998).

T lymphocytes, the cells responsible for GVHD, may be depleted from the allogeneic stem cell product. T cell depletion studies have been conducted at numerous centers. The goal in processing the cells is to remove enough of the T lymphocytes to decrease GVHD while still maintaining enough T lymphocytes to stimulate an immune response to the tumor (graft versus tumor response). Methods that have been used involve elutriation (separates the cells based on size and density) or the use of monoclonal antibodies (binds to cell surface antigens).

Future Directions

Future directions lie in improving the stem cell graft, ex vivo expansion of stem cell products, gene manipulation, using stem cell transplantation in other patient populations, and manipulation of stem cells to differentiate into other types of cells (e.g., bone, liver, heart) other than blood cells.

CD34+ cell selection of allogeneic BSC products to decrease the incidence of chronic GVHD has been reported (Brugger et al., 1996; Garcia-Conde et al., 1996; Laport et al., 1997) but must be explored in more detail. Another possibility for expanding the use of allogeneic BSCs is the use in mismatched transplants (e.g., haploidentical transplants). Graft rejection by the recipient may be reduced by infusing a large number of stem cells. However, the incidence and severity of GVHD will need to be evaluated to determine if this is a viable option (Shea, 1999).

Generation of stem cells ex vivo is another area of future interest. A small amount of BSCs may be collected and grown with the addition of a combination of growth factors. Brugger, Heimfeld, Berenson, Mertelsmann, and Kanz (1995) described the use of ex vivo grown autologous BSCs to restore hematopoietic function following high-dose chemotherapy. They suggested that BSCs produced in this manner will reduce the amount of tumor cell contamination of the stem cell product.

Other areas of future interest include the use of high-dose therapy and BCT in patients with autoimmune diseases. In autoimmune diseases such as multiple sclerosis, rheumatoid arthritis, or systemic lupus erythematosus, standard therapy fails to cure or effectively treat the patient. High-dose therapy, followed by transplant, may replace the immune system (allogeneic) or reset the immune system (autologous). Funding for transplantation and identifying patients for referrals are issues that are currently being explored.

The use of BSCs in gene therapy trials currently is under investigation. Gene therapy involves the placement of a functioning gene into a patient's cells to correct a genetic error or to add a novel ability to those cells. Hematopoietic stem cells are considered for use with gene therapy because they are able to differentiate into myeloid and lymphoid cell lines, have a long lifespan, and are capable of self-renewal. They also are easily accessible. UCB cells may be even more receptive than BSCs to genetic engineering because of the immaturity of the cells.

Gene manipulation is another area of future research in hematopoietic stem cell transplantation. There are two methods for gene transfer (Abernathy & Wilson, 2000). In the first method, the viral genome may be modified to incorporate the desired gene. The modified virus then infects the desired cell and introduces new genetic information into the cell. The second method of gene transfer used in the clinical setting involves the use of either gene marking or gene replacement therapy. Gene marking is the labeling of cells with a specific gene so that those cells can be traced. Gene replacement therapy is used to correct a genetic error (acquired or inherited). A new, healthy gene is inserted in the place of a missing or flawed gene (Abernathy & Wilson).

Conclusion

Hematopoietic stem cell transplantation is used to treat an extensive variety of diseases. Stem cells may be collected from many sources: BM, blood, and UCB. Stem cells collected from the blood currently are the preferred stem cell source for patients who receive high-dose therapy. BCT results in earlier hematologic recovery, which translates into a potential decrease in the number of transfusions, toxicities, and hospital days. Patients or donors usually are mobilized with chemotherapy and/or growth factors to increase the number of circulating stem cells. The number of UCB transplants, because of the possibility of a decreased incidence of GVHD, also may increase in the future. Once stem cells are collected, they are either transplanted within 24 hours or are cryopreserved and stored in a freezer until transplanted. As the applications for the use of stem cells expand, so will opportunities for nurses in all areas of patient care, research, and administration. Nurses must strive to keep up to date in this continuously evolving field to be able to provide appropriate care and education for patients and their families.

References

Abernathy, E., & Wilson, H. (2000). Gene therapy: Overview and implication for peripheral stem cell transplantation. In P.C. Buchsel & P.M. Kapustay (Eds.), *Stem cell transplantation: A clinical textbook* (pp. 11.1–11.17). Pittsburgh, PA: Oncology Nursing Society.

American Association of Blood Banks. (2000). *Standards for hematopoietic progenitor cell services* (2nd ed.). Bethesda, MD: Author.

Becker, P.S., Wagle, M., Matous, S., Swanson, R.S., Pihan, G., Lowry, P.A., et al. (1997). Spontaneous splenic rupture following administration of granulocyte colony-stimulating factor (G-CSF): Occurrence in an allogeneic donor of peripheral blood stem cells. *Biology of Blood and Marrow Transplantation, 3,* 45–49.

Bell, A.J., Figes, A., Oscier, D.G., & Hamblin, T.J. (1986). Peripheral blood stem cell autografting. *Lancet, 1,* 1027.

Bender, J.G., Bik, T., Williams, S., & Schwartzberg, L.S. (1992). Defining a therapeutic dose of peripheral blood stem cells. *Journal of Hematotherapy, 1,* 329–341.

Bensinger, W. (1998). Should we purge? *Bone Marrow Transplantation, 21,* 113–115.

Bensinger, W., Appelbaum, F., Rowley, S., Storb, R., Sanders, J., Lilleby, K., et al. (1995). Factors that influence collection and engraftment of autologous peripheral blood stem cells. *Journal of Clinical Oncology, 13,* 2547–2555.

Bensinger, W.I., Weaver, C.H., Appelbaum, F.R., Rowley, S., Demirer, T., Sanders, J., et al. (1995). Transplantation of allogeneic peripheral blood stem cells mobilized by recombinant human granulocyte colony-stimulating factor. *Blood, 85,* 1655–1658.

Bertolini, F., Battaglia, M., De Iulio, C., & Sirchia, G. (1995). Placental blood collection: Effects on newborns. *Blood, 85,* 3361–3362.

Bishop, M.R. (1994). Mobilization prior to the apheresis procedure. In A. Kessinger & J.D. McMannis (Eds.), *Practical considerations of apheresis in peripheral blood stem cell transplantation* (pp. 5–10). Lakewood, CO: COBE Laboratories.

Bishop, M.R., Anderson, J.R., Jackson, J.D., Bierman, P.J., Reed, E.C., Vose, J.M., et al. (1994). High-dose therapy and peripheral blood progenitor cell transplantation: Effects of recombinant human granulocyte-macrophage colony-stimulating factor on the autograft. *Blood, 83,* 610–616.

Bishop, M.R., Jackson, J.D., O'Kane-Murphy, B., Schmit-Pokorny, K., Vose, J.M., Bierman, P.J., et al. (1996). Phase I trial of recombinant fusion protein PIXY321 for mobilization of peripheral-blood cells. *Journal of Clinical Oncology, 14,* 2521–2526.

Bishop, M.R., Tarantolo, S.R., Jackson, J.D., Anderson, J.R., Schmit-Pokorny, K., Zacharias, D., et al. (1997). Allogeneic-blood stem-cell collection following mobilization with low-dose granulocyte colony-stimulating factor. *Journal of Clinical Oncology, 15,* 1601–1607.

Blume, K.G., & Thomas, E.D. (2000). A review of autologous hematopoietic cell transplantation. *Biology of Blood and Marrow Transplantation, 6,* 1–12.

Brugger, W., Bross, K.J., Glatt, M., Weber, F., Mertelsmann, R., & Kanz, L. (1994). Mobilization of tumor cells and hematopoietic progenitor cells into peripheral blood of patients with solid tumors. *Blood, 83,* 636–640.

Brugger, W., Heimfeld, S., Berenson, R., Mertelsmann, R., & Kanz, L. (1995). Reconstitution of hematopoiesis after high-dose chemotherapy by autologous progenitor cells generated ex vivo. *New England Journal of Medicine, 333,* 283–287.

Brugger, W., Scheding, S., Subklewe, M., Faul, C., Halene, S., Brandes, A., et al. (1996). Transplantation of positively selected allogeneic blood CD34+ cells [Abstract]. *Blood, 88*(Suppl. 1), 599a.

Buchsel, P.C., Leum, E., & Randolph, S.R. (1997). Nursing care of the blood cell transplant recipient. *Seminars in Oncology Nursing, 13,* 172–183.

Buckner, C.D., Petersen, F.B., & Bolonesi, B.A. (1994). Bone marrow donors. In S. Forman & E.D. Thomas (Eds.), *Bone marrow transplantation* (pp. 259–269). Boston: Blackwell Scientific.

Camp-Sorrell, D. (Ed.). (2004). *Access device guidelines: Recommendations for nursing practice and education* (2nd ed.). Pittsburgh, PA: Oncology Nursing Society.

Castaigne, S., Calvo, F., Douay, L., Thomas, F., Benbunan, M., Gerota, J., et al. (1986). Successful haematopoietic reconstitution using autologous peripheral blood mononucleated cells in a patient with acute promyelocytic leukaemia. *British Journal of Haematology, 62*, 209–211.

Cavallaro, A.M., Lilleby, K., Majolino, I., Storb, R., Appelbaum, F.R., Rowley, S.D., et al. (2000). Three to six year follow-up of normal donors who received recombinant human granulocyte colony-stimulating factor. *Bone Marrow Transplantation, 25*, 85–89.

Chan, K., & Bond, M. (1994). Pediatric issues. In A. Kessinger & J. McMannis (Eds.), *Practical considerations of apheresis in peripheral blood stem cell transplantation* (pp. 63–69). Lakewood, CO: COBE Laboratories.

Chern, B., McCarthy, N., Hutchins, C., & Durrant, S.T. (1999). Analgesic infiltration at the site of bone marrow harvest significantly reduces donor morbidity. *Bone Marrow Transplantation, 23*, 947–949.

Christopher, K. (2000). The experience of donating bone marrow to a relative. *Oncology Nursing Forum, 27*, 693–700.

Dyson, P.G., Horvath, N., Joshua, D., Barrow, L., Van Holst, N.G., Brown, R., et al. (2000). CD34+ selection of autologous peripheral blood stem cells for transplantation following sequential cycles of high-dose therapy and mobilization in multiple myeloma. *Bone Marrow Transplantation, 25*, 1175–1184.

Feremans, W.W., Bastin, G., Le Moine, F., Ravoet, C., Delville, J.P., Pradier, O., et al. (1996). Simplification of the blood stem cell transplantation (BSCT) procedure: Large volume apheresis and uncontrolled rate cryopreservation at −80°C. *European Journal of Haematology, 56*, 278–282.

Forte, K.J. (1997). Alternative donor sources in pediatric bone marrow transplantation. *Journal of Pediatric Oncology Nursing, 14*, 213–224.

Foundation for the Accreditation of Cellular Therapy. (1996). *Standards for hematopoietic progenitor cell collection, processing and transplantation.* Omaha, NE: Author.

Gale, R.P., Henon, P., & Juttner, C. (1992). Blood stem cell transplants come of age. *Bone Marrow Transplantation, 9*, 151–155.

Garcia-Conde, J., Martin-Gaitero, M.J., Arbone, C., Benet, I., Marugan, I., Terol, M.J., et al. (1996). High frequency of chronic graft-versus-host disease associated with unmodified allogeneic peripheral blood progenitor cell transplantation. Preliminary results of allogeneic CD34+ selected cell PBPCT [Abstract]. *Blood, 88*(Suppl. 1), 261a.

Gianni, A.M., Bregni, M., Siena, S., Villa, S., Sciorelli, G.A., Fravagnani, F., et al. (1989). Rapid and complete hemopoietic reconstitution following combined transplantation of autologous blood and bone marrow cells. A changing role of high dose chemotherapy? *Hematological Oncology, 7*, 139–148.

Gianni, A.M., Siena, S., Bregni, M., Tarella, C., Stern, A., Pileri, A., et al. (1989). Granulocyte-macrophage colony-stimulating factor to harvest circulating haemopoietic stem cells for autotransplantation. *Lancet, 2*, 580–585.

Gianni, A.M., Tarella, C., Siena, S., Bregni, M., Boccadoro, M., Lombardi, F., et al. (1990). Durable and complete hematopoietic reconstitution after autografting of rhGM-CSF exposed peripheral blood progenitor cells. *Bone Marrow Transplantation, 6*, 143–145.

Glaspy, J.A., Shpall, E.J., LeMaistre, C.F., Briddell, R.A., Menchaca, D.M., Turner, S.A., et al. (1997). Peripheral blood progenitor cell mobilization using stem cell factor in combination with filgrastim in breast cancer patients. *Blood, 90*, 2939–2951.

Gluckman, E., Broxmeyer, H.A., Auerbach, A.D., Friedman, H.S., Douglas, G.W., Devergie, A., et al. (1989). Hematopoietic reconstitution in a patient with Fanconi anemia by means of umbilical cord blood from an HLA-identical sibling. *New England Journal of Medicine, 321*, 1174–1175.

Golde, D.W. (1991). The stem cell. *Scientific American, 265*, 86–93.

Goldman, J. (1995). Peripheral blood stem cells for allografting. *Blood, 85*, 1413–1415.

Gorin, N.C. (1992). Cryopreservation and storage of stem cells. In E. Areman, H.J. Deeg, & R.A. Sacher (Eds.), *Bone marrow and stem cell processing: A manual of current techniques* (pp. 292–308). Philadelphia: F.A. Davis Company.

Haas, R., Ho, A.D., Bredthauer, U., Cayeux, S., Egerer, G., Knauf, W., et al. (1990). Successful autologous transplantation of blood stem cells mobilized with recombinant human granulocyte-macrophage colony-stimulating factor. *Experimental Hematology, 18*, 94–98.

Haire, W.D., Lieberman, R.P., Lund, G.B., Wieczorek, B.M., Armitage, J.O., & Kessinger, A. (1990). Translumbar inferior vena cava catheters: Safety and efficacy in peripheral blood stem cell transplantation. *Transfusion, 30*, 511–515.

Henon, P.R., Liang, H., Beck-Wirth, G., Eisenmann, J.C., Lepers, M., Wunder, E., et al. (1992). Comparison of hematopoietic and immune recovery after autologous bone marrow or blood stem cell transplants. *Bone Marrow Transplantation, 9*, 285–291.

Henslee-Downey, P.J., Abhyankar, S.H., Parrish, R.S., Pati, A.R., Godder, K.T., Neglia, W.J., et al. (1997). Use of partially mismatched related donors extends access to allogeneic marrow transplant. *Blood, 89*, 3864–3872.

International Bone Marrow Transplant Directory/Autologous Blood and Marrow Transplant Directory. (2002). *Summary slides: State-of-the-art in blood and marrow transplantation.* Retrieved May 22, 2003, from http://instruct.mcw.edu/IBMTR/BWebServer/summarysldset/summset_files/v3_document.htm

Kahn, D.G., Prilutskaya, M., Cooper, B., Kennedy, M.J., Meagher, R., Pecora, A.L., et al. (1997). The relationship between the incidence of tumor contamination and number of pheresis for stage IV breast cancer. *Blood, 90*(Suppl. 1), 565a.

Kanold, J., Halle, P., Rapatel, C., Berger, M., Gembara, P., deLumley, L., et al. (1998). Safe and efficient peripheral blood stem cell collection in the smallest of children. *Therapeutic Apheresis, 2*, 49–57.

Kapustay, P.M., & Buchsel, P.C. (2000). Process, complications, and management of peripheral stem cell transplantation. In P.C. Buchsel & P.M. Kapustay (Eds.), *Stem cell transplantation: A clinical textbook* (pp. 5.1–5.28). Pittsburgh, PA: Oncology Nursing Society.

Kessinger, A. (1993). Utilization of peripheral blood stem cells in autotransplantation. *Hematology/Oncology Clinics of North America, 7*, 535–545.

Kessinger, A., Armitage, J.O., Landmark, J.D., & Weisenburger, D.D. (1986). Reconstitution of human hematopoietic function with autologous cryopreserved circulating stem cells. *Experimental Hematology, 14*, 192–196.

Kessinger, A., Schmit-Pokorny, K., Smith, D., & Armitage, J. (1990). Cryopreservation and infusion of autologous peripheral blood stem cells. *Bone Marrow Transplantation, 5*(Supp. 1), 25–27.

Kessinger, A., & Sharp, G. (1996). Mobilization of hematopoietic progenitor cells with epoetin alfa. *Seminars in Hematology, 33*(Suppl. 1), 10–15.

Kessinger, A., Smith, D.M., Strandjord, S.E., Landmark, J.D., Dooley, D.C., Law, P., et al. (1989). Allogeneic transplantation of blood-derived, T cell-depleted hemopoietic stem cells after myeloablative treatment in a patient with acute lymphoblastic leukemia. *Bone Marrow Transplantation, 4*, 643–646.

Kline, R.M., & Bertolone, S.J. (1998). Umbilical cord blood transplantation: Providing a donor for everyone needing a bone marrow transplant? *Southern Medical Journal, 91*, 821–828.

Korbling, M., Dorken, B., Ho, A.D., Pezzutto, A., Hunstein, W., & Fliedner, T.M. (1986). Autologous transplantation of blood-derived hemopoietic stem cells after myeloablative therapy in a patient with Burkitt's lymphoma. *Blood, 67*, 529–532.

Korbling, M., Przepiorka, D., Huh, Y.O., Engel, H., van Besien, K., Giralt, S., et al. (1995). Allogeneic blood stem cell transplantation for refractory leukemia and lymphoma: Potential advantage of blood over marrow allografts. *Blood, 85*, 1659–1665.

Laport, G.F., Bensinger, W., Daugherty, C.K., Yanovich, S., Cornetta, K., Skikne, B.S., et al. (1997). A pilot study of allogeneic CD34+ peripheral blood stem cell transplantation using mismatched related donors for patients with advanced hematologic malignancies [Abstract]. *Blood, 90*(Suppl. 1), 110a.

Lee, V., Li, C.K., Shing, M.M., Chik, K.W., Li, K., Tsang, K.S., et al. (2000). Single vs. twice daily G-CSF dose for peripheral blood stem cells harvest in normal donors and children with nonmalignant diseases. *Bone Marrow Transplantation, 25,* 931–935.

Letheby, B.A., Jackson, J.D., & Warkentin, P.I. (2000). Processing, cryopreservation, and storage of peripheral blood progenitor cells. In P.C. Buchsel & P.M. Kapustay (Eds.), *Stem cell transplantation: A clinical textbook* (pp. 4.1–4.20). Pittsburgh, PA: Oncology Nursing Society.

Lobo, F., Kessinger, A., Landmark, J.D., Smith, D.M., Weisenburger, D.D., Wigton, R.S., et al. (1991). Addition of peripheral blood stem cells collected without mobilization techniques to transplanted autologous bone marrow did not hasten marrow recovery following myeloablative therapy. *Bone Marrow Transplantation, 8,* 389–392.

Mijovic, A., Fishlock, K., Pagliuca, A., & Mufti, G.J. (1998). Blast counts in blood progenitor cell (BPC) correlate with CD34+ cells and CFU-GM and are a useful predictor of haemopoietic recovery after autologous BPC transplantation collections. *Bone Marrow Transplantation, 21,* 869–872.

National Cancer Institute. (1999). *Common toxicity criteria manual.* Bethesda, MD: Author.

Pahys, J., Fisher, V., Carneval, M., Yomtovian, R., Sarode, R., & Nieder, M. (2000). Successful large volume leukapheresis on a small infant allogeneic donor. *Bone Marrow Transplantation, 26,* 339–341.

Pecora, A. (1999). Impact of stem cell dose on hematopoietic recovery in autologous blood stem cell recipients. *Bone Marrow Transplantation, 23*(Suppl. 2), S7–S12.

Pettengell, R., Morgenstern, G.R., Woll, P.J., Chang, J., Rowlands, M., Young, R., et al. (1993). Peripheral blood progenitor cell transplantation in lymphoma and leukemia using a single apheresis. *Blood, 82,* 3770–3777.

Reiffers, J., Bernard, P., David, B., Vezon, G., Sarrat, A., Marit, G., et al. (1986). Successful autologous transplantation with peripheral blood hemopoietic cells in a patient with acute leukemia. *Experimental Hematology, 14,* 312–315.

Richman, C.M., Weiner, R.S., & Yankee, R.A. (1976). Increase in circulating stem cells following chemotherapy in man. *Blood, 47,* 1031–1039.

Ringden, O., Remberger, M., Runde, V., Bornhauser, M., Blau, I.W., Basara, N., et al. (1999). Peripheral blood stem cell transplantation from unrelated donors: A comparison with marrow transplantation. *Blood, 94,* 455–464.

Roberts, M.M., To, L.B., Gillis, D., Mundy, J., Rawling, C., Ng, K., et al. (1993). Immune reconstitution following peripheral blood stem cell transplantation, autologous bone marrow transplantation and allogeneic bone marrow transplantation. *Bone Marrow Transplantation, 12,* 469–475.

Rubinstein, P., Carrier, C., Scaradavou, A., Kurtzberg, J., Adamson, J., Migliaccio, A.R., et al. (1998). Outcomes among 562 recipients of placental-blood transplants from unrelated donors. *New England Journal of Medicine, 22,* 1565–1577.

Rubinstein, P., Rosenfield, R.E., Adamson, J.W., & Stevens, C.E. (1993). Stored placental blood for unrelated bone marrow reconstitution. *Blood, 81,* 1679–1690.

Russell, N.H., & Hunter, A.E. (1994). Peripheral blood stem cells for allogeneic transplantation. *Bone Marrow Transplantation, 13,* 353–355.

Schmit-Pokorny, K., & Nuss, S. (2000). Pediatric peripheral stem cell transplantation. In P.C. Buchsel & P.M. Kapustay (Eds.), *Stem cell transplantation: A clinical textbook* (pp. 16.1–16.24). Pittsburgh, PA: Oncology Nursing Society.

Schmitz, N., Dreger, P., Suttorp, M., Rohwedder, E.B., Haferlach, T., Loffler, H., et al. (1995). Primary transplantation of allogeneic peripheral blood progenitor cells mobilized by filgrastim (granulocyte colony-stimulating factor). *Blood, 85,* 1666–1672.

Secola, R. (1997). Pediatric blood cell transplantation. *Seminars in Oncology Nursing, 13,* 184–193.

Sharp, J.G., Kessinger, A., Vaughan, W.P., Mann, S., Crouse, D.A., Dicke, K., et al. (1992). Detection and clinical significance of minimal tumor cell contamination of peripheral stem cell harvests. *International Journal of Cell Cloning, 10*(Suppl. 1), 92–94.

Shea, T.C. (1999). Introduction: Current issues in high-dose chemotherapy and stem cell support. *Bone Marrow Transplantation, 23*(Suppl. 2), S1–S5.

Shpall, E.J. (1999). The utilization of cytokines in stem cell mobilization strategies. *Bone Marrow Transplantation, 23*(Suppl. 2), S13–S19.

Siena, S., Bregni, M., Brando, B., Belli, N., Ravagnani, F., Gandola, L., et al. (1991). Flow cytometry for clinical estimation of circulating hematopoietic progenitors for autologous transplantation in cancer patients. *Blood, 77,* 400–409.

Smith, T.J., Hillner, B.E., Schmitz, N., Linch, D.C., Dreger, P., Goldstone, A.H., et al. (1997). Economic analysis of a randomized clinical trial to compare filgrastim-mobilized peripheral-blood progenitor-cell transplantation and autologous bone marrow transplantation in patients with Hodgkin's and non-Hodgkin's lymphoma. *Journal of Clinical Oncology, 15,* 5–10.

Socinski, M.A., Cannistra, S.A., Elias, A., Antman, D.H., Schnipper, L., & Griffin, J.D. (1988). Granulocyte-macrophage colony stimulating factor expands the circulating haemopoietic progenitor cell compartment in man. *Lancet, 1,* 1194–1198.

Stephens, L.C., Haire, W.D., Schmit-Pokorny, K., Kessinger, A., & Kotulak, G. (1993). Granulocyte macrophage colony stimulating factor: High incidence of apheresis catheter thrombosis during peripheral stem cell collection. *Bone Marrow Transplantation, 11,* 51–54.

Stephens, L.C., Haire, W.D., Tarantolo, S., Reed, E., Schmit-Pokorny, K., Kessinger, A., et al. (1997). Normal saline versus heparin flush for maintaining central venous catheter patency during apheresis collection of peripheral blood stem cells (PBSC). *Transfusion Science, 18*(2), 187–193.

Stiff, P.J. (1999). Management strategies for the hard-to-mobilize patient. *Bone Marrow Transplantation, 23*(Suppl. 2), S29–S33.

Stiff, P.J., Koester, A.R., Weidner, M.K., Dvorak, K., & Fisher, R.I. (1987). Autologous bone marrow transplantation using unfractionated cells cryopreserved in dimethylsulfoxide and hydroxyethyl starch without controlled-rate freezing. *Blood, 70,* 974–978.

Storek, J., Gooley, T., Siadak, M., Bensinger, W.I., Maloney, D.G., Chauncey, T.R., et al. (1997). Allogeneic peripheral blood stem cell transplantation may be associated with a high risk of chronic graft-versus-host disease. *Blood, 90,* 4705–4709.

Sugarman, J., Kaalund, V., Kodish, E., Marshall, M., Reisner, E., Wilfond, B., et al. (1997). Ethical issues in umbilical cord blood banking. *JAMA, 278,* 938–943.

Sugrue, M.W., Hutcheson, C.E., Fisk, D.D., Roberts, C.G., Mageed, A., Wingard, J.G., et al. (1998). The effect of overnight storage of leukapheresis stem cell products on cell viability, recovery, and cost. *Journal of Hematotherapy, 7,* 431–436.

Tilly, H., Bastit, D., Lucet, J.C., Esperou, H., Monconduit, M., & Piguet, H. (1986). Haemopoietic reconstitution after autologous peripheral blood stem cell transplantation in acute leukaemia. *Lancet, 2,* 154–155.

To, L.B., Roberts, M.M., Haylock, D.N., Dyson, P.G., Branford, A.L., Thorp, D., et al. (1992). Comparison of haematological recovery times and supportive care requirements of autologous recovery phase peripheral blood stem cell transplants, autologous bone marrow transplants and allogeneic bone marrow transplant. *Bone Marrow Transplantation, 9,* 277–284.

To, L.B., Shepperd, K.M., Haylock, D.N., Dyson, P.G., Charles, P., Thorp, D.L., et al. (1990). Single high doses of cyclophosphamide enable the collection of a high number of hemopoietic stem cells from the peripheral blood. *Experimental Hematology, 18*, 442–447.

Vescio, R.A., Hong, C.H., Cao, J., Kim, A., Schiller, G.J., Lichtenstein, A.K., et al. (1994). The hematopoietic stem cell antigen, CD34, is not expressed on the malignant cells in multiple myeloma. *Blood, 84*, 3283–3290.

Vose, J.M., Kessinger, A., Bierman, P.J., Sharp, G., Garrison, L., & Armitage, J.O. (1992). The use of rhIL-3 for mobilization of peripheral blood stem cells in previously treated patients with lymphoid malignancies. *International Journal of Cell Cloning, 10*(Suppl. 1), 62–65.

Watts, M.J., Sullivan, A.M., Leverett, D., Peniket, A.J., Perry, A.R., Williams, C.D., et al. (1998). Back-up bone marrow is frequently ineffective in patients with poor peripheral-blood stem-cell mobilization. *Journal of Clinical Oncology, 16*, 1554–1560.

Weaver, C.H., Hazelton, B., Birch, R., Palmer, P., Allen, C., Schwartzbert, L., et al. (1995). An analysis of engraftment kinetics as a function of the CD34 content of peripheral blood progenitor cell collections in 692 patients after the administration of myeloablative chemotherapy. *Blood, 86*, 3961–3969.

Weaver, C.H., Longin, K., Buckner, C.D., & Bensinger, W. (1994). Lymphocyte content in peripheral blood mononuclear cells collected after the administration of recombinant human granulocyte colony-stimulating factor. *Bone Marrow Transplantation, 13*, 411–415.

Weaver, C.H., Tauer, K., Zhen, B., Schwartzbert, L.S., Hazelton, B., Weaver, Z., et al. (1998). Second attempts at mobilization of peripheral blood stem cells in patients with initial low CD34+ cell yields. *Journal of Hematotherapy, 7*, 241–249.

Wiesneth, M., Schreiner, T., Friedrich, W., Bunjes, D., Duncker, C., Krug, E., et al. (1998). Mobilization and collection of allogeneic peripheral blood progenitor cells for transplant. *Bone Marrow Transplantation, 21*(Suppl. 3), S21–S24.

Transplant Course

Introduction

The transplant course begins with the preparatory regimen, followed by the hematopoietic stem cell (HSC) infusion and post-transplant engraftment. This chapter will discuss the rationale and types of preparatory regimens, the expected side effects and toxicities, acute adverse effects, the administration of autologous and allogeneic HSCs, and post-transplant engraftment.

Preparative Regimens for Hematopoietic Stem Cell Transplant

The transplant course begins with the preparative or conditioning regimen. This may be administered on an inpatient or outpatient basis dependent on the type of regimen and the institution. Regimens may include single or multiple chemotherapy drugs, with or without radiation therapy and immunosuppressive drugs. The preparative regimen is given for several reasons: to eliminate malignant or residual disease, to immunosuppress the host to allow graft acceptance, and to create room in the marrow space for the new graft (Mangan, 2000).

The types of drugs, doses, schedules, and techniques for administering the drugs and/or radiotherapy are not standardized and vary from institution to institution. Most preparatory regimens are classified into four types: high-dose chemotherapy (HDC), total body irradiation (TBI), regimens with TBI and HDC, and innovative regimens using immunosuppressive agents with or without chemotherapy or radiotherapy (Mangan, 2000).

Combinations of chemotherapy and radiation therapy are chosen in a variety of doses and schedules based on the patient's disease and the type of transplant. There may be scheduled days of rest that allow the HDC to be eliminated from the body. The scheduled days of the preparative regimen are counted as minus days, with transplant day as day 0. For example, a common regimen is cyclophosphamide/TBI. It has two days of cyclophosphamide followed by four days of TBI. Chemotherapy begins on day –7. For example, Day –7, HDC; Day –6, HDC; Day –5, TBI; Day –4, TBI; Day –3, TBI; Day –2, TBI ; Day –1, rest; Day 0, transplant. Refer to Table 4-1 for common preparative regimens.

High-Dose Chemotherapy

Most HDC regimens are combinations of the most effective agents for a particular disease given at high doses (Cagnoni, Nieto, & Jones, 2000). Few randomized trials have been published that directly compare the toxicity and efficacy of different preparatory regimens.

Two regimens that have been widely used are TBI/cyclophosphamide and busulfan/cyclophosphamide. These regimens generally are well tolerated and are useful as myeloablative regimens for the treatment of hematologic malignancies, especially leukemias (Mangan, 2000).

Multiple myeloma (MM) is commonly treated with melphalan and TBI. The preparative regimen seems ideal for this because melphalan is highly active in myeloma, and myeloma is sensitive to radiation therapy (Barlogie, 1999).

Treatment of Hodgkin's disease (HD) and non-Hodgkin's lymphoma (NHL) often includes the use of alkylating agents in the preparative regimen. Many regimens have been intensified to reduce the rate of relapse in autologous transplants for these diseases. The CBV regimen (cyclophosphamide, BCNU, and etoposide) is widely used for both HD and NHL. The cyclophosphamide and TBI combination has been widely used for NHL, particularly low-grade lymphomas. TBI-containing regimens are used less often for patients with HD because of the risk of increased pulmonary toxicity, as many of these patients have received prior radiation therapy (Bierman & Armitage, 1999). See Table 4-2 for toxicities of preparative regimens.

Total Body Irradiation

The use of TBI for preparation of patients prior to HSCT was developed in the 1940s and 1950s following the use of the nuclear bomb and accidental radiation exposures. Researchers demonstrated that transplanted hematopoietic cells could proliferate and repopulate the depleted recipient's marrow cavity after TBI in animal models (Yaholom & Fuks, 1992). This led to the first clinical applications of TBI. It is now estimated that more than 20,000 patients have received TBI as part of pretransplant conditioning.

The critical dose-limiting toxicity of TBI in a nontransplanted patient is bone marrow failure. Because successful engraftment of hematopoietic progenitor cells after BMT

Table 4-1. Common Preparative Regimens and Indications[a]

Abbreviation	Regimen/Agents	Indications/Disease
Cy/TBI	Cyclophosphamide/total body irradiation	AML, MDS, ALL, CML, CLL, MM, HD, NHL
TBI/VP	Total body irradiation/etoposide	AML, ALL, NHL, HD
Bu/Cy	Busulfan/cyclophosphamide	AML, MDS, ALL, CML, CLL, MM, HD, NHL
Bu/Cy/VP	Busulfan/cyclophosphamide/etoposide	AML, MDS, ALL, CML, CLL, MM, HD, NHL
Cy	Cyclophosphamide	Severe aplastic anemia
Cy/ATG	Cyclophosphamide/antithymocyte globulin	Severe aplastic anemia
TBI/Mel	Total body irradiation/melphalan	Multiple myeloma
Mel	Melphalan	Multiple myeloma, nonmyeloablative SCT[b]
CTCb	Cyclophosphamide/thiotepa/carboplatin	Breast cancer
CT	Cyclophosphamide/thiotepa	Breast cancer
CEC	Cyclophosphamide/etoposide/carboplatin	Breast cancer, solid tumors
CBV	Cyclophosphamide/carmustine/etoposide	NHL, HD
BEAM	Carmustine/etoposide/cytarabine/melphalan	NHL, HD
MCC	Mitoxantrone/carboplatin/cyclophosphamide	Ovarian cancer
TBI	Total body irradiation	Nonmyeloablative SCT[b]
Fludara/Bu/ATG	Fludarabine/busulfan/antithymocyte globulin	Nonmyeloablative SCT[b]
Fludara/Cy	Fludarabine/cyclophosphamide	Nonmyeloablative SCT[b]
Fludara/Cy/ATG	Fludarabine/cyclophosphamide/antithymocyte globulin	Nonmyeloablative SCT[b]
Fludara/Mel	Fludarabine/melphalan	Nonmyeloablative SCT[b]

[a] This list in not all-inclusive and serves only as examples of preparative regimens.
[b] These agents are currently used in clinical trials.

ALL—acute lymphoycytic leukemia; AML—acute myelogenous leukemia; CLL—chronic lymphocytic leukemia; CML—chronic myelogenous leukemia; HD—Hodgkin's disease; MDS—myelodysplastic syndrome; MM—multiple myeloma; NHL—non-Hodgkin's lymphoma; SCT—stem cell transplant

Note. Based on information from Armitage & Antman, 1992; Ezzone, 1997; Mangan, 2000.

overcomes this toxicity, the dose can be increased to lethal levels (Yaholom & Fuks, 1992). Another toxicity of TBI is gastrointestinal toxicity; however, treatment with IV fluids, electrolytes, antidiarrheal agents, antiemetics, and antibiotics help to protect the gastrointestinal tract and minimize this toxicity.

Pulmonary and hepatic toxicity are two additional dose-limiting effects of TBI. Attempts to increase the tumoricidal effects of the TBI dose have resulted in unacceptable pulmonary and hepatic complications of hematopoietic stem cell transplantation (HSCT) (Yaholom & Fuks, 1992). Idiopathic pneumonia syndrome occurs in 15% of all patients undergoing HSCT. The incidences have been reported to increase with the total dose and dose rate of radiation delivered to the lungs prior to transplantation (Kreit, 2000). A higher incidence of veno-occlusive disease has been reported in patients receiving regimens using high doses of TBI (Vinayek, Demetris, & Rakela, 2000). These toxicities limit the doses of TBI to a maximum of 1,500 cGy in dose-fractionated schemes (Yaholom & Fuks).

Indications for Total Body Irradiation

Because of the limitations, TBI is mostly used in the management of malignancies that exhibit a high sensitivity to

irradiation, such as leukemias and lymphomas. TBI is more widely used in allogeneic HSCT than autologous HSCT. In allogeneic HSCT, radiation also provides powerful immune suppression to prevent rejection of the donor cells as well as eradicate tumor cells. Most patients do not receive TBI alone but also receive chemotherapy drugs such as cyclophosphamide, etoposide, or melphalan (Mangan, 2000) (see Table 4-1 for common regimens).

Administration of Total Body Irradiation

There is no standard technique for the delivery of TBI, and almost every bone marrow transplant (BMT) center has developed its own approach to accommodate its radiation equipment and clinical facilities (Yaholom & Fuks, 1992). Careful measuring and treatment planning is necessary to ensure homogenous dose distribution to all sites (Yaholom & Fuks). A variety of patient positioning techniques have been used, such as standing, sitting, and lying flat. The daily positioning of the patient needs to be reproducible. The dose, dose rate, and schedule of TBI may vary by institution. Single-dose TBI delivered at high rates is more toxic to the lungs, gastrointestinal tract, and renal tissue compared with fractionated TBI. Fractionated doses of 150–200 cGy often are administered twice a day for three to four days. This allows

Table 4-2. Side Effects of Preparative Regimens by Agent and System

System	Cyclophosphamide	Busulfan	Carboplatin	Thiotepa	Melphalan	Carmustine	Cytarabine	Etoposide	Fludarabine	Mitoxantrone	ATG	TBI
Hematopoietic												
Anemia	X	X	X	X	X	X	X	X	X	X	X	X
Leukopenia	X	X	X	X	X	X	X	X	X	X	X	X
Thrombocytopenia	X	X	X	X	X	X	X	X	X	X	X	X
Gastrointestinal												
Nausea/vomiting	X	X	X	X	X		X	X	X		X	X
Anorexia	X			X	X		X	X			X	X
Mucositis/stomatitis	X	X	X	X	X		X	X	X	X	X	X
Diarrhea	X		X	X	X		X	X	X		X	
Constipation												
Hepatotoxicity	X					X	X					X
Genitourinary												
Hemorrhagic cystitis	X	X		X				X			X	
Nephrotoxicity	X	X	X			X					X	X
Electrolyte imbalances	X							X				X
Cardiovascular												
Cardiotoxicity	X						X			X		
Hypo- or hypertension								X				
Pulmonary												
Fibrosis	X		X		X	X			X			X
Pneumonitis	X								X			X
Reproduction												
Infertility	X		X	X	X	X						X
Gynecomastia		X										
Integumentary												
Dermatitis	X		X	X	X	X	X	X			X	X
Hyperpigmentation	X			X		X		X				X
Alopecia			X	X	X	X	X	X		X	X	X
Erythema			X	X			X					
Immunologic												
Fever/chills		X	X	X			X	X	X		X	X
Hypersensitivity/allergic reaction/anaphylaxis				X				X	X		X	
Neurologic												
Ototoxicity			X				X	X				
Peripheral neuropathy			X				X	X				
Seizures		X		X			X					
Headache/altered mental status	X			X								
Miscellaneous												
Secondary malignancy	X											
Cataracts								X				X
Nasal congestion	X					X		X				X
Conjunctivitis						X	X					
Parotitis												X

Note. Based on information from Ezzone, 1997; Ezzone & Camp-Sorrell, 1994; Gross & Johnson, 1994.

for total dose escalation of TBI, as the chance for administering TBI in fractionated doses increases the recovery time of normal tissue (Mangan, 2000). The lungs often are shielded for one or two days to prevent pulmonary damage. This varies from center to center.

Side Effects of Total Body Irradiation

Fractionated and hyperfractionated TBI programs are generally well tolerated. As most patients receive both HDC and TBI, it can be difficult to distinguish among the side effects. TBI side effects can be acute and long term, and most are manageable. The most common side effects of TBI are listed in Table 4-2.

Nursing Management: Administration of Preparative Regimen

Nearly all institutions have specific policies and procedures for the administration of chemotherapy. Guidelines are also available through the Oncology Nursing Society. The administration of HDC and TBI presents many unique issues. All chemotherapy and radiotherapy used in HSCT cause some degree of toxicity. An important component of nursing management is recognizing, preventing, and treating both expected and unexpected toxicities.

TBI, as well as most HDC, is considered moderately to highly emetogenic, and prophylaxis of patients with antiemetic therapy is necessary. Sedation may be needed for young children receiving TBI (Ezzone, 1997).

Many regimens contain bladder-toxic drugs such as cyclophosphamide, and measures to protect against hemorrhagic cystitis are necessary. These preventive measures *may* include vigorous intravenous (IV) hydration, placement of a Foley catheter for bladder irrigation, and forced diuresis. Mercapto-ethane sodium sulfate (mesna), a uroprotectant, may be used alone or in conjunction with bladder irrigation (Simpson, 2000).

IV hydration may be necessary because of the use of nephrotoxic agents. Because large volumes of fluid are administered, diuretics should be administered with caution when other nephrotoxins are in use (Ezzone, 1997). Frequent assessment for signs of fluid overload, congestive heart failure, pulmonary edema, and electrolyte imbalance is necessary. Recording daily weight and the patient's intake and output every four to eight hours are essential components of monitoring. The rigorous schedules for administering chemotherapy, infusion of large volumes of fluid, management of side effects, and the need for close monitoring of the patient create a busy and challenging situation for even the most experienced nurse (Reed & Franco, 1992).

Patient and Caregiver Education

Another important role of the nurse is patient and caregiver education. The education process usually begins during the pretransplant evaluation phase and continues through the entire transplant course. Many centers have an HSCT patient education handbook that assists with this process (Simpson & Burgunder, 2000). The purpose of the preparative regimen and the name, dose, schedule, and side effects of each chemotherapy agent should be taught and reinforced (Ezzone, 1997). The TBI schedule, patient positioning, and long- and short-term side effects also should be reviewed daily. It is important to discuss the differences between this treatment and previous chemotherapy treatments. Many transplant centers perform various types of transplants as outpatient procedures. This requires intense caregiver education. The caregiver should be given in-depth instruction and ongoing educational reinforcement from the HSCT

Table 4-3. Management of Adverse Effects of Cryopreserved Hematopoietic Stem Cells

Adverse Reactions by System	Management Strategies
Cardiac: Bradycardia, tachycardia, hypotension, hypertension, cardiac arrest	Slow or temporarily stop infusion; monitor vital signs; administer appropriate drug therapy (e.g., epinephrine, antihypertensives, pressor agents, diuretics); administer aggressive life support as necessary.
Pulmonary: Chest tightness, cough, dyspnea, pulmonary edema	Slow or temporarily stop infusion; monitor oxygen saturation; administer O_2 as needed; administer diuretics; decrease IV fluid rate.
Gastrointestinal: Abdominal cramps, diarrhea, nausea, vomiting	Slow or temporarily stop infusion; administer antidiarrheals, antiemetics; replace calcium.
Renal: Hemoglobinuria, oliguria, renal failure, temporary renal dysfunction, fluid overload	Monitor intake and output; administer diuretics; maintain adequate hydration; perform hemodialysis as necessary.
Immunologic: Fever, chills, allergic reaction, anaphylaxis, flushing, rash, erythema	Slow or temporarily stop infusion; administer acetaminophen, corticosteroids, antihistamines, meperidine, or aggressive life support as necessary.
Miscellaneous: Headache, unpleasant taste	Administer pain medications; have patient suck on hard candies, flavored liquids, or flavored ice pops.

Note. Based on information from Ezzone, 1997; Ezzone & Camp-Sorrell, 1994.

team (Herschl, 2000). Many centers have formal classes for caregivers with subjects such as central venous catheter care, intake and output, and emergency procedures and contacts. Written materials and support services for the caregiver also should be provided.

Infusion of Hematopoietic Stem Cells

The infusion of HSCs occurs on Day 0. Autologous cells may be infused in one to two days depending on the volume and to minimize the side effects of dimethyl sulfoxide (DMSO) (Ezzone, 1997). The hematopoietic stem cells may be infused without delay after TBI but are usually infused 48–72 hours after the last dose of chemotherapy. This is to ensure that no residual cytotoxic therapy that could harm the cells is still circulating (Kapustay & Buchsel, 2000).

Administration of Cryopreserved Hematopoietic Stem Cells

Autologous or allogeneic HSCs may be cryopreserved (frozen) and stored for infusion at a later date. The HSC product is thawed rapidly at the bedside and infused immediately; however, the process begins in the HSC laboratory. HSC laboratory personnel remove the bags of frozen cells from the freezer and place them in a dry shipper for transport to the bedside. Sterile saline or sterile water is heated in a disinfected water bath to 37°–45°C. The water bath and the shipper with the cells then are taken to the bedside (Law, 2000). Each bag is removed from the cassette, and the identity is verified by two staff members, including the nurse, physician, or HSC laboratory staff. The bag is immersed into the warm water bath. A secondary bag may be used to protect the cells in the event that breakage or leakage occurs. The cells are immediately infused by gravity drip or by using a syringe. The thawing process on the second bag should not be initiated until the infusion of the prior bag is complete, because prolonged exposure of stem cells to DMSO has been shown to decrease colony formation of cryopreserved HSCs (Law).

Little research has been conducted comparing the infusion methods of IV drip versus IV bolus. Theoretically, bolus methods result in shorter exposure of the stem cells to the toxicity of DMSO, whereas drip methods may allow better patient tolerance of the emetogenic and arrhythmogenic effects of the DMSO.

Adverse Effects

The stem cell infusion may be accompanied by many minor complications, but most resolve within 24–48 hours. Most adverse effects are caused by DMSO, the cryoprotectant used for stem cell preservation. Adverse effects also may be caused by red cell contamination and breakdown and the total volume of cells infused (Kapustay & Buchsel, 2000). This results in hemoglobinuria, which occurs secondary to the breakdown of red cells in the stem cell or bone marrow product. The patient's urine may be pink-tinged or cherry red for 24–48 hours following the infusion. Other adverse effects

that may occur include nausea, vomiting, abdominal cramping, diarrhea, facial flushing, hypertension, hypotension, bradycardia, tachycardia, cardiac arrhythmias, tachypnea, dyspnea, cough, chest tightness, fever, and chills. In addition to hemoglobinuria, other adverse effects unique to stem cell infusion are a garlic-like taste in the mouth and unusual breath odor (Reed & Franco, 1992). The garlic-like taste is caused by the DMSO and should only last 24–48 hours (Ezzone, 1997). The family and staff will notice a garlic-like odor on the patient's breath and urine.

Nursing Management

Aggressive IV hydration is begun before the transplant to increase renal perfusion and minimize renal compromise caused by inadvertent red cell contamination of the stem cell product during collection (Kapustay & Buchsel, 2000). The hydration product may include mannitol and sodium bicarbonate to promote osmotic diuresis. Premedications, such as acetaminophen, diphenhydramine, corticosteroids, diuretics, and possibly an antiemetic, may be administered (Ezzone, 1997). These medications are administered to diminish the reactions to DMSO and to manage fluid volume excess. Premedications may include lorazepam, an antianxiety medication, but caution should be taken because of the potential synergistic effects of lorazepam and DMSO, which may cause extreme drowsiness (Kapustay & Buchsel).

Preparation for the stem cell infusion and monitoring the patient for any and all of the adverse effects that may occur is important. Some centers monitor the patient's cardiac rhythm and oxygenation throughout the procedure. Cardiac monitoring equipment and oxygen support should be available at the bedside. Vital signs should be checked prior to the start of the infusion and every 10–30 minutes during the infusion. Severe reactions to the DMSO may occur, despite prophylactic medications, and continual monitoring of the patient should be conducted throughout the HSC infusion. Refer to Table 4-3 for strategies for the management of adverse events related to cryopreserved frozen stem cell infusion.

Patient and Family Education

Education of the patient and family should begin at least the day before the infusion and be repeated on the day of the infusion. This may help to decrease patient anxiety related to the events of the infusion. Education should include what to expect before, during, and after the stem cell infusion. An explanation of the room setup, use of premedications, the thawing and infusion of the stem cells, and potential adverse reactions to the infusion should be given (Simpson, 2000).

In particular, it is important to educate about the garlic-like taste the patient will experience from the DMSO. Hard candy or flavored ice pops should be offered to decrease the unpleasant taste. The family should be cautioned that they will notice a garlic-like odor on the patient's breath and urine. Explain that this is because of the DMSO and should last only 24–48 hours (Ezzone, 1997). Education should include an explanation to the patient and family regarding hemoglobin-uria, usually lasting 24–36 hours after the infusion. Assurance should be given that the red urine is not due to bleeding, but rather the red cells from the stem cell infusion breakdown are excreted from the urine. A well-educated patient and family will have less anxiety.

Fresh Hematopoietic Stem Cell Infusion

Allogeneic HSCs usually are infused fresh, immediately after apheresis or marrow harvest. Under some circumstances, they are cryopreserved and frozen. Additionally, when placental or cord blood is collected, it must be cryopreserved and stored (Rowley, 1999). If frozen, the allogeneic stem cells would be administered, as previously described. When allogeneic stem cells are infused fresh, they are taken directly from the donor to the processing lab (Simpson, 2000). If the donor and recipient have incompatible red cell phenotype, processing may include red cell depletion or plasma reduction (Stroncek et al., 1991). Other processing may include T cell depletion to reduce the incidence of graft versus host disease (GVHD) (Ezzone & Camp-Sorrell, 1994). Once the stem cell processing is completed, the allogeneic stem cells are delivered at the bedside and infused via gravity into the patient's central venous catheter (Simpson). The nurse usually infuses the allogeneic HSCs with a physician readily available, in the event that any adverse effects should occur.

Adverse Effects

Fresh HSC infusion has fewer adverse effects than frozen HSC infusion, as the product is not cryopreserved with DMSO. Potential adverse effects are similar to those seen with blood product infusions and can include shortness of breath, hypotension, hypertension, tachycardia, chills, fever, chest pain or tightness, flushing, nausea and vomiting, rash, hives, or anaphylaxis. Treatment is symptomatic and may include slowing the rate of the infusion; administering medications such as hydrocortisone, diphenhydramine, and epinephrine; and administering oxygen to relieve dyspnea (Whedon, 1991). Aggressive cardiopulmonary support may be necessary, and emergency equipment should be on hand at the bedside (Ezzone & Camp-Sorrell, 1994).

Nursing Management

IV hydration may be necessary if an ABO incompatibility exists. Sodium bicarbonate may be added to the IV fluids to alkalinize the urine and prevent renal damage from any hemolyzed cells. Premedications such as antipyretics and antihistamines should be administered to prevent a hemolytic reaction. Other premedications may include antiemetics and sedatives (Ezzone & Camp-Sorrell, 1994). Cardiac monitoring and/or pulse oximetry to monitor oxygenation may be performed. Vital signs are monitored before the start of the infusion and then every 10–30 minutes. The ABO compatible HSCs should be infused over two to four hours, depending on the volume, and must be infused with nonfiltered tubing to ensure that no stem cells are filtered out. Because ABO incompatible HSCs are plasma reduced, the infusion time may be shorter because of the decreased volume of HSC products to be infused. Upon the completion of the infusion, the catheter should be flushed with preservative-free saline to prevent damage to the stem cells.

Patient and Family Education

Review of the infusion of fresh HSCs should be performed the day before the infusion as well as the day of the infusion. Providing information early may decrease patient and family anxiety. Education of the patient and family should include the use of the cardiac monitor and premedications and facts on the frequency of vital signs and the possible adverse effects of the infusion. The patient should be encouraged to report all symptoms he or she experiences and to ask questions throughout the procedure.

Post Stem Cell Infusion

The first day post-HSC infusion is Day +1, second day is Day +2, third day is Day +3, and so on. The first few weeks following the administration of HSCs are the most critical. Patients may experience multiple toxicities from the preparative regimen and at the same time have little or no bone marrow function.

In addition to the expected toxicities from the preparative regimen listed in Table 4-2, several acute adverse events also may occur.

Acute Adverse Effects

Acute adverse effects manifested as metabolic emergencies are common in patients with malignancies as well as in patients receiving chemotherapy (Flombaum, 2000). Patients receiving preparative regimens for bone marrow or hematopoietic blood stem cell transplantation are at risk for several of them. The following sections will describe the most common.

Acute Tumor Lysis Syndrome

Tumor lysis syndrome (TLS) is typically seen during conditioning and not after stem cell infusion. The acute tumor lysis syndrome (ATLS) describes a group of metabolic complications that can occur spontaneously or in a variety of treatment settings, including during cytoreductive therapy in preparation for BMT (Fleming, Henslee-Downey, & Coffey, 1991; Przepiorka & Gonzales-Chambers, 1990).

Etiology and Risk Factors: The tumors most frequently associated with ATLS are hematologic malignancies, such as high-grade lymphomas (particularly Burkitt's lymphoma) and acute or chronic leukemias with high leukocyte counts. Other risk factors predisposing to ATLS include the presence of extensive disease, as evidenced by large tumor masses and/or high LDH levels, preexisting renal dysfunction, or acute renal failure developing after treatment. Renal clearance is the primary mechanism for excretion of uric acid, potassium, and phosphorus; thus, the metabolic complications of tumor lysis are more likely to appear and be severe in these patients (Flombaum, 2000). In addition, ATLS commonly occurs with corticosteroid use alone in patients with very sensitive lymphomas and leukemias (Dhingra & Newcom, 1988; Malik, Abubakar, Alam, & Khan, 1994; Sparano, Ramirez, & Wiernik, 1988; Tiley et al., 1992); with drugs such as tamoxifen (Cech, Block, Cone, & Stone, 1986), interferon alfa (Fer et al., 1984), amsacrine (Volger, Morris, & Winton, 1983), and cladribine (Dann et al., 1993); and during intrathecal administration of methotrexate (Simmons & Somberg, 1991).

Pathophysiology: ATLS is characterized by the rapid development of hyperuricemia, hyperkalemia, hyperphosphatemia, hypocalcemia, azotemia, or full-blown acute renal failure. These abnormalities may occur alone or together, with acute rises in blood urea nitrogen (BUN) and serum phosphorus levels being the most common. Hypocalcemia and increases in lactic dehydrogenase (LDH) also are frequently seen. These biochemical alterations are related to the acute release of intracellular products into the circulation as a result of the lysis of radiosensitive or chemosensitive rapidly proliferating cells (tumor cells) (Flombaum, 2000). Acute renal insufficiency results from the precipitation of uric acid in the renal tubules and/or calcium phosphate crystals in the renal tubules.

Diagnostic Studies: Serum electrolytes, BUN, phosphorus, calcium, magnesium, uric acid, and creatinine levels should be measured at least twice daily or more often as evidence of tumor lysis develops. When the release of uric acid occurs more slowly, uric acid stones can form in the renal pelvis and occasionally lead to ureteral obstruction.

Medical Management: The introduction of allopurinol before the initiation of chemotherapy or radiotherapy has reduced the incidence of acute renal failure secondary to acute uric acid nephropathy. Marked hyperphosphatemia is the usual precipitating factor of renal failure following chemotherapy. If allopurinol alone does not cure hyperuricemia, alkalization of the urine can be achieved by the addition of sodium bicarbonate to IV fluids. Urine pH should be kept above 7. Sodium acetate can replace sodium bicarbonate when there is a concomitant need to administer calcium or magnesium in IV fluids.

Acetazolamide, given orally or IV, also may be used to alkalinize the urine, especially in patients with metabolic alkalosis and/or with decreased renal function. Overly vigorous urinary alkalinization may increase the possibility of calcium phosphate precipitation in the renal tubules, so bicarbonate administration should be discontinued once serum uric acid is normalized (Flombaum, 2000).

Hyperkalemia is the first life-threatening abnormality appearing during ATLS and can occur during the first 6–72 hours after initiating therapy. The usual treatment includes hypertonic glucose with insulin and sodium/potassium exchange resin. Furosemide also is useful and acts by increasing urinary potassium excretion. Calcium should not be administered unless there is evidence of neuromuscular ir-

ritability. It is not unusual for patients who are at risk for developing ATLS to have some degree of renal insufficiency (either because of lymphomatous infiltration of the kidneys or from urinary obstruction before starting the chemotherapy). Treatment of the underlying malignancy may improve renal function by correcting the reason for the renal failure (Flombaum, 2000).

In the event that conservative measures are not successful, acute uric acid nephropathy responds rapidly to hemodialysis, with restoration of urine flow and improvement in renal function as hyperuricemia resolves. Hemodialysis also is effective in correcting hyperkalemia, hyperphosphatemia, and hypocalcemia, but because of the large phosphate burden present in some of these patients, it is frequently necessary to repeat the procedure at 12- to 24-hour intervals. Life-threatening hyperkalemia can recur even after dialysis has been performed; therefore, potassium levels should be checked frequently (Flombaum, 2000). Continuous arteriovenous hemodialysis with a high dialysate flow rate (Pichette et al., 1994) and continuous venovenous hemofiltration also have been used and are especially effective in removing large amounts of phosphorous (Flombaum; Sakarcan & Quigley, 1994).

Nursing Management: Identification of patients at risk for development of ATLS and monitoring of electrolyte abnormalities, fluid balance, and patients' responses to treatment are the focus of nursing management. Early recognition of signs and symptoms of hyperuricemia, hyperkalemia, hyperphosphatemia, and hypocalcemia will promote initiation of preventative therapy and minimize complications (Ezzone, 1999).

Hypercalcemia

Etiology and Risk Factors: Hypercalcemia is an acute complication that is rarely seen in the HSCT setting. It may occur in patients with hematologic complications, such as multiple myeloma or lymphoma. Other tumors associated with the occurrence of hypercalcemia are carcinomas of the breast and lung; squamous cell carcinoma of the head, neck, and uroepithelial tract; and hypernephroma. Causes of hypercalcemia include immobilization, granulomatous disease, primary hyperparathyroidism, drugs (thiazides and lithium), and Addison's disease (Flombaum, 2000).

Hypercalcemia is a common complication in patients with multiple myeloma because of the presence of extensive bone destruction (Ziegler, 1994).

Pathophysiology: Bone resorption is increased by parathyroid hormone–related protein and osteoclast-activating factors secreted from myeloma cells. In addition, related substances that possess osteoclast-activating factor properties, such as cytokines that include tumor necrosis factor-beta along with interleukin- (IL-) 1 and IL-6, also are potent inhibitors of osteoblastic bone formation (Mundy, 1990). Abnormal renal function also is common in multiple myeloma (Barnett, 1999).

Ninety-nine percent of the body's calcium is combined with phosphorus and is concentrated in the skeletal system, which serves as the body's calcium reservoir. The remaining 1% is in the serum, which is half freely ionized and the other half bound by circulating protein (primarily albumin) (Schaffer, 1997). The freely ionized form is biologically active and must be maintained within a narrow range. Homeostasis of normal calcium levels involves a balance of several body processes, including bone remodeling, renal calcium reabsorption, and gastrointestinal absorption. Hormonal factors also influence the interchange of calcium among the gut, kidney, bone, and extracellular fluid. Parathyroid hormone and calcitonin are the primary hormones that regulate extracellular calcium homeostasis. In turn, each substance is controlled by the level of serum-ionized calcium (Barnett, 1999).

Humoral hypercalcemia and local osteolytic hypercalcemia are the two main mechanisms that contribute to the occurrence of hypercalcemia in malignancy. These mechanisms disrupt the balance of calcium by producing hormones, cytokines, or growth factors that interfere with the normal physiologic functioning of the bone, kidneys, and gut (Barnett, 1999). Another humoral mediator of malignancy-related hypercalcemia is vitamin D. Although vitamin D–related hypercalcemia is not a common finding, it has been seen in human T cell leukemia, virus-related T cell lymphomas, and Hodgkin's lymphoma (Schweitzer, Hamdy, & Frolich, 1994; Warrell, 1993).

Calcium plays a role in maintaining cell membrane permeability, which, in turn, impacts the cellular activity of multiple body systems, resulting in signs and symptoms of hypercalcemia (Lang-Kummer, 1997).

Clinical Manifestations and Diagnostic Studies: Common symptoms of hypercalcemia include fatigue, anorexia, weight loss, bone pain, constipation, polydipsia, muscle weakness, nausea and vomiting, confusion, and polyuria (Shuey, 1994). In symptomatic patients with a serum calcium level of 12–14 mg/dl, the finding is serious because any event that causes a volume depletion or a decrease in the glomerular filtration rate may lead to severe hypercalcemia. Urgent treatment is required for patients with a corrected serum calcium concentration > 14 mg/dl and for patients with symptomatic moderate hypercalcemia (Raue & Pecherstorjer, 1994). Hypercalcemia is diagnosed by the use of the corrected serum calcium level. The total serum calcium level is a poor indicator of the freely ionized calcium; therefore, the use of a correction formula that considers the effect of an altered albumin concentration is important. The following formula is used: Ca (corrected mg/dl) = Ca (measured mg/dl) + [0.8 x (4–albumin concentration g/dl)] (Moore, 1994; Warrell, 1993). Other laboratory values that are important to review include serum electrolytes, ionized calcium, BUN, and creatinine. Potassium and calcium have an inverse relationship, and hypokalemia has been reported in more than half of patients with hypercalcemia whose renal function is normal (Mundy, 1990). Magnesium levels also may decrease, aggravating the neuromuscular effects (Schaffer, 1997). Hypercalcemia resulting from direct bony involvement (e.g.,

breast cancer, myeloma, renal cell carcinoma) often results in increased serum phosphorus levels (Bajournas, 1990).

Medical Management: Treatment of malignancy-induced hypercalcemia is aimed at treating the underlying disease as well as the mechanisms causing hypercalcemia. The two mechanisms of hypercalcemia (accelerated bone resorption and increased calcium reabsorption in the kidneys) are treated by initiating hydration with saline diuresis to increase the calcium excretion from the kidneys followed by antiresorptive therapy to decrease bone resorption (Chisholm, Mulloy, & Taylor, 1996). Once rehydration has been established, bisphosphonates are effective when administered orally or intravenously, depending on the severity of the hypercalcemia. Treatment also includes a review of medications that might contribute to hypercalcemia, such as thiazide diuretics, vitamins A and D, or any type of calcium supplements, including additives in hyperalimentation (Barnett, 1999).

Nursing Management: Nursing management of hypercalcemia of malignancy is directed at prevention, early detection, treatment, management, and support of the patient and family. It is important to identify patients who are at risk, assess for signs and symptoms, and monitor laboratory values (Barnett, 1999).

Disseminated Intravascular Coagulation

Definition: Disseminated intravascular coagulation (DIC) represents an overstimulation of normal coagulation in which thrombosis and hemorrhage may occur simultaneously. This results from injury to the vascular endothelium and activation of platelets and clotting factors. Depending on the severity, the syndrome may be chronic or acute, fulminating when it becomes overwhelming to the body (Gobel, 1999). In the acute form, there is dramatic microvascular thrombosis and possibly large vessel thrombosis, which leads to impairment of blood flow, ischemia, and end organ damage (Bick, 1994).

Etiology and Risk Factors: Acute DIC is seen in a variety of defined clinical situations such as sepsis, acute leukemia, and tumor lysis. Because of one of these processes, injury to the vascular endothelium occurs with activation of platelets and clotting factors (Gobel, 1999). Historically, the highest incidence of DIC (approximately 85%) has occurred in individuals with acute promyelocytic leukemia (Bunn & Ridgeway, 1993). This has been known to occur before and in conjunction with chemotherapy (Goodnough, 1991). A procoagulant substance has been identified on the promyeloblast cell that is similar to thromboplastin. It is believed that this substance is released from granules on the promyelocyte, which, subsequently, initiates the clotting response (Kurtz, 1993).

Hepatic failure secondary to primary liver disease or metastasis, or as a complication of radiation or chemotherapy, can increase the risk of DIC (Gobel, 1999). Hemolytic transfusion reactions and massive blood transfusions may be complicated by DIC. Prosthetic devices such as LeVeen or Denver shunts may be used to push excess ascitic fluid into the intravascular system. The ascitic fluid contains collagen and other procoagulant substances, and when shunted into the general circulation, they can cause DIC (Lankiewicz & Bell, 1993).

Pathophysiology: In acute DIC, there is an overstimulation of coagulation, in which the ability to control intravascular thrombin may activate both coagulation and fibrinolysis (Gobel, 1999). The initial event in acute DIC is a thrombotic diathesis, in which clotting factors and platelets are consumed (Kempin, 1997). Excess circulating thrombin separates fibrinogen, which combines with circulating fibrin degradation products (FDPs) to form an insoluble form of fibrin. These insoluble clots may become deposited in the microvasculature of various organs, with resultant multisystem failure (Bick, 1994). The lodged clots further trap circulating platelets, leading to a worsening of the thrombocytopenic state. The trapped platelets impede blood flow, leading to hypoxia, tissue ischemia, and necrosis of affected organs, along with consumption of clots and clotting factors (Gobel, 1997). Once clotting factors and platelets drop below critical levels, hemorrhage occurs (Gobel, 1999). Excess thrombin also assists in the conversion of plasminogen to plasmin, resulting in fibrinolysis that results in increased FDPs. FDPs have strong anticoagulant properties and, thus, interfere with fibrin clot formation and aid in the consumption of clotting factors and platelets. Plasmin also can activate the complement and kinin systems. Activation of these systems leads to shock, hypotension, and increased vascular permeability (Bick, 1996; Bick, Strauss, & Frenkel, 1996). The clinical presentation is generally a combination of extreme thrombosis and bleeding.

Clinical Manifestations: Bleeding is the most obvious sign of DIC. Most patients with DIC bleed from at least three unrelated sites (Bick, 1994; Marder, Martin, & Coleman, 1993). A less evident but equally dramatic sign of DIC is thrombosis. Both microvascular and large vessel thrombosis may occur, which may result in end organ damage and ischemic changes (Gobel, 1999). Subtle signs and symptoms of thrombi include red indurated areas found in multiple organ sites (Gobel, 1997).

Diagnostic Studies: Laboratory testing of DIC can be variable and complex based on the pathophysiology of this process. In DIC, the prothrombin time may be normal or even short because of interference of activating clotting factors or FDPs. The activated partial thromboplastin time is normal in approximately 40%–50% of patients with DIC. The platelet count is usually decreased in DIC, but the mere presence of thrombocytopenia is neither sensitive nor specific for DIC (Williams & Mosher, 1997). Newer modalities for testing DIC have become available, which is making the laboratory assessment of DIC more exact. One of the most reliable tests performed to assess DIC is the D-dimer assay. D-dimer is a neoantigen that is formed when plasmin digests fibrin. The D-dimer test is specific for FDPs (Bick & Baker, 1992). Another test for DIC is the FDP titre; a positive FDP titre indicates DIC. DIC is almost always associated with increased fibrinolysis,

which may result in increased levels of FDPs (Williams & Mosher). The diagnosis of DIC also may be supported by tests that demonstrate accelerated fibrinolysis. A decreased level of antithrombin III demonstrates accelerated coagulation (Gobel, 1997).

Medical Management: The basic principle of treating DIC is treating the underlying cause of DIC (Bick, 1994). If the process of DIC continues after measures aimed at treating the underlying stimulus have been attempted, some of the recent literature recommends treating the intravascular clotting process as the next step (Bick, 1996; Riewald & Riess, 1998; Staudlinger, Locker, & Frass, 1996). The reason for treating the clotting process next is that thrombosis is the process that impacts the most on the morbidity and mortality associated with DIC. The use of heparin, however, is somewhat controversial, as studies have not provided a conclusion related to survival (Gobel, 1999).

Nursing Management: Early detection of the signs and symptoms associated with DIC may allow for prompt attention, early diagnosis, and treatment of this condition. Even though the thrombosis of DIC is the strongest contributor to morbidity and mortality associated with this syndrome, bleeding is the most observable sign of DIC. Attempting to provide care in a calm and reassuring environment may help to decrease patient and family anxiety (Gobel, 1999).

Syndrome of Inappropriate Antidiuretic Hormone

Definition: Syndrome of inappropriate antidiuretic hormone (SIADH) is classified as an endocrine paraneoplastic syndrome, meaning the disorder is caused by abnormal secretion of an endocrine peptide not directly related to invasion by the primary tumor or its metastasis. SIADH results from the inappropriate production and secretion of antidiuretic hormone (ADH). ADH also is known as arginine vasopressin, the biologically active form of ADH in humans (Ferlito, Rinaldo, & Devaney, 1997). Vasopressin is synthesized in large neuronal cells located in the supraoptic and paraventricular nuclei of the hypothalamus (Guyton, 1991). After synthesis, the hormone is transported down axons that terminate in the posterior lobe of the pituitary gland (neurohypophysis) (Guyton). Vasopressin is stored in the neurohypophysis until appropriate reflexes signal secretion into the blood stream. A major physiologic action of vasopressin is to regulate water reabsorption in the renal tubules. Antidiuretic hormone acts specifically on the tubular segments of the collecting duct system. With high plasma concentrations of vasopressin, the collecting duct becomes highly permeable to water; thus, water is retained with the excretion of a small volume of concentrated urine (Vander, 1995).

Etiology and Risk Factors: A likely cause of SIADH in the transplant setting is excessive ADH release. Drugs that stimulate ADH secretion include cyclophosphamide, vincristine, morphine, and amitriptyline (Sanders, 1998). Additionally, cyclophosphamide enhances the effect of ADH on kidneys. Other nonectopic mechanisms associated with SIADH include infectious sepsis and central nervous system etiologies. Infectious causes of SIADH are frequently associated with infections in the lung or brain. Central nervous system effects secondary to head trauma, with or without fracture, also may influence the development of SIADH because of leakage of vasopressin stores (Baylis, 1997).

Diagnosis/Diagnostic Studies: The hallmark of SIADH is hyponatremia. After documentation of hyponatremia, it is necessary to confirm a water excess by measuring plasma osmolality that decreases below 275 mOsm/kg. In addition, inappropriately concentrated urine with low serum osmolality is a key diagnostic feature (Keenan, 1999).

Clinical Manifestations: The signs and symptoms of SIADH are the result of water excess and consequent hyponatremia. Signs and symptoms are typically categorized as mild, moderate, or severe and relate to the magnitude of hyponatremia as well as the rapidity of occurrence. In mild cases, patients may be asymptomatic or may complain of headache, fatigue, anorexia, difficulty in concentrating, weakness, muscle cramps, and/or weight gain. These are nonspecific signs and symptoms and are frequently observed in patients with cancer. Moderate signs and symptoms may include thirst, impaired taste, confusion, lethargy, nausea and vomiting, diarrhea, oliguria, incontinence, depressed deep tendon reflexes, and personality changes. Severe signs and symptoms may progress to coma and seizure activity (Keenan, 1999).

Medical Management: Correction of hyponatremia should not exceed 0.5 mEq/l/hr and not more than 12 mEq in any 24-hour period (Flombaum, 2000). Major therapeutic strategies used to manage hyponatremia include fluid restriction, pharmacologic agents, and IV fluids. Methods of treatment are dictated by both underlying cause and clinical presentation. To prevent progression of SIADH, the most effective approach involves therapy directed to the malignancy, if the malignancy is the cause. Beyond treating the underlying malignancy, fluid restriction is the cornerstone of therapy. Fluid intake must be less than output so that a negative water balance is achieved. If fluid restriction is not effective, demeclocycline is the drug of choice. It inhibits the action of ADH on renal tubules, thus allowing excretion of water. Patients with life-threatening hyponatremia require aggressive therapy with hypertonic saline (3%) and IV furosemide. Clinical trials are being conducted on new pharmacologic agents classified as nonpeptide vasopressin receptor antagonists (Keenan, 1999).

Nursing Management: Close attention to laboratory values, intake and output, and daily weights may help offset a severe case of SIADH. Hypovolemia manifested by postural hypotension, poor skin turgor, and increased heart rate excludes the diagnosis of SIADH. Also, hypovolemia, with signs such as dependent edema and jugular vein distension, is not found in SIADH. If antineoplastic drugs such as cyclophosphamide (common in the transplant setting) or cisplatin are required, meticulous attention to the patient's fluid status is warranted. The substantial hydration necessary with such drugs may worsen SIADH. Administration of furosemide and normal saline is monitored. Decreases in weight up to 2–3 kg over three to four days reflect excretion of excess water. Measurements of urine specific gravity, taken every four to eight hours, indicate the ability of the kidneys to concentrate urine. During reversal of hyponatremia, especially in severe chronic cases, the nurse must be aware of overcorrection. If normal sodium levels are exceeded, it may be necessary to slow or discontinue therapy (Keenan, 1999).

Sepsis

Definition: Sepsis is the systemic response to infection. This systemic response is manifested by two or more of the following conditions as a result of infection: temperature greater than 38°C; heart rate greater than 90 beats/minute for an adult; respiratory rate greater than 20 breaths/minute for an adult or PaCO2 less than 32 mmHg; white blood cell (WBC) count greater than 12,000 cells/mm³ or less than 4,000 cells/mm³ or greater than 10% immature band forms in non-neutropenic individuals (Shelton, 1999).

Risk Factors and Etiology: Risk factors for infection in the transplant recipient encompass everything from the disease itself to treatment modalities. The most common consistent risk factor for infection is the duration of neutropenia (Biagi et al., 1997; Currie, Miller, & Mitchell, 1995; Engervall & Bjorkholm, 1995; Finkbinder & Ernst, 1993; Howell, Walters, Donowitz, & Farr, 1995; Pizzo, 1993; Schaffer, Garzon, Heroux, & Korniewicz, 1996). Infection risk also may be dependent on the specific type of immune deficit the patient manifests. Deficits of granulocytes, complement proteins, macrophages, immune globulin, and lymphocytes present risks for different infecting organisms, different sites of infection, and variable morbidity (Engervall & Bjorkholm; Shelton, 1996). Patients at high risk for developing sepsis include neonates, the elderly, patients with hematologic malignancy, and those developing fever while in the hospital (Rolston, 1998). Patients receiving immunosuppressive therapy also are at risk because of normal responses being suppressed. The Hospital Infection Control Practice Advisory Committee [HICPAC] (1995) reported that more than 90% of nosocomial blood infections are related to venous access devices.

Clinical Manifestations: Sepsis by definition is a total body inflammatory response to perceived invading pathogens, and, hence, manifests with both local and systemic symptoms. The process involves neurologic, endocrine, immunologic, and cardiovascular compensatory responses that produce an integrated attempt to reject and destroy the pathogen. When compensation is present, inflammatory mediators are predominant, and a "warm hyperdynamic" clinical presentation is typical. When compensatory mechanisms fail and myocardial depression prevails, a "cold hypodynamic" (myocardial failure and perfusion deficit) clinical picture is evident. Patients with suspected sepsis require a thorough physical examination focusing on high-risk sites of infection, such as the skin and oral cavity (Shelton, 1999).

Diagnostic Studies: The diagnosis of sepsis is based on clinical indicators, laboratory tests, and a variety of other diagnostic methods, such as radiology or sonography, that provide characteristic clues in certain infections. The most important and sensitive of these tests is the culture and sensitivity of body fluids and surfaces (Chernecky & Berger, 1997; Schaffer et al., 1996). Blood cultures are a vital part of any fever workup. Although 40%–70% of febrile episodes do not yield a positive culture for any organism, the occurrence of fever is treated as infection (Pizzo, 1993; Yoshida, 1997). One study has shown that blood cultures drawn from an infected central line became culture positive an average of six hours sooner than peripheral cultures in the same patient (Blot et al., 1998). This may help with the prediction of line sepsis versus sepsis from other causes, allowing the removal of infected lines sooner (Shelton, 1999). The use of complementary diagnostic tools will vary with infection site, organism, and patient population; however, the use of radiology for diagnosis of pneumonia is well established. Almost all febrile episodes result in a screening chest x-ray, yet research demonstrates that they are rarely abnormal in the absence of respiratory symptoms (Katz, Bash, Rollins, Cash, & Buchanan, 1991; Pizzo; Volker, 1998).

Prevention of Sepsis: The single most important method of preventing infection in immunocompromised patients is recognizing risk factors and altering them whenever possible. Immunocompromised patients develop infection from environmental exposures, through reactivation of latent organisms, from normal flora (Finkbinder & Ernst, 1993), or through care-related exposures (Shelton, 1999).

Transmission of infections via blood products is infrequent, affecting less than 2% of all donated products (American Association of Blood Banks [AABB], 1998; Dodd, 1994; Labovich, 1997). Unfortunately, when it does occur with an immunocompromised patient, it can be life-threatening (Shelton, 1999). Infections transmitted unintentionally through donor blood include Chagas' disease, hepatitis C and E, malaria, babesiosis, yersinia, adenovirus, retrovirus, HIV, and cytomegalovirus (AABB; Dodd; Walter-Coleman, 1996). Infection is specific to the incubation of the infecting organism and has been reported from several days to several months after the transfusion (Dodd). Infections that are related to contamination of the blood product during harvest or preparation are almost universally bacterial and more immediately life-threatening. The most common reported organisms are *Eschericia coli*, streptococcus, and staphylococcus. Septic shock immediately after transfusion is the most common presentation and supports the practice of not sending patients off the unit when blood products are transfusing (Shelton, 1999).

Prophylactic Antibiotics: The administration of antibiotics as prophylaxis against infection in high-risk patients has been a source of controversy for many years because of the known association of microbial resistance to antimicrobial use (Finkbinder & Ernst, 1993; Goldman, 1995; Hathorn, 1993; Martino et al., 1998). Studies comparing infection rates with and without prophylactic antibiotics in high-risk individuals demonstrate that infection morbidity is reduced by prophylactic antibiotic administration (Finkbinder & Ernst; Hathorn; Martino et al.). Patient selection for prophylaxis is the most important variable (Goldman). Microorganisms for which antimicrobial prophylaxis is typically used include cytomegalovirus, herpes simplex reactivation, *Mycobacterium avium-intracellulare*, *Mycobacterium tuberculosis*, *Pneumocystis carinii*, and catheter-related coagulase-negative staphylococci (Goldman; Hathorn).

Granulocyte Transfusions: There has been a renewed interest in granulocyte transfusion for severely neutropenic, infected patients. White blood cell infusions require intensive monitoring for hypersensitivity reactions and leukoagglutination syndrome, which may occur in severe pulmonary infections (Walter-Coleman, 1996). The success of this treatment is still unclear, but it offers hope for otherwise hopelessly septic patients (Shelton, 1996; Shelton, 1998; Toney & Parker, 1996; Walter-Coleman).

Growth Factors and Immune Stimulants: Hematopoietic growth factors are used to accelerate cell regeneration and differentiation in patients with bone marrow aplasia. Early WBC return with growth factors has reduced infection-related morbidity and mortality (De Lalla, 1997; Finkbinder & Ernst, 1993; Hathorn, 1993). In any regimen with a reported incidence of neutropenic infection exceeding 40%, growth factors are considered standard adjunctive therapy (American Society of Clinical Oncology, 1994; Lieschke & Burgess, 1992; Smith, 1996). It is generally believed that short-term neutropenia, in which infections are almost always bacterial in origin, only require granulocyte stimulation (granulocyte–colony-stimulating factor [G-CSF]). Long-term neutropenia places patients at risk for additional infections, such as fungal or opportunistic disease, and some believe multilineage products (PIXY or granulocyte macrophage–colony-stimulating factor [GM-CSF]) may be more advantageous (Lieschke & Burgess). In an attempt to conserve resources, some clinicians have tried starting growth factors after the decrease in the WBC count when evidence of infection is present. Studies have not shown a benefit of starting growth factors after infection is present (Beam, 1994; Goldman, 1995), although research in this area continues (Mortsyn, Foote, & Nelson, 1997; Riikonen, 1995).

Research on immunoglobulin therapy has revealed that many patients who are chronically ill, long-term immunosuppressed (BMT recipients), or patients with renal disease, hepatic failure, multiple myeloma, or chronic lymphocytic leukemia become immunoglobulin deficient (Ambrosino, 1991; Dwyer, 1992; Pilarski et al., 1986; Pizzo, 1993; Polmar, 1992; Popa, Kim, & Heiner, 1993; Weeks, Tierney, & Weinstein, 1991; Wordell, 1987). When immunoglobulin G (IgG) deficiency is present, there is impaired response to polysaccharide encapsulated bacteria, making infections with pneumococci and *Haemophilis influenzae* more common (Shelton, 1996). IV immunoglobulin (IVIG) therapy also has been shown to be effective in the prevention of some viral infections. IVIG replacement therapy is well established and relatively safe. As with all foreign proteins, there is a risk of hypersensitivity reaction, which requires that the infusion be started slowly and the infusion rate slowly increased while the patient is monitored (Wordell).

Medical/Nursing Management: The septic patient will present with fever and either vasodilation and relative vascular volume deficiency or vasoconstriction and myocardial depression (Bone, 1991; Luce, 1987; Rice, 1991; Toney & Parker, 1996). The most important management strategy for suspected sepsis in any patient with cancer is prompt initiation of antimicrobial therapy (Shelton, 1999). When broad-spectrum antibiotics are used early, frequently, or without careful consideration, there is concern that microbial resistance to the best agents will develop (Beam, 1994; Finkbinder & Ernst, 1993; Luce). This will result in few antibiotic choices available for patients with severe infection and resistant organisms. Unless patients exhibit signs or symptoms of impending shock, the antimicrobial regimen usually is not changed for 72 hours (Volker, 1998).

Patients with hematologic malignancy or who are undergoing BMT often require a more comprehensive regimen because of prolonged neutropenia or known T lymphocyte defects (De Lalla, 1997; HICPAC, 1995; Pizzo, 1993; Trilla & Miro, 1995). These patients usually receive a fourth-generation cephalosporin or an antipseudomonal penicillin with an aminoglycoside to better cover anaerobic bacteria or atypical organisms (De Lalla; HICPAC; Pizzo).

The literature has questioned the practice of hospitalization with IV broad-spectrum antimicrobial therapy for patients with a low risk for developing sepsis (Buchanan, 1993; Freifield & Pizzo, 1996; Rapp, Perry, & Rotche, 1996; Rolston, 1998). Low-risk patients include outpatients and those with responsive malignancies, solid tumors, no comorbid conditions, short aplasia or increasing counts, and quick resolution of fever (Aquino, Tkaczewski, & Buchanan, 1997; Bash et al., 1994; Lau et al., 1994; Rolston; Talcott et al., 1994).

Patient and Caregiver Education

The site of care during the transplantation period affects the required patient and caregiver education. Because each transplant center is unique, institution-specific educational materials must be developed. These materials must provide detailed information regarding the preparative regimen, including drug, dose, route, frequency, duration, side effects, and side effect management. The anticipated time of engraftment and monitoring of transplant-related complications should be discussed, with an emphasis on patient and caregiver reporting of symptoms to the transplant team. Instructions regarding protective precautions recommended during the period of myelosuppression include dietary restrictions, infection prevention, and bleeding precautions. Eligibility criteria for discharge vary according to the site of care, time frame after transplant, and follow-up care required. Because the site of care varies among transplant centers at each phase following transplant, institution-specific criteria must be developed to ensure consistent care. If partial or complete outpatient transplant is performed, medical and nursing care may be coordinated through a homecare agency referral. Additional patient and family caregiver education will be required and may include IV fluid infusion, medication, or total parenteral nutrition; obtaining, reporting, and documenting vital signs and assessment of physical and psychological findings; oral care regimens; symptom management strategies; and obtaining emergency care (Ezzone, 2000). Patients usually are discharged from the transplant center to the care of the referring physician one to two months after transplant. Each transplant center may have unique requirements for continued follow-up care that depend on protocols and the type of transplant the patient received. The expected frequency of outpatient visits both at the transplant center and at the referring physician's office should be explained to patients and family members. Some medications and protective precautions may be continued on a long-term basis and should be explained to those involved. Successful methods of providing education to patients and caregivers are individualized to their educational levels, reading levels, attentiveness, and stated preferences (Ezzone, 2000).

Engraftment

Engraftment of HSCs refers to the state of acceptance of the infused HSCs as evidenced by a gradual but steady increase in blood counts. When the donor cells enter the bone marrow cavity and begin to reproduce, engraftment occurs.

Migration or homing of transplanted cells to the bone marrow for engraftment is a complex process that is not fully understood. After transplantation or infusion, these cells pass through a blood-marrow barrier, which appears to be facilitated by five families of adhesion molecules: integrins, immunoglobulins, selectins, mucins, and proteoglycans. The cell membranes of CD34+ cells have multiple receptors for these adhesion molecules. The receptors are highly specific but have regulatable levels of affinity, allowing them to bind molecules and then release them, enabling them to direct stem cells to move along a particular pathway. This pathway has been called the adhesion cascade (Abboud & Lichtman, 1995; Turner & Sweetenham, 1996). In the process of homing or migration, stem cells first adhere to the inner surface of the blood-marrow barrier, the endothelial cells lining the vascular sinuses in the bones. After forming a migration pore in the endothelial cell cytoplasm, stem cells penetrate the basement membrane and then pass through gaps in the adventitial reticular layer. Once stem cells pass through the barrier and into the extravascular space, components of the marrow stroma interact with the cells to direct them into their appropriate niches. Here, presumably, they are retained and/or trapped (Abboud & Lichtman; Turner & Sweetenham).

Following the transplantation, newly infused stem cells give rise to a new hematopoietic and immune system. A consistent rise in the WBC count heralds hematopoietic and immune recovery. Early evidence of engraftment is seen as the WBC count rises and the population of cells shifts from lymphocytes to neutrophils. Red blood cells, platelets, and neutrophils are all capable of functioning effectively as soon as they are generated. This is not the case, however, for T and B cells, whose effectiveness returns slowly and may never return to pretransplant levels (Atkinson, 1994).

In autologous HSCT, WBCs appear in the circulation 7–10 days following transplant. With marrow transplants, WBCs appear about two weeks later. Faster recovery sometimes allows the entire transplant procedure to be performed in the outpatient arena, thereby completely eliminating the need for hospitalization and resulting in a considerable cost savings. Faster recovery also results in an improved quality of life during the procedure. This rapid recovery is the major reason that autologous BMTs are rarely performed today and have been almost completely replaced by HSCTs (Kessinger, 1999).

Allogeneic Hematopoietic Stem Cell Transplantation

The literature that followed the initial reports on allogeneic HSCT was primarily focused on engraftment characteristics. Unfortunately, a comparative analysis of these reports is made difficult by small sample size, significant differences in terms of patient characteristics, preparative regimens, supportive care, and GVHD prophylaxis (with or without methotrexate), as well as the nonrandomized nature of these studies. Nevertheless, some general conclusions can be drawn from these data (Anderlini, 1999). Compared to historical controls, when patients received marrow allografts, the recovery of granulocytes and platelets seemed to be at least comparable and, according to most investigators, faster. This seems to be true particularly for platelet recovery. This has translated into a reduced red cell and platelet transfusion requirement. In view of the fast myeloid engraftment after allogeneic HSCT, it is unclear whether postinfusion cytokines (e.g., recombinant human granulocyte–colony-stimulating factor [rhG-CSF]) are beneficial or cost effective (Anderlini).

In the allogeneic setting, successful engraftment of donor cells in marrow is known as a chimeric state (meaning that only donor cells exist within the patient). In some patients, a mix of donor and recipient cells, referred to as mixed chimera, may exist after a transplant. Ideally, in time, only the donor cells will populate the patient's marrow. In the event of graft failure, a backup infusion of stem cells may be given.

Although engraftment is suggested by the increase of peripheral cell counts, cytogenetic studies such as chromosomal analysis may help to identify successful transplant by identifying the origin of the new marrow. If the donor and recipient are not of the same gender, engraftment is confirmed by the presence of the donor's sex chromosomes in the recipient's new bone marrow. Cytogenetic studies detect remission of disease by monitoring the disappearance of unique chromosomal abnormalities specific to the patient's malignancy. If the recipient and donor are of the same gender, erythrocyte typing, human leukocyte antigen (HLA) typing, complement typing, and immunoglobulin allele typing may confirm engraftment. However, complex methods of DNA typing tests also are commonly used to confirm engraftment (Alcoser & Burchett, 1999).

In general, hematopoietic recovery post-transplantation is more rapid following transplantation using the peripheral blood stem cell (BSC) than recovery following the use of bone marrow stem cells. On average, patients become platelet transfusion-independent approximately one week earlier with BSCs than with bone marrow. Although the exact mechanisms of this quicker recovery are not fully understood, a number of factors most likely contribute to it. A larger number of progenitor cells are collected peripherally than from marrow. A higher percentage of progenitor cells is committed to a line of differentiation, so less time is needed for these cells to traverse the differentiation compartments. The number of peripheral cells in cycle is greater than the number of cells in cycle that are collected directly from the marrow (Korbling & Champlin, 1996). It is not completely clear whether any of these differences are because of the differences between HSCs collected from the peripheral blood and those harvested directly from the marrow. The influence may be the priming process used to mobilize stem cells; if marrow was harvested following the same priming process, it is possible that it would produce the same or a more rapid reconstitution of marrow function (Korbling & Champlin).

The tempo of immune reconstitution function following HSCT is dependent on (a) the rate at which the patient's cells disappear after preparation, (b) the rate at which new cells engraft, and (c) the survival and longevity of mature lymphocytes present in the graft at the time of transplantation (Witherspoon, 1994). The survival and longevity of mature lymphocytes present in the graft at the time of transplantation greatly influence immune recovery. When stem cells are harvested by apheresis, the product typically contains 10 times more T cells than the product of a marrow harvest. This may lead to improved engraftment but also increases the possibility of GVHD (Sutherland, 1997).

Stability and Sustainment

The most conventional way to monitor the immediate hematopoietic recovery is through granulocyte recovery. It is obvious that granulocyte recovery is more rapid with blood versus bone marrow autografts, and this is detected when blood cells are collected after mobilization with chemotherapy or hematopoietic growth factors. The limitation of studying this question in humans has been the lack of an assay for stem cells responsible for long-term engraftment. Gene marking probably will be a way to follow engraftment and to study the correlation between engraftment and bone marrow recovery (Brenner, Herczeg, & Slater, 1992).

Bensinger et al. (2001) published the results of a multicenter randomized trial conducted to compare transplantation of bone marrow with peripheral blood cells from HLA-identical relatives in patients with hematologic cancers. In this trial, the peripheral blood cells were mobilized with G-CSF. The transplantation of peripheral blood cells was associated with faster recovery of neutrophils and platelets and with the transfusion of fewer units of platelets than was the transplantation of allogeneic bone marrow. Specifically, absolute neutrophil counts exceeded 500/mm^3 five days earlier in the patients assigned to receive peripheral blood cells than in the patients assigned to receive bone marrow. Platelet counts exceeded 20,000/mm³ without the need for transfusions, six days earlier in the peripheral blood cell group than in the bone marrow group, but the two groups received a similar number of units of red cells. These results are similar to those generally observed with autologous peripheral blood stem cells (Bensinger et al.).

References

Abboud, C.N., & Lichtman, M.A. (1995). Structure of the marrow. In E. Beutler, M.A. Lichtman, B.S. Collier, & T.J. Kipps (Eds.), *Williams hematology* (5th ed., pp. 25–37). New York: McGraw Hill.

Alcoser, P.W., & Burchett, S. (1999). Bone marrow transplantation: Immune system suppression and reconstitution. *American Journal of Nursing, 99*(6), 26–31.

Ambrosino, D.M. (1991). Impaired polysaccharide responses in immunodeficient patients: Relevance to bone marrow transplant patients. *Bone Marrow Transplantation, 7*(Suppl. 3), 48–51.

American Association of Blood Banks. (1998). *Facts about blood and blood banking, donor screening and referral; testing of donor blood for infectious diseases.* Retrieved August 23, 2002, from http://www.aabb.org/docs/facts.html.1998

American Society of Clinical Oncology. (1994). Recommendations for the use of hematopoietic colony-stimulating factors: Evidence-based clinical practice guidelines. *Journal of Clinical Oncology, 12,* 2471–2508.

Anderlini, P. (1999). *The role of allogeneic peripheral blood stem cell transplantation.* Retrieved August 23, 2002, from http://www.bmtinfo.org/bmt/topics/htm/paolo_1.html

Aquino, V.M., Tkaczewski, I., & Buchanan, G.R.R. (1997). Early discharge of low-risk febrile neutropenic children and adolescents with cancer. *Clinics of Infectious Disease, 25,* 74–78.

Armitage, J.O., & Antman, K.H. (1992). *High dose cancer therapy.* Philadelphia: Lippincott Williams and Wilkins.

Atkinson, K. (1994). Hematopoietic reconstitution post-transplant. In K. Atkinson (Ed.), *Clinical bone marrow transplantation: A reference textbook* (pp. 31–41). New York: Cambridge University Press.

Bajournas, D.R. (1990). Clinical manifestations of cancer-related hypercalcemia. *Seminars in Oncology, 17*(Suppl. 5), 16–25.

Barlogie, B. (1999). Autologous hematopoietic cell transplantation for multiple myeloma. In E.D. Thomas, K.G. Blume, & S.J. Forman (Eds.), *Hematopoietic cell transplantation* (2nd ed., pp. 1003–1013). Malden, MA: Blackwell Science.

Barnett, M.L. (1999). Hypercalcemia. *Seminars in Oncology Nursing, 15*(3), 190–201.

Bash, R.O., Katz, J.A., Cash, J.V., & Buchanan, G.R. (1994). Safety and cost effectiveness of early hospital discharge of lower-risk children with cancer admitted for fever and neutropenia. *Cancer, 74,* 189–196.

Baylis, P.H. (1997). Syndrome of inappropriate antidiuretic hormone secretion. In R. Sheaves, P.J. Jenkins, & J.A. Wass (Eds.), *Clinical endocrine oncology* (pp. 479–483). Cambridge, MA: Blackwell Science.

Beam, T.R. (1994). Anti-infective drugs in the prevention and treatment of sepsis syndrome. *Critical Care Nursing Clinics of North America, 6,* 275–293.

Bensinger, W.J., Martin, P., Storer, B., Clift, R., Forman, S.J., Negrin, R., et al. (2001). Transplantation of bone marrow as compared with peripheral blood cells from HLA-identical relatives in patients with hematologic cancers. *New England Journal of Medicine, 344,* 175–181.

Biagi, E., Arrigo, C., Dell'Orto, M.G., Balduzzi, A., Pezzini, C., Rovelli, A., et al. (1997). Mechanical and infective central venous catheter-related complications: A prospective non-randomized study using Hickman and Groshong catheters in children with hematologic malignancies. *Supportive Cancer Care, 5,* 228–233.

Bick, R.L. (1994). Disseminated intravascular coagulation. Objective criteria for diagnosis and management. *Medical Clinics of North America, 78,* 519–543.

Bick, R.L. (1996). Disseminated intravascular coagulation: Objective clinical and laboratory diagnosis, treatment, and assessment of therapeutic response. *Seminars in Thrombosis and Hemostasis, 22,* 69–88.

Bick, R.L., & Baker, W. (1992). Diagnostic efficacy of the D-dimer assay in DIC and related disorders. *Thrombosis Research, 65,* 785–790.

Bick, R.L., Strauss, J.F., & Frenkel, E.P. (1996). Thrombosis and hemorrhage in oncology patients. *Hematology Oncology Clinics of North America, 10,* 875–907.

Bierman, P.J., & Armitage, J.O. (1999). Autologous hematopoietic cell transplantation for Hodgkin's disease. In E.D. Thomas, K.G. Blume, & S.J. Forman (Eds.), *Hematopoietic cell transplantation* (2nd ed., pp. 952–962). Malden, MA: Blackwell Science.

Blot, F., Schmidt, E., Nitenberg, G., Tancrede, C., Leclercq, B., Laplanche, A., et al. (1998). Earlier positivity of central venous versus peripheral blood cultures is highly predictive of catheter-related sepsis. *Journal of Clinical Microbiology, 35,* 105–109.

Bone, R.C. (1991). The pathogenesis of sepsis. *Annals of Internal Medicine, 115,* 457–469.

Brenner, H.R., Herczeg, A., & Slater, C.R. (1992). Synapse-specific expression of acetylcholine receptor genes and their products at original synaptic sites in rat soleus muscle fibres regenerating in the absence of innervation. *Development, 116,* 41–53.

Buchanan, G. (1993). Approach to treatment of the febrile cancer patient with low risk neutropenia. *Hematology and Oncology Clinics of North America, 7,* 919–935.

Bunn, R.A., & Ridgeway, E.C. (1993). Paraneoplastic syndromes. In V.T. DeVita, S. Hellman, & S.A. Rosenberg (Eds.), *Cancer: Principles and practice of oncology* (4th ed., pp. 2026–2071). Philadelphia: Lippincott.

Cagnoni, P.J., Nieto, Y., & Jones, R.B. (2000). High-dose chemotherapy conditioning regimens for autologous or allogeneic hematopoietic stem cell transplantation. In E.D. Ball, J. Lister, & P. Law (Eds.), *Hematopoietic stem cell therapy* (pp. 382–402). New York: Churchill Livingstone.

Cech, P., Block, B., Cone, L.A., & Stone, R. (1986). Tumor lysis syndrome after tamoxifen flare. *New England Journal of Medicine, 315,* 263–264.

Chernecky, C.C., & Berger, B.J. (Eds.). (1997). *Laboratory tests and diagnostic procedures* (2nd ed.). Philadelphia: W.B. Saunders.

Chisholm, M.A., Mulloy, A.L., & Taylor, T.A. (1996). Acute management of cancer-related hypercalcemia. *Annals of Pharmacotherapeutics, 30,* 507–513.

Currie, I.C., Miller, E.J., & Mitchell, A. (1995). Experience of an implantable central venous access system in a district general hospital. *Journal of the Royal College of Surgeons of Edinburgh, 40,* 31–34.

Dann, E.J., Gillis, S., Poliak, A., Okon, E., Rund, D., & Rachmilewitz, E.A. (1993). Brief report: Tumor lysis syndrome following treatment with 2-chlorodeoxyadenosine for refractory chronic lymphocytic leukemia. *New England Journal of Medicine, 329,* 1547–1548.

De Lalla, F. (1997). Antibiotic treatment of febrile episodes in neutropenic cancer patients: Clinical and economic considerations. *Drugs, 53,* 789–804.

Dhingra, K., & Newcom, S. (1988). Acute tumor lysis syndrome in non-Hodgkin's lymphoma induced by dexamethasone. *American Journal of Haemotology, 29,* 115–116.

Dodd, R.Y. (1994). Adverse consequences of blood transfusion: Quantitative risk estimates. In S.T. Nance (Ed.), *Blood supply risks, perceptions and prospects for the future* (pp. 1–24). Bethesda, MD: American Association of Blood Banks.

Dwyer, J.M. (1992). Manipulating the immune system with immune globulin. *New England Journal of Medicine, 326,* 107–116.

Engervall, P., & Bjorkholm, M. (1995). Infections in neutropenic patients. I: Aetiology. *Medical Oncology, 12,* 251–256.

Ezzone, S.A. (Ed.). (1997). *Peripheral blood stem cell transplantation: Recommendations for nursing education and practice.* Pittsburgh, PA: Oncology Nursing Society.

Ezzone, S.A. (1999). Tumor lysis syndrome. *Seminars in Oncology Nursing, 15,* 202–208.

Ezzone, S.A. (2000). Patient and family caregiver teaching. In P. Bucshel, & P.M. Kapustay (Eds.), *Stem cell transplantation: A clinical textbook* (pp. 6.1–6.10). Pittsburgh, PA: Oncology Nursing Society.

Ezzone, S.A., & Camp-Sorrell, D. (Eds.). (1994). *Manual for bone marrow transplant nursing: Recommendations for practice and education.* Pittsburgh, PA: Oncology Nursing Society.

Fer, M.G., Bottino, G.C., Sherwin, S.A., Hainsworth, J.D., Abrams, P.G., Foon, K.A., et al. (1984). Atypical tumor lysis syndrome in a patient with T-cell lymphoma treated with recombinant leukocyte interferon. *American Journal of Medicine, 77,* 953–956.

Ferlito, A., Rinaldo, A., & Devaney, K.O. (1997). Syndrome of inappropriate antidiuretic hormone secretion associated with head and neck cancers: Review of the literature. *Annals of Otology, Rhinology, and Laryngology, 106,* 878–883.

Finkbinder, K.L., & Ernst, T.F. (1993). Drug therapy management of the febrile neutropenic cancer patient. *Cancer Practice, 1,* 295–304.

Fleming, D.R., Henslee-Downey, P.J., & Coffey, C.W. (1991). Radiation-induced acute tumor lysis syndrome in the bone marrow transplant setting. *Bone Marrow Transplantation, 8,* 235–236.

Flombaum, C.D. (2000). Metabolic emergencies in the cancer patient. *Seminars in Oncology, 27,* 322–334.

Freifield, A.G., & Pizzo, P.A. (1996). The outpatient management of febrile neutropenia in cancer patients. *Oncology, 10,* 599–616.

Gobel, B.H. (1997). Bleeding disorders. In S.L. Groenwald, M.H. Frogge, M. Goodman, & C.H. Yarbro (Eds.), *Cancer nursing: Principles and practice* (4th ed., pp. 604–639). Sudbury, MA: Jones and Bartlett.

Gobel, B.H. (1999). Disseminated intravascular coagulation. *Seminars in Oncology Nursing, 15,* 174–182.

Goldman, M.P. (1995). Antibiotic prophylaxis in the critical care setting. *Critical Care Clinics of North America, 7,* 667–674.

Goodnough, L.T. (1991). Management of disseminated intravascular coagulation. In E.C. Rossi, T.L. Simon, & G.S. Moss (Eds.), *Principles of transfusion medicine* (pp. 373–382). Baltimore: Lippincott Williams and Wilkins.

Gross, J., & Johnson, B.L. (Eds.). (1994). *Handbook of oncology nursing.* Sudbury, MA: Jones and Bartlett.

Guyton, A.C. (1991). Renal and associated mechanisms for controlling extracellular fluid osmolality and sodium concentration. In A.C. Guyton (Ed.), *Textbook of medical physiology* (pp. 308–319). Philadelphia: W.B. Saunders.

Hathorn, J.W. (1993). Critical appraisal of antimicrobials for prevention of infections in immunocompromised hosts. *Hematology and Oncology Clinics of North America, 7,* 1051–1099.

Herschl, J. (2000). Psychosocial considerations: A family approach to patient care. In E.D. Ball, J. Lister, & P. Law (Eds.), *Hematopoietic stem cell therapy* (pp. 672–681). New York: Churchill Livingstone.

Hospital Infection Control Practice Advisory Committee. (1995). *American Journal of Infection Control, 23,* 87–94.

Howell, P.B., Walters, P.E., Donowitz, G.R., & Farr, B.M. (1995). Risk factors for infection of adult patients with cancer who have tunneled central venous catheters. *Cancer, 75,* 1367–1375.

Kapustay, P.M., & Buchsel, P.C. (2000). Process, complications, and management of peripheral stem cell transplantation. In P.M. Kapustay, & P.C. Buchsel (Eds.), *Stem cell transplantation: A clinical textbook* (pp. 5.1–5.28). Pittsburgh, PA: Oncology Nursing Society.

Katz, J.A., Bash, R., Rollins, N., Cash, J., & Buchanan, G.R. (1991). The yield of routine chest radiography in children with cancer hospitalized for fever and neutropenia. *Cancer, 68,* 940–943.

Keenan, A.M. (1999). Syndrome of inappropriate secretion of antidiuretic hormone in malignancy. *Seminars in Oncology Nursing, 15,* 160–167.

Kempin, S.J. (1997). Hemostatic defects in cancer patients. *Cancer Investigations, 15,* 23–26.

Kessinger, A. (1999). Autologous peripheral blood stem cell transplantation. Retrieved October 3, 2002, from http://www.bmtinfo.org/bmt/topics/htm/annetech.html

Korbling, M., & Champlin, R. (1996). Peripheral blood progenitor cell transplantation: A replacement for marrow auto- or allografts. *Stem Cells, 14,* 185–195.

Kreit, J.W. (2000). Respiratory complications. In E.D. Ball, J. Lister, & P. Law (Eds.), *Hematopoietic stem cell therapy* (pp. 563–577). New York: Churchill Livingstone.

Kurtz, A. (1993). Disseminated intravascular coagulation with leukemia patients. *Cancer Nursing, 16,* 456–463.

Labovich, T.M. (1997). Transfusion therapy: Nursing implications. *Clinical Journal of Oncology Nursing, 1,* 61–72.

Lang-Kummer, J. (1997). Hypercalcemia. In S.L. Groenwald, M.H. Frogge, M. Goodman, & C.H. Yarbro (Eds.), *Cancer nursing: Principles and practice* (4th ed., pp. 684–700). Sudbury, MA: Jones and Bartlett.

Lankiewicz, M.W., & Bell, W.B. (1993). Disseminated intravascular coagulation. In W.B. Bell (Ed.), *Hematologic and oncologic emergencies* (pp. 110–121). New York: Churchill Livingstone.

Lau, R.C., Doyle, J.J., Freedman, M.H., King, S.M., & Richardson, S.E. (1994). Early discharge of pediatric febrile neutropenic cancer patients by substitution of oral for intravenous antibiotics. *Pediatric Hematology and Oncology, 11,* 417–421.

Law, P. (2000). Graft processing, storage, and infusion. In E.D. Ball, J. Lister, & P. Law (Eds.), *Hematopoietic stem cell therapy* (pp. 312–321). New York: Churchill Livingstone.

Lieschke, G.J., & Burgess, A.W. (1992). Granulocyte colony stimulating factor and granulocyte-macrophage colony stimulating factor. *New England Journal of Medicine, 327,* 99–106.

Luce, J.M. (1987). Pathogenesis and management of septic shock. *Chest, 91,* 883–888.

Malik, I.A., Abubakar, S., Alam, F., & Khan, A. (1994). Dexamethasone-induced tumor lysis syndrome in high-grade non-Hodgkin's lymphoma. *Southern Medical Journal, 87,* 409–411.

Mangan, K.F. (2000). Choice of conditioning regimens. In E.D. Ball, J. Lister, & P. Law (Eds.), *Hematopoietic stem cell therapy* (pp. 403–413). New York: Churchill Livingstone.

Marder, J.V., Martin, S.E., & Coleman, R.W. (1993). Clinical aspects of consumptive thrombohemorrhagic disorders. In R.W. Coleman, J. Hirsh, J.V. Marder, & E.W. Salzman (Eds.), *Hemostasis and thrombosis* (3rd ed., pp. 665–693). Philadelphia: Lippincott.

Martino, R., Subira, M., Altes, A., Lopez, R., Sureda, A., Domingo-Albos, A., et al. (1998). Effect of discontinuing prophylaxis with norfloxacin in patients with hematologic malignancies and severe neutropenia. A matched case control study of the effect on infectious morbidity. *Acta Haematologica, 99,* 206–211.

Moore, J.M. (1994). Metabolic emergencies. In J. Gross & B.L. Johnson (Eds.), *Handbook of oncology nursing* (2nd ed., pp. 676–691). Sudbury, MA: Jones and Bartlett.

Mortsyn, G., Foote, M., & Nelson, S. (1997). Clinical benefits of improving host defenses with rHuG-CSF. *Ciba Foundation Symposium, 204,* 78–85.

Mundy, G.R. (1990). Pathophysiology of cancer-associated hypercalcemia. *Seminars in Oncology, 17*(Suppl. 5), 10–15.

Pichette, V., Leblanc, M., Bonnardeaux, A., Ouimet, D., Geadah, D., & Cardinal, J. (1994). High dialysate flow rate continuous arteriovenous hemodialysis: A new approach for the treatment of acute renal failure and tumor lysis syndrome. *American Journal of Kidney Disease, 23,* 591–596.

Pilarski, L.M., Andrews, E.J., Mant, M.J., & Ruether, B.A. (1986). Humoral immune deficiency in multiple myeloma patients due to compromised B cell function. *Journal of Clinical Immunology, 6,* 491–501.

Pizzo, P.A. (1993). Management of fever in patients with cancer and treatment-induced neutropenia. *New England Journal of Medicine, 328,* 1323–1332.

Polmar, S.H. (1992). The role of the immunologist in sinus disease. *Journal of Allergy and Clinical Immunology, 90,* 511–515.

Popa, V., Kim, K., & Heiner, D.C. (1993). IgG deficiency in adults with recurrent respiratory infections. *Annals of Allergy, 70,* 418–424.

Przepiorka, D., & Gonzales-Chambers, R. (1990). Acute tumor lysis syndrome in a patient with chronic myelogenous leukemia in blast crisis: Role of high dose ara-c. *Bone Marrow Transplantation, 6,* 281–282.

Rapp, J.S., Perry, M.C., & Rotche, R.M. (1996). Extensive stage small cell lung cancer: Determining suitability for outpatient management of febrile neutropenia. *Seminars in Oncology, 23,* xv–xxii.

Raue, F., & Pecherstorjer, M. (1994). Drug therapy of hypercalcemia due to malignancy. *Recent Results in Cancer Research, 137,* 138–160.

Reed, E.C., & Franco, T. (1992). Nursing for patients receiving high-dose chemotherapy with hematopoietic rescue. In J.O. Armitage & K.H. Antman (Eds.), *High-dose cancer therapy: Pharmacology, hematopoietins, stem cells* (pp. 405–418). Baltimore: Williams and Wilkins.

Rice, V. (1991). Shock. A clinical syndrome. *Critical Care Nurse, 11,* 20–24, 26–27.

Riewald, M., & Riess, H. (1998). Treatment options for clinically recognized disseminated intravascular coagulation. *Seminars in Thrombosis and Hemostasis, 24,* 53–59.

Riikonen, P. (1995). Recombinant human granulocyte-macrophage colony-stimulating factor in combination with antibiotics in the treatment of febrile neutropenia in children. *Stem Cells, 13,* 201–205.

Rolston, K.V. (1998). Expanding the options for risk-based therapy in febrile neutropenia. *Diagnostic Microbiology of Infectious Disease, 31,* 411–416.

Rowley, S.D. (1999). Hematopoietic stem cell cryopreservation. In E.D. Thomas, K.G. Blume, & S.J. Forman (Eds.), *Hematopoietic cell transplantation* (2nd ed., pp. 481–492). Malden, MA: Blackwell Science.

Sakarcan, A., & Quigley, R. (1994). Hyperphosphatemia in tumor lysis syndrome. The role of hemodialysis and continuous venous-venous hemofiltration. *Pediatric Nephrology, 8,* 351–356.

Sanders, L.R. (1998). Disorders of water metabolism. In M.T. McDermott (Ed.), *Endocrine secrets* (pp. 147–162). Philadelphia: Hanley and Belfus.

Schaffer, S.D., Garzon, L.S., Heroux, D.L., & Korniewicz, L.M. (1996). *Infection prevention and safe practice.* St. Louis, MO: Mosby.

Schaffer, S.L. (1997). Oncologic complications. In S.E. Otto (Ed.), *Cancer nursing* (3rd ed., pp. 413–421). St. Louis, MO: Mosby.

Schweitzer, D.H., Hamdy, N.A., & Frolich, M. (1994). Malignancy-associated hypercalcemia: Resolution of controversies over vitamin D metabolism by a pathophysiological approach to the syndrome. *Clinical Endocrinology, 41,* 251–256.

Shelton, B.K. (1996). Neutropenia. In J. Hebra & M.A. Kuhn (Eds.), *Manual of critical care nursing* (pp. 215–227). Boston: Little, Brown, & Co.

Shelton, B.K. (1998). Leukopenia. In C.R. Ziegfeld, B.G. Lubejko, & B.K. Shelton (Eds.), *Oncology fact finder. Manual of cancer nursing* (pp. 289–306). Philadelphia: Lippincott.

Shelton, B.K. (1999). Sepsis. *Seminars in Oncology Nursing, 15,* 209–221.

Shuey, K.M. (1994). Heart, lung and endocrine complications of solid tumors. *Seminars in Oncology Nursing, 10,* 186–187.

Simmons, E.D., & Somberg, K.A. (1991). Acute tumor lysis syndrome after intrathecal methotrexate administration. *Cancer, 65,* 2062–2065.

Simpson, J.K. (2000). Specialized nursing. In E.D. Ball, J. Lister, & P. Law (Eds.), *Hematopoietic stem cell therapy* (pp. 683–687). New York: Churchill Livingstone.

Simpson, J.K., & Burgunder, M.R. (2000). Coordination and data collection. In E.D. Ball, J. Lister, & P. Law (Eds.), *Hematopoietic stem cell therapy* (pp. 688–696). New York: Churchill Livingstone.

Smith, T.J. (1996). Economic analysis of the clinical use of the colony stimulating factors. *Current Opinion in Hematology, 3,* 175–179.

Sparano, J., Ramirez, M., & Wiernik, P.H. (1988). Increasing recognition of corticosteroid induced tumor lysis syndrome in non-Hodgkin's lymphoma. *Cancer, 65,* 1072–1073.

Staudlinger, T., Locker, G.J., & Frass, M. (1996). Management of acquired coagulation disorders in emergency and intensive care medicine. *Seminars in Thrombosis and Hemostasis, 22,* 93–104.

Stroncek, D.F., Fautsch, S.K., Lasky, L.C., Hurd, D.D., Ramsay, N.K., & McCullough, J. (1991). Adverse reactions in patients transfused with cryopreserved marrow. *Transfusion, 31,* 521–526.

Sutherland, C.W. (1997). The hematology and immunology of peripheral stem cell transplantation. In P.C. Buchsel (Ed.), *Advanced concepts in peripheral stem cell transplantation* (pp. 8–16). Pittsburgh, PA: Oncology Education Services, Inc.

Talcott, J.A., Whalen, A., Clark, J., Rieker, P.P., & Finberg, R. (1994). Home antibiotic therapy for low-risk cancer patients with fever and neutropenia: A pilot study of 30 patients based on a validated prediction rule. *Journal of Clinical Oncology, 12,* 107–114.

Tiley, C., Grimwade, D., Findlay, M., Treleaven, J., Height, S., Catalano, J., et al. (1992). Tumor lysis following hydrocortisone prior to a blood product transfusion in T-cell acute lymphoblastic leukemia. *Leukemia and Lymphoma, 8,* 143–146.

Toney, J.F., & Parker, M.M. (1996). New perspectives on the management of septic shock in the cancer patient. *Infectious Disease Clinics of North America, 10,* 239–253.

Trilla, A., & Miro, J.M. (1995). Identifying high risk patients for Staphylococcus aureus infections: Skin and soft tissue infections. *Journal of Chemotherapy, 3*(Suppl. 7), 37–43.

Turner, M.L., & Sweetenham, J.W. (1996). Hemopoietic progenitor homing and mobilization. *British Journal of Haematology, 94,* 592–596.

Vander, A.J. (1995). Control of sodium and water excretion: Regulation of plasma volume and osmolarity. In A.J. Vander (Ed.), *Renal physiology* (5th ed., pp. 116–144). New York: McGraw-Hill.

Vinayek, R., Demetris, J., & Rakela, J. (2000). Liver disease in hematopoietic stem cell transplant recipients. In E.D. Ball, J. Lister, & P. Law (Eds.), *Hematopoietic stem cell therapy* (pp. 541–556). New York: Churchill Livingstone.

Volger, W.R., Morris, J.G., & Winton, E.F. (1983). Acute tumor lysis syndrome in T-cell leukemia induced by amsacrine. *Archives of Internal Medicine, 143,* 165–166.

Volker, D. (1998). Fever of unknown origin. *Nursing Practice Forum, 9,* 170–176.

Walter-Coleman, S. (1996). Transfusion therapy for patients critically ill with cancer. *AACN Clinical Issues in Critical Care, 7,* 37–45.

Warrell, R.P. (1993). Metabolic emergencies. In V.T. DeVita, S. Hellman, & S.A. Rosenberg (Eds.), *Cancer: Principles and practice of oncology* (4th ed., 251–256). Philadelphia: Lippincott.

Weeks, J.C., Tierney, M.R., & Weinstein, M.C. (1991). Cost effectiveness of prophylactic intravenous immune globulin in chronic lymphocytic leukemia. *New England Journal of Medicine, 325,* 81–86.

Whedon, M.B. (1991). Autologous bone marrow transplantation: Clinical indications, treatment process, and outcomes. In M.B. Whedon (Ed.), *Bone marrow transplantation: Principles, practice, and nursing insights* (pp. 20–48). Sudbury, MA: Jones and Bartlett.

Williams, E.C., & Mosher, D.F. (1997). Disseminated intravascular coagulation. In V.T. DeVita, S. Hellman, & S.A. Rosenberg (Eds.), *Cancer: Principles and practice of oncology* (5th ed., pp. 1758–1769). Philadelphia: Lippincott.

Witherspoon, R.P. (1994). Immunological reconstitution after allogeneic marrow, autologous marrow or autologous peripheral blood stem cell transplantation. In K. Atkinson (Ed.), *Clinical bone marrow transplantation: A reference textbook* (pp. 62–72). New York: Cambridge University Press.

Wordell, C.J. (1987). Intravenous immune globulin: Dosage and administration. *Pharmacotherapy, 7,* 827–830.

Yaholom, J., & Fuks, Z.Y. (1992). Strategies for the use of total body irradiation as systemic therapy in leukemia and lymphoma. In J.O. Armitage, & K.H. Antman (Eds.), *High-dose cancer therapy: Pharmacology, hematopoietins, stem cells* (pp. 61–83). Baltimore: Williams and Wilkins.

Yoshida, M. (1997). Infections in patients with hematologic diseases: Recent advances in serological diagnosis and empiric therapy. *International Journal of Hematology, 66,* 279–289.

Ziegler, R. (1994). Clinical picture of humoral hypercalcemia of malignancy. *Recent Results in Cancer Research, 137,* 107–113.

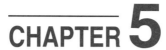

CHAPTER 5

Joyce J. Adams, RN, MN
Kathleen Clifford, RN, MSN, FNP, CS, AOCN®
Debra Adornetto, RN, MS

Considerations in Hematopoietic Stem Cell Transplant Program Development and Sites of Care Delivery

Introduction

In the 1970s, allogeneic bone marrow transplantation (BMT) began as a cancer treatment in specialized research and university centers around the world. The evolution of stem cell technologies based on this work has rapidly developed. Initially, the majority of care for the transplant recipient was provided in a specialized hospital setting. With technological advances, shifts in care sites have allowed for additional settings. Between 1990 and 1995, the number of both allogeneic and autologous hematopoietic marrow and blood stem cell transplants (HSCT) rose from 12,000 to 30,000 worldwide (Rowlings, 1996). At present, more than 300 centers worldwide report data to the International Bone Marrow Transplant Registry (IBMTR).

Beginning in 1985, the use of autologous transplant therapy accelerated with the use of blood stem cells (BSCs) (Horowitz, 1995). The use of autologous BSC has resulted in more rapid engraftment with decreased infection rates and improvement in treatment-related mortality for autologous transplant. This has increased the application of autologous BSC therapy to more tumor types. By 1990, the number of autologous procedures equaled the number of allogeneic transplants. In 1998, it was nearly double, with an estimated 17,000 allogeneic and more than 30,000 autologous transplants performed (Bredeson, 2000). More than 200 autologous transplant centers in North and South America contributed to the Autologous Blood and Marrow Transplant Registry (ABMTR), providing data on approximately 50% of autologous transplants performed.

Despite the growth of autologous transplantation, post-HSCT relapse remains a major cause of death. This and the limited ability to use autologous HSCT in leukemias because of tumor contamination of the stem cell product make allogeneic HSCT the treatment of choice for many diseases. Development of nonmyeloablative HSCT has allowed more patients to receive the benefits of allogeneic therapies. The advantages of BSCs are currently being applied in the allogeneic setting, expanding the application of allogeneic transplants to a broader age range and more disease types (Bensinger et al., 2001).

Administrative Issues in Hematopoietic Stem Cell Transplant Program Development

Planning and organizing an HSCT program for the adult or pediatric population is a serious endeavor that requires a dedicated multidisciplinary planning team, financial/organizational support, and internal and external analyses regarding feasibility of the program as part of the strategic plan for an organization. Key members of the planning team should include the medical director, inpatient and outpatient hospital and nursing administrator, financial officer, nurse manager, advanced practice nurse, patient coordinator, and infectious disease physician. Other members or representatives to include at various times during the planning process would be the laboratory director, pharmacist, dietitian, social worker, and plant operations and housekeeping personnel (Abramovitz & Link, 1995; Nelson, 1997). Foundation for the Accreditation of Cellular Therapy (FACT) program accreditation standards address the recommended HSCT professional team composition (see Table 5-1).

The first phase in the program development assessment is an evaluation of the feasibility of a transplant program. This evaluation includes an assessment of both the internal and external environments. The external environment includes the community at large, whereas the internal environment should include an evaluation of the organization, available resources, and commitment to the development and support of a transplant program. The purpose of the assessment is to provide a comprehensive and realistic review of the variables that would impact program development. Based on the information garnered from this process, a decision as to whether to proceed with a HSCT program is determined by the planning team and key members of the organization. Figure 5-1 identifies commonly asked feasibility questions. Once this assessment has been completed and evaluation of the data indicates that the development and implementation of a HSCT program would be beneficial to the community without creating a financial burden for the organization, the planning process is ready to begin.

Table 5-1. Staff Requirements for the Transplant Team

Position	Education and Experience
Program director	• Licensed physician in the United States or Canada • Responsible for administrative and clinical operations • Board certified in one of the following specialties: hematology, oncology, immunology, or pediatric hematology/oncology • A minimum of one year of training in hematopoietic progenitor cell transplantation or two years experience as an attending physician responsible for the management of patients undergoing hematopoietic progenitor cell transplantation

Other attending physicians	• Licensed physician in the United States or Canada
	• Board certified or eligible in hematology, oncology, immunology, or pediatric hematology/oncology
	• Minimum of one year experience in the management of transplant recipients
	• Specific training and competency in a number of clinically relevant transplant areas, such as
	  - Indications for transplant
	  - Pre- and post-transplant evaluation and care
	  - Marrow or stem cell harvesting, apheresis, or stem cell processing
	  - Management of neutropenia and thrombocytopenia
	  - Diagnosis and management of graft failure
	  - Investigational protocol, documentation, and reporting
	• Additional training and competency required if allogeneic hematopoietic stem cell accreditation is being sought

Consulting physician services	• Surgery • Pulmonary medicine • Intensive care medicine • Gastroenterology • Nephrology • Infectious disease • Cardiology • Pathology • Psychiatry • Radiation therapy (experience with total body or total lymphoid irradiation treatment protocols)

Nursing services	• Experienced nursing staff and supervisors in the management of patients receiving hematopoietic progenitor cell transplant, including
	  - Administration of high-dose therapy and growth factors
	  - Management of severely neutropenic patients
	  - Administration of blood products
	  - Appropriate degree of intensive medical/oncology nursing

Clinical support services	• Transplant coordinator • Apheresis facilities with trained personnel • Laboratory services, including 24-hour blood bank facilities, with the ability to provide cytomegalovirus-negative and irradiated blood components • HLA testing facilities • Pharmacy • Dietary • Physical therapy • Psychosocial services • Information systems management

Note. From "Peripheral Stem Cell Transplantation Program Development Using the Foundation for the Accreditation of Hematopoietic Cell Therapy Standards" (p. 26) by P. Kapustay in P. Buchsel (Ed.), *Advanced Concepts in Peripheral Stem Cell Transplantation*, 1997, Pittsburgh, PA: Oncology Education Services, Inc. Copyright 1997 by Oncology Education Services, Inc. Adapted with permission.

The next step would include establishing the mission, goals, and objectives of the program. A mission statement will facilitate the identification of types of patients to be treated and research and treatment protocols to be used. Goals and objectives will establish individual accountability and realistic timelines for project completion. Timelines may include construction plans, equipment purchases, staff recruitment, and education of staff. During this process the formal business plan is written, incorporating all individuals and departments that will be affected by the new program (Campbell & Foody, 1995).

Physical space and providing care will depend upon whether the program is primarily outpatient or inpatient or a combination of both clinical settings. Figure 5-2 addresses

Figure 5-1. Feasibility Review of the Internal and External Organizational Environment

External Environment

- What are the specific needs of the community?
- What is our business? Can we do it well?
- What types of patients will we treat, and what types of transplants will we perform?
- What change to the physical plant will be required to accommodate this service?
- What additional resources will be needed to support the program?
- Are the expenditures reasonable and recoverable through the administration of the program?
- What are the patient referral patterns to the organization? What strategies can be utilized to increase referrals with the introduction of a hematopoietic stem cell transplant (HSCT) program?
- What is the availability of similar services within the community?

Internal Environment

- What is the organization's commitment to an HSCT program?
- How does the HSCT program fit within the mission and goals of the organization?
- What support services are currently available (e.g., physician consultants across all disciplines, technology support)?
- What is the organization's current market share (analysis of financial impact of program)?
- What are the organization's weaknesses and strengths?

Note. Based on information from Campbell & Foody, 1995.

many regulatory planning considerations for both inpatient and outpatient units; it is not all-inclusive and should not be considered a comprehensive list.

Staff Development and Education in Program Development

Leadership and Management

The administrative and clinical aspects of developing a transplant program have been extensively reviewed (Buchsel & Kapustay, 2000; Buchsel & Whedon, 1995; Kapustay, 1997; Kelleher, 1991; Nelson, 1997; Rettger, 1992). One of the key factors to a successful HSCT program is the leadership and management of an expert staff. Recruitment of a nurse manager or director is a critical first step. An RN prepared at the master's level with both HSCT experience and management and business experience is desired (Campbell & Foody, 1995). The nurse manager or director must lead, mentor, and develop staff while creating, maintaining, and expanding a demanding transplant program. The HSCT program is resource intensive, and the leader must prioritize these resources to achieve goals (Farley & Jones, 1995). The nurse manager or director develops a vision with a focus and a mission (a reason for the vision) that is congruent with the values, mission, and goals of the institution and communicates this information to the staff. Other aspects of the role are the development of a quality management plan and establish-

ing the scope of service of the HSCT program in collaboration with the medical director and other members of the multidisciplinary care team. The nurse manager/director must role model professional behavior as well as motivate and empower staff. The management role entails tasks such as preparing budgets, overseeing special projects, facilitating staff performance, and monitoring quality improvement indicators. The successful HSCT program needs an individual who can both lead and manage, one that others will follow, and one who can manage the unit from a business perspective (Jeffries, 1996).

Staffing

The first step in determining inpatient staffing requirements is to identify the nursing model of care: primary/case management, functional, team, or modular- and patient-focused care. The model of care also will be dependent upon whether intensive care services will be offered on the HSCT

Figure 5-2. Facility Design With Program Development

Inpatient Unit

- Evaluate requirements of Joint Commission on the Accreditation of Healthcare Organizations (JCAHO), State Health Department, Occupational Safety and Health Administration (OSHA), and Foundation for the Accreditation of Cellular Therapy (FACT) guidelines.
- Unit with private rooms and HEPA or positive airflow filtration, critical care monitoring equipment if unit has the capability. An ability for nursing to easily monitor patients
- Centralized nursing station
- Charting area
- Conference area
- Storage and utility areas
- Satellite pharmacy
- Nourishment preparation area
- Visitors/family lounge
- Equipment: bed, chair, overbed table, commode, infusion pumps, weight scale, personal care items
- Grounded electrical outlets and nursing call system
- Staff areas: lounge/locker room, bathrooms, conference room
- Administrative offices: staff, business office, medical records
- Public areas: waiting rooms, bathrooms

Outpatient Clinic

- Evaluate requirements of JCAHO, State Health Department, OSHA, and FACT guidelines.
- Treatment areas: chemotherapy and blood administration areas (chairs, beds), special procedure area (per FACT: any ability to provide an environment that protects patients from infectious agents and allows for prolonged infusions)
- Ability to promptly evaluate and treat the HSCT recipient on a 24-hour basis (FACT recommendation)
- Ancillary areas: nursing station, pharmacy, laboratory and imaging diagnostics, waste disposal area, and housekeeping
- Equipment planning: medical equipment/supplies, ambulatory pumps, furniture, lighting and air system, as well as storage for equipment and supplies
- Staff areas: lounge/locker room, bathrooms, conference room
- Administrative offices: staff, business office, medical records
- Public areas: waiting rooms, bathrooms

Note. Based on information from Campbell & Foody, 1995; FACT, 2002; Lamkin, 1993.

unit. The next step in the initial staffing process is determining the number of different personnel that will be required to meet the HSCT recipient's needs. Staffing needs can be predicted through an industrial engineering approach. With this approach, nursing tasks are identified and timed, workflow is analyzed, and tasks are arranged for greatest efficiency. These measurements, along with projected patient census, will determine staffing requirements. Nurse-patient ratios are calculated on task frequency and difficulty. Nursing standards of care for the HSCT recipient will assist in identifying and validating the staffing needs. Management engineering methods to determine staffing ratios may not be the initial approach to determine staffing needs. Using a descriptive method, prescribed nurse-patient ratios and forecasted patient census data may be used to determine the number of nursing personnel required to provide care on the HSCT unit (Gillies, 1989). A new developing program will have a projected census for which the unit will be budgeted. HSCT recipients will be cared for in an established oncology unit or outpatient clinic; additional nursing and ancillary resources (secretarial support and certified nursing assistants) will need to be added to the existing staffing plan.

A high ratio of RNs with a complement of certified nursing assistants is recommended for the HSCT recipient. An RN-to-patient ratio of one to two is recommended, especially in an intensive care setting. One certified nursing assistant for every 6–8 patients during the day and one for every 10–12 patients at night should be adequate. Secretarial staff, especially during the busier hours of the day (7 am–7:30 pm), is essential for the seamless functioning of the unit (Campbell & Foody, 1995).

Another tool to establish and validate inpatient or outpatient care staffing requirements is a patient acuity tool specific to the HSCT recipient. Many institutions have specific tools that are used universally, for all patients, and may not be specific to the unique needs of the HSCT patient. Campbell and Foody (1995) have identified an inpatient tool specific for the transplant recipient. Patient classification systems identify the level of care intensity, establish staffing requirements, and require the establishment of validity and reliability of the tool (Gillies, 1989). Figure 5-3 is a sample of an inpatient HSCT-specific acuity tool, identifying therapeutic indicator categories.

Outpatient care for the HSCT recipient requires consideration of the following needs: complexity of the patient assessment; intravenous (IV) therapies, including blood transfusions; complex chemotherapy; and procedures such as bone marrow biopsies. Determining the outpatient operating hours, projected number of patients to be served, or additional patients to be served in an established clinic are crucial. Numerous methods can be used to determine outpatient staffing levels: direct patient care hours, direct and indirect patient care hours, established nurse and patient ratios, number of procedures, number of patient visits, or the utilization of an acuity system (Houston & Houston, 1995). Ambulatory patient classi-

fication systems can be based on patient acuity, staff-to-patient ratios, and time factors for specific nursing tasks (Houston & Houston).

Recruitment and Retention

The initial step in recruitment is selecting a team of experienced nurses. Careful selection of nursing staff will assist in the retention of the staff in the future. The best way to ensure quality staff is to hire quality people (Campbell & Foody, 1995; Jeffries, 1996). Nurses with oncology backgrounds are the targeted group, but other specialties such as critical care, pediatrics, and medical-surgical also should be considered. A diversified staff with different levels of experiences and skills will provide a strong clinical care environment. When it is determined that adequate staff are hired to provide quality patient care, the second step is developing the orientation program.

Recruitment of staff may be difficult in light of the current nursing shortage, so emphasis should be placed on retention of those employees currently on staff. Job satisfaction is key, and a leader must consider the individual employee's interests, motivators, stressors, and goals. An environment of professional participation, collaboration, autonomy, and respect also is vital. Staff participation needs to be fostered through unit-based committees and task forces, where ideas and opinions are valued. Opportunities for professional growth need to be encouraged by way of tuition reimbursement, educational in-services, and involvement in research projects. A professional practice team atmosphere with access to clinical ladders and yearly performance appraisals is essential to a satisfied workforce. Cohen and Musgrave (1998) discussed the utilization of a preceptorship program in an HSCT unit for both experienced and student nurses. One of the positive benefits noted upon evaluation of the program was recruitment of nursing staff to the unit.

Retaining valued employees requires the leaders of the HSCT program to communicate expectations, listen to employees' needs, and acknowledge accomplishments in caring for a population undergoing extremely stressful therapy with a high mortality. Providing recognition verbally and through a variety of incentives will demonstrate to employees that they are appreciated. Fostering creativity and accountability will empower the employee. The manager or director needs to encourage goal setting and explore with the employees their desired career paths. Retention of members of the transplant team is essential to the growth of the program and the professional development of new team members.

Orientation

Orientation is defined by the American Nurses Association (1990) council on continuing education (CE) and staff development as "the means by which new staff members are introduced to the philosophy, goals, policies, procedures, role expectations, physical facilities, and special services in a specific work setting" (Abruzzese & Quinn-O'Neal, 1992, p. 1209).

Figure 5-3. Sample Hematopoietic Stem Cell Transplant Acuity Tool Indicators

Neurologic
- Stable: requiring a minimum of one assessment each shift
- Unstable: hepatic encephalopathy or suicidal requiring q one hour or greater nursing intervention

Cardiac
- Stable: stable hemodynamics, no requirements for vasopressive agents
- Unstable: vasoactive/antiarrhythmic medication requirement with cardiac monitoring

Respiratory
- Stable: no requirement of supplemental oxygen or room air
- Unstable: progressive respiratory distress requiring frequent suctioning or requirements for continuous pulse oximetry and frequent changes in supplemental oxygen therapy up to and including intubation

Renal
- Stable: balanced fluid status, no evidence of renal compromise
- Unstable: decreasing renal function with the requirement of short-term hemodialysis

Psychological
- Stable: appropriate coping skills, adequate family or caregiver support
- Unstable: patient or family crisis requiring frequent psychosocial intervention and referral

Teaching or Discharge Planning
- Stable: patient/caregiver able to demonstrate or perform required procedures (central venous catheter care) and identify symptoms to report to healthcare team
- Unstable: patient/caregiver requiring intensive interventions because of language or cultural obstacles or educational or developmental barriers. Further follow-up with homecare or home infusion therapy

Infection
- Stable: on antimicrobial and antifungal therapies without evidence of infection
- Unstable: positive fungal or bacterial cultures, temperature unresponsive to antipyrogens. Requiring 6 or greater IV meds per 12-hour shift.

Integument
- Stable: mucositis controlled by oral treatment regimen and pain medications. For allotransplant grade 0 or I skin graft versus host disease (GVHD).
- Unstable: mucositis impairing airway, requiring frequent suctioning, Grade II–IV skin GVHD requiring frequent skin care and pain management intervention

Self-Care
- Stable: able to perform activities of daily living and mobility exercises and activities with minimal assistance
- Unstable: unstable gait, altered mental status, risk for bleeding

Fluid and Electrolytes
- Stable: < 3 IV medications, no total parenteral nutrition (TPN), no requirements for multiple electrolyte boluses. Daily labs only. Grade 0 or I gastrointestinal (GI) GVHD.
- Unstable: TPN, lipids, > 2 electrolyte boluses. GI GVHD grade II–IV > 250 ml of stool/24 hours. Severe abdominal cramping requiring narcotic analgesia

Hematology
- Stable: no evidence of active bleeding; blood product support needs to be assessed every other day until engraftment.
- Unstable: active bleeding requiring multiple blood products, infusing blood products seven hours or more in a 24-hour period

Note. Based on information from Campbell & Foody, 1995.

Caring for the transplant population is highly complex and requires staff to complete a comprehensive orientation program. The program may extend for a period of six weeks but may vary for individual nurses learning about available needs and resources. Orientation combines didactic content from the classroom with clinical experience at the bedside. Figure 5-4 addresses the recommended didactic content for orientation.

Orientation should be based on adult learning principles; therefore, orientation content should be introduced in a variety of ways to enhance the learning process. The didactic portion should be provided in lecture format with audiovisuals, handouts, and reference articles. The clinical "hands on" portion should include direct patient care and a variety of skills laboratories (Campbell & Foody, 1995).

With a new program, the clinical nurse specialist or nurse educator will be instrumental in training the initial staff members of the HSCT team. This staff will become the future preceptors of the program. Together, under the daily guidance and support of the manager or director and identified HSCT educator, the novice HSCT staff will grow into

an expert staff. Having an experienced HSCT RN on staff or a nurse with several years of experience can provide a new staff with encouragement and direction. Consulting with another experienced or established HSCT center also can be an excellent resource for the newly developed HSCT team. A positive orientation program can set the tone for future learning experiences and can influence employees' attitudes toward the work environment.

Continuing Education

CE is required so the HSCT nurse can continue to develop and expand on the knowledge base and skills associated with advancing technology. The ultimate goal is to be able to provide up-to-date, cost-effective nursing care to the HSCT recipient (Swansburg, 1995). HSCT is continually undergoing changes and new developments in treatments. To maintain expertise in this field, CE is required. An employee's annual assessment can help to evaluate learning needs for CE program development. Also recommended are periodic in-services on pertinent clinical topics and mandatory in-services regarding research protocols to keep staff up-to-date on cur-

---

Figure 5-4. Didactic Course Content for Orientation of Hematopoietic Stem Cell Transplant Nurses

- Overview of transplantation (allogeneic or autologous)
- Pathophysiology, diseases treated
- Review of immunologic or hematopoietic system
- Side effects of therapy, immunosuppressive therapy, or agents used
- Complications of therapy
- Infectious complications, infection prevention
- Radiation therapy
- Transfusion therapy
- Psychosocial issues
- Discharge planning

rent treatments (Campbell & Foody, 1995). Staff must be required to attend in-services or view recorded instructional sessions on new research protocols that will be used for patient care on the unit. This recorded attendance is a demonstration of staff knowledge and competency and is required for regulatory purposes.

Multidisciplinary Team

Advanced Practice Nursing

The care of the HSCT recipient is complex and requires the coordinated efforts of the primary care providers (medical and nursing), as well as members of a multidisciplinary team. Advanced practice nurses have played a variety of roles in the care and management of the HSCT recipient. Lin (1994) described the role of the advanced practice clinical nurse specialist (CNS) in the transplant coordinator role. The CNS in this role is involved in all aspects of the patient's care across the continuum from pre- to post-transplant and was able to incorporate the CNS roles of direct care, education, consultation, and research into practice. In some centers, the transplant coordinator is an RN who is non–master's prepared and is involved primarily during the pretransplant and post-transplant phases. The primary role responsibilities are gathering medical information, obtaining insurance clearance, scheduling pretransplant diagnostic tests, and coordinating post-transplant clinic visits. Education about the transplant process may be part of the role responsibility of a coordinator as well. A hospital-based HSCT CNS may be involved with patient as well as staff education and may rotate between the inpatient and outpatient setting. Neumann (2000) explained the role of the advanced practice clinical program coordinator in an HSCT Compliance Task Force that includes an HSCT physician, psychiatrist, social worker, case manager, and both inpatient and outpatient nurses. The team works primarily with patients in regard to compliance and caregiver issues.

The nurse practitioner (NP) or physician assistant (PA) in the HSCT program may rotate between inpatient and outpatient services. Typically, the NP or PA has a caseload similar to the physician and may work with one primary transplant physician. The NP or PA who will be following the patient in the outpatient setting customarily will see the patient several days prior to discharge to meet the patient and review the discharge plan. A collaborative approach is facilitated between the NP or PA and transplant physician. Patient visits that are conducted independently are reviewed with the transplant physician. Communication between the transplant physician and the PA or NP includes abnormal laboratory values, changes in physical findings, and treatment plan alterations. Those patients that require immediate consultation may need a clinic visit with the physician. Cases requiring inpatient admission are discussed with the physician prior to admission (Griffith, 1999). Multidisciplinary rounds help to facilitate communication regarding patient care issues and enhance the patient care plan across the continuum of care.

Dietary

The role of the dietitian in either the inpatient or outpatient setting requires an initial nutritional assessment of the HSCT recipient and can include monitoring of the patient's nutritional intake by using anthropometric, biochemical, and clinical data. The dietitian works collaboratively with the HSCT team by participating in daily rounds and making nutritional recommendations based on the patient's diagnosis and current clinical problems. Other role responsibilities include quality assurance and documentation of the dietary plan of care, patient counseling, and education. It is recommended that the dietitian be registered with the American Dietetic Association and have two to three years of critical care, nutrition support, or oncology experience (Stern & Lenssen, 1995).

Pharmacy

Pharmacy, as with dietary, requires pharmacists familiar with the care management of either oncology or HSCT patients. Pharmaceutical costs are one of the primary expenses for the individual undergoing HSCT (Kline, Merman, Tarantino, Herzig, & Bertolone, 1998; Yoder, 1998). Clinical pharmacy activities, such as assessment of therapeutic appropriateness of the prescribed therapies, evaluation of drug efficacy, toxicity, side effects, and participation in drug use evaluation and quality assurance, are key activities (Chan, 2000). Participation in working multidisciplinary rounds provides an opportunity to educate the transplant team about the prescribed drug therapies and make specific therapeutic recommendations for the patient undergoing HSCT (Wilkins, 1995).

Laboratory

A dedicated laboratory, which is available 24 hours a day to provide crucial diagnostic and blood product support, is necessary to provide care for the HSCT recipient. Laboratory personnel are frequently medical technologists (MTs) with blood bank or hematology experience. The importance of having a qualified clinical processing laboratory is evident by the emphasis that FACT places on the qualifications of the laboratory. Laboratory accreditation can be for the clinical program including the laboratory or separately as an independent laboratory that processes and collects hematopoietic progenitor cells (FACT, 2002). Extensive training in the various procedures of processing and cryopreservation of the peripheral blood progenitor cells (PBPCs) is crucial. Proficiency testing is performed at regular intervals, and documentation of formal training, certification, and CE are extremely important (Letheby, Jackson, & Warkentin, 2000). The MT is involved in all phases of PBPC collection and processing, such as apheresis, cell-counting techniques, progenitor cell assays, maintenance of records, and quality control at all stages of the stem cell process.

Psychosocial

The psychosocial concerns and demands for the patient undergoing transplantation require team members skilled in social service, psychology or psychiatry, and spiritual care. Programs vary in how extensive their services are. Some programs are involved with the patient from pretransplant to discharge. Other programs become involved only during a crisis. It is recommended that transplant programs assess and meet the following needs of HSCT recipients (Syrjala, 1995).

- Legal competence and ability to adhere to a treatment plan
- Screening of preexisting psychological and social problems (e.g., substance abuse)
- Tangible resource needs (e.g., housing, financial assistance, transportation)
- Family interventions for those with high conflict or situational stressors
- Liaison consultation with nursing and medical staff that interact with the patient

Another key member of the HSCT professional care team may be the clinical-based clergy. More than 60% of patients identified a clergy person in the community whom they can contact if they wish (Van de Creek, 1997). Pastoral care involves spiritual counseling in keeping with the beliefs of patients and their families. Spiritual care may be provided through a hospital-based chaplaincy program or by the patient's own pastor, priest, or rabbi. Having a clearly defined referral system and using guidelines for pastoral care services allows team members to access spiritual care for patients.

Rehabilitation

In 1989, the Oncology Nursing Society (ONS) defined cancer rehabilitation as "a process by which individuals, within their environments, are assisted to achieve optimal functioning within the limits imposed by cancer" (p. 433) (Mayer & O'Connor, 1989). Dietz (1980) defined four functional rehabilitative goals that can be applied to the HSCT recipient. First, preventative goals focus on pretransplant and transplant process instruction by physical therapy in an exercise program to minimize weakness and fatigue and enhance functional status. Second, restorative goals may be developed by occupational therapy to assist the post-transplant patient with issues of energy conservation, homemaking, work skills, and activities of daily living. Third, supportive goals include physical and occupational therapy assistance for patients following allogeneic transplant with

chronic graft versus host disease (GVHD) who experience myositis and contractures. A treatment plan that addresses range of motion, fine motor skills, and exercise is developed. Last, an example of palliative goals may include the patient with breast cancer who has metastatic bony disease following autologous HSCT. Goals for a patient who is semi-bedridden may include teaching passive range of motion to minimize stiffness and promote comfort. Caregivers are instructed in bedside transfers of the patient to the commode or wheelchair. Integrating the work of multiple team members is crucial for the rehabilitation and adaptation of the HSCT recipient prior to and following transplant.

The complex care needs of the HSCT patient require the skills and expertise of multiple individuals in this team effort. Team members may be involved in patient care at any time during the HSCT treatment phases of (a) preparation and evaluation, (b) mobilization, (c) apheresis or collection of BSCs or bone marrow, (d) administration of the preparative regimen, (e) reinfusion of BSCs or bone marrow, (f) engraftment, and (g) long-term recovery and rehabilitation (Buchsel & Kapustay, 1995). Collaboration and coordination of care are essential to maintain quality patient outcomes and assist in developing a cohesive and comprehensive HSCT program (Ezzone, 1997).

Sites of Care

Inpatient Care

Historically, much of the care of the HSCT recipient was performed in a traditional hospital setting. Technological advances and cost-containment issues have brought alternative sites of care to the forefront. With the rapid recovery period now seen with the HSCT recipient and the transition to short stay and outpatient care, bed space is less a factor in determining the transplant program size. There is the ability to use flexible staffing patterns to care for patients across clinical settings. A shift in care has occurred, and the family or designated caregiver is taking an increased responsibility in all sites of care. The role of professional nursing provides for complex assessments, care planning, and patient management throughout the HSCT process. Care maps and case management are helpful approaches to managing this complex patient population in any clinical setting (Burns, Tierney, Long, Lambert, & Carr, 1995; Holecek & Sellards, 1997; Madden & Ponte, 1994; Neumann & De Jesus, 1998).

Inpatient care in the autologous and allogeneic HSCT program may occur in designated rooms within a general oncology unit as a subset of the patient census. Most tertiary care or university care settings have a dedicated transplant unit. A core of knowledgeable staff is necessary to meet the special needs of the transplant recipient.

Intensive Care

The use of high-dose myeloablative therapy may cause complex side effects and complications that often require transfer to an intensive care unit (ICU) (Shivnan, Shelton, & Onners, 1996). Studies report critical illness in 20%–36%

CHAPTER 5. CONSIDERATIONS IN HEMATOPOIETIC STEM CELL TRANSPLANT PROGRAM DEVELOPMENT

of patients. Both autologous and allogeneic transplant recipients are at risk for life-threatening complications. The acuity of the allogeneic population has led many centers to provide critical care within the inpatient transplant unit. Toxicities associated with autologous HSCT have decreased, but significant treatment-related mortality and relapse rates still remain (Bredeson, 2000; Shorr, Moores, Edenfield, Christie, & Fitzpatrick, 1999). All patients undergoing transplantation need access to intensive care services provided by physician consultants and nurses knowledgeable in the complications of this therapy (FACT, 2002).

The general definition of intensive care in this high-risk population is the provision of invasive monitoring and ventilator support (Shapiro, 1995). Patients may require intensive care for a variety of complications that can affect multiple organ systems with potentially fatal outcomes. The preparative regimen of high-dose therapy results in the potential for respiratory and cardiac complications, veno-occlusive disease, renal dysfunction, and central and peripheral nervous system toxicities. These occur in the setting of marrow aplasia with subsequent infectious risks. Adverse effects of the treatment may extend for several weeks (Shivnan et al., 1996). Factors that contribute to the use of intensive care services and subsequent mortality in the transplant population have been identified to assist in treatment decisions (Hitt, 2001; Rubenfeld & Crawford, 1996). The cost of intensive care services may add as much as $100,000 to this already expensive treatment (Shapiro). The related issues of resource allocation in light of the poor outcome are best addressed with a medical ethics approach.

Focusing on continuity of care for the patient and family regardless of changes in acuity requires a team approach. Support systems (medical, psychological, nursing, social, and pastoral care) that understand the psychosocial needs of patients and families must be involved across the sites of care. Critically ill HSCT recipients continue to need specialized isolation, air handling, and staff who understand the unique risks of the immune-compromised patient. Established care standards, medical consultation, pharmacy, respiratory support, and appropriate ancillary services are essential to the provision of intensive care (Hitt, 2001; Shapiro, 1995).

Intensive care is delivered in a number of models: (a) provision of ventilator support and invasive monitoring on the HSCT unit, (b) transfer of patients to a designated ICU, which may or may not have designated HSCT beds, or (c) a HSCT specialty unit capable of one-to-one nursing care and frequent noninvasive monitoring with transfers of patients requiring more monitoring and mechanical ventilation. The choice of a model for providing the appropriate level of care must be based on how best to meet the special needs of the patient and institutional resources.

The university and tertiary care centers that perform allogeneic transplants usually have HSCT ICU capabilities integrated on the transplant unit. In 1991, 52% of centers reported keeping their critically ill patients on the HSCT unit. This survey was conducted prior to the advent of community HSCT programs and primarily represents allogeneic

programs (Shapiro, 1995). With the increase in the number of transplant programs by 1998, 40% of participating programs provided some level of intensive care on the unit. Programs have used creative solutions to meet patient care needs. Nursing staff may be cross-trained in critical care to accompany the patient when transfer to an ICU is required. The HSCT team continues to be involved in the clinical management and support of the patient and family, whether the patient is on the inpatient transplant unit or in an intensive care setting. The appropriate provision of intensive care services requires strategic planning and communication among areas (Clifford, 2000; Shapiro).

Outpatient Care

The success in developing efficacious high-dose regimens that are relatively safe and can be administered in outpatient settings has been critical to the outpatient movement (Meisenberg et al., 1997; Peters et al., 1994; Schiffman et al., 1996; Schwartzberg et al., 1998; Weaver et al., 1997). Advances in symptom management with more effective antiemetics and home infusion devices have facilitated outpatient management (Meisenberg, Gollard, Brehm, McMillian, & Miller, 1996). During the managed care expansion in the 1980s and 1990s, programs focused on cost-containment efforts. One method to decrease cost has been to shift care to the outpatient, ambulatory care arena. This has resulted in a 25% reduction in overall cost of care without adverse effect in selected populations (Farah, Aquino, Munoz, & Sandler, 1998; Meisenberg et al., 1998; Rizzo et al., 1999).

Numerous studies support the outpatient approach and suggest strategies for care delivery. Although the term "outpatient transplant" is frequently used, the transplant recipient continues to use support services requiring IV therapy and a 24-hour caregiver (Dix et al., 1999; Freeman et al., 1999; Gluck et al., 1997; Meisenberg et al., 1997, 1998; Schmit-Pokorny, Hruska, & Ursick, 1998; Schwartzberg et al., 1998; Westermann et al., 1999). Some transplant programs use a treatment room on an inpatient unit for outpatient services by establishing an observation or outpatient charge system. With flexible staffing, continuity of care is maintained, with inpatient HSCT nurses providing the assessment and treatment for outpatients. Outpatient charge systems for hospital rooms can expand the availability to 24 hours a day and provide for short-stay use. Use of specific regimens, aggressive antiemetic therapy, hydration, and standards for infection prophylaxis facilitate outpatient management. HSCT team involvement and communication with consistent care standards across all clinical settings are required. Each area must have access to medical records and provide appropriate documentation of encounters. Eligibility criteria for outpatient care (see Figure 5-5) and use of established treatment guidelines, protocols, and critical pathways are essential (see Figure 5-6) (Buchsel & Parchem, 1988; Burns et al., 1995; Centers for Disease Control and Prevention, 2000; Chielens & Herrick, 1990; Dix et al.; Dix & Geller, 2000).

Three basic models have been developed to provide outpatient-based care: early discharge, delayed admission, and

Determining Eligibility
- Clinic eligibility—disease staging, organ function, performance status
- Psychosocial assessment
- Insurance review
- Dedicated/trained caregiver on a 24-hour/day basis
- Appropriate housing within 30–60 minutes proximity
- Reliable transportation
- Informed consent process
- Access to 24-hour outpatient care

Continuation of Outpatient Status
- No evidence of active, ongoing, or uncontrolled infection
- Responsive to antiemetic and antibiotic regimens
- Ability to maintain fluid and electrolyte balance
- Appropriate level of pain control
- Performance status greater than 60%
- Homecare services may be required to supplement trained caregiver.

Note. Based on information from Dix & Geller, 2000.

comprehensive or total outpatient care delivery (Dix & Geller, 2000). The Duke University Medical Center Bone Marrow Transplant Program led the nation in the late 1980s with the use of an early discharge model that administered the high-dose therapy in the hospital then discharged patients to a nearby cooperative residential hotel for housing following stem cell reinfusion. Patients were required to have a responsible caregiver staying with them and were followed at an outpatient clinic with extended hours. The program addressed administrative and logistic barriers. The program had the ability to provide emergency inpatient care, if required, by maintaining an open bed on the HSCT unit. This model was found to lower cost and increase patient satisfaction (Peters et al., 1994).

The delayed admission model, used in many autologous transplant programs, allows for the administration of high-dose therapy and HSC reinfusion in an outpatient setting. Patients then are admitted for supportive care when they develop febrile neutropenia, have pain management issues secondary to mucositis, or require IV hydration and electrolyte replacement for vomiting and/or diarrhea. The inpatient stay may or may not be shortened by this model (Dix & Geller, 2000; Weaver et al., 1997).

The total outpatient model is a comprehensive approach whereby the high-dose therapy, HSC reinfusion, and supportive care all occur outpatient. This requires close proximity, with patients staying within 30 minutes of the center. Tertiary care centers have found that nearby or adjacent housing is advantageous for their population. Allogeneic patients should have dedicated environments versus staying in their own home. Nearby contracted residential hotels or on-campus housing is used with frequent clinic visits or home-health services (Pisseri, 1998). Many insurance companies will provide a housing stipend for patients who travel to a referral center, thus saving the patients out-of-pocket housing costs (Peters et al., 2000). All of these models have the ability to

provide emergency inpatient care, if required, by having a bed reserved on the HSCT unit.

The recent use of non–marrow-ablative conditioning regimens reduces the toxicities from the chemotherapy, with subsequent decreased inpatient admissions and lengths of stays. These outpatient models have grown to meet the needs of the nonablative HSCT group for more complex ambulatory care services. The Hope Village at the City of Hope National Medical Center (www.bmt.cityofhope.org) provides on-campus housing, using small houses with individual suites for a patient and a caregiver. These have emergency contacts to the program. The Johns Hopkins Oncology Center (www.hopkinscancercenter.org) developed a care delivery model it termed "IPOP" or Inpatient/Outpatient Care Continuum. This includes intensive ambulatory support with a dedicated caregiver in a residential living facility adjacent to the inpatient HSCT unit. There is access to care 24 hours a day with the continuity of a team approach. The inpatient length of stay for IPOP participating patients is less than 10 days .

Community Setting

High-dose therapy with HSC support in the community remains a high-risk, intensive therapeutic process requiring multidisciplinary involvement and a structured program (Clifford, 2000). Community cancer centers can successfully care for the patient undergoing autologous HSCT with necessary laboratory and blood bank support and with careful preparation. Many community sites are associated with regional medical centers that provide a full range of oncology services to a large service area. One or more community physician oncology practices treat patients from the existing oncology service population base. Community-based programs report that only 10% of patients come from outside their state (Appel, 2001). Although autologous HSCT centers may have been initially developed to treat solid tumors, they also treat patients with lymphoma, myeloma, and leukemia. Many patients treated in community settings, in contrast to those seen in tertiary settings, are of middle to low economic status. They are high risk and may lack the resources necessary to travel to a metropolitan center (Clifford; Stetz, McDonald, & Compton, 1996).

Research consortiums have improved availability of high-dose clinical trials in community transplant programs. Schiffman et al. (1996) reported on autologous HSCT recipients treated in academic centers or in one of 10 participating community cancer centers. The study reviewed the outcomes and compared the regimen-related toxicity and mortality between the two types of centers. They found no sig-

Figure 5-6. Communication Tools Across Sites of Care

- Standard care plans
- Teaching flow sheets
- Critical pathways
- Care records or diaries
- Checklists or worksheets

Note. Based on information from Burns et al., 1995.

CHAPTER 5. CONSIDERATIONS IN HEMATOPOIETIC STEM CELL TRANSPLANT PROGRAM DEVELOPMENT

nificant difference between the centers. Transplant-related deaths occurred in 10% of patients in the academic center and in 7% of those treated in their community center. In another study, the 100-day mortality in 1,000 consecutive patients treated with high-dose therapy and autologous HSCT in a community-based, multicenter clinical trials program was 5.9% (Weaver et al., 1997). These statistics demonstrated that high-dose therapy and autologous HSCT could be performed in community cancer centers with comparative safety. Many community programs are limited to chemotherapy-based regimens because high-dose radiation requires a specialized radiation therapy facility.

The community transplant program is a referral center within its region that also must address the issues of caregivers and affordable housing close to the center. Resource utilization is ongoing as the family and home system and long-term care issues are considered as part of the spectrum of care. Community programs have the ability to provide this treatment option in an individualized care program where the patient can have maximum family and social support. A community hospital can provide cost-effective, high-quality care to select patients with high patient and family satisfaction (Amato et al., 1998).

Home Care

Home care of the HSCT recipient has been influenced by the growth and application of autologous and allogeneic HSCT for a variety of disease processes, technological advances, changing practice patterns, and managed care (Kelley, Randolph, & Leum, 2000). Homecare providers for the transplant population can be part of a large tertiary care network or an independent, privately operated agency that offers services to the oncology or transplant population.

The homecare provider often is determined by contracts with the patient's medical insurance provider, not the treatment center. The selection of a homecare agency requires an assessment of the agency's internal capabilities, resources, and commitment to the transplant population. An evaluation of the following will assist the transplant program or team in determining if the homecare agency will meet the needs of the HSCT recipient (Kelley et al., 2000).
- Ability of homecare provider to complement existing services
- Agency's understanding of the transplant process and ability to provide knowledgeable care pre- and post-transplant
- Scope of geographic coverage
- Ability to provide 24-hour care
- Timely response to changes in therapy
- Ability to educate family or caregiver on changing therapies

Standardized policy and procedures and guidelines for discharge to the home setting are essential for a smooth transition of the HSCT recipient to home. Involvement of homecare nurses in care conferences encourages understanding of the needs of the HSCT recipient (Lonergan, Kelley, McBride, & Randolph, 1996).

Following the return to home and referring physicians, the patient may need home-health services for infusion therapies, such as total parenteral nutrition, antibiotics, antifungals, and antiviral therapies. Homecare agencies can assist in central venous catheter care and laboratory monitoring as needed.

Although homecare agencies supported the shift to the outpatient setting, studies have not found the use of these services to decrease the overall cost of care (Peters et al., 2000). The move to outpatient care and designated on-campus housing has decreased the need for homecare services. Some centers have eliminated the need for using home-health agencies through expanded clinical services and training of care providers (family caregivers) (Franco, 1999; Peters et al., 2000). In Australia, a model was implemented that kept autologous patients in their homes and brought the care team to them. Although oncology or transplant-trained nurses provided the care, the authors identified the need for an advanced practice oncology or transplant nurse to assess the patient and provide care, given the autonomy of the nursing role in the homecare setting. Costs of inpatient versus home care were evaluated and found to be almost equal. Inpatient hospital admissions were facilitated if needed. As with most patient-centered models, they reported high patient and family satisfaction (Hermann, Leather, Leather, & Leen, 1998).

Home care is another viable alternative care site for the patient undergoing HSCT. The transplant team, in collaboration with the transplant-trained homecare nurse, can evaluate the impact and stressors of early discharge and outpatient care on the HSCT recipient and caregivers (Kelley & Randolph, 1998).

Referring Physician's Office

Reduction in the time patients remain at the tertiary care centers for outpatient monitoring has expanded the role of referring physicians in post-transplant patient monitoring and treatment. In the past, patients were asked to remain in the area for 100 days post-transplant. Care advances have lead to allogeneic patients staying at the center to day +50 to +70, whereas autologous patients remain an average of 30 days (Buchsel, Leum, & Randolph, 1996). The criteria for returning patients to the referring physicians may depend on their experience with transplant recipients and the clinical stability of the HSCT recipient. Patients may be required to return to the transplant center for periodic evaluations. Complex long-term follow-up needs are met in the community where healthcare providers must be knowledgeable in assessment and treatment of the growing transplant population. The primary oncologist encounters chronic GVHD, long-term toxicities, secondary malignancies, and prolonged immune suppression with the resulting need for prophylaxis, monitoring, and frequent visits. The transplant care coordinator must provide the nurses at the referring physician's office with information necessary to safely care for the patient (Whedon, 1995).

Clinical trials looking at the outcomes of transplant earlier in the disease process and use of immune therapy post-

HSCT are extending the time period that the primary oncology setting is involved in transplant-related protocols. Data collection for periodic restaging and long-term follow-up often is conducted in the patient's community. If a data management system is not in place, the ambulatory care nurse in the referring physician's office or cancer clinic often coordinates compliance with protocols and transfer of information back to the transplant center. Patients are rarely referred back to the tertiary care center for relapse or progressive disease. End-of-life care traditionally occurs in the community setting. Nurses provide front-line care to the patient and family across all settings (Lilleby, 2000) and can proactively improve care by educating themselves and sharing their knowledge to bridge the gap between sites of care.

Caregiver Role

Caregiver Selection

Identification of a dedicated caregiver during the transplant process is crucial. The variety of care settings in which HSCT occurs requires a supportive and able individual to assist the patient undergoing transplantation. Parents and spouses are usually the primary caregivers across the disease trajectory. Occasionally, extended family members or friends are available to stay with the patient during varying stages—someone who can relocate and stay with the patient. The caregiver is identified prior to the transplant and will be used in the acute phase, for outpatient care, and once the patient is discharged from the center for recovery care. Although one caregiver is ideal, patients often have a series of family members or friends who assume this role through the transplant process on a rotating basis.

Caregiver Needs

Studies have looked at the role of caregivers and their perceived needs during the acute phase of the transplant process, the recovery period, and long-term follow-up period. All studies point to the need for intensive education and support for the caregiver across the care continuum (Boyle et al., 2000; Foxall & Gaston-Johansson, 1996; Franco, 1999; McDonald, Stetz, & Compton, 1996). Caregivers' information needs and experiences before and during the acute phase of the transplant process have been categorized as preparing for caregiving, managing the care, facing challenges, developing supportive strategies, and discovering unanticipated rewards and benefits (Stetz et al., 1996). Preparing for care begins prior to arrival at the transplant center. As soon as the consult visit is scheduled, there is a need for information about the program and specific educational materials (McDonald et. al.).

Patient and Caregiver Education

A comprehensive and ongoing educational program is essential during each step of the HSCT process (Ezzone, 2000). Patient and caregiver education is an individualized process that is based on an assessment of learning needs (Tarzian, Iwata, & Cohen, 1999). The assessment of the potential caregiver includes the status of the caregiver's energy reserves, emotional fragility, and psychosocial stressors (De Koster & McLaughlin, 2001). Studies on learning needs in the transplant process point to the importance of being realistic about side effects and potential toxicity, while focusing on the positive aspects as well. During the acute phase, there is a need for intensive one-to-one involvement with physical care. The caregiver needs basic knowledge and technical skills to provide safe care of the patient whose condition is complex and can change rapidly (Ezzone, 2000; Jassak & Porter, 1995). The COPE (creativity, optimism, planning, and expert information) model of education is a prospective problem-solving approach to prepare caregivers. They are taught how to develop and carry out a plan of care in coordination with the healthcare professional's plans. These plans address both medical and psychosocial problems to help to reduce stress and empower the caregiver (Houts, Nezu, Nezu, & Bucher, 1996).

Many centers have developed their own teaching materials and use a variety of approaches (Ezzone & Fliedner, 1997). Throughout the HSCT process, education of the patient, family, and caregiver must be provided; and recommendations include the use of written materials, videotapes, posters, and flipcharts. Individualized discussions may be appropriate as well as classroom discussions. Written materials are essential to help to reinforce verbal instructions. Whatever method is used, to be successful, the patient's educational level, reading level, barriers to learning, and attentiveness must be assessed. The appropriate reading level of written educational materials also must be reviewed (Ezzone, 2000). Informational and psychological needs of patients and family caregivers depend on the site of care delivery for each phase of treatment. The flow between each treatment phase can be confusing to patients and must be explained. Education must begin at the pretransplant evaluation and continue through the mobilization, collection, transplantation, discharge, and follow-up stages of the patient's treatment. Table 5-2 addresses the stages of patient and caregiver education throughout the transplant process.

Each member of the interdisciplinary HSCT team must work together to educate the patient, family, and caregiver through each step of the transplant process, with nurses assuming the overall coordination. The type of education provided will depend on the site of care delivery, complications experienced by the patient, and the individual needs of the patient and caregiver.

Caregiver Roles and Responsibilities

The caregivers manage care by assisting with daily activities, self-medication regimens, central line care, transportation, and monitoring of temperature and intake and output (Ezzone, 2000; Franco, 1999; Peters et al., 1994). Education and training for the caregiver role has resulted in greater satisfaction of patients and caregivers, with increased patient privacy and autonomy in the care process.

The challenges of transplant for the patient and caregivers and the development of strategies to meet their needs in-

Table 5-2. Stages of Patient and Caregiver Education

Stage	Education
Pretransplant	Transplant overview: explanation of the procedure and potential adverse effects
Mobilization	Process and rationale for mobilization agents to be used by the donor and/or autologous recipient. Instruction on the administration of subcutaneous injection in the home setting. Referral to homecare is an excellent resource for follow-up teaching.
Central venous catheter placement	Management of central line, flushing techniques, and dressing changes are required.
Apheresis	Review of procedure, equipment used, duration of apheresis (dependent on CD 34+ cell count). On-site visit to apheresis area, process of cryopreservation, freezing, and storage of cells.
Transplant	
Transplantation	Admission to the inpatient unit, outpatient clinic, or day hospital. On-site visit to area with a review of day-to-day routines. Institution-specific educational materials that review • Preparative regimen (e.g., chemotherapy regimen, radiation therapy) • Daily hygiene (oral care) • Infection control precautions • Dietary restrictions • Blood product administration • Side effects of therapy • Engraftment • Post-transplant complications • Psychosocial support for patient and family
Post-transplant	
Discharge	Review and follow-up with home care or home infusion therapy. Multidisciplinary involvement with pharmacy and dietary, if intravenous (IV) nutritional support is needed. Potential for rehabilitation services as well for enhancing endurance and activity • Outpatient care • Central venous catheter care • Emergency care • Protective precautions • Taking a temperature • Managing IV therapy in the home setting
Follow-up care	Long-term follow-up care should address • Return to school or work issues • Sexuality issues • Management of fatigue and long-term complications related to transplant • Outpatient follow-up • Referring physician follow-up.

Note. Based on information from Ezzone, 2000.

fluences the ability to adjust in the post-transplant process. Studies of the family caregiver found there was a perception of difficulty in communicating with healthcare professionals, requiring a consistent care coordinator or case manager who is present across the care continuum (Stetz et al., 1996).

Caregiver Burden

The potential for chronic effects from transplant can result in long-term demands on the family system (Buchsel et al., 1996). Patients may experience psychological distress, psychiatric symptoms, and mood disturbances such as anxiety and depression. Many report disruptions in sexual function for several months following transplant (Neitzert et al., 1998).

The shift in care to the outpatient setting has not had a negative impact on the financial cost to the patient. Rizzo et al. (1999) studied the economic and social cost of outpatient

care models for the patient and caregiver and found no significant difference between settings (inpatient and outpatient). The observational study in Canada by Summers, Dawe, and Stewart (2000) looked at the psychosocial impact of outpatient autologous HSCT on the patient and caregiver. Caregiver burden was evident. The outpatient caregiver, when compared to a caregiver whose significant other was an inpatient, experienced the greatest impact on their schedules, reduced work hours, change in employment status, and childcare issues. Emotional well-being of the caregiver was low, as measured by depression and anxiety. The financial impact on the family or caregiver unit was a concern and included lost wages, costs for accommodations during the transplant, and large expenses such as travel, medications, and parking.

Surveys of the post-transplant recovery process have found that at six months, caregiver burden continued to be high, as the loved one had not returned to the former roles and responsibilities and because of financial concerns and fatigue. Unexpected and intense demands continue to affect family roles, leaving them feeling inadequate in meeting continued care needs. Information and ongoing support is essential to the adjustment of patients and caregivers who may have role changes for years post-transplant (Boyle et al., 2000).

Development of Standards of Care for Hematopoietic Stem Cell Transplant

To ensure excellent patient care by a trained transplant staff, policy and procedures, standards of care, and unit expectations or guidelines should be instituted. Staff accountability should be established and monitored via performance and quality audits.

Nursing standards of care for the oncology nurse and the advanced practice oncology nurse have been identified. A collaborative effort between ONS and the American Nurses Association have established professional practice standards and professional performance standards for both the oncology nurse and the advanced practice oncology nurse. The practice standards address structure, process, and outcome standards in the following areas: theory, data collection, nursing diagnoses, planning, intervention, and evaluation. Performance standards address professional development, multidisciplinary collaboration, quality assurance, ethics, and research (American Nurses Association & ONS, 1996). HSCT nursing as a subspecialty of oncology nursing can use these practice and performance standards in developing behavioral outcomes and standards for transplant nursing and advanced practice transplant nursing.

Two landmark documents regarding nursing practice, education, and standards of care in the area of marrow and peripheral stem cell transplantation are the *Manual for Bone Marrow Transplant Nursing* and *Peripheral Blood Stem Cell Transplantation: Recommendations for Nursing Education and Practice*. These manuals were a collaborative effort between members of the ONS BMT Special Interest Group, ONS members active in HSCT nursing, and the ONS Clinical Practice Committee (Ezzone, 1997; Ezzone & Camp-Sorrell, 1994). Both manuals address recommendations for education and practice that provide guidance for developing educational programs in HSCT and establishing standards of care, including policies, procedures, and care pathways to promote quality care for the HSCT recipient. Table 5-3 addresses the six recommendations for education and practice for HSCT nursing.

Establishing standards of care includes development of policies and procedures to promote quality care for the HSCT recipient. ONS manuals and books by Buchsel and Kapustay, 2000; Buchsel and Whedon, 1995; and Whedon and Wujcik, 1997, are excellent resources to use in standard of care and policy and procedure development when establishing a transplant program in either the community or tertiary care setting. FACT standards for clinical practice are addressed under the section on accreditation of HSCT programs. Standards should address accountability in adhering to policies and procedures. Standards should state the program's patient or family education plans, management of symptoms and complications, discharge planning, and outpatient management. HSCT resource manuals should be provided and readily available for staff on the unit. Standards should be discussed on a frequent basis and reviewed annually by staff with a commitment to adhere to them (Ezzone, 1997).

Policy and Procedure Development

Determining a list of specific policies or standard operating procedures (SOPs) needed for the transplant program or unit should be a multidisciplinary team effort. It may be helpful to review existing policy and procedures in the institution and in other patient care units that provide specialized care. Policies should reflect specific practices of the team

---

Table 5-3. Recommendations for Hematopoietic Stem Cell Transplant Education and Practice

Recommendation	Procedure
I	Nurses must be knowledgeable about peripheral blood stem cell transplant (PBSCT) and be able to meet the needs of recipients, donors, and their families. Focus on the physical, psychosocial, cultural, spiritual, and educational needs.
II	Standards of care that cover all phases of the transplant process must be developed to ensure effective, safe, and cost-effective care.
III	Nurses using the nursing process should evaluate patient outcomes throughout the PBSCT treatment phases.
IV	Focus on quality of life (QOL) of the patient and caregiver; four domains of QOL issues should be assessed.
V	Nurses should maintain current knowledge in the rapidly developing field of hematopoietic stem cell transplant.
VI	Nursing should promote evidence-based practice and participate in nursing and medical research.

Note. Based on information from Ezzone, 1997.

that include but are not limited to administration of high-dose chemotherapy, reinfusion of hematopoietic stem cells, isolation or neutropenic precautions, special dietary needs or restrictions, and post-transplant rehabilitation. Written policies and procedures should be referenced with current research and evidence-based practice, and staff should be educated on how to access and use the available policies. Nurses need to be encouraged to question how policies and procedures are influencing patient outcomes (Mooney, 2001).

Unit Guidelines

Unit guidelines or expectations for the HSCT team should be developed. Unit standards should include behavioral expectations to guide the interpersonal interactions of the staff and include working together, supporting each other, and being kind and friendly. Demonstrating respect in a professional environment of trust encourages a team atmosphere. The development of standards of care, policies and procedures, and unit expectations directs the HSCT staff to deliver excellent, consistent patient care. Unit or program behavioral expectations provide direction, identify group expectations, and provide a way to measure the performance of team members.

Quality Improvement

A well-defined quality program is required by regulatory agencies such as the Joint Commission on Accreditation of Healthcare Organizations (JCAHO), FACT, and other accrediting bodies. The HSCT program scope of care should be reviewed with staff yearly, with attention to high-risk, high-volume indicators. In continual quality improvement, an organization or unit analyzes its processes to reduce unnecessary variation and improve the quality of its services. A systematic and scientific approach is used to continually improve and control the organization or unit processes.

Focus-PDCA (Plan, Do, Check, Act) is one of the recommended systematic methods for improving processes and evaluating improvement. A process improvement team uses Focus-PDCA as an extension of the PDCA cycle, called the Shewhart cycle, which was first developed in the 1930s (Deming, 1986). PDCA alone is the scientific method. Figure 5-7 describes the Focus-PDCA process.

The transplant staff should be instructed on the use of this process for identifying issues and systematically working through them with the goal of improving patient care. Quality improvement teams should be multidisciplinary when appropriate. Examples of quality improvement projects are improving patient education materials or the process of obtaining patient satisfaction surveys. If the process change was an improvement, the change would then be built into the system, the staff educated, and policies changed to standardize the new process. A data collection plan is created for ongoing monitoring of the new process. If the process change was not an improvement, the change is abandoned, and what was learned becomes input for further process improvements.

Figure 5-7. Focus-PDCA

F: find a process to improve.
O: organize a team to improve the process.
C: clarify the current knowledge of the process.
U: understand sources of process variation.
S: select the process improvement.
P: plan the improvement and data collection.
D: do the improvement and the data collection.
C: check the results of the implementation.
A: act to hold the gain and continue the improvement.

To illustrate the improvement process, Focus-PDCA storyboards can be created by the teams and displayed on the nursing units (Executive Learning, Inc., 1993). Encouraging a culture of process improvement by a team approach through Focus-PDCA gives the transplant staff the opportunity to enhance patient care by improving processes and developing new and improved standards of care.

Accreditation of Hematopoietic Stem Cell Transplant Centers

Both the American Society of Hematology (ASH) and the American Society of Clinical Oncology (ASCO) identified the necessary criteria for the safe and successful performance of BMT. The five areas identified were patient volume, facilities, personnel (physicians and nurses trained in the management of autologous or allogeneic transplant recipients), treatment outcomes, and data reporting to available registries, such as IBMTR (ASCO & ASH, 1990). The European Group for Blood and Marrow Transplantation subcommittee also has identified recommended standards for the performance of HSCT that closely parallel ASH's and ASCO's recommendations. The subcommittee identified standards for patient volume (minimum of 20 patients over two years for newly established programs), clinical facilities, staff requirements, data collection, and support facilities for centers desiring to develop or maintain a HSCT program (Link, Schmitz, Gratwohl, & Goldman, 1995).

In a continuation of their initial study of autologous transplantation for treatment of lymphoid malignancies, the University of Nebraska (2001) validated in their 1999 study that (a) centers that perform a large volume of transplants are more advanced on the learning curve and use resources more efficiently; (b) a referral system or screening criteria promote admission of patients who are better candidates; (c) improved supportive technologies are likely to lead to decreased costs of care and improved survival rates (Bennett et al., 1995; Freeman et al., 1999). The type of scientific support for the expertise of a HSCT center validates the need for standards of performance for all HSCT programs.

Based on the initial recommendations for standards of practice, the International Society for Hematotherapy and Graft Engineering (ISHAGE) and ASBMT merged their standards in 1994, covering all aspects of hematopoietic cell therapy. The two societies formed FACT to develop a voluntary inspection and accreditation process using the established standards.

International Bone Marrow Transplant Registry and Autologous Blood and Marrow Transplant Registry

Prior to the recommendation for accreditation of HSCT programs, IBMTR, organized in 1972, gathered data on both allogeneic and syngeneic transplants worldwide. IBMTR and ABMTR are voluntary organizations that gather data to address important issues in blood and marrow transplantation (both allogeneic and autologous). FACT recommendations and standards strongly encourage participation with IBMTR or ABMTR as a method of recording and sharing patient data. The 12 working committees of IBMTR/ABMTR provide oversight of the use of the data from both registries and help to establish priorities for the utilization of resources. Some of the identified working groups include leukemia, breast cancer, multiple myeloma, and pediatric cancers (IBMTR & ABMTR, 2001).

National Marrow Donor Program

The National Marrow Donor Program (NMDP) was founded in 1986 and is an international leader in the facilitation of unrelated marrow and BSCT. The NMDP has an extensive network of national and international affiliates and facilitates more than 100 transplants each month. Criteria for transplant centers wishing to participate with NMDP identify facility, transplant team, support services, and administrative services required. The requirements include many of the identified FACT standards, such as transplant team composition and expertise in the area of HSCT, number of allogeneic transplants performed, an HLA laboratory accredited by the American Society of Histocompatibility and Immunogenetics or the European Foundation for Immunogenetics. SOPs are required, and use of an NMDP donor requires data submission to the NMDP. A quality improvement program is crucial as well. Administratively, computer information systems are required, which allow links between transplant and donor centers and the NMDP (NMDP, 2001).

In 2002, FACT began the voluntary accreditation of transplant programs. In 1996, FACT established national standards for clinical programs, stem cell collection centers, and processing laboratories. While defining the minimal requirements for the number of transplants to maintain competency and provide for quality patient care, these standards allow for varied program designs to meet the needs of this specialized population.

To apply for FACT accreditation, an HSCT program must have completed a minimum of 10 transplants the year prior to application. The type of transplants performed will determine the request for accreditation. If both autologous and allogeneic transplantation accreditation is being requested, a minimum of 10 transplants of each type must have been completed. The standard for program volume does not differentiate between the pediatric or adult population transplant team.

Few of the FACT standards specifically address nursing practice issues. Key phases of hematopoietic cell therapy in which nursing plays a role, such as the collection of stem cells and the reinfusion of cells, are very clear from a technical standpoint but are vague in providing direction for nursing practice. FACT standards include the establishment of nurse-to-patient ratios based on patient acuity. In an era of continued healthcare cost containment, there is a tremendous need for patient acuity systems that reflect and measure accurately the productivity of nurses in both the inpatient and outpatient clinical setting (Kapustay, 1997).

Recommendations and standards regarding the clinical environment address physical plant requirements for the inpatient and outpatient unit (see Figure 5-2). Trained staff must be available on a 24-hour basis (FACT, 2002). Whatever the care setting, staff must be integrated and able to provide care across a variety of settings. Multidisciplinary rounds are a method of communicating patient care needs across all care delivery settings (Kapustay, 1997).

The FACT standard recommends a quality management program that covers all aspects of the transplant program: staff training and education, proficiency testing, and record management. Each aspect of the program must be evaluated through some form of a quality assurance audit (FACT, 2002). A continuous quality improvement process using Focus-PDCA, as previously discussed, can be used to look at FACT recommendations for auditing and evaluating adverse or sentinel events as part of the quality improvement program. The specific standards address a process for development, review, and evaluation of SOPs. Figure 5-8 is an example of an SOP. Of note, FACT standards do not address outcomes, which often are an area of marked importance for third-party payors.

FACT Donor and Cell Collection Standards

A standardized procedure should be developed for donor selection, and consideration must be given to donors who do not meet the established standard criteria. Figure 5-9 identifies basic donor evaluation criteria.

A rationale for using a less-than-suitable donor must be documented. The transplant physician's decision to use a donor that does not meet criteria is complex. It can be dependent on the recipient's prognosis, if there is a delay, or the possibility of finding another donor, as well as other variables (FACT, 2002).

Once it has been established that a donor is appropriate, informed consent must be obtained. Cultural sensitivity is increasingly important; informed consent must be obtained in the language and at the level of understanding of the donor and prior to the initiation of high-dose therapy for the stem cell recipient. A donor, whether an adult or minor, must be given the opportunity to refuse to donate if he or she chooses to do so.

Collection Facility

The collection facility of the hematopoietic progenitor cells must be affiliated with an accredited and licensed labo-

Figure 5-8. Policy and Procedure

Title: Administration of Frozen Autologous Hematopoietic Progenitor Cells

Number: 000.000.000

Purpose: To ensure safe administration of the maximum viable hematopoietic progenitor cells to facilitate recovery following marrow aplasia from high-dose therapy.

Objectives:
1. Thawing will be completed safely with minimal damage and/or loss of hematopoietic progenitor cells.
2. Administration of hematopoietic progenitor cells will be completed safely with minimal damage and/or loss of hematopoietic progenitor cells.

Outcomes:
1. Patient will experience minimal adverse effects during the administration of hematopoietic progenitor cells.
2. Patient will exhibit evidence of marrow engraftment and recovery within an acceptable period of time.

Equipment:
1. Water bath
2. Ethanol 70%
3. Sterile water (approximately 3,000 ml)
4. Laboratory thermometer
5. Portable cooler
6. Dry ice
7. Sterile plastic bags
8. Sterile 60 ml syringe
9. 18-gauge needle
10. Macrodrip IV tubing without filter (primary and secondary)
11. Extension tubing
12. Three-way stopcock
13. Sodium chloride 0.9% IV solution (50 ml, 250 ml, and 1,000 ml bags)
14. Diphenhydramine hydrochloride 25 mg diluted in 50 ml sodium chloride IV solution
15. Hydrocortisone 50 mg diluted in 50 ml sodium chloride IV solution
16. Sphygmomanometer and stethoscope
17. Standby oxygen and nasal cannula
18. Emergency drug cart (diphenhydramine hydrochloride, mannitol, meperidine hydrochloride, lorazepam, furosemide, hydrocortisone)

Procedure:
1. Coordinate anticipated time for infusion with physician, nursing staff, and processing laboratory.
2. Verify the number of units to be infused with the processing laboratory and physician.
3. Obtain physician orders for premedication and hydration.
4. Clean water bath with ethanol 70% and fill with sterile water.
5. Using a laboratory thermometer, allow temperature to equilibrate to 38°–40°C.
6. Explain procedure to patient.
7. Have patient void.
8. Obtain patient's weight and baseline vital signs.
9. Place blood pressure cuff on patient.
10. Position patient comfortably.
11. Begin IV hydration as ordered using primary macrodrip IV tubing, three-way stopcock, and extension tubing.
12. Contact physician and processing laboratory.
13. Transport hematopoietic progenitor cells to bedside in a portable cooler containing dry ice.
14. Administer premedication as ordered.
15. Remove one unit of cells from the cooler and place in a sterile bag.
16. Thaw unit thoroughly in water bath by gently rotating the bag while observing for evidence of any leakage.
17. Verify patient identification armband with label on unit.
18. Infuse cells over 5–10 minutes via secondary macrodrip IV tubing, piggybacked into primary IV line while normal saline is turned off. If infusion is slow, cells can be drawn from bag via an 18-gauge needle into a 60 ml syringe and pushed through the port of the three-way stopcock under the direction of the physician.
19. Monitor blood pressure, pulse, respirations, and intake and output every 5–10 minutes throughout the infusion.
20. Observe patient for reaction (e.g., fever, chills, dyspnea, urticaria, back pain, chest pain, painful tingling) and provide comfort measures, reassurance, oxygen, and/or medication as indicated.
21. Resume normal saline infusion when unit completed.
22. Repeat steps 15–21 until designated number of units are infused.
23. Continue to hydrate and monitor patient for two to four hours following completion of infusion.

Documentation:
Record the following information in the progress notes:
1. Baseline vital signs
2. IV solution and rate of hydration
3. Time cell infusion initiated and completed
4. Personnel present during infusion
5. Patient response to infusion, including any adverse reactions or side effects
6. Vital signs throughout the infusion
7. Intake and output, including amount and number of units infused

References: _____

Prepared (date): _____

Approved by (transplant director): _____

Approved date: _____

Reviewed (date): _____

Revised (date): _____

Note. From "Peripheral Stem Cell Transplantation Program Development Using the Foundation for the Accreditation of Hematopoietic Cell Therapy Standards" (p. 25) by P. Kapustay in P. Buchsel (Ed.), *Advanced Concepts in Peripheral Stem Cell Transplantation*, 1997, Pittsburgh, PA: Oncology Education Services, Inc. Copyright 1997 by Oncology Education Services, Inc. Reprinted with permission.

Figure 5-9. FACT Donor Evaluation Criteria

Medical history
Physical examination
Laboratory testing:
- Infectious disease studies: HbsAG, Anti-HBC, Anti-HCV, CMV, Anti-HIV-1, including an evaluation for high-risk behavior for HIV infection
- ABO and Rh type
- HLA-A, -B, -DR (if an allogeneic transplant)
- Pregnancy screening for females of childbearing age

Note. Based on information from FACT, 2002.

ratory that is able to perform all the diagnostic tests required for a donor. In addition for marrow or peripheral HSC collections (either autologous or allogeneic), there must be a transfusion facility or blood bank that is able to provide 24-hour blood component support as well as emergency and intensive care services. The medical director of the collection facility must be licensed in the state or province (Canada) where the facility is located and have performed a minimum of 10 collection procedures of each type (marrow or BSCs).

Cell Processing and Cryopreservation

The clinical and administrative management of the cell processing facility is under the direction of a laboratory medical director. Day-to-day supervision of laboratory personnel working in the HSC processing facility is the responsibility of the laboratory manager or director. The HSC processing standards address procedures according to the type of com-

ponent collected and manipulation techniques needed. Table 5-4 describes three types of HSC manipulation.

The processing standards address the importance of SOPs for component labeling, infection control, biochemical and radiological safety measures, biohazard waste disposal, and emergency response systems in the event of exposure to communicable diseases or biohazardous spills (Kapustay, 1997). Other aspects of the standards include recommendations for storage, security, and transportation of product between centers and disposal of the stem cell components that are unused.

FACT Accreditation

The accreditation team consists of members from ISHAGE and ASBMT who meet the qualifications that have been established for the inspectors. The process consists of the initial inspection, renewal inspection that occurs every three years, and a reinspection if deficiencies are found. A center seeking accreditation completes and submits a registration form for evaluation and consideration. If the center does not meet the minimum criteria for number of procedures performed and the medical staff does not meet the minimum qualifications, the transplant facility will be deemed ineligible for accreditation. FACT accredited 112 transplant facilities in the United States as of March 2003. Accreditation is increasingly recognized as a measure of the quality and expertise of an HSCT program. Recognition by a national accrediting body enhances a program's credibility in the community, attracts third-party payors, and provides patients seeking transplantation services a measurement tool to evaluate transplant programs.

Table 5-4. Types of Hematopoietic Progenitor Cell Manipulation

Component	Definition
Unmanipulated components	Components not subject to any form of manipulation (additives limited to heparin, citrate-based anticoagulants, and appropriate electrolyte solutions to maintain cell integrity), such as • Bone marrow • Peripheral blood progenitor cells • Cord blood • Cadaveric marrow
Minimally manipulated components	Limited to procedures that do not subject components to ex vivo procedures that would remove, enrich, expand, or functionally alter cell populations, such as • Plasma depletion • Red cell depletion • Buffy coat preparations • Cryopreservation
Manipulated components	Components subject to procedures that selectively remove, enrich, expand, or functionally alter specific cell populations, such as • Purging • Positive selection • Ex vivo expansion • Gene manipulation

Note. Based on information from Foundation for the Accreditation of Hematopoietic Cell Therapy, 1997. From "Peripheral Stem Cell Transplantation Program Development Using the Foundation for the Accreditation of Hematopoietic Cell Therapy Standards" (p. 30) by P. Kapustay in P. Buchsel (Ed.), *Advanced Concepts in Peripheral Stem Cell Transplantation,* 1997, Pittsburgh, PA: Oncology Education Services, Inc. Copyright 1997 by Oncology Education Services, Inc. Adapted with permission.

Financial Considerations in Program Development

Initial Program Startup Costs

A preliminary budget for the HSCT program should include the capital and operating costs for the first year of the program and should be part of the initial feasibility study. Such costs include recruitment, orientation, and retention of staff; identification of a model of patient care; and any physical plant alterations that must be made to accommodate the patients, including necessary equipment to provide patient care. Support services such as blood bank, pharmacy, radiology, and dietary must be considered as well. Figure 5-10 is a sample of an initial startup budget for an HSCT program; this budget is not all-inclusive and contains fixed expenses (costs not impacted by volume) and variable expenses (costs impacted by volume). Pretransplant diagnostic evaluation tests are not included. Frequently, these diagnostic tests are not performed at the transplant center.

Another important factor to consider is payor mix, which will influence the types and number of patients that will be served by the program. Payor mix ultimately will influence the financial status of the program if the operating costs exceed revenues (Abramovitz & Link, 1995).

Reimbursement Methodologies

There are numerous reimbursement methodologies for transplant services, including fee for service, case rates, and capitation (see Table 5-5). The majority of methods involve some financial risk sharing between the transplant facility and the third-party payor. Risk sharing and the potential for financial exposure require accurate and reliable cost versus charge data for services provided through the transplant course. This information is necessary for a center to negotiate a reasonable contract for HSCT services (Bedell & Mroz, 1997; Nelson, 1995).

Technology and Hematopoietic Stem Cell Transplant Costs

Innovative and new care technologies in the area of HSCT have impacted and will continue to impact the cost of this therapy. Managed care and the rising costs of health care also have placed demands on the healthcare system. Transplant programs, in order to stay viable and cutting edge, must develop or consider alternative care settings, review treatment algorithms, and develop a more evidence-based practice of care to validate their treatment protocols. Care pathway development is one way to monitor and validate care. Pathways can be multidisciplinary program-specific or based on diagnosis-related groups and offer an opportunity to review patient variance from what is expected (DeMeyer, 2000). The three highest areas of expense in a transplant program reported have been pharmacy, blood bank, and nursing care (Yoder, 1998). Costs are not static, and the introduction of a change, such as changes in a protocol, can affect costs.

Knowledge and understanding of what drives the program costs can impact clinical practice and facilitate changes. In a review of five papers that address cost and cost-effectiveness of HSCT, Westerman and Bennett (1996) concluded that further advances that would minimize GVHD and cytomegalovirus infections would increase the cost-effectiveness of allogeneic transplantation. An analysis of pediatric HSCT charges over a three-year period at a large pediatric hospital in the eastern part of the United States noted that pharmaceutical costs comprised the largest component of hospital charges, followed by room charges, central supply, transfusion services, and laboratory. These findings influenced the overall costs of the program. Based on the data gathered, alteration in clinical practice occurred that did not directly impact the quality of care of the pediatric transplant recipient but reduced cost. The changes included IV tubing change every three days versus every day; reevaluation of the use of total parenteral nutrition in patients who were well nourished; and modification in protective isolation practices (Kline et al., 1998).

The use of BSCs cells versus bone marrow stem cells also has impacted the care and cost of transplantation. Enhancement of the number of BSCs (CD34+ cells) greater than or equal to 5×10^6/kg has been associated with decreased supportive needs and decreased costs of HSCT (Glaspy, 1999). A retrospective cost identification analysis noted that patients receiving allogeneic peripheral blood stem cell transplants had an initial median total cost of $18,000 less when compared to the group that received allogeneic BMT. The investigators did not follow patients beyond the initial discharge and identified that their data only identified short-term cost savings (Bennett et al., 1999). Outpatient care and subsequent readmission were not addressed. Outpatient costs may constitute as much as 20%–45% of the total treatment costs (Waters, 1997).

It has been noted that specific to breast cancer, the frequent use of autologous HSCT prior to 1999 had brought significant financial gain to hospitals, physicians, and commercial enterprises. Thus, too many autologous HSCTs have been performed without defined scientific goals. The need for following the usual scientific process of evaluating new technologies in HSCT by phase I–II and subsequent phase III trials is crucial (Bennett et al., 1999). A commitment to high-quality clinical investigations by healthcare providers, insurers, and federal funding agencies (e.g., National Cancer Institute, National Institutes of Health) will produce valid research and enhance scientific knowledge regarding this treatment modality and, ultimately, will produce cost-efficient quality care (Blume & Thomas, 2000).

Centers of Excellence and Stem Cell Transplant Network Development

Initial steps toward developing Centers of Excellence (COE) (i.e., Institutes of Quality or HSCT networks) for transplantation were undertaken in 1986 by the Prudential Insurance Company of America. Using information from a

Figure 5-10. Startup Budget for a Hematopoietic Stem Cell Transplant Program

FIXED EXPENSES			YEAR 1
Staffing			$x,xxx.xx
Benefits			$x,xxx.xx
Overtime			$x,xxx.xx
Maintenance			$x,xxx.xx
Equipment depreciation			$x,xxx.xx
Construction depreciation			$x,xxx.xx
Medical director fee			$x,xxx.xx
Nursing director fee			$x,xxx.xx

Total Fixed Expenses			$x,xxx.xx

VARIABLE EXPENSES	Frequency	Costs/Unit	Total/Transplant
Stem cell procurement	xx	$x.xx	$x,xxx.xx
G-CSF 10 mcg/kg	xx	$x.xx	$x,xxx.xx
Reagents	xx	$x.xx	$x,xxx.xx
CBC	xx	$x.xx	$x,xxx.xx
Mononuclear cell count	xx	$x.xx	$x,xxx.xx
CD34 assay	xx	$x.xx	$x,xxx.xx
CFU-GM	xx	$x.xx	$x,xxx.xx
Stem cell storage	xx	$xx.xx	$x,xxx.xx

Total Stem Cell Harvest			$x,xxx.xx

Other Stem Cell Harvest Costs	Frequency	Costs/Unit	Total/Transplant
Epinephrine	xx	$x.xx	$x.xx
Vitamin K 10 mg	xx	$x.xx	$xx.xx
Heparin flushes 2 lumens	xx	$xx.xx	$xxx.xx

Total Drugs			$xxx.xx

Radiology and Lab	Frequency	Costs/Unit	Total/Transplant
Chest X-ray	xx	$xx.xx	$xx,xxx.xx
EKG	xx	$xx.xx	$xx,xxx.xx
Type and screen	xx	$xx.xx	$xx,xxx.xx
Blood cultures (bacterial & fungal)	xx	$xx.xx	$xx,xxx.xx
CBC	xx	$xx.xx	$xx,xxx.xx
Chem 20	xx	$xx.xx	$xx,xxx.xx
PT/PTT	xx	$xx.xx	$xx,xxx.xx
Bone marrow biopsy	xx	$xx.xx	$xx,xxx.xx

Total Lab and Radiology			$xx,xxx.xx

Blood Products	Frequency	Costs/Unit	Total/Transplant
PRBCs	xx	$xx.xx	$xx,xxx.xx
Filter	xx	$xx.xx	$xx,xxx.xx
Irradiation	xx	$xx.xx	$xx,xxx.xx
Platelets	xx	$xx.xx	$xx,xxx.xx
Pack	xx	$xx.xx	$xx,xxx.xx
Filter	xx	$xx.xx	$xx,xxx.xx
Irradiation	xx	$xx.xx	$xx,xxx.xx

Total Blood Products			$xx,xxx.xx

Pharmacy	Frequency	Costs/Unit	Total/Transplant
Conditioning regimen	xx	$xx.xx	$xx,xxx.xx
Cytoxan 120 mg/kg IV	xx	$xx.xx	$xx,xxx.xx
Mesna 120 mg/kg IV	xx	$xx.xx	$xx,xxx.xx

(Continued on next page)

Etoposide 30 mg/kg IV	xx	$xx.xx	$xx,xxx.xx
Busulfan 16 mg/kg po	xx	$xx.xx	$xx,xxx.xx
Ondansetron 10 mg IV	xx	$xx.xx	$xx,xxx.xx
Lorazepam 2 mg IV	xx	$xx.xx	$xx,xxx.xx
Metoclopramide 2 mg/kg	xx	$xx.xx	$xx,xxx.xx

Total Conditioning			**$xx,xxx.xx**

Post-Transplant Drug Therapy	**Frequency**	**Costs/Unit**	**Total/Transplant**
G-CSF 10 mcg/kd/d	xx	$xx.xx	$xx,xxx.xx
Ondansetron 10 mg IV	xx	$xx.xx	$xx,xxx.xx
Compazine	xx	$xx.xx	$xx,xxx.xx
Lorazepam 2 mg IV	xx	$xx.xx	$xx,xxx.xx
Norfloxacillin	xx	$xx.xx	$xx,xxx.xx
Nystatin	xx	$xx.xx	$xx,xxx.xx
Imipenum 500 mg qid	xx	$xx.xx	$xx,xxx.xx
Vancomycin 900 mg bid	xx	$xx.xx	$xx,xxx.xx
Amphotericin	xx	$xx.xx	$xx,xxx.xx
D51/2NS	xx	$xx.xx	$xx,xxx.xx
Diphenhydramine	xx	$xx.xx	$xx,xxx.xx

Total Transplant Pharmacy Costs			**$xxx,xxx.xx**

TOTAL VARIABLE EXPENSES	**$X,XXX,XXX.XX**
TOTAL FIXED EXPENSES	**$X,XXX,XXX.XX**
TOTAL COSTS	**$X,XXX,XXX.XX**

COST ANALYSIS FOR AUTOLOGOUS HEMATOPOIETIC STEM CELL TRANSPLANT

review by the U.S. Office of Technology Assessment, which correlated experience with a procedure and clinical outcome, Prudential initially developed a network of transplant centers of expertise for solid organ transplantation. This was followed by marrow transplantation, and in 1990, they developed their autologous HSC transplantation program (Draglin, Perkins, & Plocher, 1990). With the estimated first-year charges for an autologous HSCT being $144,400 and an allogeneic HSCT costing $232,600, healthcare insurers, employer groups, and individuals considering transplant as a treatment option are concerned about quality outcomes and cost (Haulboldt & Roberts, 1999). Managed care concerns related to quality clinical outcomes and cost have lead to the development of transplant networks of expertise on a regional and national basis.

The COE process starts with a request for proposal (RFP). This document is an application provided by the insurance carrier to the transplant center, which desires to become part of the insurer's network of providers of transplant services (see Table 5-6). Unfortunately, for transplant centers applying to become part of several insurers' transplant network of providers, the RFP will differ from insurer to insurer. Figure 5-11 addresses the COE process and reasons for agreements between transplant centers and insurers.

New and developing HSC transplant programs frequently do not meet the volume criterion nor have the clinical outcome data that are acceptable for the COE network initially.

In addition, the program may not be needed by the insurer's network because other comparable centers are available in the same service area. In developing a new program, it is important to assess not only the community's needs, but also the insurer base to determine if they mandate a COE facility for transplant services for their insured lives. This mandate will impact a new center's volume of clients. It could take several years for a new program to meet volume and outcome criteria of third-party payors.

For-Profit Corporations

Early in the 1990s, for-profit corporations focusing on outpatient autologous HSCT developed treatment centers in community settings across the United States. These groups established or supported community-based centers and urban freestanding clinics that competed directly with traditional programs. These centers were provided with equipment and training for nursing, pharmacy, and laboratory staff. Protocols, practice guidelines, standardized care plans, and data management are centrally developed and monitored to ensure quality. National practice management services such as Pro Med and US Oncology also have developed the capacity to assist physician practice groups and hospitals with the development and operation of HSCT programs on a national basis.

The competition for patients led research and academic centers to pursue relationships with community programs.

Table 5-5. Marrow and Stem Cell Transplant Financial Reimbursement Methods

Service	Reimbursement Methodologies
Fee for service	Can be traditional indemnity insurance type of arrangement or managed care arrangement. With managed care fee for service, there are negotiated fees between the provider and the managed care plan based on services defined by the Current Procedural Terminology (CPT) codes. Another managed care arrangement identified as fee for service is global fees. A global fee is an arrangement in which a negotiated fee is all-inclusive (one fee is paid for the entire episode of care, such as pretransplant evaluation). Adjustments can be made for care that is less costly or more costly than the determined fee.
Capitation	A per member per month single payment arrangement to cover costs of all services provided for a defined period of time. Payment is made in advance of the delivery of healthcare service.
Case rates	Similar to a global fee, it is a negotiated fixed fee rate for a specific service, such as HSCT. Case rates can be adjusted for those situations requiring more intensive care (outlier).
Per diem	Fixed rate of payment per day for services rendered, usually used in the inpatient hospital setting. Per diem rates for HSCT and ICU are much higher than per diem rates for general medical-surgical care.
RBRVS	HCFA (Health Care Financing Administration) method of payment for physicians that encourages the use of primary care services. Method may be used to reimburse specialists
DRG	Prospective payment plan, which is a flat fee for all inpatient services related to a diagnosis and a single episode of care.

Note. Based on information from the Patient Advocate Foundation, 1997.

Although they may or may not be financially linked, such relationships involve sharing of protocols and consultation services in the community with referral of allogeneic patients and more difficult cases to the larger partner center (academic tertiary care centers) (Clifford, 2000).

Conclusion

HSCT is a constantly evolving and ever-changing treatment modality. As this oncology subspecialty has grown and matured over the last 30 years, innovations in care delivery sites have occurred, based on client and economic demands. Standards regarding the delivery of nursing and multidisciplinary care have developed, and recommendations for accreditation of HSCT programs to acknowledge expertise of established and new programs have evolved. An organization considering the development of a transplant program needs to review multiple variables that will impact the success and solvency of a program.

Figure 5-11. Certificate of Excellence Components and Requirements

Factors that impact inclusion of an HSCT program in a COE
- Identified need of third-party payors for an HSCT center in that region
- Ability of the transplant center and insurer to develop a working and effective partnership
- Quality in both transplant process and outcomes

Requirements by state or federal regulation
- Provide assurances of transplant service availability.
- Provide a basis for managing costs and utilizing transplant services.
- Minimize misunderstandings and liability of exposure for the insurer and the transplant facility.

Note. Based on information from Burke, 1998.

Table 5-6. Sample Request for Proposal for Center of Excellence Designation

Services	Data
Information about transplant team and the areas of expertise of the team members, as well as support persons	Number and types of transplants performed (e.g., adult, pediatric, autologous, allogeneic)
Program development and areas of current clinical research protocols that would be offered to potential transplant candidates	Survival data of transplant recipients and post-transplant complications
Continuing education programs for the transplant team and education offered to the community	Patient selection criteria
Quality improvement program	Facility or hospital-specific information

Note. Based on information from Nelson, 1995.

References

Abramovitz, L., & Link, L. (1995). Administrative issues of an inpatient BMT unit. In P.C. Buchsel & M.B. Whedon (Eds.), *Bone marrow transplantation: Administrative and clinical strategies* (pp. 95–111). Sudbury, MA: Jones and Bartlett.

Abruzzese, R.S., & Quinn-O'Neal, B. (1992). Orientation for general and specialty areas. In R.S. Abruzzese (Ed.), *Nursing staff development* (pp. 259–282). Philadelphia: Mosby.

Amato, J.J., Williams, M., Greenberg, C., Bar, M., Lo, S., & Tepler, I. (1998). Psychological support to an autologous bone marrow transplant unit in a community hospital: A pilot experience. *Psycho-Oncology, 7*(2), 121–125.

American Nurses Association & Oncology Nursing Society. (1996). *Statement on the scope and standards of oncology nursing practice.* Washington, DC: American Nurses Association.

American Society of Clinical Oncology & American Society of Hematology. (1990). ASCO/ASH recommended criteria for the performance of bone marrow transplantation. *Blood, 75,* 1209.

Appel, P. (2001, February 16). *Transplant program organization and key relationships*. Lecture and slide presentation given at the ASBMT BMT Center Administrative Directors Conference, Keystone, CO.

Bedell, M.K., & Mroz, W.T. (1997). The bone marrow and stem cell transplant marketplace. In M.B. Whedon & D. Wujcik (Eds.), *Blood and marrow stem cell transplantation: Principles, practice, and nursing insights* (pp. 475–483). Sudbury, MA: Jones and Bartlett.

Bennett, C.L., Armitage, J.L., Armitage, G.O., Vose, J.M., Bierman, P.J., Armitage, J.O., et al. (1995). Costs of care and outcomes for dose therapy and autologous transplantation for lymphoid malignancies: Results from the University of Nebraska 1987–1991. *Journal of Clinical Oncology, 13*, 969–973.

Bennett, C.L., Stinson, T., Amagor, O., Pavletic, Z., Tarantolo, S., & Bishop, M. (1999). Valuing clinical strategies early in development: A cost analysis of allogeneic peripheral blood stem cell transplantation. *Bone Marrow Transplantation, 24*, 555–560.

Bensinger, W.I., Martin, P.J., Storer, B., Clift, R., Forman, S.J., Negrin, R., et al. (2001). Transplantation of bone marrow as compared with peripheral-blood cells from HLA-identical relatives in patients with hematologic cancers. *New England Journal of Medicine, 344*, 175–181.

Blume, K.G., & Thomas, E.D. (2000). A review of autologous hematopoietic cell transplantation. *Biology of Blood and Marrow Transplantation, 6*, 1–12.

Boyle, D., Blodgett, L., Gnesdiloff, S., White, J., Bamford, A.M., Sheridan, M., et al. (2000). Caregiver quality of life after autologous bone marrow transplantation. *Cancer Nursing, 23*, 193–203.

Bredeson, C. (2000). Report on the state of the art in blood and marrow transplantation. *IBMTR/ABMTR Newsletter, 7*, 3–10.

Buchsel, P.C., & Kapustay, P.M. (1995). Peripheral stem cell transplantation. *Oncology Nursing: Patient Treatment and Support, 2*(2), 1–14.

Buchsel, P.C., & Kapustay, P.M. (Eds.). (2000). *Stem cell transplantation: A clinical textbook*. Pittsburgh, PA: Oncology Nursing Society.

Buchsel, P.C., Leum, E.W., & Randolph, S.R. (1996). Delayed complications of bone marrow transplantation: An update. *Oncology Nursing Forum, 23*, 1267–1291.

Buchsel, P.C., & Parchem, C. (1988). Ambulatory care of the bone marrow transplant patient. *Seminars in Oncology Nursing, 4*(1), 41–46.

Buchsel, P.C., & Whedon, M.B. (1995). *Bone marrow transplantation: Administrative and clinical strategies*. Sudbury, MA: Jones and Bartlett.

Burke, J.W. (1998). Selective medical provider contracting. In J.J. Stein (Ed.), *Managed care: Integrating the delivery and financing of health care, part B* (pp. 21–37). Washington, DC: Health Insurance Association of America.

Burns, J.M., Tierney, D.K., Long, G.D., Lambert, S.C., & Carr, B.E. (1995). Critical pathway for administering high-dose chemotherapy followed by peripheral blood stem cell rescue in the outpatient setting. *Oncology Nursing Forum, 22*, 1219–1224.

Campbell, L.R., & Foody, M.C. (1995). Administrative issues of an inpatient BMT unit. In P.C. Buchsel & M.B. Whedon (Eds.), *Bone marrow transplantation: Administrative and clinical strategies* (pp. 39–68). Sudbury, MA: Jones and Bartlett.

Centers for Disease Control and Prevention. (2000). *Guidelines for preventing opportunistic infections among hematopoietic stem cell transplant recipients*. Retrieved August 20, 2003, from http://www.cdc.gov/mmwr/preview/mmwrhtml/rr4910a1.htm

Chan, B. (2000). The pharmacology of peripheral stem cell transplantation. In P.C. Buchsel & P.M. Kapustay (Eds.), *Stem cell transplantation: A clinical textbook* (pp. 8.1–8.23). Pittsburgh, PA: Oncology Nursing Society.

Chielens, D., & Herrick, E. (1990). Recipients of bone marrow transplants: Making a smooth transition to an ambulatory care setting. *Oncology Nursing Forum, 17*, 857–862.

Clifford, K. (2000). Peripheral stem cell transplantation in the community setting. In P.C. Buchsel & P.M. Kapustay (Eds.), *Stem cell transplantation: A clinical textbook* (pp. 12.1–12.13). Pittsburgh, PA: Oncology Nursing Society.

Cohen, C., & Musgrave, C.F. (1998). A preceptorship program in an Israeli bone marrow transplant unit. *Cancer Nursing, 21*, 259–262.

De Koster, D., & McLaughlin, B. (2001). Fred Hutchinson nurses offer a perspective on pediatric transplants in the ambulatory setting. *Blood and Marrow Stem Cell Transplant Special Interest Group Newsletter, 12*(1), 4.

DeMeyer, E.S. (2000). Care paths in peripheral stem cell transplantation. In P.C. Buchsel & P.M. Kapustay (Eds.), *Stem cell transplantation: A clinical textbook* (pp. 7.1–7.16). Pittsburgh, PA: Oncology Nursing Society.

Deming, W.E. (1986). *Out of the crisis*. Cambridge, MA: Center for Advanced Engineering Study, Massachusetts Institute of Technology.

Dietz, J.H. (1980). Adaptive rehabilitation in cancer. *Postgraduate Medicine, 68*, 145–153.

Dix, S.P., Cord, M.K., Howard, S.J., Coon, J.L., Belt, R.J., & Geller, R.B. (1999). Safety and efficacy of a continuous infusion, patient-controlled antiemetic pump to facilitate outpatient administration of high-dose chemotherapy. *Bone Marrow Transplantation, 24*, 561–566.

Dix, S.P., & Geller, R.B. (2000). High-dose chemotherapy with autologous stem cell rescue in the outpatient setting. *Oncology, 6*, 185–186.

Draglin, D., Perkins, D., & Plocher, D.W. (1990). Institutes of quality: Prudential's approach to outcomes management for specialty procedures. *Quality Review Bulletin, 16*(3), 111–115.

Executive Learning, Inc. (1993). *Continual improvement handbook: A quick reference guide for tools and concepts*. Nashville, TN: Author.

Ezzone, S.A. (Ed.). (1997). *Peripheral blood stem cell transplantation: Recommendations for nursing education and practice*. Pittsburgh, PA: Oncology Nursing Society.

Ezzone, S.A. (2000). Patient and family caregiver teaching. In P.C. Buchsel & P.M. Kapustay (Eds.), *Stem cell transplantation: A clinical textbook* (pp. 6.1–6.10). Pittsburgh, PA: Oncology Nursing Society.

Ezzone, S., & Camp-Sorrell, D. (1994). *Manual for bone marrow transplant nursing: Recommendations for practice and education*. Pittsburgh, PA: Oncology Nursing Society.

Ezzone, S.A., & Fliedner, M. (1997). Transplant networks and standards of care: International perspectives. In M.B. Whedon & D. Wujcik (Eds.), *Blood and marrow stem cell transplantation: Principles, practice, and nursing insights* (pp. 474–496). Sudbury, MA: Jones and Bartlett.

Farah, R.A., Aquino, V.M., Munoz, L.L., & Sandler, E.S. (1998). Safety and cost-effectiveness of outpatient total body irradiation in pediatric patients undergoing stem cell transplantation. *Journal of Pediatric Hematology/Oncology, 20*, 319–321.

Farley, S., & Jones, M. (1995). Leadership. In R.C. Swansburg & L.C. Swansburgh (Eds.), *Nursing staff development—A component of human resources development* (pp. 303–324). Sudbury, MA: Jones and Bartlett.

Foundation for the Accreditation of Cellular Therapy. (2002). *FACT accreditation manual*. Omaha, NE: Author.

Foundation for the Accreditation of Hematopoietic Cell Therapy. (1997). *FAHCT accreditation manual*. Omaha, NE: Author.

Foxall, M.J., & Gaston-Johansson, F. (1996). Burden and health outcomes of family caregivers of hospitalized bone marrow transplant patients. *Journal of Advanced Nursing, 24*, 915–923.

Franco, M. (1999). Cooperative care is the future of transplantation at the University of Nebraska Medical Center. *Blood and Marrow Stem Cell Transplant Special Interest Group Newsletter, 10*(2), 3.

Freeman, M.B., Vose, J.M., Bennett, C.L., Anderson, J.R., Kessinger, A., Turner, K., et al. (1999). Costs of care associated with high-dose therapy and autologous transplantation for non-Hodgkin's lymphoma: Results from the University of Nebraska Medical Center 1989–1995. *Bone Marrow Transplantation, 24,* 679–684.

Gillies, D.A. (1989). *Nursing management: A systems approach* (2nd ed.). Philadelphia: W.B. Saunders.

Glaspy, J.L. (1999). Economic considerations in the use of peripheral blood progenitor cells to support high-dose chemotherapy. *Bone Marrow Transplantation, 23*(Suppl. 2), S21–S27.

Gluck, S., des Rochers, C., Cano, C., Dorreen, M., Germond, C., Gill, K., et al. (1997). High-dose chemotherapy followed by autologous blood cell transplantation: A safe and effective outpatient approach. *Bone Morrow Transplantation, 20,* 431–434.

Griffith, K.A. (1999). Holism in the care of the allogeneic bone marrow transplant population: Role of the nurse practitioner. *Holistic Nurse Practitioner, 13,* 20–27.

Haulboldt, R.H., & Roberts, S.A. (1999). *Cost implications of human organ and tissue transplantations.* Albany, NY: Milliman and Roberston.

Hermann, R.P., Leather, M., Leather, H.L., & Leen, K. (1998). Clinical care for patient's receiving autologous hematopoietic stem cell transplantation in the home setting. *Oncology Nursing Forum, 25,* 1427–1432.

Hitt, D. (2001). A team approach benefits pediatric bone marrow transplant recipients in the intensive-care unit. *Blood and Marrow Stem Cell Transplant Special Interest Group Newsletter, 12*(1), 1–6.

Holecek, R.A., & Sellards, S.M. (1997). Use of a detailed clinical pathway for bone marrow transplant patients. *Journal of Pediatric Oncology Nursing, 14,* 252–257.

Horowitz, M. (1995). New IBMTR/ABMTR slides summarize current use and outcomes of allogeneic and autologous transplants. *IBMTR Newsletter, 2*(1), 1–8.

Houston, D.A., & Houston, G.R. (1995). Administrative issues and concepts in ambulatory care. In P.C. Buchsel & C.H. Yarbro (Eds.), *Oncology nursing in the ambulatory setting: Issues and models of care* (pp. 1–19). Sudbury, MA: Jones and Bartlett.

Houts, P.S., Nezu, A.M., Nezu, C.M., & Bucher, J.A. (1996). The prepared family caregiver: A problem-solving approach to family caregiver education. *Patient Education and Counseling, 27,* 63–73.

International Bone Marrow Transplant Registry & Autologous Blood and Marrow Transplant Registry. (2001). *Mission statement.* Retrieved August 20, 2003, from www.ibmtr.org

Jassak, P.F., & Porter, N.L. (1995). Strategies for education of the BMT patient. In P.C. Buchsel & M.B. Whedon (Eds.), *Bone marrow transplantation: Administrative and clinical strategies* (pp. 353–363). Sudbury, MA: Jones and Bartlett.

Jeffries, E. (1996). *The heart of leadership.* Dubuque, IA: Kendall/Hunt.

Kapustay, P. (1997). Peripheral stem cell transplantation program development using the Foundation for the Accreditation of Hematopoietic Cell Therapy Standards. In P. Buchsel (Ed.), *Advanced concepts in peripheral stem cell transplantation* (pp. 23–31). Pittsburgh, PA: Oncology Education Services, Inc.

Kelleher, J. (1991). Developing a bone marrow transplant program: Planning, environmental and personnel challenges. In M.B. Whedon (Ed.), *Bone marrow transplantation: Principles, practice and nursing insights* (pp. 378–395). Sudbury, MA: Jones and Bartlett.

Kelley, C.H., & Randolph, S. (1998). The role of the homecare nurse throughout the continuum of blood stem cell transplantation. *Journal of Intravenous Nursing, 21,* 361–366.

Kelley, C.H., Randolph, S.R., & Leum, E. (2000). Home care of peripheral stem cell transplant recipients. In P.C. Buchsel & P.M. Kapustay (Eds.), *Stem cell transplantation: A clinical textbook* (pp. 13.3–13.6). Pittsburgh, PA: Oncology Nursing Society.

Kline, R.M., Merman, S., Tarantino, M.D., Herzig, R.H., & Bertolone, S.J. (1998). A detailed analysis of charges for hematopoietic stem cell transplantation at a children's hospital. *Bone Marrow Transplantation, 21,* 195–203.

Lamkin, L. (1993). The new oncology ambulatory clinic. In P.C. Buchsel & C.H. Yarbro (Eds.), *Oncology nursing in the ambulatory setting: Issues and models of care* (pp. 107–131). Sudbury, MA: Jones and Bartlett.

Letheby, B.A., Jackson, J.D., & Warkentin, P.I. (2000). Processing, cryopreservation, and storage of peripheral blood progenitor cells. In P.C. Buchsel & P.M. Kapustay (Eds.), *Stem cell transplantation: A clinical textbook* (pp. 4.3–4.20). Pittsburgh, PA: Oncology Nursing Society.

Lilleby, K. (2000). A nursing history of bone marrow and peripheral stem cell transplantation. In P.C. Buchsel & P.M. Kapustay (Eds.), *Stem cell transplantation: A clinical textbook* (pp. 15.1–15.8). Pittsburgh, PA: Oncology Nursing Society.

Lin, E.M. (1994). A combined role of clinical nurse specialist and coordinator: Optimizing continuity of care in an autologous bone marrow transplant program. *Clinical Nurse Specialist, 8*(1), 48–55.

Link, H., Schmitz, N., Gratwohl, A., & Goldman, J. (1995). Standards for specialist units undertaking blood and marrow stem cell transplants. Recommendations from the EBMT. *Bone Marrow Transplantation, 16,* 733–736.

Lonergan, J.N., Kelley, C.H., McBride, L.H., & Randolph, S.R. (1996). *Home care management of the bone marrow transplant patient* (2nd ed.). Sudbury, MA: Jones and Bartlett.

Madden, M.J., & Ponte, P.R. (1994). Advanced practice roles in the managed care environment. *Journal of Nursing Administration, 24*(1), 56–62.

Mayer, D., & O'Connor, L. (1989). Rehabilitation of persons with cancer: An ONS position statement. *Oncology Nursing Forum, 16,* 433.

McDonald, J.C., Stetz, K.M., & Compton, K. (1996). Educational interventions for family caregivers during marrow transplantation. *Oncology Nursing Forum, 23,* 1432–1439.

Meisenberg, B.R., Feffan, K., Hoflenbach, K., Brehm, T., Jollon, T., & Piro, L.D. (1998). Reduced charges and costs associated with outpatient autologous stem cell transplantation. *Bone Marrow Transplantation, 21,* 927–932.

Meisenberg, B.R., Gollard, R., Brehm, T., McMillian, R., & Miller, W. (1996). Prophylactic antibiotics eliminate bacteremia and allow safe outpatient management following high-dose chemotherapy and autologous stem cell rescue. *Supportive Care in Cancer, 4,* 364–369.

Meisenberg, B.R., Miller, W.E., McMillan, R., Callaghan, M., Sloan, C., Brehm, T., et al. (1997). Outpatient high-dose chemotherapy with autologous stem cell for hematologic and non-hematologic malignancies. *Journal of Clinical Oncology, 15,* 11–17.

Mooney, K.H. (2001). Advocating for quality cancer care: Making evidence-based practice a reality. *Oncology Nursing Forum, 28*(Suppl. 2), 17–21.

National Marrow Donor Program. (2001). *NMDP transplant center participation criteria.* Retrieved August 20, 2003, from http://www.marrow.org

Neitzert, C.S., Ritvo, P., Dancey, J., Weiser, K., Murray, C., & Avery, J. (1998). The psychosocial impact of bone marrow transplantation: A review of the literature. *Bone Marrow Transplantation, 22,* 409–422.

Nelson, J.P. (1995). Centers of excellence for marrow transplantation. In P.C. Buchsel & M.B. Whedon (Eds.), *Bone marrow transplantation: Administrative and clinical strategies* (pp. 443–462). Sudbury, MA: Jones and Bartlett.

Nelson, J.P. (1997). The blood cell transplant program. *Seminars in Oncology, 13,* 208–215.

Neumann, J.L. (2000). Compliance Task Force. *Oncology Nursing Forum, 26,* 683.

Neumann, J.L., & De Jesus, A.Y. (1998). Use of collaborative pathway to manage neutropenic fever in bone marrow transplant patients. *Nursing Interventions in Oncology, 10,* 15–19.

CHAPTER 5. CONSIDERATIONS IN HEMATOPOIETIC STEM CELL TRANSPLANT PROGRAM DEVELOPMENT

Patient Advocate Foundation. (1997). *The managed care answer guide.* Newport News, VA: Author.

Peters, W.P., Baynes, R.B., Cassells, L., Dansey, R., Klein, J., Hamm, C., et al. (2000). The Dix/Geller article reviewed. *Oncology, 6,* 191–192.

Peters, W.P., Ross, M., Vredenburgh, J.J., Hussein, A., Rubin, P., Dukelow, K., et al. (1994). The use of clinic support to permit outpatient autologous bone marrow transplantation of breast cancer. *Seminars in Oncology, 21*(4 Suppl. 7), 25–31.

Pisseri, H. (1998). Institution studies use of autologous stem cell transplants for patients with advanced ovarian cancer. *Bone Marrow Transplant Special Interest Group Newsletter, 9*(1), 1–5.

Rettger, B.L.C. (1992). Setting up an autologous bone marrow transplant program. *Nursing Management, 23*(5), 96L–96M.

Rizzo, J.D., Vogelsang, G.B., Krumm, S., Frink, B., Mock, V., & Bass, E.B. (1999). Outpatient-based bone marrow transplantation for hematologic malignancies: Cost savings or cost shifting? *Journal of Clinical Oncology, 17,* 2811.

Rowlings, P.A. (1996). Summary slides show current use and outcome of blood and marrow transplantation. *IBMTR/ABMTR Newsletter, 3*(1), 6–12.

Rubenfeld, G.D, & Crawford, S.W. (1996). Withdrawing life support from mechanically ventilated recipients of bone marrow transplants: A case for evidence-based guidelines. *Annals of Internal Medicine, 125,* 625–633.

Schmit-Pokorny, K., Hruska, M., & Ursick, M. (1998). Peripheral blood stem cell transplantation: Outpatient strategies. *Innovations in Breast Cancer Care, 3*(3), 52–56.

Schiffman, K.S., Bensinger, W.I., Appelbaum, F.R., Rowley, S., Lilleby, K., Clift, R.A., et al. (1996). Phase II study of high-dose busulfan, melphalan, and thiotepa with autologous peripheral blood stem cell support in patients with malignant disease. *Bone Marrow Transplantation, 17,* 943–950.

Schwartzberg, L.S., Birch, R., West, W.H., Tauer, K.W., Wittlin, F., Leff, R., et al. (1998). Sequential treatment including high-dose chemotherapy with peripheral blood stem cell support in patients with high-risk stage II–III breast cancer. *American Journal of Clinical Oncology, 21,* 523–531.

Shapiro, T.W. (1995). Intensive care management of the BMT patient: Administrative and clinical issues. In P.C. Buchsel & M.B. Whedon (Eds.), *Bone marrow transplantation: Administrative and clinical strategies* (pp. 443–462). Sudbury, MA: Jones and Bartlett.

Shivnan, J., Shelton, B.K., & Onners, B.K. (1996). Bone marrow transplantation: Issues for critical care nurses. *AACN Clinical Issues, 7*(1), 95–108.

Shorr, A.F., Moores, L.K., Edenfield, W.J., Christie, R.J., & Fitzpatrick, T.M. (1999). Mechanical ventilation in hematopoietic stem cell transplantation: Can we effectively predict outcomes? *Chest, 116,* 1012–1018.

Stern, J.M., & Lenssen, P. (1995). Food and nutrition services for the BMT patient. In P.C. Buchsel & M.B. Whedon (Eds.), *Bone marrow transplantation: Administrative and clinical strategies* (pp. 113–136). Sudbury, MA: Jones and Bartlett.

Stetz, K.M., McDonald, J.C., & Compton, K. (1996). Needs and experiences of family caregivers during marrow transplantation. *Oncology Nursing Forum, 23,* 1422–1427.

Summers, N., Dawe, U., & Stewart, D.A. (2000). A comparison of inpatient and outpatient ASCT. *Bone Marrow Transplantation, 26,* 389–395.

Swansburg, R.C. (1995). *Implications for the future: Nursing staff development.* Sudbury, MA: Jones and Bartlett.

Syrjala, K. (1995). Meeting the psychosocial needs of recipients and families. In P.C. Buchsel & M.B. Whedon (Eds.), *Bone marrow transplantation: Administrative and clinical strategies* (pp. 283–301). Sudbury, MA: Jones and Bartlett.

Tarzian, A.J., Iwata, P.A., & Cohen, M.Z. (1999). Autologous bone marrow transplantation: The patient's perspective of information. *Cancer Nursing, 22,* 103–110.

University of Nebraska. (2001). *FACT accredited programs. 1–5.* Lincoln, NE: Author.

Van de Creek, L. (1997). Collaboration between nurses and chaplains for spiritual caregiving. In E.J. Taylor & J.R. Mickley (Eds.), *Spirituality and cancer* (pp. 279–280). Philadelphia: W.B. Saunders.

Waters, T.M. (1997). Economic analyses of new technologies: The case of stem cell transplantation. *Journal of Clinical Oncology, 15,* 2–4.

Weaver, C.H., Schwartzberg, L.S., Hainsworth, F.A., Greco, F.A., Li, W., Buchner, C.D., et al. (1997). Treatment-related mortality in 1,000 consecutive patients receiving high-dose chemotherapy and peripheral blood progenitor cell transplantation in community cancer center. *Bone Marrow Transplantation, 19,* 671–678.

Westermann, A.M., Holtkamp, M.M., Linthorst, G.A., van Leeuwen, L., Willemse, E.J., van Dijk, W.C., et al. (1999). At home management of aplastic phase following high-dose chemotherapy with stem-cell rescue for non-hematological malignancies. *Annals of Oncology, 10,* 493–494.

Westerman, I.L., & Bennett, C.L. (1996). A review of the costs, cost-effectiveness, and third-party charges of bone marrow transplantation. *Stem Cells, 14,* 312–319.

Whedon, M.B. (1995). Bone marrow transplantation nursing: Into the twenty-first century. In P.C. Buchsel & M.B. Whedon (Eds.), *Bone marrow transplantation: Administrative and clinical strategies* (pp. 3–18). Sudbury, MA: Jones and Bartlett.

Whedon, M.B., & Wujcik, D. (Eds.). (1997). *Blood and marrow stem cell transplantation: Principles, practice, and nursing insights* (2nd ed.). Sudbury, MA: Jones and Bartlett.

Wilkins, V.J. (1995). Pharmaceutical services for a BMT program. In P.C. Buchsel & M.B. Whedon (Eds.), *Bone marrow transplantation: Administrative and clinical strategies* (pp. 137–151). Sudbury, MA: Jones and Bartlett.

Yoder, L.H. (1998). Costs and outcomes of a military bone marrow transplant program. *Military Medicine, 163,* 661–666.

CHAPTER 6

Graft Versus Host Disease

Overview and Significance of the Problem

Early human transplants of allogeneic marrow often were complicated by graft versus host disease (GVHD), and GVHD remains one of the most serious transplant-related complications adversely affecting the overall success of allogeneic hematopoietic stem cell transplantation (HSCT). As the treatment of infections and procedure-related complications has improved, GVHD has emerged as the main factor limiting the wider application of allogeneic HSCT. Despite improved immunosuppression, the overall incidence of GVHD has remained between 30% and 60% and still caries a mortality of up to 50% (Ringden & Deeg, 1997). Strategies to reduce the risk of developing GVHD include selecting a histocompatible hematopoietic stem cell donor, T cell depletion of the stem cell product, and post-transplant immunosuppression and immune modulation. Although GVHD can be a major cause of morbidity and mortality in allogeneic HSCT and may significantly affect the quality of life of long-term survivors, strategies aimed at completely eliminating GVHD can have effects that are just as devastating, resulting in an increased incidence of disease relapse, fatal infections, and graft failure (Ringden, 1993). The goal of current and future research is to design graft engineering and immunomodulatory approaches that achieve rapid and durable engraftment and limit the development of severe GVHD while preserving a graft versus tumor effect (Appelbaum, 2002; Barrett, 1995; Bittencourt et al., 2002; Haddad, Saade, & Safieh-Garabedian, 2003; Morton, Hutchins, & Durant, 2001; Noga & O'Donnell, 1998; Talmadge, 2003).

Definitions

GVHD occurs when immunologically competent donor-derived T lymphocytes (the *graft*) recognize as foreign the antigens and cells in the transplant recipient (or *host*) and mount an immunologic attack. The attack of these donor-derived T lymphocytes causes damage of varying degrees of severity to recipient or host tissues (*disease*). Thus, the term is given, *graft versus host disease*, to describe the result of this immunologic assault.

As first proposed by Billingham (1966), three conditions are required for the development of GVHD. First, the graft must contain a sufficient number of *immunologically competent* cells. Second, the host or recipient must possess tissue antigens that are not present in the donor *so that the host appears foreign to the graft*. Third, the host must be *incapable of mounting an effective immunologic response to destroy the transplanted cells*.

GVHD is clinically divided into acute and chronic GVHD based on the time of onset, distinct pathophysiology, and different clinical presentations (Goker, Haznedaroglu, & Chao, 2001). The term *acute GVHD* is used to a describe a distinctive syndrome affecting the liver, skin, gastrointestinal (GI) tract, and immune system that occurs within 100 days of allogeneic HSCT. The term *chronic GVHD* describes a syndrome that is more variable in its manifestations and develops after day +100.

The distinction of acute and chronic GVHD based on the time frame of before or after day +100 may be less applicable in the era of cord blood transplantation and nonmyeloablative transplantation and subsequent donor lymphocyte infusion (DLI). These and other novel approaches to allogeneic HSCT are changing the time frames for the development and perhaps even the character of the presenting symptoms of acute and chronic GVHD (Akpek et al., 2002; Michallet et al., 2001; Sanz et al., 2001; Sanz & Sanz, 2002; Schetelig et al., 2002; Silberstein et al., 2001). However, the clinical and sometimes histopathologic features of acute and chronic GVHD, regardless of the time frame in which they develop, may help in distinguishing each form of GVHD (Heymer, 2002).

Since the criteria for the development of GVHD were first identified (Billingham, 1966), they have been revised somewhat, in that scientists and clinicians have recognized that a GVHD syndrome can occur with autologous and syngeneic HSCT (Hess, 1997; Miura et al., 2001) and with infusion of nonirradiated blood products in immunoincompetent individuals (Anderson, 1997).

Biology and Pathogenesis of Acute Graft Versus Host Disease

Much has been learned about the pathogenesis of GVHD. This improved understanding of the biology of GVHD will bring new directions for therapies to prevent and treat GVHD, while preserving the beneficial aspects of the phenomenon (Ordemann et al., 2002; Reddy et al., 2003; van Leeuwen, Guiffre, Atkinson, Rainer, & Sewell, 2002).

GVHD occurs when T lymphocytes contained in an allogeneic hematopoietic stem cell graft proliferate and differentiate in vivo in response to antigens present on host tissue that are recognized by the graft as foreign. Directly, and through the secretion of inflammatory cytokines (Ferrara, 1998), these donor T lymphocytes attack host tissues, thus producing the signs and symptoms of acute GVHD. A three-phase conceptual model for the pathogenesis of GVHD has been proposed by Ferrara and Antin (1999), Ferrara, Levy, and Chao (1999), and Goker et al. (2001) and is depicted in Figure 6-1. The first phase involves tissue damage second-

ary to the conditioning regimen, while the second phase consists of donor T cell activation, stimulation, and proliferation. In the third phase, these donor T cells produce, either directly or indirectly, tissue damage within the target organs.

Phase One—Host Tissue Damage Facilitates Antigen Presentation

The first phase in the development of GVHD is initiated even before donor cells are infused. The transplant conditioning regimen of chemotherapy and radiation therapy damages and activates host tissues, including the intestinal mucosa, the liver, and the skin. In response to this tissue damage, inflammatory cytokines are secreted, including tumor necrosis factor (TNF)-α, interleukin (IL)-1, transforming growth factor (TGF)-ß, IL-12, and many others. These cytokines cause the damaged tissues to attract and retain white blood cells. They also upregulate major histocompatibility complex (MHC) and minor histocompatibility antigens (mHAs) present on host tissues. This upregulation of MHC and mHA antigens makes it easier for the mature donor T cells contained in the stem cell graft to recognize the host's tissues as foreign and mount an inflammatory response.

Phase Two—Donor T Cell Activation and Cytokine Production

In this second phase, the donor T lymphocytes contained in the stem cell graft recognize recipient or host tissues as foreign and mount a series of responses. These responses include recruitment of donor and residual host antigen-presenting cells, activation and stimulation of T lymphocytes, and proliferation and differentiation of these activated T cells.

The stem cell transplant graft that is infused into the circulation of the recipient contains both the pluripotent stem cells, which are necessary to establish engraftment, and mature T lymphocytes. These donor-derived mature T lymphocytes circulate in the recipient's blood stream, coming into extensive contact with many minor antigens expressed on the surface of the recipient's cells. Even in related transplants, where the major histocompatibility antigens are matched, the donor T cells will recognize one or more of the recipient's minor antigens as foreign, and they will bind to the antigen. Once bound to the antigen-presenting cell, co-stimulatory signals direct a subset of T lymphocytes— T-helper or Th-1 lymphocytes—to begin producing several pro-inflammatory cytokines, including IL-12, IL-2, and interferon-γ (IFN-γ), and to increase expression of receptors for these cytokines on the surface of the T cell. These cytokines recruit cytotoxic T lymphocyte (CTL) and natural killer (NK) cell responses and stimulate both donor and residual host monocytes to produce IL-1 and TNF-α. The activated T cells expand and differentiate over the three to five days following antigen recognition, producing the specific cytokines that result in the recruitment of CTLs and NK cells to enact the cell and tissue destruction in target organs

Figure 6-1. Pathophysiology of Graft Versus Host Disease

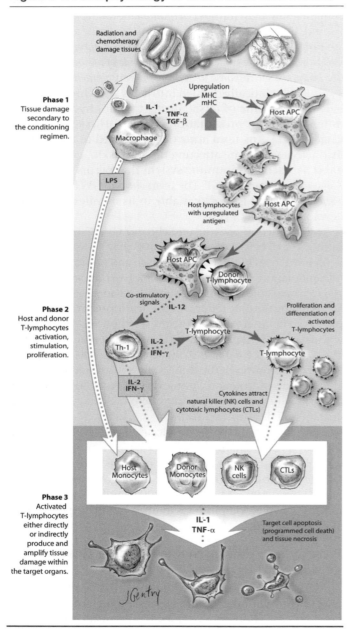

HEMATOPOIETIC STEM CELL TRANSPLANTATION: A MANUAL FOR NURSING PRACTICE

that is postulated to occur in the final phase of the graft versus host reaction.

Phase Three—Graft Versus Host Disease Target Tissues Destroyed

It is hypothesized that the tissue destruction and end-organ dysfunction that produce the signs and symptoms of GVHD result from several additive and synergistic mechanisms. First, there is direct cytolytic damage in the target organs of the skin, gut, and liver caused by CTLs that are recruited by the cytokines (IL-2 and IFN-γ) released by the Th-1 lymphocytes in phase II. The Th-1 lymphocytes also stimulate CTLs and NK cells to increase their secretion of inflammatory cytokines, including TNF-α and IL-1. TNF-α plays an important role in the pathophysiology of acute GVHD, and studies have demonstrated elevated levels of TNF-α in the serum of patients with acute GVHD (Lindgren et al., 1997). TNF- α can cause direct tissue damage by inducing necrosis of target cells, or it may induce tissue destruction through apoptosis or programmed cell death. In addition to these proinflammatory cytokines, excess nitric oxide produced by activated CTLs may contribute to the deleterious effects of the cytokines on GVHD target tissues (Ferrara, 1995; Nestel, Greene, Kichian, Ponka, & Lapp, 2000). It is also thought that the damage to intestinal cells caused by the conditioning regimen, as discussed for phase I, results in the release of lipopolysaccharide (LPS), an endotoxin. LPS subsequently may stimulate gut-associated lymphocytes and macrophages to increase their secretion of TNF-α and IL-1 (Hill et al., 1997; Hill & Ferrara, 2000). LPS reaching skin tissues also may stimulate keratinocytes, dermal fibroblasts, and macrophages to produce similar cytokines in the dermis and epidermis. Thus, monocytes that have been primed by Th-1 cytokines to secrete TNF-α and IL-1 receive a second triggering signal to increase their secretion of TNF-α and IL-1 from LPS; this is a result of damage to intestinal cells caused by the conditioning regimen (Hill & Ferrara). In phase III, inflammatory cytokines intensify the cellular damage caused by CTLs and NK cells, amplifying local tissue injury and further promoting an inflammatory response, all of which ultimately lead to the observed target tissue destruction in the HSCT host.

Ferrara and Antin (1999) and Ferrara et al. (1999) summarized the pathogenesis of acute GVHD as an exaggerated and undesirable manifestation of a normal physiologic inflammatory mechanism. When donor cells are transplanted into the recipient, they encounter a host that has been profoundly damaged, and they react in a fashion that would foster the control or resolution of an invasion of foreign substances under ordinary circumstances (Ferrara & Antin). The net effects of this complex interaction among T lymphocytes and other inflammatory cells, cytokines, and their resultant cellular targets are the severe inflammatory manifestations we recognize as clinical GVHD (Ferrara, 1995).

The role of inflammatory cytokines in GVHD may explain a number of unique and seemingly unrelated aspects of GVHD (Ferrara, 1995; Ferrara et al., 1999). For example, the principal target organs of acute GVHD all share an extensive exposure to endotoxins and other bacterial products that can trigger and amplify local inflammation. These target organs also have large populations of antigen-presenting cells that may facilitate the graft versus host reaction (Ferrara et al.). Further, a number of studies have noted that an increased risk of GVHD is associated with certain intensive conditioning regimens and with viral infection (Goker et al., 2001). The reduction in GVHD seen in certain groups of patients undergoing transplantation in laminar airflow environments with gut decontamination may be explained by the reduction of bacterial endotoxins on the skin and gut. Viral infections also are commonly associated with GVHD. They are more frequent in patients with GVHD, and a viral illness may cause the initiation of GVHD or worsening of established GVHD. Cytomegalovirus infection has a particularly close association with GVHD (Einsele et al., 1994), as does herpes simplex virus (Adler et al., 1998; Gratama, Sinnige, & Weijers, 1987) and possibly human herpes virus-6 (Appleton, Sviland, Peiris, Taylor, & Wilkes, 1995). Although the precise pathophysiology of this connection remains uncertain, it may be that cellular damage to the intestine or liver as a result of these infections may result in the release of endotoxins. Alternatively, GVHD may result because of either a virus-induced activated T cell or an NK cell attack (Matzinger, 1994). It also may be that viral infections flare in the setting of GVHD, either as a result of the intensified immunosuppressive therapy or as a result of the intrinsic immunosuppression of GVHD.

Based on the roles postulated for donor T lymphocytes, IL-1, IL-2, and TNF-α, a wide variety of immunomodulatory approaches to the prevention or control of GVHD have been designed or are in development (Chao, 1999b; Gaziev, Galimberti, Lucarelli, & Polchi, 2000; Przepiorka, 2000; Teshima & Ferrara, 2002). For example, corticosteroids interfere with antigen processing and presentation and induce apoptosis of activated lymphocytes. Monoclonal antibodies have been developed targeting activated T lymphocytes with overexpression of TNF-α receptor (infliximab, Remicade®, Centocor, Malvern, PA) or IL-2 receptors (daclizumab, Zenapax®, Roche Pharmaceuticals, Nutley, NJ). T cell depletion strategies attempt to remove T lymphocytes from the stem cell product prior to transplantation or to remove T lymphocytes from the circulation through the use of a monoclonal antibody that destroys lymphocytes (Kottaridis et al., 2000). Cyclosporine and tacrolimus are potent inhibitors of early phases of T cell activation, and antimetabolites, such as mycophenolate mofetil (MMF), interfere with T lymphocyte proliferation. Studies of keratinocyte growth factor suggest that it may limit the severity of GVHD in the GI tract by reducing LPS and TNF-α levels (Krijanovski et al., 1999). These and other approaches for the prevention or treatment of GVHD are discussed in more detail later in this chapter.

Predictive Factors for Acute Graft Versus Host Disease

Some of the factors associated with a greater incidence and severity of GVHD include pretransplant splenectomy, more advanced disease at the time of transplantation, inclusion of more than 1,200 cGy of total body irradiation in the conditioning regimen, early engraftment, viral serology in the donor or recipient (higher risk of GVHD when recipient is cytomegalovirus [CMV] or Epstein-Barr virus [EBV] seropositive; higher risk when donor is herpes simplex virus [HSV] or CMV seropositive or EBV seronegative), and specific human leukocyte antigen (HLA) groups (Chao, 1999a; Deeg & Henslee-Downey, 1990; Ringden, 1993; Ringden & Deeg, 1997; Socie & Cahn, 1998). Whether the use of peripheral blood stem cells instead of bone marrow leads to more GVHD remains controversial. Studies suggest that although the use of peripheral blood stem cells (PBSCs) is associated with significantly better overall survival, it also may be associated with a higher incidence of both acute and chronic GVHD (Couban et al., 2002; Cutler et al., 2001; Schmitz & Barrett, 2002). In contrast, other studies have shown that there is no increased risk of GVHD associated with the use of PBSCs, even in unrelated donor transplants (Remberger et al., 2001; Ustun et al., 1999). It has been hypothesized that there should be less GVHD associated with nonmyeloablative HSCT because there is less tissue injury with these reduced-intensity conditioning regimens and because there should be less GVHD in a state of mixed chimerism. However, to date, studies have not consistently demonstrated a reduced risk of GVHD in these recipients (Anagnostopoulos & Giralt, 2002; Schetelig et al., 2002). The factors that are associated with a higher risk of acute GVHD are summarized in Table 6-1.

Clinical and Histopathologic Features of Acute Graft Versus Host Disease

The classic target organs of acute GVHD are the skin, intestinal tract, and liver. Any one organ or combination of these organs may be affected. Involvement of each organ system is assessed clinically and pathologically, and staging is generally summarized in the form of an overall grade, as discussed later in this chapter.

Dermatitis

A maculopapular skin rash, usually occurring at or near the time of the white blood cell engraftment, is the first and most common clinical manifestation of acute GVHD. Early stages of the rash may be pruritic or painful and may be described as a sunburn. Classically, the first areas involved include the nape of the neck, ears, and the shoulders, as well as the palms of the hands and the soles of the feet. The rash may spread, becoming more confluent and involving the whole integument. In severe GVHD, the maculopapular rash can evolve into generalized erythroderma and bullous lesions, often progressing to desquamation and epidermal necrolysis (Goker et al., 2001) (see Figure 6-2).

Differential diagnosis of a post-transplant skin rash includes chemoradiotherapy effects, drug allergy, and viral infection. Careful history and physical examination, consultation with dermatology, and skin biopsy are helpful in establishing the diagnosis. Biopsy of the skin rash will reveal classic dermal and epidermal changes, including exocytosed lymphocytes, dyskeratotic epidermal keratinocytes, follicular involvement, satellite lymphocytes adjacent to or surrounding dyskeratotic epidermal keratinocytes, and dermal perivascular lymphocytic infiltration (Darmstadt, Donnenberg, Vogelsang, Farmer, & Horn, 1992). However, histopathologic confirmation may be limited by the fact that similar changes also can be seen within the first few months after chemotherapy or radiation therapy and may occur with infection (Chao, 1999a; Heymer, 2002; Norton, 1995). Serial biopsies and careful observation of the features of the skin rash help establish the diagnosis and severity of GVHD. Viral studies for CMV and human herpes virus-6 may help to differentiate GVHD from a viral exanthem.

Hepatitis

The liver is the second most commonly involved organ in acute GVHD. The earliest and most common abnormality is a rise in the direct bilirubin, alkaline phosphatase, and aminotransferases, reflecting a nonspecific cholestatic picture. Differential diagnoses include hepatic veno-occlusive disease, the effects of the preparatory regimen, total parenteral nutrition, viral infection, sepsis, and drug toxicity, including the drugs cyclosporine A, tacrolimus, and methotrexate, which are used for GVHD prophylaxis (Chao, 1999a; Sullivan, 1999; Vinayek, Demetris, & Rakela, 2000).

Hepatotoxicity caused by tacrolimus or cyclosporine A usually improves within several days of modifying the dose. Transjugular liver biopsy may be performed, revealing bile duct atypia and degeneration, cholestasis, lymphocytic infiltration of portal tracts, degeneration and destruction of small bile ducts, periportal fibrosis, and hepatocyte degeneration (Chao, 1999a; Strasser & McDonald, 1999). A hepatitic variant of GVHD of the liver, characterized by markedly elevated transaminases and histologic evidence of lobular hepatitis, has been described following DLI (Akpek et al., 2002).

Gastrointestinal Tract

The third main organ system to be affected by GVHD is the gut, and it is often the most severe. Symptoms of acute GVHD of the distal small bowel and colon include profuse diarrhea, intestinal bleeding, crampy abdominal pain, distention, and paralytic ileus. The diarrhea is often green, mucoid, watery, and mixed with exfoliated cells and tissue shreds. Paralytic ileus may develop associated with the GVHD or with the increased use of narcotics to control the physical discomfort. Voluminous secretory diarrhea may persist even with cessation of oral intake and can be in excess of 10 liters per day (Goker et al., 2001). The diarrhea

Table 6-1. Factors Influencing the Incidence and Severity of Acute Graft Versus Host Disease

Factor	Less GVHD	More GVHD
Degree of donor-recipient histocompatibility	Human leukocyte antigen (HLA)-identical related donors	HLA-matched unrelated donors HLA-mismatched related donors (haploidentical, one or two antigen mismatches), with increasing degrees of histoincompatibility associated with more GVHD
Source of stem cells	Bone marrow Umbilical cord blood	Peripheral blood
CD34+ cell dose		Suggestion that higher CD34+ cell dose that often occurs with peripheral blood stem cell collection associated with more acute GVHD
Type of pretransplant conditioning regimen	Nonmyeloablative preparative regimens are hypothesized to produce less acute GVHD; however, to date, there is no evidence that these preparative regimens are associated with a lower incidence or severity of GVHD. Incidence of chronic GVHD with these regimens is not yet known.	Regimens that include intense, myeloablative conditioning chemotherapy and total body irradiation are associated with more GVHD.
Cellular composition of the graft	T cell depleted	Unmanipulated T cell repleted
Intensity of GVHD prophylaxis used	Broader prophylaxis with one or more agents at full doses FK 506 may be more potent than cyclosporine A for prevention of acute GVHD.	Prophylaxis with single agent or reduced dose/attenuated course of prophylaxis (e.g., reduced dose of cyclosporine or tacrolimus; omission of one or more post-transplant methotrexate doses) associated with increased GVHD
Donor-recipient sex match	Male to male Male to female	Female to male
Donor-recipient viral serologies		Donor and recipient cytomegalovirus seropositivity
Donor parity	Nulliparous female	Parous female
Donor transfusion status	Donor never received blood transfusions.	Donor previously transfused
Age of recipient/donor	Younger	Older
Host microenvironment	Protective environment, including skin and gut decontamination	No special protective environment; no skin and gut decontamination
History of prior splenectomy		Splenectomy before transplantation may increase GVHD risk.

Note. Based on information from Anagnostopoulos & Giralt, 2002; Chao, 1999a, 1999b; Cutler et al., 2001; Flowers et al., 1999; Goker et al., 2001; Kanfer, 1995; Passweg et al., 1998; Przepiorka, 2000; Przepiorka, Smith, et al., 1999; Ringden & Deeg, 1997; Sanz & Sanz, 2002; Schetelig et al., 2002; Socie & Cahn, 1998.

initially may be watery, but often becomes progressively bloodier, with increasing transfusion requirements. Hypoalbuminemia, at times severe, can occur secondary to GVHD-associated intestinal protein leak and negative nitrogen balance. Patients also may present with upper GI symptoms, including nausea, vomiting, anorexia, food intolerance, and dyspepsia (Goker et al.).

GVHD of the gut should be considered among the differential diagnoses whenever an HSCT recipient experiences abdominal pain, nausea and vomiting, diarrhea, or hyperbilirubinemia (Williams, 1999). Other possible etiologies for these GI symptoms include residual effects of chemotherapy and radiation therapy and intestinal infection, primarily CMV, *Candida* species, or *Clostridium difficile* in the lower GI

Figure 6-2. Acute Graft Versus Host Disease of the Skin

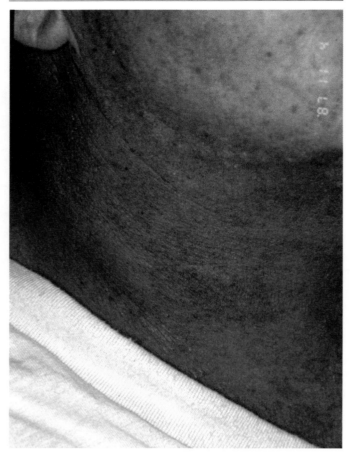

Fine, discrete, and confluent erythematous, blanchable macules and papules involving the upper trunk. Lesions may be pruritic or slightly tender with palpation. Earliest skin findings usually seen on face, palms/soles, and upper trunk.

Note. Photo courtesy of Ontario Cancer Institute, Toronto, Canada. Used with permission.

tract and CMV, HSV, or *Candida* species in the upper GI tract (Heymer, 2002). Lower or upper endoscopy or both may be required to evaluate the patient's symptoms. Enteric cultures are needed to rule out infection.

Endoscopic findings suggestive of GVHD include mucosal erythema, edema, and mucosal sloughing involving the cecum, ileum, ascending colon, stomach, duodenum, and rectum (Sullivan, 1999) (see Figure 6-3). Whole areas may be denuded, similar to the loss of epithelium that is observed in the skin (Chao, 1999a; Ponec, 1999). Histopathologic confirmation of enteric GVHD includes crypt-cell apoptosis and drop out, accumulation of cellular debris within crypts, variable lymphocytic infiltration of the epithelium, and, in severe cases, total epithelial denudation (Chao, 1998; Norton, 1995; Ponec; Sullivan). As with biopsies of skin, early after HSCT, it may be difficult to distinguish GVHD from the effects of chemoradiotherapy conditioning (Norton).

Imaging of the bowel with CT scanning typically includes mucosal enhancement, diffuse bowel involvement, and

fluid-filled dilated bowel loops (Donnelly & Morris, 1996). Bowel wall thickening often is absent in acute GVHD but may be present in chronic GVHD (Benya & Goldman, 1997). An uncommon complication is formation of a stricture and subsequent obstruction of the small bowel (Benya & Goldman). Klein et al. (2001) described the use of high-resolution ultrasonography and color Doppler imaging as useful tools for detecting acute GVHD of the lower intestine even before clinical symptoms occur. This modality may have use in defining the severity of acute GVHD in a noninvasive fashion in those patients who do not have clinical symptoms of acute GVHD of the GI tract and in following a patient's response to immunosuppressive therapy.

Other Manifestations of Acute Graft Versus Host Disease

Subtle effects on hematopoiesis and immune functioning also can occur with acute GVHD. These include hypogammaglobulinemia; a decline in white blood cells, hematocrit levels, and platelet counts; increased risk of infection, especially CMV infection; and decreased responsiveness to immunization (Chao, 1999a). Other findings that may be noted in patients with acute GVHD include photophobia, hemorrhagic conjunctivitis (Saito et al., 2002), scleritis (Kim et al., 2002), infectious and noninfectious pneumonia, and serositis (Przepiorka & Cleary, 2000). Endothelialitis may present as microangiopathic hemolytic anemia, involving microangiopathy, hemolysis, and thrombocytopenia

Figure 6-3. Acute Graft Versus Host Disease of the GI Tract

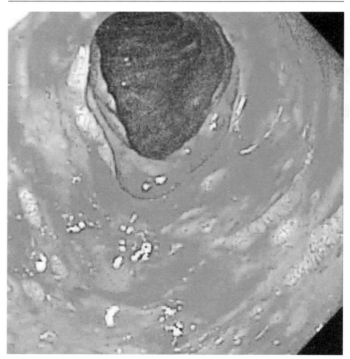

Images obtained during endoscopy demonstrate tissue edema, extensive erythema, and mucosal ulcerations.

Note. Photo courtesy of Dr. Bruce Greenwald, University of Maryland Medical Center, Baltimore. Used with permission.

(Daly, Hasegawa, Lipton, Messner, & Kiss, 2002; Przepiorka & Cleary; Sullivan, 1999). A case of acute GVHD presenting with an acquired lupus anticoagulant also has been described (Kharfan-Dabaja, Morgensztern, Santos, Goodman, & Fernandez, 2003).

Hyperacute GVHD is a severe fulminant form of acute GVHD that is frequently fatal but, fortunately, is rare in the setting of GVHD prophylaxis. It develops 7–14 days after transplantation, and its manifestations include fever, generalized erythroderma, desquamation, severe hepatitis, noncardiogenic pulmonary edema, and vascular leakage (Sullivan, 1999).

Grading and Staging Systems for Acute Graft Versus Host Disease

The severity of GVHD is determined both histologically and clinically. The Glucksberg grading and staging of GVHD involves the assessment of the degree of skin, liver, and gut involvement, with the staging of each organ system, then the summarization in the form of an overall grade. Approximating the daily amount of diarrhea, identifying the level of hyperbilirubinemia, and distinguishing maculopapular rashes from erythroderma with bullous formation are the factors that are considered in determining the stage and grade of GVHD (see Table 6-2). As illustrated in Figure 6-4, the Rule of Nines method is used to estimate the extent of skin involvement. Clinically significant acute GVHD usually is defined as overall grades II–IV. Although the hematopoietic and immune systems are a sensitive target for acute GVHD, they are not included in the grading.

Several problems with the Glucksberg et al. (1974) staging and grading system for acute GVHD have been identified, and additional work is needed to refine current systems or develop new ones. Some of the limitations include a failure to consider the kinetics of GVHD (e.g., subclinical disease); the variability in interobserver stage or grade assignment; the requirement that patients with different patterns of skin, liver, and gut involvement (who also have significantly different risks of treatment-related mortality and treatment failure) may be assigned the same summary grade; and the fact that additional target organs such as the conjunctivae and immune system are not addressed (Deeg & Henslee-Downey, 1990). Recently, the International Bone Marrow Transplant Registry (IBMTR) designed a new staging system from a large data set of adult patients receiving an HLA-identical sibling transplant (Rowlings et al., 1997). The IBMTR Severity Index appeared to be more predictive of the risk of transplant-related mortality and treatment failure than the Glucksberg criteria (Martino et al., 1999). The IBMTR Severity Index is presented in Table 6-2.

Onset and Incidence of Acute Graft Versus Host Disease

The onset of acute GVHD generally occurs between 14 and 60 days post-transplantation; however, if methotrexate is not used for GVHD prophylaxis, the onset may be as early as the first week post-transplantation (Przepiorka & Cleary, 2000). Neutrophil recovery is not necessary for GVHD to occur, and the signs of GVHD may be noted prior to hematopoietic engraftment (Przepiorka & Cleary). Acute GVHD also may occur after DLI for the prevention or treatment of disease relapse after transplantation. The clinical manifestations of acute GVHD following DLI are the same as when GVHD develops post-transplant. The median time to onset of GVHD is approximately one month after DLI (Przepiorka & Cleary).

Even with intensive immunosuppression, clinically significant acute GVHD, defined as grade II–IV or higher, occurs in 9%–50% of patients who receive an HLA-identical sibling HSCT, and the incidence in unrelated HLA-matched HSCT may approach 70%. The development of grade II, III, or IV GVHD significantly affects the outcome of HSCT, with only 40%–50% of those patients who develop grade II–IV GVHD experiencing long-term survival (Chao, 1999a; Fleming, 2002).

Chronic Graft Versus Host Disease

Chronic GVHD remains the most common late complication of allogeneic HSCT. Although there have been significant improvements in the prevention and treatment of acute GVHD, these advancements have not substantially reduced the incidence of chronic GVHD. Moreover, as the demographics of HSCT shift to include more unrelated donor transplants, older transplant recipients, and more heavily pretreated recipients, the incidence of GVHD is expected to increase (Marcellus & Vogelsang, 2000).

Pathogenesis of Chronic Graft Versus Host Disease

Although less is known about the pathogenesis of chronic GVHD, it is hypothesized that it includes all of the mechanisms outlined previously for acute GVHD, as well as an autoimmune aspect. In chronic GVHD, the T lymphocytes come to recognize as foreign not only the minor histocompatibility antigens (those antigens that are not able to be matched between recipient and donor) but also the major histocompatibility antigens (those antigens that are generally completely matched between patient and donor) (Ferrara & Antin, 1999). The development of these self- or autoreactive T cells is thought to be related to impaired functioning of the thymus (Sullivan, 1999; Teshima et al., 2003; Vogelsang & Hess, 1994). When the thymus is functioning normally, it is capable of eliminating autoreactive T lymphocytes before they can mount a response against the host (Sykes & Strober, 1999). When the thymus is damaged, whether by age, injury from the chemotherapy and radiation therapy used in the conditioning regimen, or acute GVHD, its ability to delete these autoreactive T cells may be impaired. This can result in circulating T lymphocytes programmed to recognize the host as foreign and stimulate the cytokine cascade similar to that described for

Table 6-2. Staging and Grading Systems for Acute Graft Versus Host Disease

Consensus Criteria for Clinical Staging and Grading of Acute GVHD

Organ	Grade	Description
Skin	+1	Maculopapular eruption over < 25% of body area
	+2	Maculopapular eruption over 25%–50% of body area
	+3	Generalized erythroderma
	+4	Generalized erythroderma with bullous formation and often with desquamation
Liver	+1	Bilirubin 2–3 mg/dl
	+2	Bilirubin 3.1–6 mg/dl
	+3	Bilirubin 6.1–15 mg/dl
	+4	Bilirubin > 15 mg/dl
Gut	+1	Diarrhea > 500 ml/day or > 30 ml/kg
	+2	Diarrhea > 1,000 ml/day or > 60 ml/kg
	+3	Diarrhea > 1,500 ml/day or > 90 ml/kg
	+4	Diarrhea > 2,000 ml/day or > 120 ml/kg

Overall Stage

Stage	Skin	Liver	Gut	Performance Status
I	+1 to +2	0	0	No decrease
II	+1 to +3	+1	and/or +1	Mild decrease
III	+2 to +3	+2 to +3	and/or +2 to +3	Marked decrease
IV	+2 to +4	+2 to +4	and/or +2 to +4	Extreme decrease

If no skin disease is present, the overall grade is the higher, single organ stage.

Criteria for International Bone Marrow Transplant Register Severity Index for Acute GVHD

Index*	Extent of Rash		Total Bilirubin		Volume of Diarrhea
A	< 25%	or	< 2 mg/dl	or	< 500 ml/day
B	25%–50%	or	2–6 mg/dl	or	500-1,500 ml/day
C	> 50%	or	6.1–15 mg/dl	or	> 1,500 ml/day
D	Bullae	or	> 15 mg/dl	or	Severe pain or ileus

*Index assigned based on maximum organ involvement.

Note. Based on information from Glucksberg et al., 1974.

acute GVHD (Vogelsang & Hess). Thymic damage also results in the formation of autoantibodies, similar to those noted in other chronic autoimmune disorders. Autoantibody formation has been noted in experimental models of chronic GVHD, and clinical reports replicate these findings (Lister, Messner, Keystone, Miller, & Fritzler, 1987). Thymic damage also may help to explain GVHD that develops in the setting of autologous transplant or syngeneic transplant, where autoreactive T cells have been identified as well. Newer research also has suggested that the manifestations of chronic GVHD may be a reflection of the progressive loss of the microvasculature and resultant replacement fibrosis in target tissues, such as the skin, lung, and liver—a reaction that was initially mediated by cytotoxic T lymphocytes (Biedermann et al., 2002).

Incidence and Predictive Factors

Among patients who survived 150 days after allogeneic stem cell transplantation, chronic GVHD was observed in 33%–49% of HLA-identical related transplant and in 64% of matched unrelated donor transplants (Przepiorka et al., 2001; Sullivan et al., 1991). Chronic GVHD may be as high as 60% following DLI (Collins, Shpilberg, & Drobyski, 1997; Mackinnon et al., 1995; Peggs & Mackinnon, 2001).

Risk factors for chronic GVHD include previous acute GVHD, older recipient age, and female donor to male recipient (Carlens et al., 1998). The incidence of chronic GVHD also may be higher in recipients of PBSCs versus recipients of bone marrow derived stem cells (Couban et al., 2002; Cutler et al., 2001), although this issue has not been fully resolved. A continuing need for corticosteroids

Figure 6-4. Rule of Nines

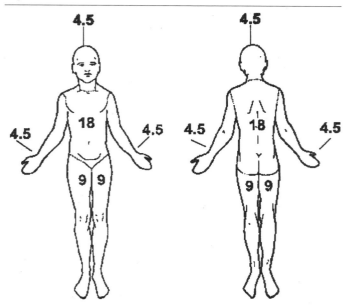

The Rule of Nines body surface area diagram is used to estimate the percentage of body surface involved with graft versus host disease of the skin.

for control of GVHD by day +100 was also a significant risk factor for the development of chronic GVHD (Wagner et al., 1998).

Subacute chronic GVHD detected by skin biopsy or buccal mucosal biopsy has been shown to be a strong predictor for subsequent development of chronic GVHD (Wagner et al., 1998). A recent preliminary report also suggested that lip and skin biopsies with histologic evidence of GVHD and a positive Schirmer's test at day +100 are associated with an increased risk of mortality (Wagner, Flowers, Longton, Storb, & Martin, 2001). In some transplant programs, periodic skin and buccal mucosal biopsies are part of the routine post-transplant surveillance of allogeneic HSCT recipients (Loughran et al., 1990). However, no data exist to suggest that treatment should be initiated in the absence of clinically evident GVHD (Vogelsang, 2001). Patients with a history of acute GVHD, patients who received HSCT from matched unrelated or mismatched related donors, and those with histopathologic or other evidence of subclinical chronic GVHD on surveillance studies should be closely monitored for the development of chronic GVHD (Marcellus & Vogelsang, 2000).

Clinical and Histopathologic Features of Chronic Graft Versus Host Disease

Clinical manifestations of chronic GVHD resemble those of progressive systemic sclerosis, systemic lupus erythematosus, lichen planus, Sjogren's syndrome, and rheumatoid arthritis. The manifestations of chronic GVHD are seen in the skin, liver, eyes, oral cavity, lungs, GI system, neuromuscular system, and a variety of other body systems.

Cutaneous

The skin is the most commonly involved organ in chronic GVHD. Two types of cutaneous involvement have been described: sclerodermatous (similar to scleroderma) and lichenoid (similar to lichen planus). The onset of skin involvement may be generalized erythema, with plaques and extensive areas of desquamation. This can progress, without treatment, to a skin that is hyper- and/or hypopigmented with tightening (hide-like skin), atrophy, and telangiectasias. Joint contractures similar to scleroderma can occur as a result. The skin involvement can occur anywhere and does not show the typical distribution of acute GVHD. Localized chronic GVHD of the skin demonstrates nodular induration and dyspigmentation, whereas the generalized type frequently exhibits severe poikiloderma (atrophy of the skin with associated pigmentation changes, erythema, and telangiectasias) with diffuse areas of hypo- and hyperpigmentation and, if progressive, contractures, alopecia, damage or loss of nails, and skin ulcerations (Heymer, 2002) (see Figures 6-5, 6-6, 6-7, 6-8, and 6-9). Skin damaged from either acute GVHD, sun exposure, or herpes zoster infection may be more susceptible to chronic GVHD.

Skin biopsy is helpful in establishing the diagnosis. Histomorphologically, lichenoid lesions show slight epidermal hyperplasia and a band-like lymphocytic infiltration of the upper dermis, close to the dermo-epidermal junction (Heymer, 2002). Occasionally, individual apoptotic keratinocytes are seen, and the changes bear a striking resemblance to lichen planus. With increasing deposition of collagen, the changes acquire a scleroderma-like picture. The overlying epidermis becomes diffusely atrophic, and the rete ridges disappear. There also is atrophy and fibrosis of adnexal structures. In contrast to acute GVHD, involvement of the eccrine glands is a characteristic of chronic GVHD (Heymer).

Figure 6-5. Lichenoid Chronic Graft Versus Host Disease of the Lumbar Region

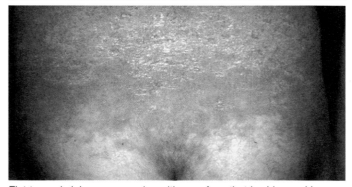

Flat-topped violaceous papules with a surface that is shiny and has a lacy white pattern. The eruption is confluent in some areas, and hypertrophic plaques have developed.

Note. Photo courtesy of T.L. Diepgen & G. Yihune, Dermatology Online Atlas (www.dermis.net/doia/). Used with permission.

Figure 6-6. Lichenoid Chronic Graft Versus Host Disease of the Abdomen and Inguinal Fold

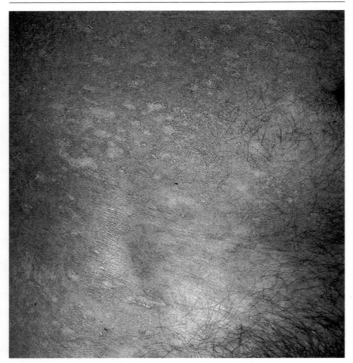

Flat-topped violaceous papules with a lacy white appearance. Many of the lesions are sharply demarcated from noninvolved tissue and are annular (oval or circular) in shape. Note the postinflammatory hyperpigmentation that has developed in some areas.

Note. Photo courtesy of T.L. Diepgen & G. Yihune, Dermatology Online Atlas (www.dermis.net/doia/). Used with permission.

Hepatic

Liver function tests manifest predominantly cholestatic abnormalities, with moderate elevations in alkaline phosphatase, bilirubin, and transaminases. Clinically, patients typically have few symptoms referable to their liver until their hepatic disease becomes severe. The differential diagnosis of late hepatic abnormalities is broad and includes viral infection, hepatotoxic drug reactions, gallstones, and fungal infection (Vinayek et al., 2000).

Liver biopsies are helpful in establishing the diagnosis. Pathology demonstrates a marked reduction or complete absence of small bile ducts, cholestasis, and a dense plasmacytic infiltration in portal areas (Sviland, 2000). Differential diagnosis of GVHD of the liver from viral infections such as CMV and hepatitis is important because immunosuppressive therapy following an erroneous diagnosis of chronic GVHD is likely to alleviate the clinical manifestations of both processes and mask an underlying viral hepatitis infection or reactivation (Schubert & Sullivan, 1990; Seth et al., 2002). The presence of cytologically atypical and destructive bile ducts on pathologic review favors the diagnosis of GVHD, whereas mononuclear cell infiltration of portal tracts and sinusoids and spotty hepatocellular necrosis suggest viral infection (Sviland).

Gastrointestinal

The small bowel and colon also may be involved in chronic GVHD. Diarrhea, abdominal pain, and cramping may be present, but the more common manifestations are of a "wasting syndrome," with malabsorption, weight loss, poor performance status, and increasing GI symptoms, such as dysphagia and early satiety, suggestive of progression of GVHD (Akpek, Chinratanalab, et al., 2003). Esophageal involvement in chronic GVHD results in dysphagia and retrosternal pain from mucosal desquamation and peptic esophagitis, with resultant fibrosis, esophageal webs, and stricture (Ratanatharathorn, Ayash, Lazarus, Fu, & Uberti, 2001). Endoscopy may reveal diffuse mucosal sloughing, with histologic examination demonstrating fibrosis and significant crypt distortion, or features more characteristic of acute GVHD of the intestine, with apoptosis—with or without cryptitis (Akpek, Chinratanalab, et al.). Pancreatic insufficiency may accompany or complicate chronic GVHD of the GI tract or liver (Akpek, Valladares, Lee, Margolis, & Vogelsang, 2001; Grigg, Angus, Hoyt, & Szer, 2003).

Ocular

Ocular involvement occurs in approximately 60% of patients with chronic GVHD (Ratanatharathorn et al., 2001). Ophthalmic symptoms of keratoconjunctivitis sicca include burning, irritation, photophobia, excessive tearing (an early manifestation), and pain. Tear function is evaluated by Schirmer's testing and fluorescein biomicroscopy of the cornea. Even in the absence of symptoms, patients should be screened for ocular sicca and started on artificial tear replacement, if indicated. Patients should be advised to wear protective eyewear outdoors, especially on windy days (Ratanatharathorn et al., 2001).

Oral

The oral mucosa is involved in more than 80% of patients with chronic GVHD. Patients develop dryness, sensitivity to acidic or spicy foods, and increasing oral pain. Lichenoid reactions range from fine white lace-like striae on buccal surfaces to large plaques on the buccal surface or the lateral tongue. Mucosal surfaces may become atrophic, with resultant gingival and buccal stippling (Schubert & Sullivan, 1990) (see Figures 6-10 and 6-11). In patients displaying sclerodermatous GVHD, a decreased oral opening due to perioral fibrosis may be seen.

Oral pain (either continuous or occurring with the stimulation of eating or oral hygiene) often is reported by patients with chronic GVHD and may be one of the first symptoms associated with the onset of chronic GVHD of the oral cavity or heralding a flare-up of disease (Schubert & Sullivan, 1990). Xerostomia also is associated with chronic GVHD, and studies of patients more than one year post-HSCT have demonstrated that chronic GVHD adversely influences salivary flow rates (Schubert & Sullivan). However, in the first four to six months after HSCT, it may be difficult to differentiate GVHD-related oral dryness from radiation-induced salivary gland dysfunction. Xerostomia is uncomfortable,

Figures 6-7 and 6-8. Chronic Graft Versus Host Disease of the Skin With Irregularly Shaped, Deeply Hyperpigmented Macular Lesions

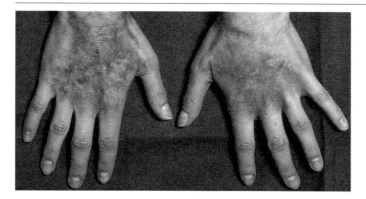 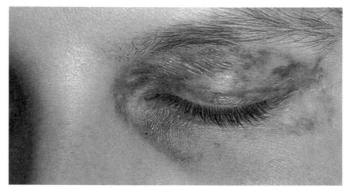

Note the atrophy of dermal and subcutaneous tissues, with paper-thin skin giving an easily wrinkled and/or shiny appearance and a prominence to the small blood vessels visible just beneath the skin surface. The term *poikiloderma* is used to describe the classic features of patchy hypopigmentation and hyperpigmentation, dermal atrophy, and telangiectasias (small diameter linear blood vessels seen on the skin's surface).

Note. Photos courtesy of T.L. Diepgen & G. Yihune, Dermatology Online Atlas (www.dermis.net/doia/). Used with permission.

may interfere with nutrition, and places patients at greater risk for dental caries. Patients with GVHD involving the oral cavity benefit from regular thorough evaluation of the oral mucosa and close follow-up because they are at greater risk for dental caries and second malignancies involving the oral mucosa (Abdelsayed et al., 2002). Fluoride treatments may be beneficial in patients at increased risk for dental caries because of xerostomia (Schubert & Sullivan).

Sino-Pulmonary

Obstructive lung disease, called bronchiolitis obliterans, is a clinical feature of chronic GVHD. In bronchiolitis obliterans, there is progressive obstruction of small bronchioles because of proliferation of the peribronchiolar tissue. This can progress to pulmonary fibrosis that often is related to cofactors such as the long-term pulmonary toxicity of total body irradiation or chemotherapy or interstitial fibrosis resulting from viral infection (Afessa, Litzow, & Tefferi, 2001; Wolff et al., 2002). A bronchodilator-resistant decrement is noted in the DLCO, FEV 1/FVC, and FEF on pulmonary function tests. Accompanying symptoms may include dry cough, dyspnea, and wheezing. Because there is also a high prevalence of sinusitis in patients with GVHD who are on immunosuppression, radiographic assessment of the paranasal sinuses is recommended (Thompson, Couch, Zahurak, Johnson, & Vogelsang, 2002). Video-assisted thoracoscopic lung biopsy is required to make a definitive histologic diagnosis. Lung biopsies show small airway involvement with fibrinous obliteration of the lumen. Peribronchiolar inflammatory cellular infiltrates consisting of neutrophils and lymphocytes also may be present (Afessa et al.).

Musculoskeletal

Myositis and myopathy have been described in patients with chronic GVHD (Couriel et al., 2002; Kaushik, Flagg, Wise, Hadfield, & McCarty, 2002; Leano, Miller, & White,

2000). Patients with GVHD frequently complain of muscle cramps, although the exact etiology of these cramps remains unclear. Patients may develop limited range of motion of joints secondary to involvement of the deeper fascia or because of thickening or sclerosis of the skin (Marcellus & Vogelsang, 2000).

Neurologic

Neurologic conditions have been reported in patients with chronic GVHD, including peripheral neuropathy and myasthenia gravis; in animal models, there is evidence of cerebral

Figure 6-9. Sclerodermatous Graft Versus Host Disease of the Skin

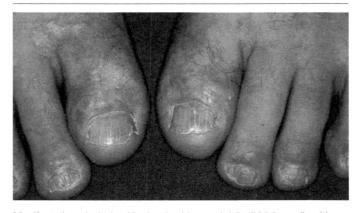

Manifestations include skin that is shiny and tight (hidebound), with edema, erythema, and fibrosis. Also seen are the nail changes (onychodystrophy) typical of chronic GVHD. These may include splitting, nail fragility and roughness, longitudinal striations/ridging, periungual erythema and edema, and onycholysis (separation of the nail plate starting at the distal-free margin and progressing proximally).

Note. Photo courtesy of T.L. Diepgen & G. Yihune, Dermatology Online Atlas (www.dermis.net/doia/). Used with permission.

Figure 6-10. Erosive Oral Lichen Planus

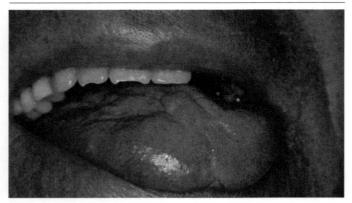

Erosive oral lichen planus, with edematous, erythematous, and eroded lateral tongue surfaces.

Note. Photo courtesy of Ontario Cancer Institute, Toronto, Canada. Used with permission.

involvement with GVHD (Padovan et al., 2001). Nerve biopsy and autoantibody studies may help in diagnosing these complications. Patients with chronic GVHD are also at risk for opportunistic infections of the central nervous system, such as toxoplasmosis. Neuropathy is frequently associated with treatment for GVHD, including thalidomide and occasionally tacrolimus or cyclosporine (Ratanatharathorn et al., 2001).

Hematopoietic

Suppression of peripheral blood counts is a common occurrence in patients with chronic GVHD. Patients with chronic GVHD also sometimes have eosinophilia (Marcellus & Vogelsang, 2000). It is not clear whether these hematopoietic abnormalities are a direct result of chronic GVHD or a specific autoimmune manifestation.

Autoimmune Manifestations

Nearly all known autoimmune syndromes have been reported as part of chronic GVHD. Aspects of GVHD may mimic systemic lupus erythematosus, scleroderma, progressive systemic sclerosis, lichen planus, sicca syndrome, eosinophilic fasciitis, rheumatoid arthritis, polymyositis, myasthenia gravis, idiopathic thrombocytopenic purpura, and hemolytic anemia (Chao, 1998; Sevilla & Gonzalez-Vicent, 2001). In patients with chronic GVHD, autoantibodies such as antinuclear antibody also can be detected in a similar fashion to those found in connective tissue diseases (Lister et al., 1987).

Effects of Chronic Graft Versus Host Disease on Immunologic Reconstitution

Multiple deficiencies in the functioning of the immune system are observed in patients with chronic GVHD. Thymic injury, impaired mucosal defense, chemotactic defects, functional asplenia, T cell alloreactivity, and qualitative and quantitative B cell abnormalities contribute to the suscepti-

bility to infection in patients with chronic GVHD (Parkman & Weinberg, 1999). The presence of an abnormal Schirmer's test (less than 5 mm of wetting), an elevated alkaline phosphatase level, and a platelet count of less than 100,000 at day +100 were correlated with an increased risk of mortality, suggesting that even a low level of undetected chronic GVHD may be associated with an immune deficiency (Wagner et al., 2001).

Other Findings

Vaginal sicca and vaginal stenosis and stricture have been noted in women with chronic GVHD. Lichenoid nail changes (Palencia, Rodriguez-Peralto, Castano, Vanaclocha, & Iglesias, 2002) and recurrent sterile effusions, including polyserositis and pericardial effusion, also have been reported as manifestations of chronic GVHD (Silberstein et al., 2001).

Classification and Grading of Chronic Graft Versus Host Disease

Chronic GVHD may occur as either an extension of acute GVHD (progressive chronic GVHD), after resolution of acute GVHD (quiescent onset), or without preceding acute GVHD (de novo onset). A fourth pattern of onset, explosive GVHD, was described by Vogelsang, Altomonte, and Farmer (1993) and manifests as diffuse erythroderma, involvement of liver and/or gut, and chronic GVHD changes of the mouth and eyes. Many of these patients have had no prior acute GVHD but may have known chronic GVHD. Explosive GVHD may be associated with abrupt cessation of immunosuppressive medication, often because of noncompliance, or severe skin injury secondary to sunburn or

Figure 6-11. Oral Lichen Planus Changes

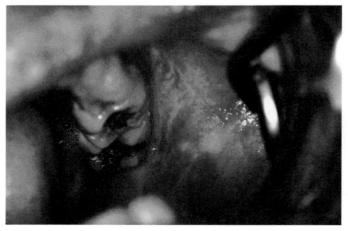

Oral lichen planus changes in a patient with graft versus host disease more than 130 days post-allogeneic peripheral blood stem cell transplant. Note the confluent, smooth, white papules that create a lacy pattern on the buccal mucosa.

Note. Photo courtesy of Dr. Jane Fall-Dickson, National Institutes of Health, Bethesda, MD. Used with permission.

herpes zoster infection (Marcellus & Vogelsang, 2000). Although progressive chronic GVHD is the most common pattern of onset, the increasing use of DLIs and nonmyeloablative conditioning regimens has increased the incidence of quiescent onset or de novo onset chronic GVHD (Baron & Beguin, 2002; Fleming, 2002; McCarthy & Bishop, 2000; Porter et al., 1999).

Patients with chronic GVHD also can be classified, based on the extent of their disease, as having either limited or extensive chronic GVHD. This classification system for chronic GVHD is presented in Table 6-3. Patients also may be classified according to their primary clinical and histologic pattern as having lichenoid or sclerodermatous disease. These three models for categorizing patients with chronic GVHD are summarized in Table 6-4. Similar to acute GVHD, biopsies of skin, oral cavity, and sometimes liver are used to diagnose the disease and gauge response to therapy. Akpek, Lee, et al. (2003) evaluated the performance of a new clinical grading system for chronic GVHD based on a prognostic model designed to predict overall survival of patients with chronic GVHD. They found that three risk factors, specifically extensive skin involvement, thrombocytopenia, and chronic GVHD that evolves as an extension of acute GVHD, if present at the time of diagnosis of chronic GVHD, were associated with increased, nonrelapse mortality. Efforts are under way to evaluate and refine this predictive clinical grading system for chronic GVHD (Akpek, Lee, et al., 2003).

The spectrum, character, and timing of onset of abnormalities in chronic GVHD may be affected by newer treatment approaches including nonmyeloablative transplantation (Schetelig et al., 2002), use of DLI (Lewalle et al., 2003; Raiola et al., 2003), and new regimens for the prevention/treatment of acute GVHD. Table 6-5 summarizes the clinical features, screening/evaluation tests, and interventions recommended for patients with chronic GVHD.

Table 6-3. Classification of Chronic Graft Versus Host Disease

Classification	Extent of Disease
Limited chronic GVHD	Either or both: • Localized skin involvement • Hepatic dysfunction because of chronic GVHD
Extensive chronic GVHD	Either: • Generalized skin involvement • Localized skin involvement and/or hepatic dysfunction because of chronic GVHD Plus: • Liver histology showing chronic aggressive hepatitis, bridging necrosis, or cirrhosis • Involvement of eye (Schirmer's test with less than 5 mm wetting) • Involvement of minor salivary glands or oral mucosa demonstrated on labial biopsy • Involvement of any other target organ

Note. Based on information from Sullivan, 1999.

Major Therapeutic Options for Preventing and Treating Acute and Chronic Graft Versus Host Disease

Advances in the development of medications and other therapies to prevent and treat GVHD have played a key role in improving the outcomes of allogeneic transplantation. Our knowledge of the optimal combinations and sequencing of GVHD therapies is continuing to evolve (Vogelsang, Lee, & Bensen-Kennedy, 2003). The wide range of therapeutic options aimed at preventing and treating acute and chronic GVHD is presented in Figure 6-12. These therapies and modalities are used in different combinations and sequences with the goal of either preventing or treating

Table 6-4. Models for Classifying Chronic Graft Versus Host Disease

Model	Type of Chronic GVHD	Characteristics
Pattern of onset	De novo	No antecedent acute GVHD
	Quiescent	Onset after complete resolution of acute GVHD
	Progressive	Direct evolution from acute GVHD
	Explosive	Acute and chronic GVHD features occur aggressively and concomitantly at the time of onset.
Extent of disease	Limited	Localized skin involvement with absent to mild liver involvement
	Extensive	Generalized skin involvement and/or severe liver, eye, mouth, or any other target organ involvement
Clinical/histologic pattern	Lichenoid	Maculopapular rash, skin thickened and rough, common oral and ocular involvement. Can evolve to sclerodermatous involvement.
	Sclerodermatous	Thickening and tautness of the skin, usually patchy, occasional blisters and ulcers. Associated or isolated involvement of the underlying fascia can cause severe limitation in range of motion.

Note. From "Chronic Graft-Versus-Host Disease" (p. 616) by D.C. Marcellus and G.B. Vogelsang in E.D. Ball, J. Lister, and P. Law (Eds.), *Hematopoietic Stem Cell Therapy*, 2000, Philadelphia: Elsevier. Copyright 2000 by Elsevier. Adapted with permission.

Table 6-5. Chronic Graft Versus Host Disease: Clinical Manifestations, Screening and Evaluation, and Interventions

System	Clinical Manifestations	Screening Studies/Evaluation	Interventions
Dermal	Dyspigmentation, xerosis (dryness), erythema, hyperkeratosis, pruritus, scleroderma, lichenification, onychodystrophy (nail ridging/nail loss), alopecia, second malignancies	Clinical examination, skin biopsy—3 mm punch biopsy from forearm and posterior iliac crest areas	• Immunosuppressive therapy • Psoralen and ultraviolet irradiation (PUVA); extracorporeal photopheresis • Topical tacrolimus ointment (Prograf® ointment) • Topical with steroid creams, moisturizers/emollient, antibacterial ointments to prevent superinfection; aggressive lubrication of the skin • If the sweat glands are affected, avoid overheating because heat prostration and heat stroke can occur. • Avoid sun light exposure; use sunblock lotion and a large hat that shades the face when outdoors.
Oral	Lichen planus, xerostomia, ulceration, second malignancies	Oral biopsy from inner lower lip	• Steroid mouth rinses, oral PUVA, pilocarpine and anetholetrithione for xerostomia, fluoride gels/rinses to decrease caries • Careful attention to oral hygiene; regular dental evaluations
Ocular	Keratitis, sicca syndrome Increased risk for cataracts secondary to protracted use of post-transplant steroids	Schirmer's test, ophthalmic evaluation	• Regular ophthalmologic follow-up • Preservative-free tears and moisturizing ophthalmic ointments • Temporary or permanent lacrimal duct occlusion • Consider therapy with retinoic acid. • Consider trial of cyclosporine A ophthalmic emulsion.
Hepatic	Jaundice, abdominal pain	Liver function tests—SGOT, SGPT, alkaline phosphatase, bilirubin	• Consider bile acid displacement therapy with ursodeoxycholic acid (Actigall®) 300 mg po tid
Pulmonary	Obstructive/restrictive pulmonary disease, shortness of breath, cough, dyspnea, wheezing, fatigue, hypoxia, pleural effusion	Pulmonary function studies, peak flow, arterial blood gas, CT of the chest	• Prevent and treat pulmonary infections, including *Pneumocystis carinii* and *Streptococcus pneumoniae*. • Aggressively investigate changes in pulmonary function, as these may represent GVHD of lung/bronchiolitis obliterans. • Encourage smoking cessation.
Gastrointestinal	Nausea, odynophagia, dysphagia, anorexia, early satiety, malabsorption, diarrhea, weight loss	Stool cultures, esophagogastroduodenoscopy, colonoscopy, nutritional assessment, fecal fat excretion studies, serum amylase, D-xylose absorption test, CT of the abdomen	• Refer to gastroenterologist; consult with nutritionist; suggest nutrition support. • Consider empirical trial of pancreatic enzyme supplementation. • Aggressive management of gastrointestinal symptoms, such as nausea and vomiting • Consider the use of cholestyramine (Questran®) in the management of diarrhea. • Consider a trial of oral beclomethasone.
Nutritional	Protein and calorie deficiency, malabsorption, dehydration, weight loss, muscle wasting	Weight, fat store measurement, pre-albumin	• Nutritional monitoring, supplementation, symptom-specific interventions • Trial of Megace® or other approaches to appetite stimulation (e.g., Remeron® or similar antidepressants, Marinol®)
Genitourinary	Vaginal sicca, vaginal atrophy, stenosis or inflammation	Pelvic examination	• Consider trial of mucosal application of corticosteroid ointment, cyclosporine ointment, or tacrolimus ointment. • Suggest use of vaginal lubricants. • Suggest sexual counseling.

(Continued on next page)

Table 6-5. Chronic Graft Versus Host Disease: Clinical Manifestations, Screening and Evaluation, and Interventions *(Continued)*

System	Clinical Manifestations	Screening Studies/Evaluation	Interventions
Immunologic	Hypogammaglobulinemia, autoimmune syndromes, recurrent infections, including CMV, HSV, VZV, fungus, PCP, and encapsulated bacteria	Quantitative immunoglobulin levels, CD4/CD8 lymphocyte subsets	• Intravenous immunoglobulin supplementation, as indicated, and prophylactic antimicrobials (rotating antibiotics for recurrent sinopulmonary infections, PCP prophylaxis, topical antifungals) • Screening for CMV and other opportunistic infection with frequent surveillance cultures and antigen detection • Consider vaccination against influenza and *pneumococcus.*
Musculoskeletal	Contractures, debility, muscle cramps/aches, carpal spasm	Performance status, formal quality-of-life evaluation (e.g., FACT-BMT), formal evaluation of rehabilitation needs (CARES)	• Physical therapy • Correct electrolyte imbalances • Consider clonazepam treatment for muscle cramping or myalgias.

Note. Based on information from Abdelsayed et al., 2002; Akpek, Valladares, et al., 2001; Aristei et al., 2002; Baker et al., 2003; Buchsel et al., 1996; Chao, 1998; Gold et al., 1998; Grigg et al., 2003; Lash, 2001; Lee et al., 2003; Loughran et al., 1990; Seber & Vogelsang, 1998; Treleaven, 1995; Vogelsang, 2001.

GVHD. The selection of these therapies is as much an art as it is an evolving science, as there exists a fine balance between too much or too little immunosuppression. As will be discussed in a subsequent section of the chapter, the therapeutic regimen selected will vary based on whether the goal is prevention or treatment, whether the patient has acute or chronic GVHD, what organ systems are involved, and the patient's response to alternate therapies (Ratanatharathorn et al., 2001; Vogelsang et al., 2003). Each transplant center follows center-specific protocols for the prophylaxis and treatment of acute and chronic GVHD as well as their supportive care management. After a discussion of each of these therapeutic modalities, the current approach to combining these therapies to prevent and treat acute and chronic GVHD is reviewed. Table 6-6 illustrates the mechanism of action for the major categories of immunosuppressive agents used in the treatment of GVHD.

Systemic Immunosuppression

A wide variety of systemic immunosuppressive therapies may be used to prevent or treat GVHD, including nonspecific immunosuppressive agents (e.g., corticosteroids, methotrexate), specific T cell immunosuppressive drugs (e.g., cyclosporine A, tacrolimus, mycophenolate mofetil), and monoclonal or polyclonal antibodies.

Corticosteroids have broad immunosuppressive effects, including induction of apoptosis of activated lymphocytes, downregulation of cytokine expression in lymphocytes and phagocytes, decreased antigen processing and presentation, and decreased phagocytosis (Przepiorka, 2000). As a single agent, corticosteroids are not effective in preventing GVHD. Further, although they may be used as a component of combination regimens for GVHD prophylaxis, they are of uncertain efficacy in preventing acute GVHD and may increase the morbidity of allogeneic HSCT and the frequency of chronic GVHD (Ancin et al., 2001; Deeg et al., 1997; Ross et al., 1999). However, corticosteroids are an important compo-

nent of the treatment of both acute and chronic GVHD and may be given at high doses (Akpek, Lee, Anders, & Vogelsang, 2001). Side effects of corticosteroids include hyperglycemia,

---

Figure 6-12. Options for Graft Versus Host Disease Prevention and Treatment

Systemic Immunosuppression
- Corticosteroids
- Cyclosporine
- Tacrolimus
- Mycophenolate mofetil
- Methotrexate
- Rapamycin

Polyclonal or Monoclonal Antibody-Based Therapies
- Antithymocyte globulin
- Daclizumab
- Infliximab
- Etanercept
- Alemtuzumab

Other Systemic Therapies
- Intravenous immunoglobulin
- Thalidomide
- Octreotide
- N-acetylcysteine
- Pentoxifylline
- Beclomethasone
- Hydroxychloroquine

Phototherapy
- 8-methoxypsoralen plus ultraviolet A irradiation (PUVA)
- UVB phototherapy
- Extracorporeal photopheresis

Local and Topical Therapy
- Topical corticosteroids
- Intralesional steroid injections (mouth only)
- Topical tacrolimus
- Corticosteroid mouthwash
- Vaginal cyclosporine or tacrolimus ointment/gel
- Ophthalmic cyclosporine

Other
- T cell depletion pretransplant
- Total lymphoid irradiation

Table. 6-6. Side Effects and Nursing Implications of Selected Immunosuppressants Used in Allogeneic Stem Cell Transplantation

Agent/Drug	Mechanism of Action	Dosing/Administration	Side Effects	Nursing Implications
Cyclosporine A (Sandimmune®, Neoral®, Novartis Pharmaceuticals, East Hanover, NJ)	Prevents IL-2 gene expression, thus impairs IL-2 synthesis and activation of T lymphocytes	Total daily dose is usually 1.5 mg/kg IV q 12h, 0.75 mg/kg q 6 h, or 3 mg/kg/day as a continuous infusion, with dosage adjusted to achieve therapeutic levels IV to po conversion is approximately 1:3. Dosage is dependent on achieving and sustaining therapeutic blood levels based on laboratory evaluation. Therapeutic monitoring is not required once drug is being tapered.	Metabolic: hyperkalemia and hyperglycemia, hypomagnesemia, hyperlipidemia, hyperuricemia, diabetes mellitus Neurotoxicity: headache, tremor, insomnia, paresthesia, dizziness, seizures Gastrointestinal (GI): diarrhea, nausea, constipation, anorexia, vomiting, abdominal pain, ascites, elevated liver function tests Renal: elevated creatinine, nephrotoxicity Cardiovascular: hypertension, chest pain Hematologic: anemia Cutaneous: acneform rash, striae Other: peripheral edema, infection, impaired wound healing, osteoporosis, gingival hyperplasia, flushing, sweating, hirsutism	• Bioavailability differs between oral solution and capsule formulation. Once a regimen is established, patients should be instructed not to change their formulation or brand. • Take with food. • Instruct patient on importance of strict adherence to the administration schedule and to notify the healthcare team immediately if unable to take because of GI side effects. • Monitor serum creatinine, BUN, potassium, magnesium, glucose, and triglyceride levels. • Avoid potassium-sparing diuretics. • Replete electrolytes as indicated. • Co-administration with grapefruit juice may increase cyclosporine A levels and should be avoided. • Drug-drug interactions can lead to subtherapeutic or toxic cyclosporine A levels. Drugs that inhibit or induce cytochrome P450 are most responsible. • Cyclosporine A trough levels to be drawn prior to administration of morning dose. Therefore, doses are usually timed for 10 am and 10 pm to allow trough blood draw at morning clinic visit. Instruct patient to bring dose to clinic and to administer once trough level is drawn. • Should not be used simultaneously with tacrolimus. • Tacrolimus should be discontinued 24 hours prior to starting cyclosporine A. In the presence of increased tacrolimus levels, initiation of cyclosporine A usually should be further delayed. • Doses should be adjusted for renal dysfunction. • Monitor levels carefully in patients with renal or hepatic dysfunction.
Tacrolimus (Prograf®, Fujisawa, Chantilly, VA)	Impaired synthesis of IL-2 prevents T lymphocyte proliferation; interferes with the gene transcription for a variety of cytokines, including IFN-γ, TNF-α.	Total daily dose is usually 1–2 mg po q 12 hours; 0.05–0.1 mg/kg/day as a continuous infusion, with dosage adjusted to achieve therapeutic levels. IV to po conversion is approximately 1:4. Dosage dependent on achieving and sustaining therapeutic blood levels based on laboratory evaluation. Therapeutic monitoring not required once drug is being tapered.	Metabolic: hyperkalemia and hypokalemia, hyperglycemia, hypomagnesemia, hyperlipidemia, hypophosphatemia, diabetes mellitus Neurotoxicity: headache, tremor, insomnia, paresthesia, dizziness, seizures GI: diarrhea, nausea, constipation, anorexia, vomiting, abdominal pain, ascites, elevated liver function tests Renal: elevated creatinine, nephrotoxicity Cardiovascular: hypertension, chest pain Hematologic: anemia, leukocytosis, thrombocytopenia	• Take on an empty stomach. • Instruct patient on importance of strict adherence to the administration schedule and to notify the healthcare team immediately if unable to take because of GI side effects. • Monitor serum creatinine, BUN, potassium, magnesium, phosphorus, glucose, and triglyceride levels. • Avoid potassium-sparing diuretics. • Replete electrolytes as indicated. • Co-administration with grapefruit juice may increase tacrolimus levels and should be avoided. • Drug-drug interactions can lead to subtherapeutic or toxic tacrolimus levels. Drugs that inhibit or induce cytochrome P450 are most responsible. • Tacrolimus trough levels to be drawn prior to administration of morning dose. Therefore, doses usually are timed for 10 am and 10 pm to allow trough blood draw at morning clinic

(Continued on next page)

Table. 6-6. Side Effects and Nursing Implications of Selected Immunosuppressants Used in Allogeneic Stem Cell Transplantation *(Continued)*

Agent/Drug	Mechanism of Action	Dosing/Administration	Side Effects	Nursing Implications
Tacrolimus (Prograf®, Fujisawa, Chantilly, VA) *(cont.)*			Cutaneous: pruritus, acneform rash Pulmonary: pleural effusion, atelectasis, dyspnea Other: peripheral edema, infection, impaired wound healing, osteoporosis	visit. Instruct patient to bring dose to clinic and to administer once trough level is drawn. • Should not be used simultaneously with cyclosporine A. • Tacrolimus should be discontinued 24 hours prior to starting cyclosporine A. In the presence of elevated cyclosporine A levels, initiation of tacrolimus should usually be further delayed. • Doses should be adjusted for renal dysfunction. • Monitor levels carefully in patients with renal or hepatic dysfunction.
Steroids	The immunosuppressive properties of steroids are related to their ability to decrease cytotoxic T cell proliferation, inhibit production of IL-1 and IFN-γ, prevent production of IL-2, and inhibit neutrophil function by stabilization of leukocyte lysosomal membrane and inhibiting chemotaxis.	Dosage varies according to institutional protocols. Dosage ranges from 0.5–2 mg/kg/day q12h, with tapering schedule based on starting dose and patient response.	Metabolic: fluid and electrolyte imbalance, diabetes mellitus, hyperlipidemia Neurotoxicity: tremors, seizures, headache, difficulty concentrating, insomnia GI: GI irritation Cardiovascular: hypertension, arrhythmias Cutaneous: bruising, fragile skin Neurotoxicity: tremors, seizures, headache Other: hunger, peripheral edema, infection, impaired wound healing, hirsutism, osteoporosis, weight gain, steroid myopathy, cataracts/glaucoma, Cushingoid changes, psychiatric disturbances (steroid psychosis, mood changes, confusion)	• Usually used in combination with cyclosporine A or tacrolimus • Consult physical therapy for proximal muscle strengthening exercise program. • Instruct patient in strategies to prevent or treat hyperglycemia and in diabetic self-management. • Administer oral corticosteroids with food/milk to minimize GI upset. • Administer H$_2$ blockers as ordered. • May increase tacrolimus or cyclosporine A levels. • Report complaints of visual changes and consult ophthalmology. • For patients on long-term steroids or otherwise at risk for or experiencing osteopenia (e.g., patients with acute lymphocytic leukemia, post-menopausal), ensure regular DEXA scans, calcium and vitamin D supplementation, and specific treatment for osteopenia with antiresorptive agents such as pamidronate and alendronate. • A tapering calendar specifying the dosage to be taken each day can help to facilitate adherence in patients who are on tapering doses of steroids or an alternate day steroid regimen.
Mycophenolate mofetil (MMF) (CellCept®, Roche, Nutley, NJ)	Antimetabolite that selectively inhibits the proliferation of T and B lymphocytes by interfering with purine nucleotide synthesis	Dosage ranges from 1–1.5 grams IV or po every 12 hours depending upon institutional guidelines.	Metabolic: hyperkalemia and hypokalemia, hyperlipidemia, hypophosphatemia, hyperglycemia Neurotoxicity: headache, insomnia, tremors, seizures GI: diarrhea, nausea, constipation, anorexia, vomiting, abdominal pain, hepatotoxicity Renal: elevated creatinine, nephrotoxicity Cardiovascular: hypertension, hypotension, arrhythmias	• MMF should be taken on an empty stomach. • Monitor complete blood count at regular intervals and adjust dosage for pancytopenia, as ordered. • Monitor liver function tests (bilirubin and serum transaminases) at regular intervals, and adjust dosage for liver function abnormalities, as ordered. • Monitor serum levels of the MMF metabolic to guide treatment in patients with renal dysfunction. • In the setting of renal impairment, or when co-administered with probenecid, acyclovir, or ganciclovir, the drug concentrations of MMF and of these drugs may increase.

(Continued on next page)

Agent/Drug	Mechanism of Action	Dosing/Administration	Side Effects	Nursing Implications
Mycophenolate mofetil (MMF) (CellCept®, Roche, Nutley, NJ) *(cont.)*			Hematologic: anemia, leukocytosis, thrombocytopenia Cutaneous: acneform rash Pulmonary: cough, dyspnea Other: fever, edema, pain, infection, muscle weakness, anxiety, depression	• There may be decreased MMF absorption when co-administered with magnesium oxide, aluminum or magnesium-containing antacids, or cholestyramine.
Azathioprine (Imuran®, Prometheus Laboratories, San Diego, CA)	Antimetabolite that selectively inhibits the proliferation of T and B lymphocytes by interfering with purine nucleotide synthesis	Usual dose is 2–2.5 mg/kg/day. Oral and IV doses are the same.	Alopecia, myelosuppression, hepatotoxicity, infection, nausea, vomiting, diarrhea, mucosal ulceration, esophagitis, second malignancies	• Dose decrement required when given with allopurinol. • May lead to anemia and leukopenia when given with ACE (angiotensin-converting enzyme) inhibitors; synergistic with other bone marrow suppressants • Use with caution in patients with hepatic or renal impairment. • Teratogenic; advise patient and partner about the need for contraception.
Methotrexate	Antimetabolite that inhibits dihydrofolate reductase, thereby hindering DNA synthesis and cell reproduction, and thus inhibiting lymphocyte proliferation	Institutional protocols vary. Usual dose is 5–15 mg/m² given IV on days +1, +3, +6, and +11 after transplantation.	Myelosuppression, mucositis, photosensitivity, interstitial pneumonitis, hepatotoxicity, nephrotoxicity	• Dose and schedule for methotrexate prophylaxis for GVHD varies by institution. A common regimen is methotrexate 5–15 mg/m² on days 1, 3, 6, and 11 post-transplant. • Doses may be adjusted or held for severe mucositis and renal or liver insufficiency. Doses may need to be adjusted for hypoalbuminemia. • Wait until at least 24 hours following stem cell infusion to give day +1 dose.
Daclizumab (Zenapax®, Roche)	Monoclonal antibody against the IL-2 receptor expressed on activated T cells. Daclizumab binds to the IL-2 receptor in a nonactivating fashion, competing with IL-2 and thereby inhibiting IL-2 driven proliferation of the activated T lymphocyte. IL-2 induced proliferation of activated (antigen stimulated) T lymphocytes is a critical step in proliferation and, ultimately, tissue destruction.	Institutional protocols vary; usual dose is 1 mg/kg by IV administration.	Constipation, nausea, vomiting, diarrhea, abdominal pain, abdominal distention, edema, tremor, headache, dizziness, nephrotoxicity, chest pain, tachycardia, fever, pain, fatigue, hypertension, hypotension, dyspnea, pulmonary edema, coughing, musculoskeletal pain, back pain	• Anaphylactoid reactions following the administration of daclizumab have not been observed but can occur following the administration of proteins. Medications for the treatment of severe hypersensitivity reactions should be available for immediate use. • The calculated volume of daclizumab should be mixed with 50 ml of sterile 0.9% sodium chloride solution and administered via a peripheral or central vein over a 15-minute period. Once the infusion is prepared, it should be administered intravenously within four hours. If it must be held longer, it should be refrigerated between 2°–8°C (36°–46°F) for up to 24 hours. After 24 hours, the prepared solution should be discarded. • No incompatibility between daclizumab and polyvinyl chloride or polyethylene bags or infusion sets has been observed. • No dosage adjustment is necessary for patients with severe renal impairment.

(Continued on next page)

Agent/Drug	Mechanism of Action	Dosing/Administration	Side Effects	Nursing Implications
Infliximab (Remicade®, Centocor, Malvern, PA)	Monoclonal antibody against TNF-α. It binds to soluble and membrane-bound TNF-α, producing reduction in serum IL-1 and reduced levels of nitric oxide synthase	Institutional protocols vary; usual dose is 10 mg/kg by IV administration. Administer over at least two hours. Must be given with a low protein binding filter of 1.2 microns or less	Headache, nausea, abdominal pain, fatigue, fever, and coughing Infusion reactions including fever, chills, chest pain, hypotension, headache, and urticaria can occur during the infusion and for up to two hours after the infusion is complete. There was no increase in the incidence of reactions after the initial infusion. Delayed serum sickness-like reactions, including myalgias, arthralgias, fever, rash, sore throat, dysphagia, and hand and facial edema, can be seen 3–12 days after infusion. Patients may develop human antichimeric antibody (HACA).	• Monitor patient for development of infusional toxicities. • Consider premedication with acetaminophen and Benadryl®. Initiate therapy at 10 ml/hr x 15 minutes, increase to 20 ml/hr x 15 minutes, and then increase to 40 ml/hr x 15 minutes, then 80 ml/hr x 15 minutes, then 150 ml/hr x 30 minutes, and then 250 ml/hr x 30 minutes to complete infusion in two hours. • Stop or slow infusion and give Benadryl, acetaminophen, or Solu-Cortef® to treat mild to moderate infusion reaction. Resume infusion at 10 ml/hour once reaction is controlled or abated. • Medications for treating hypersensitivity reactions (e.g., acetaminophen, antihistamines, corticosteroids, epinephrine) and supplemental oxygen should be available for immediate use in the event of a reaction. • Incompatible with PVC equipment or devices. Use glass infusion bottles and polyethylene-lined administration sets.
Antithymocyte globulin (ATGAM®, Pfizer Inc., New York) (equine) (Thymoglobulin®, SangStat, Menlo Park, CA) (rabbit)	Polyclonal immunoglobulin composed of horse or rabbit antibodies capable of destroying human leukocytes	Institutional protocols vary; usual dose is 10–40 mg/kg/day for equine ATG, and 2.5 mg/kg/day for rabbit ATG.	Adverse reactions include fever, chills, seizures, laryngospasm, anaphylaxis, pulmonary edema, leukopenia, and thrombocytopenia. Because ATG is a foreign xenogeneic protein and an antibody, serum sickness can occur, including myalgias, arthralgias, fever, rash, sore throat, dysphagia, and hand and facial edema.	• Monitor patient closely, both during and following infusion, for signs of serum sickness and anaphylaxis. Consider premedication with corticosteroids, acetaminophen, and H₁ and H₂ blockers. • Medications for treating hypersensitivity reactions (e.g., acetaminophen, antihistamines, corticosteroids, epinephrine) and supplemental oxygen should be available for immediate use in the event of a reaction. • Because transient and at times severe thrombocytopenia may occur following ATG administration in patients with platelet counts less than 100,000, monitor platelet count one hour following ATG administration and transfuse platelets as indicated.
Alemtuzumab (Campath-1®, Berlex Laboratories, Montville, NJ)	Monoclonal antibody directed against the cell surface antigen CD52, which is expressed on B and T lymphocytes	Institutional protocols vary; usual dose is 20 mg/day IV given over several hours for five days, beginning before transplantation.	Infusional toxicities may be severe and include fever and rigors in more than 80% of patients. Other adverse effects include neutropenia, anemia, thrombocytopenia, nausea, vomiting, rash, fatigue, and hypotension.	• Premedicate patient with acetaminophen and Benadryl. • Medications for treating hypersensitivity reactions (e.g., acetaminophen, antihistamines, corticosteroids, epinephrine) and supplemental oxygen should be available for immediate use in the event of a reaction. • Consider treatment with meperidine to control infusional rigors. • Administer fluid bolus as ordered to treat hypotension. • Produces profound and rapid lymphopenia; therefore, patients require broad antifungal, antibacterial, antiviral, and antiprotozoal prophylaxis for at least four months following treatment, and ongoing surveillance for cytomegalovirus and adenovirus infection.

(Continued on next page)

H_1 and H_2 blockers (as noted in text).

Table 6-6. Side Effects and Nursing Implications of Selected Immunosuppressants Used in Allogeneic Stem Cell Transplantation *(Continued)*

Agent/Drug	Mechanism of Action	Dosing/Administration	Side Effects	Nursing Implications
Rapamycin (Sirolimus®, Wyeth Laboratories, Madison, NJ)	Structurally similar to tacrolimus and cyclosporine A; however, it has a distinct immunosuppressant activity. Sirolimus inhibits response of B and T lymphocytes to cytokine stimulation by IL-2 and inhibits antibody production by B cells.	Long half-life permits once-daily dosing. Monitor trough blood levels.	Hyperlipidemia, thrombocytopenia, leukopenia, headache, nausea, anorexia, dizziness	• May suppress hematopoietic recovery if used in patients who have recently undergone high-dose therapy • Oral bioavailability is variable and is improved with high-fat meals. • Like tacrolimus and cyclosporine A, it is metabolized through the cytochrome P450-3A system.
N-acetylcysteine	Inhibits B7-1/CD28 expression in vitro; thought to interfere with T cell/antigen presenting cell co-stimulator pathways. May also counterbalance tissue damage from free radicals and oxidative stress.	Bolus of 150 mg/kg intravenously, followed by continuous IV infusion of 50 mg/kg/day over at least 7–21 days		• Monitor vital signs every 15 minutes during initial bolus infusion. • Compatibilities with other therapies such as TPN are unknown. Should be infused on separate IV access.
Thalidomide (Thalomid®, Celgene, Warren, NJ)	Immunosuppressive and anti-inflammatory properties include impaired neutrophil phagocytosis and chemotaxis; reduced antibody production in response to antigenic stimulation; increased T suppressor cells and reduced T helper cells; inhibition of TNF-α production by monocytes	100 mg po qhs, increasing gradually to 400–600 mg po qhs	Neutropenia, skin rash, skin ulceration, peripheral neuropathy, somnolence, lightheadedness, constipation, bradycardia, hypothyroidism, hypotension	• Thalidomide is a potent teratogen and is contraindicated in patients who are, or are likely to become, pregnant. A systematic counseling and education program, written informed consent, and participation in a confidential survey program at the start of treatment and throughout treatment is required for all patients receiving thalidomide. Both men and women who are of childbearing potential must practice protected sex while on this drug. • Perform pregnancy test prior to initiating treatment with thalidomide. • The combination of thalidomide with certain antibiotics, HIV protease inhibitors, rifampin, griseofulvin, phenytoin, or carbamazepine may decrease the effectiveness of oral contraceptives. • Obtain baseline EKG prior to treatment. • Thalidomide should not be started if the ANC is less than 750/mm³, and therapy should be reevaluated if the ANC drops below this level. • Always administer doses in the evening to minimize their impact of drowsiness on lifestyle and safety. • Teach patient to use caution when taking thalidomide with other drugs that can cause drowsiness or neuropathy. • Teach patient to rise slowly from a supine position to avoid lightheadedness. • Teach patient to report immediately signs or symptoms suggestive of peripheral neuropathy, including numbness or

(Continued on next page)

Table 6-6. Side Effects and Nursing Implications of Selected Immunosuppressants Used in Allogeneic Stem Cell Transplantation (Continued)

Agent/Drug	Mechanism of Action	Dosing/Administration	Side Effects	Nursing Implications
Thalidomide (Thalomid®, Celgene, Warren, NJ) (cont.)				tingling in the hands or feet or the development of skin rash or skin lesion. These may require immediate cessation of the drug until the patient can be evaluated for the neuropathy or skin rash. • Teach patient to use protective measures (e.g., sunscreens, protective clothing) against exposure to ultraviolet light or sunlight. • Control/manage constipation with a stool softener or mild laxative.
Methoxsalen (Oxsoralen®, ICN Pharmaceuticals, Costa Mesa, CA)	When photoactivated by ultraviolet light exposure, inhibits mitosis by binding covalently to pyrimidine bases in DNA	400 mcg/kg po 1.5–2 hours prior to exposure to ultraviolet light		• Patients who have received cytotoxic chemotherapy or radiation and who are taking methoxsalen (Oxsoralen) are at increased risk for skin cancers, and long-term use may increase the risk of skin cancer. • Toxicity increases with concurrent use of phenothiazines, thiazides, and sulfanilamides. • Severe burns may occur from sunlight or UVA exposure if dose or treatment frequency is exceeded. • Pretreatment eye examinations are indicated to evaluate for the presence of cataracts. Repeat eye examinations should be performed every six months while patients are undergoing PUVA.

Note. Based on information from Abo-Zena & Horwitz, 2002; Bush, 1999; Cather, 2001; Chao, 1998, 1999b; Charuhas, 2000; Cronin et al., 2000; Gaziev et al., 2000; Goldman, 2001; Lanuza & McCabe, 2001; Lazarus et al., 1997; National Home Infusion Association, 2001; Rudy et al., 2001; Seeley & DeMeyer, 2002; Simpson, 2001, 2003; Solimando, 1998.

hypertension, edema, myopathy, headaches, psychiatric disturbances, nausea, and gastric ulceration or bleeding. In addition, they may accelerate the development of cataracts, osteoporosis, and aseptic necrosis. In patients receiving high-dose corticosteroids, consideration should be given to the need for gastric cytoprotection with a proton pump inhibitor, such as omeprazole, and for antimicrobial prophylaxis.

Cyclosporine A and tacrolimus inhibit calcineurin, thereby preventing transcription of the earliest activation genes in T lymphocytes. Neither cyclosporine A nor tacrolimus has any effect on activated T lymphocytes. Studies comparing cyclosporine A to tacrolimus have suggested that tacrolimus is more effective in preventing acute GVHD; however, the patients who received cyclosporine A had significantly better long-term survival (Ratanatharathorn et al., 1998) and may have a lower incidence of relapse (Hiraoka et al., 2001). Commonly encountered side effects of cyclosporine A include renal insufficiency, magnesium wasting, hirsutism, hypertension, hyperkalemia, glucose intolerance, and tremor. Other side effects include headache, hyperchloremic metabolic acidosis, gingival hyperplasia, hyperuricemia, hyperlipidemia, microangiopathic hemolytic anemia, hemolytic-uremic syndrome, seizures, confusion, cortical blindness, and palmar-plantar dysesthesia. The side effect profile of tacrolimus is similar to that of cyclosporine except that tacrolimus does not cause hirsutism, gingival hyperplasia, or hyperlipidemia, and it is associated with less hypertension. Some toxic events are idiosyncratic or precipitated by rapid infusion of the drug, but the risk of nephrotoxicity is increased with elevated blood concentrations of either cyclosporine A or tacrolimus (Wingard et al., 1998). The clearance of both cyclosporine A and tacrolimus is through hepatic metabolism. Cyclosporine A and tacrolimus-induced liver dysfunction can mimic veno-occlusive disease of the liver or acute GVHD of the liver, resulting in jaundice, hepatorenal syndrome, elevated transaminases, and hepatic encephalopathy (Chao, 1998).

Both tacrolimus and cyclosporine A require therapeutic monitoring, although there is a lack of consensus on the target drug levels to be achieved (Wingard et al., 1998). The target range for tacrolimus whole blood concentrations is 10–20 ng/ml (Przepiorka, Devine, Fay, Uberti, & Wingard, 1999; Przepiorka, Nash, et al., 1999), although some centers use a range of 5–15 ng/ml (Chao, 1998). Commonly used cyclosporine assays measure either parent compound or parent compound plus metabolite; however, the therapeutic target range for cyclosporine using either assay method has not been firmly established (Chao, 1998). It is important to note that the different oral preparations of cyclosporine A are not bioequivalent, and the conversion ratio from the intravenous to the oral route depends on which formulation is used.

Doses of tacrolimus and cyclosporine A should be modified for renal toxicity, with changes made for as little as a 25% increase from baseline creatinine (Przepiorka, Devine, et al., 1999). Because cyclosporine A and tacrolimus are metabolized mainly by the CYP3A enzyme systems, substances known to inhibit these enzymes may decrease the metabolism of cyclosporine A or tacrolimus with resultant increases in whole blood or plasma concentrations. Drugs known to induce these enzyme systems may result in an increased metabolism of cyclosporine A or tacrolimus, with resultant decreases in whole blood or plasma concentrations. Monitoring of blood concentrations and appropriate dosage adjustments are essential when such drugs are used concomitantly, as is often the case in HSCT (Przepiorka, Devine, et al.). Drugs that may alter tacrolimus and cyclosporine A levels are presented in Table 6-7. Care also be should exercised when drugs that are nephrotoxic or that are metabolized by CYP3A (e.g., ritonavir) are administered concomitantly with cyclosporine A or tacrolimus. In addition, grapefruit juice affects CYP3A-mediated metabolism and should be avoided in patients taking cyclosporine A or tacrolimus. Dose adjustment of tacrolimus, cyclosporine, and methotrexate is required in patients with renal or liver dysfunction. These dose adjustments can be found in Table 6-8.

The schedules for tapering tacrolimus and cyclosporine A are protocol specific or institutionally derived and vary from 5% per week starting on day +50 post-transplant to 10% per week starting on day +180. Early discontinuation of cyclosporine or tacrolimus is generally reserved for patients at high risk for relapse, with HLA-identical donors, and in the absence of acute GVHD but carries with it the risk for the onset of chronic GVHD that may be severe. It is important to follow patients carefully during tapering to avoid missing a flare of acute GVHD or the onset of chronic GVHD.

Methotrexate inhibits T lymphocyte function by blocking purine synthesis and DNA replication. The most common toxic events associated with methotrexate use are mucositis, hypotoxicity, and myelosuppression. Routine use of leucovorin does not abrogate the immunosuppressive effect of methotrexate and may reduce toxicity. Methotrexate is cleared renally, and in patients with renal insufficiency, a dose modification is required, as illustrated in Table 6-8. Doses of methotrexate may have to be reduced or omitted if the patient develops severe oral mucositis or liver function abnormalities prior to completing a planned course of methotrexate prophylaxis. Unfortunately, attenuating a planned course of methotrexate prophylaxis increases a patient's risk of acute GVHD (Kumar et al., 2002). Sample guidelines for methotrexate dose modification in patients with hyperbilirubinemia are given in Table 6-8.

MMF also blocks purine synthesis. Absorption of MMF is variable, and co-administration with magnesium oxide, aluminum- or magnesium-containing antacids, or cholestyramine decreases MMF absorption. In patients with renal dysfunction, therapeutic monitoring of MMF metabolite levels may be helpful in directing therapy. Although MMF has been shown to be both effective and well tolerated, it is associated with a high rate of opportunistic or serious viral or bacterial infections (Baudard et al., 2002).

Systemic immunosuppressive agents have many long-term effects, including hypertension, renal insufficiency, hyperlipidemia, metabolic complications (e.g., hyperglycemia, electrolyte abnormalities), and osteoporosis. Nurses working in HSCT should be skilled in the assessment, prevention, and management of these complications (Augustine, 2000; Cronin et al., 2000; Hilton, Williams, & Nesbitt, 2000). The side effects and nursing implications of the systemic immunosuppressive agents commonly used in allogeneic stem cell transplantation are presented in Table 6-6.

Monoclonal or Polyclonal Antibody Therapies

Based on an understanding of the role of various cellular and cytokine effectors in the evolution of GVHD, monoclonal or polyclonal antibodies directed against specific cellular components of the immune system or the cytokines implicated in the pathogenesis of GVHD are now coming into increasing use in the treatment and prevention of GVHD. Daclizumab is a humanized monoclonal antibody directed against the alpha chain of the IL-2 receptor. Daclizumab binds to the IL-2 receptor in a nonactivating fashion, competing with IL-2 and thereby inhibiting IL-2 driven proliferation of the activated T lymphocyte. IL-2-induced proliferation of activated (antigen stimulated) T lymphocytes is a critical step in proliferation and, ultimately, tissue destruction. Studies have shown that daclizumab has substantial activity for the treatment of acute GVHD (Przepiorka et al., 2000). Etanercept (Enbrel®, Immunex,

---

Table 6-7. Drugs That May Alter Tacrolimus and Cyclosporine A Levels

Drugs That May Increase Cyclosporine A or Tacrolimus Blood Concentrations	Drugs That May Decrease Cyclosporine A or Tacrolimus Blood Concentrations	Drugs That May Have Synergistic Nephrotoxicity With Cyclosporine A or Tacrolimus
Calcium channel blockers: diltiazem, nicardipine, nifedipine, verapamil Antifungal agents: clotrimazole, fluconazole, itraconazole, ketoconazole Antibiotics: clarithromycin, erythromycin troleandomycin, norfloxacin, doxycycline Prokinetic agents: metoclopramide Other agents: acyclovir, bromocriptine, cimetidine, danazol, estrogens, methylprednisolone, protease inhibitors, sertra; sertraline hydrochloride, mycophenolate mofetil, allopurinol	Anticonvulsants: carbamazepine, phenobarbital, phenytoin Antibiotics: rifampin, nafcillin, isoniazid, IV trimethoprim and sulfamethoxazole Other agents: octreotide	Nonsteroidal anti-inflammatory agents Melphalan Diuretics: furosemide, thiazides Antibiotics: erythromycin, amphotericin B, aminoglycosides, cephalosporins Ganciclovir

Table 6-8. Sample Dose Adjustments of Tacrolimus, Cyclosporine, and Methotrexate in Patients With Renal or Hepatic Dysfunction

Renal Function (creatinine in mg/dl)	Percentage Cyclosporine A/ Tacrolimus Dosage	Percentage Methotrexate Dosage
< 1.5	100%	100%
1.5–1.7	75%	75%
1.8–2	50%	50%
> 2	hold dose	hold dose
Hepatic Function (bilirubin mg/dl)		
< 2	—	100%
2.1–3	—	75%
3.1–5	—	50%
> 5	—	hold dose

Note. Based on information from Chao, 1998; Goker et al., 2001.

Seattle, WA) and infliximab (Remicade) are being studied as components of the treatment of acute GVHD (Couriel, Hicks, Giralt, & Champlin, 2000; Simpson, 2003). Infliximab and etanercept are monoclonal antibodies that produce immunosuppression by neutrolizing soluble TNF-α and blocking cell membrane-bound cytokine (LaDuca & Gaspari, 2001). Both agents are fairly well tolerated, although they may induce the formation of antibodies to the drug that limit the effectiveness of continued administration (LaDuca & Gaspari).

Antithymocyte globulin (ATG) is a polyclonal antibody directed primarily against circulating T lymphocytes, although it does contain antibodies against other formed elements of the blood, such as platelets and red blood cells. It is used as a component of GVHD prophylaxis regimens and is very effective in reducing the incidence of severe acute GVHD following HSCT (Bacigalupo et al., 2001). However, in at least one study, inclusion of ATG in the prophylaxis regimen resulted in an increased risk of lethal infection, especially fungal and viral infections (Bacigalupo et al.). ATG, using a variety of dose schedules, is also commonly used as a salvage therapy for steroid-refractory acute GVHD (Hsu, May, Carrum, Krance, & Przepiorka, 2001). ATG can produce objective responses in patients with steroid-refractory acute GVHD, especially when used in patients with skin GVHD and early signs of steroid resistance (MacMillan et al., 2002). Unfortunately, a positive effect on long-term survival of salvage therapy with ATG has not been demonstrated (Arai, Margolis, Zahurak, Anders, & Vogelsang, 2002). The information needed for rational design of a dose schedule is not available because studies of the pharmacokinetics and pharmacodynamics of ATG in blood and marrow transplant recipients are lacking. Dose schedules reported to be active in the treatment of GVHD range from 15–40 mg/kg/day for equine ATG and 2.5 mg/kg/day for rabbit ATG. Adverse reactions include fever and chills, seizures, laryngospasm, anaphylaxis, pulmonary edema, leukopenia, and thrombocytopenia. Because ATG is a foreign xenogeneic protein and an antibody, serum sickness can occur, including myalgias, arthralgias, fever, rash, sore throat, dysphagia, and hand and facial edema. One of the complications of prophylaxing or treating GVHD with ATG is graft failure, and long-term, these patients are at risk for EBV-associated lymphomas (Loren, Porter, Stadtmauer, & Tsai, 2003).

Alemtuzumab (Campath-1) is a monoclonal antibody directed against the cell surface antigen CD52, which is expressed on B and T lymphocytes. It is a potent immunosuppressive agent and provides rapid and complete eradication of B and T lymphocytes. It currently is being tested for the prevention of acute GVHD in both myeloablative (Hale, Zhang, & Bunjes, 1998) and nonmyeloablative (Chakraverty et al., 2002) conditioning regimens and for the treatment of severe acute GVHD refractory to conventional immunosuppressive therapy (Simpson, 2003). It is given over several hours daily for five days beginning before transplantation. The most common side effects of Campath-1 are infusional toxicities or rigors/chills, fever and headache, neutropenia and thrombocytopenia, and a profound and long-lasting immunosuppression with markedly increased risk for infections, especially viral infection (Chakrabarti et al., 2002).

Other Systemic Therapies

Intravenous immunoglobulin (IVIG) given at a dose of 500 mg/kg/week until day +90 post-HSCT has been associated with a reduced incidence of acute GVHD, fewer infections, and less interstitial pneumonia (Sullivan et al., 1990). Its immunomodulatory properties may be explained, in part, by the fact that when IgG is bound to macrophages, IL-1 receptor antagonist production is preferentially increased over the production of the cytokine IL-1, resulting in lower levels of IL-1—one of the cytokines responsible for GVHD. Data from animal models also indicate that IVIG may induce apoptosis of donor-derived Th-1 cytokine producing T lymphocytes (Caccavelli et al., 2001).

IVIG has been hypothesized to inhibit the cytokines that mediate GVHD; therefore, it has been used in some transplant programs to help to reduce or modulate the severity of acute GVHD. However, rigorous scientific data supporting the use of IVIG therapy in prevention and treatment of GVHD is lacking (Sokos, Berger, & Lazarus, 2002). Some data exist to suggest a potential beneficial effect of IVIG on reducing acute GVHD, particularly in patients older than 20 years of age (Sokos et al.). However, studies also suggest that the use of IVIG may have long-term adverse effects on immune reconstitution. One study of the effect of IVIG on the incidence and severity of late post-transplant complications demonstrated that extending IVIG treatment beyond three months post-transplant was associated with delayed recovery of humoral immunity, as demonstrated by lower serum IgG and IgA levels (Sullivan et al., 1996).

Thalidomide has been found to have immunosuppressive and immunomodulating properties and may be useful in patients with chronic GVHD who do not respond to other therapies. It is thought to function as a downregulator of donor T cells at the antigen recognition level (Wood & Proctor, 1990). Therapy is initiated at 100 mg po nightly and increased gradually to 400–600 mg per day. Studies suggested that thalidomide offers no clinical benefit when incorporated into the initial treatment of chronic GVHD (Arora et al., 2001), and it has no benefit when used as a prophylactic measure for chronic GVHD (Chao, Parker, & Niland, 1996). Thalidomide may have value as a salvage therapy for chronic progressive GVHD. Phase I–II trials of thalidomide for chronic GVHD resulted in a 48% survival among high-risk patients. Infection was the major cause of death (Parker, Chao, & Nademanee, 1995). Thalidomide also is being investigated as an adjunct to treatment with corticosteroids and either cyclosporine or tacrolimus as initial therapy for clinically extensive chronic GVHD (Koc et al., 2000). Side effects include somnolence, skin rash, constipation, and peripheral neuropathy. There is an increased risk of severe cutaneous ulcerations in patients being treated with thalidomide, and patients with chronic GVHD who are on thalidomide should be monitored carefully for skin breakdown (Schlossberg, Klumpp, Sabol, Herman, & Mangan, 2001).

Octreotide, a synthetic somatostatin analog, is useful in managing the severe diarrhea caused by acute intestinal GVHD (Ippoliti et al., 1997; Ippoliti & Neumann, 1998; Kornblau et al., 2000). Octreotide decreases gastropancreatic secretions, stool volume, intestinal motility, and luminal fluids; it inhibits electrolyte secretion and stimulates water, chloride, and sodium reabsorption. Potential side effects include nausea, abdominal cramps, flatulence, constipation, and, rarely, ileus. Biliary sludge and cholestasis, as well as hyperglycemia or hypoglycemia, also may occur. A dose of 100–150 mcg every eight hours may be given as initial therapy and the dose titrated up to 500 mcg IV every eight hours until symptom control is achieved. Beckman, Siden, Yanik, and Levine (2000) reported the effective use of a continuous infusion of octreotide in managing diarrhea caused by acute intestinal GVHD. Ippoliti and Neumann recommended that if a benefit is not seen after four to seven days of maximal treatment, continuing octreotide therapy is neither cost-effective nor beneficial. Octreotide should be tapered over three to five days, depending on tolerance, to prevent rebound of the diarrhea.

Phototherapy

Several therapeutic approaches to the treatment of acute and chronic GVHD, all of which involve the use of ultraviolet (UV) A or B irradiation, have been described and may have an important role as an adjunct to systemic immunosuppression. These approaches include extracorporeal photopheresis (ECP), psoralen and UVA irradiation (PUVA), UVB irradiation, and UVA_1 irradiation. All of these therapies have the advantage of being relatively nontoxic, particularly when compared to systemic immunosuppression, and may allow for a reduction in the intensity of systemic immunosuppression, thus sparing the patient some of the deleterious effects of maximal systemic immunosuppression. The procedures, therapeutic rationale, toxicities and side effects, and outcomes that have been described for each of these approaches are briefly reviewed later in this chapter.

ECP, also sometimes termed extracorporeal photochemotherapy, is a therapeutic approach based on the biological effect of methoxypsoralen and UV light on mononuclear cells collected by apheresis and reinfused into the patient. ECP is performed by a standard apheresis procedure. In each treatment, 150–200 ml of buffy coat is collected, and 200 mcg of methoxypsoralen is injected into the bag containing the white blood cells diluted with plasma or plasmalyte. The cell solution then is exposed to UV light and reinfused into the patient. Patients usually are treated on two consecutive days at two-to-four week intervals (Oliven & Shechter, 2001). The mechanism of action of ECP is not well delineated, although it appears to involve a shift in cytokine profiles from a Th1 to a Th2 response and inactivation and apoptosis of T lymphocytes (French & Rook, 2002; Klosner, 2001). In patients demonstrating a response to ECP, treatment continues every two weeks for an extended period, with progressively longer intervals between treatments. The optimal duration of ECP treatment for GVHD is unclear; however, several reports have indicated that more than six months of ECP treatment may be necessary (Kanold et al., 2003). Abrupt termination of ECP is avoided because symptoms may rebound (Oliven & Schechter). Reports of the application of ECP for the treatment of acute and chronic GVHD have shown variable outcomes and are confounded by differences in patient selection, entry criteria, additive immunosuppressive treatment, and differing ECP treatment frequency, but some substantial responses have been described (Alcindor et al., 2001; Apisarnthanarax et al., 2003; Foss, Gorgun, & Miller, 2002; Greinix et al., 2000; Smith et al., 1998). In general, ECP is well tolerated, although complications such as catheter infection and thrombosis, related to the long-term indwelling central venous apheresis catheters needed to maintain the vascular access required for the treatment, may occur. Patients receiving ECP also may experience minor and self-limiting treatment-related side effects, such as transient hypotension during the procedure or postreinfusion fever and erythema (Apisarnthanarax et al.).

PUVA has been used for many years to treat a variety of dermatologic diseases, including vitiligo, lichen planus atopic dermatitis, and eczema. Although the photobiological effects of PUVA and the mechanisms involved in the generation of immunosuppression are not fully understood, UV irradiation has profound effects that can prevent or inhibit allorecognition between donor and host cells and tissues (Furlong et al., 2002). PUVA may be used to treat both acute and chronic GVHD of the skin (Bonanomi et al., 2001; Grundmann-Kollmann et al., 2000; Stander, Schiller, & Schwarz, 2002) and the oral manifestations of chronic GVHD (Elad, Garfunkel, Enk, Galili, & Or, 1999; Vogelsang et al., 1996; Wiesmann et al., 1999) and can be highly effective in some patients, although response may be difficult to predict. Several weeks of treatment may be required until improvement is noted. Patients are given methoxypsoralen, a photosensitizing medication, approximately two hours before controlled exposure to the UV light. PUVA is given three to four times per week until symptoms resolve and then slowly tapered thereafter. Serious side effects such as severe phototoxicity are rare, although many patients do experience slight redness, dryness, burning, and peeling.

Local or Topical Therapy

Although virtually all patients with extensive disease require systemic therapy, many patients also will derive symptomatic relief from local or topical therapy (Currie, Ludvigsdottir, Diaz, & Kamani, 2002). Decadron elixir 10 ml (0.5 mg/5 ml) can be swished and spit four times per day and may be effective in controlling oral manifestations of chronic GVHD (Marcellus & Vogelsang, 2000; Schubert & Sullivan, 1990) and help with oral mucosal pain and irritation. Betamethasone enemas have been shown to have some effect in improving diarrhea and/or abdominal pain in patients with refractory or severe intestinal GVHD (Rai, Hendrix, Moskaluk, Levine, & Pasricha, 1997; Wada et al., 2001), and the use of oral beclomethasone has been described in the treatment of intestinal GVHD (Sudan et al., 2002). Tacrolimus ointment 0.1% has been shown in a small case series of patients to be effective in treating the erythema and pruritus of steroid-refractory, chronic cutaneous GVHD and may be a useful therapeutic bridge to other therapies that have a slower onset, such as PUVA or ECP (Choi & Nghiem, 2001). Topical cyclosporine and corticosteroid eye drops may be helpful in controlling ocular symptoms and inflammation (Kiang, Tesavibul, Yee, Kellaway, & Przepiorka, 1998).

Other Strategies for Graft Versus Host Disease Prevention

T cell depletion is an approach to prevent GVHD in which T lymphocytes are removed from the stem cell graft. It is an attractive and highly effective method of preventing acute GVHD because it offers the potential for prevention of GVHD without the morbidity associated with immunosuppressive drugs (Talmadge, 2003).

Several approaches have been developed to deplete donor T cells from the allogeneic hematopoietic stem cell graft, including physical separation methods, immunologic separation methods, and combined physical and immunologic

separation methods (Ho & Soiffer, 2001). Physical separation techniques may be divided into negative and positive selection techniques. Negative selection techniques are designed to select out of the graft the unwanted components. Examples include density gradient fractionation or soybean lectin agglutination followed by rosetting with sheep red blood cells. Positive selection techniques are designed to select out of the graft only the desired components, thereby eliminating the undesired components. Immunoadsorption columns are an example of a positive selection technique. Immunologic methods include monoclonal antibodies directed against T cell antigens. Examples of immunologic methods of T cell depletion include immunotoxins (e.g., anti-CD5-ricin) and the set of antibodies known as Campath-1. Sometimes both physical and immunologic methods are combined; for example, soybean agglutination may be followed by treatment of the graft with a monoclonal antibody.

Although T cell depletion reduces the incidence of GVHD, it is associated with several adverse effects, including poorer engraftment, increased risk of disease relapse, delayed immune reconstitution, and an increased risk of infections, especially CMV and adenoviral infections, and secondary malignancies in the post-transplant period (Chakrabarti et al., 2002; Ho & Soiffer, 2001). Newer approaches to the evaluation of chimerism hold the potential to predict those individuals at greatest risk for disease relapse following a T cell–depleted transplant, thus permitting earliest intervention with strategies such as DLI to treat minimal residual disease (Fernandez-Aviles et al., 2003). Despite the limitations associated with current approaches to T cell depletion, great interest remains in developing and improving this technology, particularly for recipients of HLA-mismatched grafts.

Clinical Application of Strategies for Prophylaxis and Treatment of Graft Versus Host Disease

Prophylaxis of Acute Graft Versus Host Disease

There are two major approaches to the prophylaxis of GVHD following HSCT: T cell depletion of the graft and pharmacologic therapy. Prevention of GVHD may be achieved with single-agent immunosuppression (often tacrolimus or cyclosporine A) or with multiple-agent immunosuppression (methotrexate, tacrolimus, cyclosporine A, steroids, ATG), sometimes in combination with T cell depletion and/or IVIG administration (Chao, 1999b; Sullivan, 1999). More intensive strategies for GVHD prevention are required for patients at higher risk for GVHD, especially those undergoing matched unrelated HSCT.

The variety of immunosuppressive agents, alone or in combination, that may be used as prophylaxis for acute GVHD were discussed previously. Prospective randomized trials have demonstrated that combination therapy is superior to single-agent therapy in the prevention of acute GVHD;

however, to date, no one regimen of prophylaxis has consistently been shown to be superior in preventing acute GVHD or improving overall outcomes (Chao et al., 2000; Locatelli et al., 2000; Nash et al., 2000; Ogawa et al., 2002). The most widely used pharmacologic regimen for the prophylaxis of acute GVHD is a combination of methotrexate and either cyclosporine or tacrolimus. Other pharmacologic agents included in some GVHD prophylaxis regimens include corticosteroids, ATG, daclizumab, alemtuzumab, and MMF. Examples of some commonly used drug regimens for the prevention of acute GVHD are shown in Table 6-9.

Treatment of Acute Graft Versus Host Disease

Despite measures to prevent GVHD, 30%–60% of patients will still develop some degree of acute GVHD that must be treated (Arai & Vogelsang, 2000). Treatment is generally required for grade II–IV acute GVHD, and therapy generally involves the same agents as used for prophylaxis. Corticosteroids are the main component of therapy for established GVHD, along with continuing treatment with the immunosuppressive agent used for prophylaxis (tacrolimus or cyclosporine A). High doses of methylprednisolone are used, varying from 1–50 mg/kg/day. Ultra high-dose regimens are associated with fatal opportunistic infections and cannot be administered for more than a few days. Most clinicians reduce the dose rapidly to 2 mg/kg/day in divided doses. Once maximal improvement is achieved, the steroids are tapered over 8–20 weeks, based on patient response. Concomitant prophylactic antibiotic, antiviral, and antifungal therapy is recommended.

For patients in whom initial therapy has failed (commonly defined as progression after 3 days, no change after 7 days, or incomplete response after 14 days of steroid treatment), there are a variety of salvage or secondary regimens, including MMF (Basara et al., 1998), infliximab (Couriel et al., 2000; Kobbe et al., 2001), etanercept (Andolina, Rabusin, Maximova, & Di Leo, 2000; Simpson, 2001), daclizumab (Przepiorka et al., 2000), alemtuzumab (Campath-1) (Simpson, 2003; Varadi, Or, Slavin, & Nagler, 1996), pentoxifylline (Margolis, Phelps, & Chen, 2000), N-acetylcysteine (Colombo et al., 1999), sirolimus (Abo-Zena & Horwitz, 2002; Chen, Morris, & Chao, 2000; Murphy & Krensky, 1999; Simpson, 2001), and ECP (Greinix et al., 2000; Kanold et al., 2003; Richter et al., 1997).

The outcome of treatment of acute GVHD is predicted by the overall grade of acute GVHD, with higher overall grades associated with poorer outcomes (MacMilan et al., 2002). Response to treatment is another key determinant of outcome, with mortality and morbidity highest in patients who do not achieve a complete response to the initial treatment strategy for acute GVHD (Sullivan, 1999). Opportunistic infections, including CMV disease, invasive aspergillosis, and disseminated varicella zoster infection, are a particular risk in patients who have received second and third line treatment of acute GVHD (Zupan, Zver, & Pretnar, 2002).

Treatment of Chronic Graft Versus Host Disease

The diversity of organ involvement with chronic GVHD, as well as the hematologic and immunologic dysfunction associated with the syndrome, all contribute to the difficulties in successfully treating chronic GVHD (Ratanatharathorn et al., 2001). Limited chronic GVHD is generally not treated, while extensive chronic GVHD may be treated with a variety of regimens (Akpek, Lee, et al., 2001; Chao, 1998; Vogelsang, 2001). Patients with limited chronic GVHD at presentation require careful follow-up because they may progress to a more extensive category (Marcellus & Vogelsang, 2000).

Table 6-9. Examples of Commonly Used Drug Regimens for Prevention of Acute Graft Versus Host Disease

Regimen	Dosing Schedule
Cyclosporine/steroids	*Cyclosporine 3 mg/kg/day IV infusion from day −2, taper 10% weekly starting day +180 Methylprednisolone 0.25 mg/kg bid days +7 to +14, 0.5 mg/kg bid days +15 to +28, 0.4 mg/kg bid days +29 to +42, 0.25 mg/kg bid days +59 to +119, and 0.1 mg/kg daily days +120–180
Cyclosporine/methotrexate/steroids	*Cyclosporine 5 mg/kg/day IV infusion from Day −2, taper 20% every two weeks starting day +84 Methotrexate 15 mg/m^2 on day +1, 10 mg/ m^2 on days +3 and +6 Methylprednisolone 0.25 mg/kg bid days +7 to +14, 0.5 mg/kg bid days +15 to +28, 0.4 mg/kg bid days +29 to +42, 0.25 mg/kg bid days +59 to +119, and 0.1 mg/kg daily days +120–180
Tacrolimus/mini-methotrexate	*Tacrolimus 0.03 mg/kd/day infusion from day −2, taper 20% every two weeks starting day +180 Methotrexate 5 mg/m^2 on days +1, +3, +6, and +11
ATG/cyclosporine/methotrexate	ATG 20 mg/kg IV days −3, −2, and −1 *Cyclosporine 5 mg/kg/day IV infusion from day −1, taper 10% weekly starting day +180 Methotrexate 10 mg/m^2 on day +1, +3, +6, and +11

*Tacrolimus and cyclosporine have been used interchangeably with this methotrexate or steroid dose schedule.

Note. Based on information from Chao, 1998; Goker et al., 2001; Przepiorka, 2000.

HEMATOPOIETIC STEM CELL TRANSPLANTATION: A MANUAL FOR NURSING PRACTICE

The current standard treatment for extensive chronic GVHD in high-risk patients is a regimen of alternate day cyclosporine or tacrolimus and prednisone (Goerner et al., 2002; Marcellus & Vogelsang, 2000; Vogelsang, 2000). However, a recently published randomized trial comparing cyclosporine A and prednisone with prednisone alone demonstrated reduced survival in patients receiving the two-drug regimen (Koc et al., 2002). In patients with newly diagnosed extensive chronic GVHD, initial treatment consists of prednisone at 1 mg/kg/day and daily cyclosporine or tacrolimus. Treatment is continued until there is objective evidence of improvement in manifestations of chronic GVHD. Tapering of prednisone by 25%–50% per week should begin within two weeks after the first evidence of improvement, even if manifestations have not resolved entirely. Tapering should continue to achieve a dose of 1 mg/kg every other day, as long as there is no exacerbation of chronic GVHD manifestations (Flowers, Lee, & Vogelsang, 2003; Marcellus & Vogelsang). Afer reaching an every other day dosing schedule, the prednisone dose is held constant until all reversible manifestations of chronic GVHD have resolved. The prednisone taper schedule can then be resumed and prednisone subsequently discontinued after at least two weeks of treatment at a dose of 0.15 mg/kg every other day. The calcineurin inhibitor then can be tapered slowly. A sample tapering schedule utilizing these concepts is illustrated in Table 6-10.

For chronic GVHD that is refractory to steroids and calcineurin inhibitors, such as tacrolimus and cyclosporine A, or is not well controlled, a variety of secondary therapies have been tried, with variable success (Carpenter & Sanders, 2003; Gaziev, Galimberti, Lucarelli, & Polchi, 2000; Vogelsang, 2001). These include thalidomide (Browne et al., 2000; Rovelli et al., 1998); PUVA (Grundmann-Kollmann et al., 2000); ECP (Apisarnthanarax et al., 2003; Bisaccia et al., 2003; Girardi, 2000; Smith et al., 1998; Zic, Miller, Stricklin, & King, 1999); MMF (Basara et al., 1998; Mookerjee, Altomonte, & Vogelsang, 1999); etretinate (Vogelsang, 2001; Marcellus et al., 1999); hydroxychloroquine (Gilman, Beams, Teftt, & Mazumbder, 1996; Goldman et al., 2000); azathioprine (Penas et al., 2002); total lymphoid irradiation (Socie, Devergie, & Cosset, 1990); intravenous lidocaine (Voltarelli et al., 2001); and clofazimine (Lee, Wegner, McGarigle, Bierer, & Antin, 1997). Akpek, Lee, et al. (2001) presented an algorithm for controlling active chronic GVHD by combining high-dose steroids with one or more of these approaches.

For patients with liver GVHD and associated cholestasis, administration of ursodeoxycholic acid (Actigall®, Novartis, New York) has been shown to be effective in improving liver function (Strasser, Shulman, & McDonald, 1999). The mechanisms underlying the beneficial effects of Actigall in liver GVHD are not well understood but may include protection of cholangiocytes against cytotoxicity of bile acids, stimulation of hepatobiliary secretion, and protection against bile acid-induced hepatocyte cell death (Paumgartner & Beuers, 2002). When used prophylactically from the day preceding the conditioning until day +90 after transplantation, Actigall also has been shown to be effective in reducing the overall severity of acute GVHD, possibly mediated by inhibiting production of IL-2, IL-4, and IFN-γ by peripheral blood mononuclear cells (Ruutu et al., 2002). Actigall is inexpensive, given orally, and extremely well tolerated. The only side effect reported is diarrhea, which is seen in less than 5% of patients (Kowdley, 2000). The optimal dosage of Actigall is unknown; however, a dosage of 12 mg/kg/day in a divided dose has been shown to be effective, and co-administration with food may enhance absorption (Ruutu et al.).

For pulmonary manifestations of chronic GVHD, including bronchiolitis obliterans and bronchiolitis obliterans organizing pneumonia, corticosteroids along with intensified immunsuppression with tacrolimus or MMF may be necessary (Afessa et al., 2001). Macrolide antibiotics, such as erythromycin, also have been shown to improve outcomes (Ishii et al., 2000).

Oral GVHD manifestations can be managed with dexamethasone mouth rinses (Marcellus & Vogelsang, 2000; Schubert & Sullivan, 1990), tacrolimus ointment to lips, or oral UV phototherapy (Elad et al., 1999; Vogelsang, 2001). In patients with oral and ocular dryness, pilocarpine 5 mg po every six hours can reduce dryness and may be beneficial in treating these symptoms (Nagler & Nagler, 1999; Vivino et al., 1999). Oral beclomethasone may be helpful in the management of enteritis (Baehr, Bouvier, & Stern, 1994; Rai et al., 1997; Sudan et al., 2002). Tacrolimus ointment, corticosteroid ointment, or cyclosporine ointment can be helpful in the management of vaginal sicca and stricture formation. Ocular sicca symptoms resulting from GVHD may benefit from ophthalmic cyclosporine or tacrolimus (Ahmade, Stegman, Fruchthman, & Asbell, 2002) or the insertion of punctal plugs.

It should be noted that in patients with oral manifestations of GVHD and who are on immunosuppression, oral infections caused by herpes simplex virus and *Candida* species can occur simultaneously (Schubert & Sullivan, 1990). Careful evaluation of the oral cavity and cultures of the lesion is key to an accurate diagnosis and treatment of oral cavity infections. Good oral hygiene and prevention of tissue trauma are also important.

Systemic immunosuppression is the basis of treatment of chronic GVHD, yet there is a delicate balance between controlling chronic GVHD symptoms and increasing susceptibility to infections, a major cause of death in these patients. Central to managing chronic GVHD is the ability to recognize its initial manifestations and establish the diagnosis; assess its severity, trajectory, and response to therapy; and gauge its impact on survival and quality of life (Lee, Vogelsang, et al., 2002). The presentation of chronic GVHD is varied, and its symptoms may mimic other disease entities (Jacobsohn, Montross, Anders, & Vogelsang, 2001). Furthermore, because the therapy for chronic GVHD can have significant toxicities, accurate and prompt recognition of chronic GVHD is essential for optimal management and to avoid under- or overtreatment of disease manifestations

Table 6-10. Sample Treatment Plan for Alternate-Day Steroids/Tacrolimus/Cyclosporine in the Management of Extensive Chronic GVHD

Treatment Week of Therapy	Prednisone (mg/kg/day po) (Given as a single am dose)		Tacrolimus (mg/kg/day po) (in a divided dose)+ (Based on ideal weight or actual weight, whichever is less)		Cyclosporine (mg/kg/day po) (in a divided dose)+ (Based on ideal weight or actual weight, whichever is less)	
	Day A	Day B	Day A	Day B	Day A	Day B
1	1	1	0.12	0.12	10	10
2	1	1	0.12	0.12	10	10
3*	1	0.75	0.12	0.12	10	10
4	1	0.50	0.12	0.12	10	10
5	1	0.25	0.12	0.12	10	10
6	1	0.12	0.12	0.12	10	10
7	1	0.06	0.12	0.12	10	10
After resolution of all clinical manifestations	1	0	0.12	0.12	10	10
↓	1	0	0.12	0.12	10	10
20	0.7	0	0.12	0.12	10	10
22	0.55	0	0.12	0.12	10	10
24	0.35	0	0.12	0.12	10	10
26	0.25	0	0.12	0.12	10	10
28	0.20	0	0.12	0.12	10	10
30	0.15	0	0.12	0.12	10	10
32	0.15	0	0.12	0.12	10	10
34	Discontinue prednisone.	Discontinue prednisone.	May begin tapering tacrolimus.	May begin tapering tacrolimus.	May begin tapering cyclosporine.	May begin tapering cyclosporine.

* Prednisone taper begins within two weeks of objective improvement.
+ Monitor tacrolimus or cyclosporine levels.

(Jacobsohn et al., 2001). A recent study suggested that there is major practice variation in the diagnosis of chronic GVHD and assessment of disease severity (Lee, Vogelsang, et al., 2002). Classification systems for chronic GVHD are rudimentary, and development of a more refined approach to classification, grading, and prognostication for patients with chronic GVHD, which might allow for more specific therapy, is an important area of ongoing research (Akpek, Lee, et al., 2003; Akpek, Zahurak, et al., 2001; Lee, Cook, Soiffer, & Antin, 2002). There is also an urgent need to define the most appropriate diagnostic approaches for evaluating chronic GVHD, establish criteria for disease activity, and develop and test new approaches to treating chronic GVHD (Goerner et al., 2002; Lee, Vogelsang, & Flowers, 2003).

Components of Supportive Care for Patients With Acute and Chronic Graft Versus Host Disease

GVHD is a cause of significant morbidity following allogeneic stem cell transplantation. Supportive care measures, such as infection prophylaxis, nutritional management, multidisciplinary team involvement, and coordination and continuity of care, are essential to improving the length and quality of life for patients with GVHD (Arai & Vogelsang, 2000).

Earliest Detection and Prophylaxis Against Infection

There is increased susceptibility to bacterial, fungal, and viral infections in patients with acute and chronic GVHD because of the immunosuppressive effects of GVHD itself and to its treatment with potential immunosuppressive agents (Adler et al., 1998; Arai & Vogelsang, 2000; Gaziev et al., 2000; Ratanatharathorn et al., 2001). In the presence of GVHD, immune defects involving both cellular and humoral immunity lead to poor secondary immune responses and failure of interaction between T helper and B cells. Immunosuppression with corticosteroids and other potent immunosuppressive agents intensifies these risks (Rantanatharathorn et al., 2001). Infections, including *Pneumocystis carinii* pneumonia, viral infections (e.g., CMV, polyoma virus, adenovirus), pneumococcal infections, and the common pathogens founds in the upper airways are a major cause of morbidity and mortality in these patients. Guidelines for antimicrobial prophylaxis of patients with GVHD tend to be institution or protocol specific, and controversy remains in several areas, particularly with regard to routine prophylaxis for bacterial infections (Sepkowitz, 2002) and vaccination against infectious diseases (Goldberg, Cicogna, Rowley, & Pecora, 2003). The Centers for Disease Control and Prevention (CDC), in collaboration with numerous professional societies, recently has published guidelines for preventing and treating opportunistic infections among HSCT recipients (CDC, Infectious Diseases Society of America, and American Society of Blood and Marrow Transplantation, 2000). These guidelines provide evidence-based recommendations for preventing exposure to and disease from opportunistic pathogens, including bacteria, viruses, fungi, and protozoa, after HSCT.

Marcellus and Vogelsang (2000) recommended that patients with chronic GVHD receive prophylaxis for *Pneumocystis carinii* with sulfamethoxazole and trimethoprim (Bactrim DS®, Roche Pharmaceuticals) twice daily two to three times per week. Inhaled pentamidine, dapsone, or atovaquone also may be used in patients with an allergy to sulfa agents or who cannot tolerate treatment with Bactrim. Prophylaxis continues for at least six months following the completion of GVHD therapy. In all individuals with chronic GVHD, Sepkowitz (2002) recommended prophylaxis against *Streptococcus pneumoniae* using penicillin or, given the increasing *S. pneumoniae* resistance rates, an alternative agent, such as levofloxacin. Vogelsang recommended lifelong prophylaxis with penicillin for all patients with chronic GVHD. In addition, patients should receive antibiotic prophylaxis for dental and other invasive procedures according to the prophylaxis recommendations of the American Heart Association. Topical antifungal prophylaxis with clotrimazole troches or nystatin swishes should be used in all patients receiving local steroid therapy. Highly immunosuppressed transplant recipients also may be systematically prophylaxed with azole antifungal. Because many patients with chronic GVHD have low serum IgG levels, additional infection protection may be afforded by supplemental IVIG. The goal of such therapy is to keep the IgG level greater than 500 mg/dl (Marcellus & Vogelsang, 2000), and the usual dosage is 500 mg/kg given weekly or twice monthly. Consideration should be given to vaccination against *pneumococcus*, *Haemophilus influenzae* type B, and seasonal immunization against influenza to establish pathogen-specific immunity, although vaccination does not diminish the need for close follow-up and antimicrobial prophylaxis, particularly in those patients with chronic GVHD and those on immunosuppressive therapies (CDC et al., 2000; Goldberg et al., 2003).

CMV antigen surveillance should be performed weekly or at least twice monthly while patients are receiving GVHD treatment (Vogelsang, 2001). Patients with previous CMV reactivation or infection may require closer surveillance and may be maintained on ganciclovir, valganciclovir, or foscarnet prophylaxis while receiving steroids or when they have active GVHD (Seber & Vogelsang, 1998). Patients and their families should be educated about the importance of taking prophylactic antimicrobials as ordered and calling their healthcare team immediately if they experience fever or malaise. In order to minimize morbidity and mortality in chronic GVHD, healthcare providers must have a high index of suspicion for and aggressively investigate potential infections in patients with chronic GVHD. Patients with acute or chronic GVHD who are co-infected with hepatitis

B require careful monitoring, particularly as their immunosuppression is tapered. In their case series of HSCT recipients co-infected with hepatitis B, Seth et al. (2002) observed that 14% of patients experienced reactivation and clinical flare of their hepatitis B infection during tapering of immunosuppression or after withdrawal of immunosuppressive therapy. Strasser and McDonald (1999) recommended that all HSCT recipients co-infected with hepatitis B should be monitored for hepatitis B virus (HBV) DNA beginning two weeks post-transplant. Early initiation of pre-emptive antiviral therapy with lamivudine (Efremov, Georgievski, Cevreska, Pivkova, & Panovska, 2003; Picardi et al., 1998) may suppress HBV replication during the window post-transplant when patients are intensively immunosuppressed and limit hepatocellular damage at the critical time of immune recovery and immunosuppressive therapy withdrawal (Strasser & McDonald).

Nutritional Management

The clinical manifestations of GI GVHD, including nausea, vomiting, severe abdominal pain and cramping, voluminous diarrhea, and intestinal bleeding, all can affect nutritional intake, digestion and absorption of nutrients, and the enjoyment of food. Malabsorption and intestinal protein losses also are characteristic of the mucosal degeneration and resultant diarrhea associated with intestinal GVHD (Charuhas, 2000). Multiple coexisting nutrition-related problems are associated with chronic GVHD, including oral sensitivity/stomatitis, xerostomia, anorexia/poor oral intake, altered taste, fatigue, reflux symptoms, dysgeusia, weight loss and steroid-induced nitrogen loss, weight gain, diabetes, and fluid retention (Lenssen et al., 1990; Rock, 2000). It also has been suggested that the weight loss noted in patients with GVHD may be related to a higher resting energy expenditure and elevated serum level of TNF-α (Jacobsohn, Margolis, Doherty, Anders, & Vogelsang, 2002). Moreover, many of the medications used to prevent or treat GVHD also have nutritional implications (Charuhas; Nunes & Lucey, 1999). Close monitoring of nutritional status and optimal nutritional support are important complements to the therapy of acute or chronic GVHD and therefore are crucially important following allogeneic HSCT (Iestra, Fibbe, Zwinderman, van Staveren, & Kromhout, 2002).

A five-phase dietary regimen is outlined in Table 6-11 and should be instituted with the onset of clinical signs consistent with intestinal GVHD, such as more than 500 ml of watery diarrhea (Rock, 2000). The first phase consists of bowel rest with complete reliance on total parenteral nutrition to meet the needs for energy, protein, and micronutrients. Advancement through the stages from gut rest to the resumption of normal diet is based on improvement of clinical symptoms and diet tolerance. Clinical symptoms of diet intolerance include increased stool volume or diarrhea, increased emesis, and increased abdominal cramping (Rock). Lactose intolerance is common in patients with intestinal GVHD because lactose is one of the last disaccharidases to return following villous atrophy (Charuhas,

Table 6-11. Graft Versus Host Disease Progressive Diet Regimen

Stage	Diet Principles	Examples of Foods to Suggest
1	Bowel rest	NPO (nothing by mouth), consider need for total parenteral nutrition (TPN).
2	Liquids, isotonic, lactose-free, low residue, no caffeine, allow 60 ml every two to three hours. If diarrhea or cramps recur or persist, return to bowel rest. Continue TPN.	Water, decaffeinated tea, decaffeinated coffee, caffeine-free diet soft drinks, caffeine-free and sugar-free imitation fruit drinks (e.g., Crystal Light®), sugar-free Jell-O®, sugar-free Popsicles®, clear broth, consommé, bouillon, sugar-free or dietetic hard candy that does not contain sorbitol or xylitol
3	Introduce solid foods, choosing low-fiber, lactose-free, fat-free, starchy foods. Sugar is introduced during this phase. Small portions only. No meat or meat products are allowed. Low total acidity; no gastric irritants such as caffeine. Introduce one food at a time. Each new food may be tried with foods taken previously. Discontinue the most recently added food if diarrhea or abdominal pain increases. If symptoms persist, return to bowel rest. Continue TPN until calorie and protein counts are adequate and fluid intake is adequate. May drink water, decaffeinated tea, decaffeinated coffee, caffeine-free diet soft drinks, and caffeine-free and sugar-free imitation fruit drinks (e.g., Crystal Light), in addition to foods chosen from list.	Plain white bread/toast, bagel, English muffin Soda crackers, melba toast, matzo, graham crackers Cream of Wheat®, crisped rice, cornflakes, Cheerios® White rice, plain noodles Arrowroot cookies, social tea cookies Fruit juices (less than 60 ml serving/may try half strength): apple, cranberry, grape, pineapple, orange, grapefruit, or tomato juice (no more than two servings/day) Mashed or boiled potato without skin or butter Clear chicken, meat, or vegetable broth; consommé; broth containing noodles or rice Jell-O, Popsicles
4	Solid foods as in stage III but with fat intake slowly increased	Lactose-free milk Plain white bread/toast, bagel, English muffin, soda crackers, melba toast, matzo, graham crackers Cream of Wheat, crisped rice, cornflakes, Cheerios White rice, plain noodles Arrowroot cookies, social tea cookies Fruit juices (half strength or less than 60 ml serving): apple, cranberry, grape, pineapple, orange, grapefruit, or tomato juice (may increase to four servings/day) Mashed or boiled potato without skin or butter Trimmed lean meats, fish, and poultry baked, broiled, boiled, poached, roasted, or stewed Maximum one egg per day, boiled or poached Tuna or salmon packed in water or broth Cooked vegetables one to two servings/day (asparagus, carrots) Clear chicken, meat, or vegetable broth; consommé; broth containing noodles or rice Cream soups prepared with lactose-free milk Natural hard, low-fat cheese (skim-milk mozzarella, parmesan) Jell-O, Popsicles, peaches or pears canned in juice or water (maximum of half cup or two halves)
5	Advance to regular diet by adding restricted foods, one per day, to assess tolerance.	Gradually add maximum of 1 Tbsp. of butter, margarine, oil, smooth peanut butter, or mayonnaise or 2 Tbsp. of reduced-calorie salad dressing or mayonnaise Last foods to be tried include high-fiber foods, food or drinks that contain caffeine (e.g., coffee, chocolate, soft drinks with caffeine), and lactose-containing foods, including ice cream, custard, milk, and cottage cheese.

Note. Based on information from Bergerson, 1998; Charuhas, 2000; Gavreau et al., 1981; Vickers, 1994.

2000). In severe intestinal GVHD, the majority of a patient's calories and protein may need to be provided parenterally (Weisdorf & Schwarzenberg, 1999). Protein-losing enteropathy may require increased protein administration to improve nitrogen balance and maintain lean body mass.

Even when total parenteral nutrition is needed to support nutritional status, in general, some enteral nutrition should be maintained, if possible (Lenssen, Bruemmer, Aker, & McDonald, 2001). Enteral nutrition has a trophic effect on the intestinal mucosa, reducing bacterial translocation into the blood stream (Weisdorf & Schwarzenberg, 1999). It also stimulates gall bladder function, reducing cholestatic complications (Weisdorf & Schwarzenberg). Nutrition interventions should be tailored to the patient's specific problems and symptoms (Dobbin & Hartmuller, 2000). Consultation and ongoing follow-up with a clinical dietitian should be a part of the standard of care for these patients (Iestra et al., 2002). Further research is needed to determine the impact of nutritional interventions, such as glutamine supplementation, lipid supplementation, enteral feeding, and the administration of antioxidants, on GVHD and the outcomes of HSCT (Lenssen et al., 2001; Muscaritoli, Grieco, Capria, Iori, & Fanelli, 2002).

Avoidance of Sun Exposure

Sun exposure may activate or exacerbate GVHD of the skin. UV radiation may damage epidermal cells leading to increased antigen expression or increased cytokine release (Chao, 1998). Patients should be advised about appropriate methods for minimizing sun exposure, as outlined in Figure 6-13.

Multidisciplinary Team Involvement

Frequent multidisciplinary interventions, including dentistry or oral medicine, endocrinology, gynecology, ophthalmology, pulmonology, rheumatology, nutrition support, physical therapy and occupational therapy, and psychosocial oncology, are essential in caring for patients with acute and chronic GVHD. For example, because GVHD may affect the skin, eyes, mouth, and genitourinary tract, regular follow-up with dermatology, ophthalmology, dentistry, and gynecology for surveillance and treatment is an important component of the supportive care of these patients. Careful ophthalmologic follow-up is important to prevent long-term damage to the eyes in patients with ocular sicca syndrome and to ensure a successful outcome should surgery for cata-

racts (a common complication of long-term steroids and total body irradiation) be needed (Aristei et al., 2002; Penn & Kaz Soong, 2002). Patients with oral sicca syndrome are at increased risk for dental caries, so close dental follow-up is essential. The high prevalence of endocrine dysfunction in long-term survivors of HSCT, including gonadal dysfunction in men and women, adrenal insufficiency, thyroid dysfunction, and bone complications as a result of the conditioning therapy, immunosuppressive treatments, and immune system derangement (Schimmer, Minden, & Keating, 2000; Tauchmanova et al., 2002, 2003) suggest an important role for consultation with specialists in endocrinology. Physical therapy is important to prevent the limitations in range of motion, joint contractures, and impaired functional status that can result from sclerodermatous skin changes (Chao, 1998) and to minimize the proximal muscle weakness that results from long-term therapy with corticosteroids.

Support groups, individual and family psychotherapy, physical therapy, occupational therapy, and preventive and pre-emptive rehabilitation measures may help to prevent functional decline and emotional distress, thereby improving quality of life (Gillis & Donovan, 2001; Harder et al., 2002). Nurses have an important role in monitoring patients for symptoms that could benefit from the expertise of another discipline and in coordinating timely and appropriate referrals.

Coordination and Continuity of Care

Chronic GVHD is a primary factor in late transplant-related morbidity, including abnormalities of growth and development in children, quality of life, functional performance status, somatic symptoms, psychological functioning, sexual satisfaction, and employment in adults (Broers, Kaptein, LeCessie, Fibbe, & Hengeveld, 2000; Harder et al., 2002). Nurses have an important role in coordinating multidisciplinary involvement in the management of patients with GVHD, assessing and managing symptoms, and ensuring continuity of care. Supportive care and symptom management for the patient experiencing acute GVHD is a key nursing role. A standard of care for the patient with GVHD is presented in Figure 6-14.

Ongoing monitoring of patients for the rest of their life is critical for the prevention of late complications and disability (Baker et al., 2003; Kiss et al., 2002). At the time that chronic GVHD often develops, patients may be back in their local communities, at distance from healthcare providers with expertise in the identification and management of the diverse manifestations of chronic GVHD. Long-term follow-up contact by telephone, fax, or letter to patients and contact with primary care physicians, combined with regular evaluations at the transplant center, is crucial. Documentation of the development, features, severity, course, and management of GVHD is important to ensure quality of care and for outcomes evaluation. A tool for documenting the risk factors, features, severity, prevention, and management of GVHD is provided in Figure 6-15. The components of good long-term follow-up post-transplant have been outlined by Sullivan and Siadak (1997).

Figure 6-13. Counseling Guidelines for Limiting Sun Exposure

Ways to Protect Yourself From the Sun
- Limit outdoor activities between the hours of 10 am and 4 pm.
- Stay in the shade. Do not visit tanning salons.
- Routinely and liberally use a sunscreen with an SPF of 15 or higher. Apply the lotion one half-hour before you go out in the sun. Apply a generous amount and cover all exposed skin. Reapply at least every two hours, and reapply after swimming or perspiring.
- Use a lip balm with an SPF 15 sunscreen. Apply sunscreen on your face, even if you wear a hat.
- Some sunscreens may cause allergic reactions. If a sunscreen irritates your skin, change to another brand or consult your physician.
- Always apply sunscreen or cover your skin if you will have any sun exposure. Remember that you have sun exposure even on cloudy or hazy days. Water, sand, snow, and concrete can all reflect large amounts of sunlight onto the skin.
- Wear a wide-brimmed hat and sunglasses and cover all exposed areas of skin. Dark-colored, long-sleeved shirts and slacks with tightly woven fabrics offer the most protection
- The risk of sunburn is greater at high altitudes. The thinner atmosphere at high altitudes absorbs lesser amounts of damaging UV rays than at sea level.
- Some drugs and cosmetics may increase susceptibility to sunburn. These "photosensitivity reactions" may be caused by some antibiotics and by several other medications that transplant recipients commonly take.

Figure 6-14. Standard of Care for the Patient With Graft Versus Host Disease

Goals/Outcome Standards
- Patient will exhibit the absence of or control of signs and symptoms of potential physiologic and psychosocial problems listed below.
- Patient or significant other will verbalize an understanding of graft versus host disease (GVHD) and its potential impact on lifestyle and present and future health status.
  1. State the signs and symptoms of common potential complications and the appropriate action to be taken.
  2. Describe risk factors for GVHD and measures the patient can take to reduce the risk of GVHD.
  3. Describe measures to minimize the complications of GVHD, including altered skin integrity, nausea/vomiting, diarrhea, liver function abnormalities, fluid and electrolyte abnormalities, malnutrition, infection, pain, body image changes, weakness/activity intolerance, inadequate or impaired self-monitoring/health maintenance/treatment adherence.
  4. Describe the rationale for the diagnostic tests used to evaluate the signs and symptoms of GVHD.
  5. State the name, purpose, scheduling, and major side effects of the treatment approach currently being used to manage GVHD.
  6. State appropriate resources for support in coping with GVHD.

Nursing Interventions/Process Standards
Assess, monitor, and detect
- Risk factors for the development of acute and chronic GVHD.
- The impact of other preexisting health problems.
- And prevent the following potential problems and implement nursing interventions as appropriate.

Altered skin integrity, as evidenced by
- Erythematous, macular, papular skin rash involving the palms, soles, trunk, ears, face, and extremities. Bullae, desquamation, and epidermal necrosis may occur, with progression to generalized desquamation of the skin. The skin rash may be painful, burning, or itchy.
  1. Monitor skin daily for the development of findings suggestive of GVHD of skin and for the development of infection in areas of skin involved with GVHD.
  2. Keep skin lubricated with gentle moisturizing lotions.
  3. Consider use of antipruritic or steroid topical agents to manage symptoms.
  4. If skin breakdown occurs, consult enterostomal therapist or wound management specialist concerning nonadherent, absorptive dressings and the role of special beds/mattresses.
  5. Monitor patient for dehydration if there are increased insensible losses of fluid through skin with bullae and desquamation.
  6. Provide patient and family education regarding skin biopsy.
  7. Teach patient and family the importance of avoiding direct sun exposure and the importance of using sunblock and protective clothing when outdoors.
  8. Consider the need for antimicrobial prophylaxis or topic antimicrobial ointments to minimize secondary infection of open skin lesions.

Anorexia/nausea/vomiting, as evidenced by
- Lack of appetite; vague uneasiness/discomfort in the epigastrium, throat, or abdomen; forceful expulsion of stomach contents through the mouth; taste alteration
  1. Provide a calm, well-ventilated, aesthetic environment.
  2. Discuss approaches to use when experiencing taste changes, early satiety, nausea, or mucositis.
  3. Maintain hydration; consider need for total parenteral nutrition.
  4. Provide antiemetics.
  5. Modify diet to eliminate hot and spicy foods; offer cool, bland foods; provide small, frequent feedings.
  6. Absorption of oral medications may be severely impaired. Monitor blood levels of medications carefully and consider switching patient to parenteral formulation.
  7. Provide patient and family education regarding endoscopy.

Diarrhea, as evidenced by
- Profuse, green, mucoid watery stools mixed with exfoliated cells and tissue shreds, hypoalbuminemia, electrolyte imbalance, fluid imbalance, intestinal bleeding, crampy abdominal pain, and ileus
  1. Evaluate history of onset and duration of diarrhea, description of the number of stools and stool composition; review medication profile and dietary intake to identify any diarrheogenic agents/foods. Review pretreatment history, including usual bowel pattern, usual stool characteristics, and any history of recent travel or family members with diarrhea.
  2. Measure the amount of daily diarrhea and assess for the presence of hematochezia, abdominal cramping, and bowel sounds.
  3. Evaluate for dehydration, including weight loss, fluid balance, urine specific gravity, blood urea nitrogen and creatinine (BUN/Cr), and the presence of symptoms such as dizziness or lethargy.
  4. Absorption of oral medications may be severely impaired. Monitor blood levels of medications carefully and/or consider switching patient to parenteral formulation, if available.
  5. Stop all lactose-containing products and high-osmolar food supplements such as Ensure Plus®, laxatives, bulk fiber, and stool softeners.
  6. Instruct patient to avoid caffeine and alcohol and to consume a low-fat, low-fiber diet. Implement the five-phase diet outlined in Table 6-11, as appropriate.
  7. Encourage adequate oral fluids; consider the need for IV fluids to prevent dehydration.

(Continued on next page)

HEMATOPOIETIC STEM CELL TRANSPLANTATION: A MANUAL FOR NURSING PRACTICE

8. Check stool workup, including presence of blood, fecal leukocytes, *C. difficile* toxin, *Salmonella* species, *Campylobacter* species, VRE, and viruses.
9. Administer loperamide two capsules after every loose stool (MDD: 16 mg or 8 capsules) or two capsules every six hours around the clock.
10. If symptoms persist, consider tincture of opium at 0.3–1 ml po q 2–6 hours prn (MDD: 6 ml). May titrate upward, as needed.
11. If persistent diarrhea, consider octreotide 100–150 mcg tid. Consider escalating dose if no response.
12. Consider a trial of oral beclomethasone.
13. For chronic diarrhea, consider a trial of pancreatic enzyme replacement or lactase enzyme replacement.
14. Consider antibiotic prophylaxis against infection with organisms commonly found in the gut.
15. Assess perirectal skin integrity q shift and provide water-barrier ointment to areas to limit skin breakdown.
16. Consider enterostomal therapy consultation for input regarding measures to prevent or treat perirectal skin breakdown.
17. Provide patient and family education regarding endoscopy.

Liver function abnormalities, as evidenced by
- Increased bilirubin, alkaline phosphatase, AST, ALT, GGT, 5'NT, hepatomegaly, jaundice, ascites
  1. Monitor liver function tests and drug levels of cyclosporine or tacrolimus at regular intervals.
  2. Use caution when prescribing multiple hepatotoxic medications, or, where possible, select medications that are less likely to cause hepatotoxicity.
  3. Provide patient and family education regarding invasive procedures, such as liver biopsy.
  4. Administer Actigall® as ordered.

Fluid and electrolyte abnormalities, as evidenced by
- Hypokalemia, hypoalbuminemia, hypomagnesemia, orthostatic hypotension, orthostatic tachycardia, increased BUN/Cr
  1. Reinforce the importance of oral hydration of two to three liters per day, if not currently on bowel rest. If patient is NPO (nothing by mouth), administer IV fluids as ordered.
  2. Rehydrate with three to four liters of normal saline over a 24-hour period.
  3. During aggressive hydration, monitor for fluid overload and pulmonary edema through careful intake and output, serial weights, and clinical assessment.
  4. Ensure adequate replacement of fluid lost through diarrhea, third spacing, or desquamation of skin.
  5. Replete electrolytes lost through diarrhea.

Malnutrition, as evidenced by
- Inadequate carbohydrate, protein, or fat intake for needs, weight loss, low prealbumin levels
  1. Ensure regular and comprehensive evaluation of nutritional status. Follow GVHD diet, as outlined in Table 6-11, or as per institutional standards or recommendations from clinical dietitian.
  2. Monitor calorie counts and fluid intake to assess adequacy of nutritional intake.
  3. Discuss approaches to use when experiencing taste changes, thick/viscous saliva and mucus, xerostomia, early satiety, nausea/vomiting, mucositis or esophagitis, and other troubling symptoms.
  4. If patient is receiving high-dose steroids, ensure increased protein intake, calcium, and vitamin D supplementation. Consider restricted concentrated carbohydrate intake if hyperglycemia is present. Consider restricted sodium intake if fluid retention is especially problematic.
  5. Administer multiple vitamins without iron (to prevent iron overload), folic acid 1 mg po daily.
  6. Consider repletion of zinc and supplemental vitamin C if patient presents with extensive skin or gastrointestinal GVHD.
  7. Increase protein intake in patients with extensive skin or gastrointestinal GVHD.

Infection, as evidenced by
- Fever, chills, cough, dyspnea, shortness of breath, chest pain, diarrhea, dysuria, frequency, swelling, drainage, odor, perirectal pain, change in mental status
  1. Teach patient and family self-care strategies that can minimize the risk of infection.
  2. Administer prophylactic and empiric antibiotics, as ordered.
  3. Consider IV immunoglobulin therapy, if recurrent, life-threatening infections occur.
  4. Consider immunization against influenza and *Pneumococcus*, particularly for patients with chronic GVHD.

Pain, as evidenced by
- Verbalization or expression of pain/discomfort; may report abdominal cramping, muscle aches, oral mucosal pain, or skin pain
  1. Reduce diarrhea and associated cramping with loperamide, octreotide.
  2. Consider codeine, morphine, dicyclomine hydrochloride, belladonna, and opium, or deodorized tincture of opium in the management of spasmodic abdominal pain.
  3. Consider role of special bed/mattress to reduce pressure if skin is painful to touch.
  4. Administer narcotic analgesics as indicated.

Body image changes, as evidenced by
- Guilt, shame, denial, anger, hostility, despair, avoidance of social interactions, depression, inactivity, verbalized disgust with body
  1. Assess/build upon patient's strengths, appropriate socialization patterns, and coping skills.

(Continued on next page)

2. Encourage maintenance of role responsibilities.
3. Encourage therapeutic interactions with others.
4. Provide for continuity of care with minimal changes in caregiver.
5. Provide privacy to discuss feelings of self-esteem, body image, role performance, and personal identity.
6. Encourage discussion about condition, treatment, and prognosis.
7. Assist with personal grooming.

Weakness/activity intolerance, as evidenced by
- Focal muscle weakness, fatigue, dyspnea/shortness of breath
    1. Refer to physical and occupational therapy for assessment and treatment.
    2. Encourage focus exercises that provide proximal muscle strengthening to reduce proximal muscle weakness that occurs secondary to treatment with corticosteroids.
    3. Encourage patient to maintain maximal independence in activities of daily living (ADLs) and self-care.
    4. Assess which activities are most important, rewarding, and the patient's priority.
    5. Determine a schedule that allows adequate rest by coordinating all activity and treatments (e.g., ADLs, meds, health team rounds, patient's habits).
    6. Discuss parameters of assessment for tolerance and set goals for improving tolerance/endurance in activities.

Inadequate or impaired self-monitoring/health maintenance/treatment adherence, as evidenced by
- Missed appointments, unused/overused medications, questioning need for further treatment, depression, difficulty problem solving, difficulty demonstrating desired skills, inadequate knowledge base, nonadherence/noncompliance with nursing and/or medical recommendations
    1. Establish trust and congruence in goals and objectives.
    2. Provide information in a timely and specific manner.
    3. Serve as liaison between the physician and patient in interpreting medical jargon and helping patient to acquire needed information.
    4. Use positive reinforcement.
    5. Allow patient as much choice and control as appropriate and feasible.
    6. Encourage self-care whenever possible. Involve patient and family in problem-solving process.
    7. Demonstrate care, respect, and concern for the patient.
    8. Avoid the use of approaches that foster dependency (e.g., coercion, persuasion, manipulation).

Note. Based on information from Charuhas, 2000; Rosenzweig, 1998; Wesorick, 1990; Williams, 1999.

Developmental Strategies for the Prophylaxis, Treatment, and Control of Graft Versus Host Disease

A wide variety of approaches to the prevention, treatment, and control of GVHD are currently undergoing development and preclinical and clinical evaluation (Carpenter & Sanders, 2003; Cavazzana-Calvo et al., 2002; Reddy et al., 2003; Simpson, 2001, 2003). These include the application of cytokine shields to decrease the inflammatory tissue responses thought to promote acute GVHD (Hill & Ferrara, 2000), selective T cell depletion (Soiffer et al., 2001), the use of new agents with immunosuppressive properties for conditioning (Alcindor et al., 2000; Liesveld et al., 1999; Margolis et al., 2000; Proujansky, 1999), and modification of donor T cells through incorporation of suicide genes (Bonini et al., 1997), or the infusion of tumor-specific T cell clones (Patterson & Korngold, 2001).

An ability to predict which patients are at greatest risk for GVHD or to identify those patients with only biochemical serologic evidence of developing GVHD is important both for clinical trials design and clinical management. Although patients at higher risk for acute GVHD may benefit from special treatment or intensified immunosuppression, at present, one cannot precisely anticipate the degree of GVHD that will occur in an individual patient. Research efforts are ongoing to develop in vitro testing methods and sensitive predictive assays that can be used to estimate an individual patient's likelihood of developing GVHD and provide a clinically useful early indicator of evolving GVHD and a biologic measure of response to treatment (Chao, 1999a; Kayaba et al., 2000; Kokalj et al., 2002; Nakamura, 2000; Okamoto et al., 2001; Schots et al., 1998). For example, Kayaba et al. have shown in a small patient series that serum TNF-α levels were significantly higher in patients with acute GVHD, compared with those patients without acute GVHD.

Efforts are being made to determine the role of potent new immunosuppressive agents in the prevention of GVHD. Rapamycin, a macrolide produced by a filamentous bacterium, has been shown to be highly effective in preventing GVHD. It works to block signal transduction mediated by IL-2 and has long-lasting immunosuppressive effects, despite the drug's short half-life (Chen et al., 2000).

Keratinoycte growth factor (KGF) administered prior to transplantation in animal models has been shown to act as a cytokine shield (Hill et al., 1997), limiting GVHD while preserving a graft versus tumor effect (Filicko, Lazarus, and Flomenberg, 2003; Krijanovski et al., 1999; Panoskaltsis-Motari, Lacey, Vallera, & Blazar, 1998). KGF also has been shown to provide cytoprotection to thymic epithelial cells, thereby indirectly promoting normal functioning of the thymus in GVHD animal models and reducing GVHD-induced immune dysfunction (Rossi et al., 2002). Given the

Figure 6-15. Summary Record of Graft Versus Host Disease Prophylaxis and Treatment

Type of transplant:
❏ Related, fully matched ❏ Haploidentical ❏ Matched, unrelated ❏ Other: _____

❏ Ablative ❏ Nonmyeloablative

Disease:
❏ Acute myelogenous leukemia ❏ Acute lymphocytic leukemia ❏ Chronic myelogenous leukemia ❏ Aplastic anemia

❏ Hodgkin's disease ❏ Non-Hodgkin's lymphoma ❏ Multiple myeloma

Therapy:
Conditioning regimen: _____

❏ T cell depleted ❏ T cell repleted

Cell dose: _____ CD34+ cells/kg: _____CD3+ cells/kg

Date of transplant: _____

Donor CMV status: ❏ Reactive ❏ Non-reactive

Recipient CMV Status: ❏ Reactive ❏ Non-reactive

Date of initial engraftment of WBC (ANC > 1,000 for two days): _____

Dates and dose of donor lymphocyte infusion:

_____ _____ cells/kg
_____ _____ cells/kg
_____ _____ cells/kg
_____ _____ cells/kg

Initial GVHD Prophylaxis:
❏ Cyclosporine ❏ Tacrolimus ❏ Methotrexate ___mg/m^2 on days _____, _____, _____

❏ Methylprednisolone/Methylprednisolone sodium succinate: _____

Extent of GVHD:

Date	Site(s) of GVHD	Biopsy Findings	Stage/Grade Acute/Chronic	Performance Status

(Continued on next page)

GVHD Management Plan:

Therapy/ Treatment	Date Therapy Initiated/ Modified	Reason Initiated/Modified	Maximum Overall GVHD Grade	Other Findings/Comments

favorable clinical toxicity profile of KGF, this suggests that KGF may be a helpful adjunct to standard GVHD prophylaxis.

Increasingly, graft-engineering approaches may be a component of the prevention or control of GVHD (Cavazzana-Calvo et al., 2002; Noga & O'Donnell, 1998; Talmadge, 2003). For example, in animal models, the addition to the graft of a subset of regulatory (CD4+ CD25+) donor T cells that were exposed to recipient antigens and then expanded ex vivo delayed or even prevented the onset of GVHD without altering post-transplant immune reconstitution (Cohen, Trenado, Vasey, Klatzmann, & Salomon, 2002). Investigators also are focused on attempts to remove from the graft only the alloreactive T cells, the ones presumed to be major effectors of GVHD (Andre-Schmutz et al., 2002; Fehse, Frerk, Goldmann, Bulduk, & Zander, 2000). Efforts are also under way to develop methods of deactivating, rather than removing, T cells within the graft, thus inducing a state of tolerance (Chen, Cui, Liu, & Chao, 2002). Researchers are exploring whether GVHD can be controlled through insertion of a suicide gene into donor T cells at the time of engraftment. With this method, donor T cells are transfected with a gene-encoding herpes simplex type I thymidine kinase (TK) prior to transplant, and patients are then subsequently given a short course of ganciclovir. In this system, ganciclovir selectively kills dividing but not quiescent TK-transfected T cells. When the TK-gene-transfected donor T cells proliferate and divide to create GVHD, they are selectively eliminated by the ganciclovir. The pool of nonreactive, nondividing T cells is spared, thus contributing to recipient immune system reconstitution and graft versus tumor effect (Litvinova et al., 2002; Maury et al., 2002).

The success of DLI for the treatment of post-transplant relapse of CML has led researchers to explore the role of combining T cell depletion with a preplanned course of DLI post-transplant (Alyea et al., 2001; Baron & Beguin, 2002; Johnson, Becker, & Truitt, 1999; Lewalle et al., 2003; Talmadge, 2003). This approach is potentially attractive in that one can reap the benefits of T cell depletion early after transplantation by minimizing acute GVHD, yet be able to restore the graft versus tumor effect at a later time with DLI (Peggs & Mackinnon, 2001). In nonmyeloablative transplantation, early patterns of chimerism may allow clinicians to predict the time frame following HSCT at which the individual is at greatest risk for GVHD, and this information can be used to guide decisions about post-transplantation immunosuppression and about the dose and timing of post-transplantation DLI (Antin et al., 2001; Billiau, Fevery, Rutgeerts, Landuyt, & Waer, 2002; Fernandez-Aviles et al., 2003; Valcarcel et al., 2003). Currently, however, GVHD remains a major complication of DLI even when DLI is administered at a time when the patient is removed from the conditioning therapy and its associated inflammatory cytokine milieu (Akpek et al., 2002; Lee et al., 1999; Marks et al., 2002).

Induction of Graft Versus Host Disease— Preserving the Graft Versus Tumor Effect

Strategies for preventing GVHD are designed to limit the capacity of the newly grafted immune system to mount an immunologic response. These strategies have reduced the severity of GVHD; however, they also are associated with higher rates of graft failure and disease relapse (Mavroudis, 1998). It is now apparent that patients who develop GVHD have a lower risk of recurrent disease than patients without GVHD. This so-called graft versus tumor effect was first described in 1979 and has been shown to be crucial for long-term remission, particularly in patients with leukemia. Indirect evidence of a graft versus tumor effect includes the observations that T cell depletion of the HSCT graft and syngeneic HSCT are associated with a higher risk of relapse than allogeneic HSCT. It has been demonstrated clinically that graft versus tumor responses occur with DLI in 60%–80% of patients with chronic myelogenous leukemia and, to a lesser extent, with acute myelogenous leukemia, chronic lymphocytic leukemia, multiple myeloma (Alyea et al., 2001; Martino et al., 2002), non-Hodgkin's lymphoma, and renal cell carcinomas (Champlin et al., 1999; Collins et al., 1997; Dazzi, Szydlo, & Goldman, 1999). Both GVHD and the graft versus tumor effect are thought to be mediated by alloreactive donor T cells and NK cells recognizing host histocompatibility antigens. This hypothesis has subsequently led to the use of DLIs as well as other methods to augment the graft versus host response in an effort to treat or prevent disease relapse.

The initial step in promoting a graft versus tumor response to treat disease relapse involves immediate withdrawal of immunosuppressants. The allogeneic stem cell donor then is contacted for collection of lymphocytes by leukaphereses. The lymphocytes are infused into the patient, often as an outpatient procedure. There are few immediate effects of DLI; however, DLI has a 20% incidence of treatment-related mortality, mainly because of life-threatening GVHD and pancytopenia (Porter et al., 1999). Between 40%–55% of patients experience severe acute GVHD (grades II–IV) following DLI, and pancytopenia occurs in approximately 20% of patients (Collins et al., 1997). Pancytopenia may resolve spontaneously but also may require an infusion of donor stem cells to reestablish hematopoiesis. Following DLI, patients require close follow-up to monitor their disease response to DLI; determine the need for escalating DLI doses; ensure the earliest identification and appropriate treatment of signs of GVHD; and receive comprehensive supportive care to prevent and manage the effects of pancytopenia.

Escalating doses of DLI, as measured by the DLI product's CD34+ cell dose/kg of the patient's body weight, may be used to achieve an adequate graft versus tumor effect without producing life-threatening GVHD (Dazzi et al., 2000; Lewalle et al., 2003). Recent studies suggested that patients with greater tumor cell burdens, as in the case of a hematologic relapse, require greater DLI cell doses than do patients in cytogenetic or molecular relapse (Carlens, Remberger, Aschan, & Ringden, 2001; Dazzi et al., 2000).

It is possible for patients to have an allogeneic graft versus tumor effect that is not associated with clinically evident GVHD. Research is ongoing to find ways to augment the graft versus tumor effect while minimizing or separating it from GVHD (Fefer, 1999; Talmadge, 2003). These attempts include selective depletion of alloactivated donor T lymphocytes from the DLI (Andre-Schmutz et al., 2002) and escalating the lymphocyte cell dose infused to establish a dose that will stimulate graft versus tumor effect but that is below the threshold that produces severe GVHD (Lewalle et al., 2003; Mackinnon et al., 1995). Studies in animal models have demonstrated that the administration of human recombinant KGF before conditioning therapy ameliorates GVHD but does not reduce the graft versus tumor effect (Krijanovski et al., 1999; Panoskaltsis-Mortari et al., 1998). Studies also are exploring the potential to transfect donor lymphocytes with a suicide or "knock out" gene, such as herpes simplex virus TK, which confers sensitivity of the transfected lymphocytes to ganciclovir. These lymphocytes are capable of producing a graft versus tumor response; however, if moderately severe GVHD develops, it can be treated promptly with ganciclovir, resulting in lysis of the transfected lymphocytes. This novel approach may allow for extinction of T cells after they have produced the beneficial graft versus tumor effect but before they can cause life-threatening GVHD.

Conclusion

GVHD is a direct result of one of the principal functions of the immune system: the distinction of self from non-self. The pathophysiology of GVHD involves recognition of epithelial target tissues within the host as foreign by immunocompetent cells contained in the graft, resulting in an inflammatory response and eventual apoptotic death of the target tissue. Although an improved understanding of the pathogenesis of GVHD continues to evolve and despite new approaches to immunosuppression, graft engineering, and adoptive immunotherapy that are emerging at a rapid pace, GVHD remains a major cause of morbidity and mortality after HSCT.

Oncology and bone marrow transplant nurses have important roles in the care of patients experiencing this complication. Key nursing responsibilities include (a) safely and effectively administering a multidrug regimen to prevent or treat GVHD; (b) monitoring the patient for the effectiveness and side effects of treatment; (c) providing patient and family education to ensure adherence with therapy and effective self-management of expected side effects; (d) assessing and managing symptoms such as infection risk, fluid and electrolyte imbalance, nutritional compromise, altered skin integrity, and discomfort; and (e) facilitating coordination and continuity of care and appropriate ongoing multidisciplinary follow-up.

The author gratefully acknowledges the assistance and contributions of the following individuals: Dr. Howard Fine, National Cancer Institute, for his support of this project; Dr. Bruce Greenwald (University of Maryland at Baltimore), Dr. Jane Fall-Dickson (National Institutes of Health), Dr. Gabriel Yihune (University Hospitals Heidelberg), and the Online Atlas of Dermatology (www.dermis.net/doia) for providing selected photographs and endoscopic images; Donald F. Bliss, II, Medical Illustrator, Medical Arts and Photography Branch, National Institutes of Health, Office of Research Services, and Jennifer Gentry, Gentry Visualizations, for assistance with the preparation of images and illustrations; and Robert and Vera Mitchell for bibliographic assistance. A debt of gratitude also is owed to the many patients who have shared their experiences so that we may improve the care we provide.

References

Abdelsayed, R.A., Sumner, T., Allen, C., Treadway, A., Ness, G., & Penza, S. (2002). Oral precancerous and malignant lesions associated with graft-versus-host disease: Report of two cases. *Oral Surgery, Oral Medicine, Oral Pathology, 93*, 75–80.

Abo-Zena, R., & Horwitz, M. (2002). Immunomodulation in stem cell transplantation. *Current Opinion in Pharmacology, 2*, 452–457.

Adler, H., Beland, J.L., Kozlow, W., Del-Pan, N.C., Kobzik, L., & Rimm, I.J. (1998). A role for transforming growth factor-beta 1 in the increased pneumonitis in muric allogeneic bone marrow transplant recipients with graft versus host disease after pulmonary herpes simplex virus type 1 infection. *Blood, 92*, 2581–2589.

Afessa, B., Litzow, M., & Tefferi, A. (2001). Bronchiolitis obliterans and other late onset non-infectious complications in hematopoietic stem cell transplantation. *Bone Marrow Transplantation, 28*, 425–434.

Ahmade, S.M., Stegman, Z., Fruchtman, S., & Asbell, P.A. (2002). Successful treatment of acute ocular graft versus host disease with tacrolimus (FK 506). *Cornea, 21*, 432–433.

Akpek, G., Boitnott, J.K., Lee, L.A., Hallick, J.P., Torbenson, M., Jacobsohn, D.A., et al. (2002). Hepatitic variant of graft-versus-host disease after donor lymphocyte infusion. *Blood, 100*, 3903–3907.

Akpek, G., Chinratanalab, W., Lee, L.A., Torbenson, M., Hallick, J.P., Anders, V., et al. (2003). Gastrointestinal involvement in chronic graft versus host disease. A clinicopathologic study. *Biology of Blood and Marrow Transplantation, 9*, 46–51.

Akpek, G., Lee, S., Anders, V., & Vogelsang, G.B. (2001). A high-dose pulse steroid regimen for controlling active chronic graft-versus-host disease. *Biology of Blood and Marrow Transplantation, 7*, 495–502.

Akpek, G., Lee, S.J., Flowers, M.E., Pavletic, S.Z., Arora, M., Lee, S., et al. (2003). Performance of a new clinical grading system for chronic graft versus host disease: A multi-center study. *Blood, 102*, 802–809.

Akpek, G., Valladares, J.L., Lee, L., Margolis, J., & Vogelsang, G. (2001). Pancreatic insufficiency in patients with chronic graft versus host disease. *Bone Marrow Transplantation, 27*, 163–166.

Akpek, G., Zahurak, M., Piantadosi, S., Margolis, J., Doherty, J., Davidson, R., et al. (2001). Development of a prognostic model for grading chronic graft–versus–host disease. *Blood, 97*, 1219–1226.

Alcindor, T., Chan, G., Al-Olama, A., Miller, K., Roberts, T., Schenkein, D., et al. (2000). Engraftment and immunologic effects of a novel less myeloablative allogeneic transplant conditioning regimen of continuous infusion pentostatin, photopheresis, and low dose TBI [Abstract]. *Blood, 96*, 327a.

Alcindor, T., Gorgun, G., Miller, K., Roberts, T., Sprague, K., Schenkein, D., et al. (2001). Immunomodulatory effects of extracorporeal photochemotherapy in patients with extensive chronic graft-versus-host disease. *Blood, 98*, 1622–1625.

Alyea, E., Weller, E., Schlossman, R., Canning, C., Webb, I., Doss, D., et al. (2001). T-cell depleted allogeneic bone marrow transplantation followed by donor lymphocyte infusion in patients with multiple myeloma: Induction of graft-versus-myeloma effect. *Blood, 98,* 934–939.

Anagnostopoulos, A., & Giralt, S. (2002). Critical review on non-myeloablative stem cell transplantation (NST). *Critical Reviews in Oncology/Hematology, 44,* 175–190.

Ancin, I., Ferra, C., Gallardo, D., Petris, J., Berlanga, J., Gonzalez, J., et al. (2001). Do corticosteroids add any benefit to standard GVHD prophylaxis in allogeneic BMT? *Bone Marrow Transplantation, 28,* 39–45.

Anderson, K.C. (1997). Transfusion-associated graft-versus-host disease. In J.L.M. Ferrara, H.J. Deeg, & S.J. Burakoff (Eds.), *Graft-vs.-host disease* (2nd ed., pp. 587–605). New York: Marcel Dekker.

Andolina, M., Rabusin, M., Maximova, N., & Di Leo, G. (2000). Etanercept in graft versus host disease. *Bone Marrow Transplantation, 26,* 929.

Andre-Schmutz, I., Le Deist, F., Hacein-Abina, S., Vitetta, E., Schindler, J., Chedeville, G., et al. (2002). Immune reconstitution without graft-versus-host disease after haemopoietic stem cell transplantation: A phase I/II study. *Lancet, 360,* 130–137.

Antin, J., Childs, R., Filipovich, A., Giralt, S., Mackinnon, S., Spitzer, T., et al. (2001). Establishment of complete and mixed donor chimerism after allogeneic lymphohematopoietic transplantation: Recommendations from a workshop at the 2001 tandem meetings. *Biology of Blood and Marrow Transplantation, 7,* 473–485.

Apisarnthanarax, N., Donato, M., Korbling, M., Couriel, D., Gajewski, J., Giralt, S., et al. (2003). Extracorporeal photopheresis therapy in the management of steroid-refractory or steroid-dependent cutaneous chronic graft-versus-host disease after allogeneic stem cell transplantation: Feasibility and results. *Bone Marrow Transplantation, 31,* 459–465.

Appelbaum, F.R. (2002). Graft versus disease versus graft-versus-host disease: Improving the therapeutic index. *ASCO 2002 Spring Education Book,* 62–67.

Appleton, A., Sviland, L., Peiris, J.S.M., Taylor, C.E., & Wilkes, J. (1995). Human herpes virus-6 infection in marrow graft recipients: Role in pathogenesis of graft versus host disease. *Bone Marrow Transplant, 16,* 777–782.

Arai, S., Margolis, J., Zahurak, M., Anders, V., & Vogelsang, G. (2002). Poor outcome in steroid-refractory graft-versus-host disease with antithymocyte globulin treatment. *Biology of Blood and Marrow Transplantation, 8,* 155–160.

Arai, S., & Vogelsang, G.B. (2000). Management of graft versus host disease. *Blood Review, 14,* 190–204.

Aristei, C., Alessandro, M., Santucci, A., Aversa, F., Tabillo, A., Carottia, A., et al. (2002). Cataracts in patients receiving stem cell transplantation after conditioning with total body irradiation. *Bone Marrow Transplantation, 29,* 503–507.

Arora, M., Wagner, J., Davies, S., Blazar, B., Defor, T., Enright, H., et al. (2001). Randomized clinical trial of thalidomide, cyclosporine, and prednisone versus cyclosporine and prednisone as initial therapy for chronic graft versus host disease. *Biology of Blood and Marrow Transplantation, 7,* 265–273.

Augustine, S.M. (2000). Long-term management related to immunosuppression, complications and psychosocial adjustment. *Critical Care Nursing Clinics of North America, 12,* 69–77.

Bacigalupo, A., Lamparelli, T., Bruzzi, P., Guidi, S., Allessandrino, E., Bartolomeo, P., et al. (2001). Antithymocyte globulin for graft-versus-host disease prophylaxis in transplants from unrelated donors: Two randomized studies from Gruppo Italiano Trapianti Midollo Osseo. *Blood, 98,* 2942–2947.

Baehr, P., Bouvier, M.E., & Stern, J. (1994). Oral beclomethasone for enteritis caused by graft versus host disease. *Gastroenterology, 106,* A648.

Baker, K.S., DeFor, T.E., Burns, L., Ramsay, N., Neglia, J., & Robison, L. (2003). New malignancies after blood or marrow stem cell transplantation in children and adults: Incidence and risk factors. *Journal of Clinical Oncology, 21,* 1352–1358.

Baron, F., & Beguin, Y. (2002). Preemptive cellular immunotherapy after T-cell-depleted allogeneic hematopoietic stem cell transplantation. *Biology of Blood and Marrow Transplantation, 8,* 351–359.

Barrett, J.A. (1995). Strategies to enhance the graft versus malignancy effect in allogeneic transplants. In R. Sackenstein, W. Janssen, & G. Elfenbein (Eds.), *Bone marrow transplantation: Foundations for the 21st century* (pp. 203–212). New York: New York Academy of Sciences.

Basara, N., Blau, W., Romer, E., Rudolphi, M., Bischoff, M., Kirsten, D., et al. (1998). Mycophenolate mofetil for the treatment of acute and chronic GvHD in bone marrow transplant patients. *Bone Marrow Transplantation, 22,* 61–65.

Baudard, M., Vincent, A., Moreau, P., Kergueris, M.F., Harousseau, J.L., & Milpied, N., (2002). Mycophenolate mofetil for the treatment of acute and chronic GvHD is effective and well tolerated but induces a high risk of infectious complications; A series of 21 BM or PBSC transplant patients. *Bone Marrow Transplantation, 30,* 287–295.

Beckman, R., Siden, R., Yanik, G.A., & Levin, J.E. (2000). Continuous octreotide infusion for the treatment of secretory diarrhea caused by acute intestinal graft-versus-host disease in a child. *Journal of Pediatric Hematology Oncology, 22,* 344–350.

Benya, E.C., & Goldman, S. (1997). Bone marrow transplantation in children: Imaging assessment of complications. *Pediatric Clinics of North America, 44,* 741–761.

Bergerson, S. (1998). Nutritional support in bone marrow transplant recipients. In R.K. Burt, H.J., Deeg, S. Lothian, & G.W. Santos (Eds.), *Bone marrow transplantation* (pp. 343–356). Austin, TX: Landes Bioscience.

Biedermann, B.C., Sahner, S., Gergor, M., Tsakiris, D., Jeanneret, C., Pober, J., et al. (2002). Endothelial injury mediated by cytotoxic T-lymphocytes and loss of microvessels in chronic graft versus host disease. *Lancet, 359,* 2078–2083.

Billiau, A., Fevery, S., Rutgeerts, O., Landuyt, W., & Waer, M. (2002). Crucial role of timing of donor lymphocyte infusion in generating dissociated graft versus host and graft versus leukemia responses in mice receiving allogeneic bone marrow transplants. *Blood, 100,* 1894–1902.

Billingham, R.E. (1966). The biology of graft-versus-host reactions. *Harvey Lectures, 62,* 21–78.

Bisaccia, E., Palangio, M., Gonzalez, J., Adler, K., Rowley, S., & Goldberg, S. (2003). Treating refractory chronic graft-versus-host disease with extracorporeal photochemotherapy. *Bone Marrow Transplantation, 31,* 291–294.

Bittencourt, H., Rocha, V., Chevret, S., Socie, G., Esperou, H., Devergie, A., et al. (2002). Association of CD 34 cell dose with hematopoietic recovery, infections, and other outcomes after HLA-identical sibling bone marrow transplantation. *Blood, 99,* 2726–2733.

Bonanomi, S., Balduzzi, A., Tagliabue, A., Biagi, E., Rovelli, A., Corti, P., et al. (2001). Bath PUVA therapy in pediatric patients with drug-resistant cutaneous graft-versus host disease. *Bone Marrow Transplantation, 28,* 631–636.

Bonini, C., Ferrari, G., Verzeletti, S., Servida, P., Zappone, E., Ruggieri, L., et al. (1997). HSV-TK gene transfer into donor lymphocytes for control of allogeneic graft versus leukemia. *Science, 276,* 1719–1724.

Broers, S., Kaptein, A., LeCessie, S., Fibbe, W., & Hengeveld, M. (2000). Psychological functioning and quality of life following bone marrow transplantation: A three-year follow-up study. *Journal of Psychosomatic Research, 48*(1), 11–21.

Browne, P.V., Weisdorf, D., DeFor, T., Miller, W., Davies, S., Filipovich, A., et al. (2000). Response to thalidomide therapy in refractory chronic graft versus host disease. *Bone Marrow Transplantation, 26,* 865–869.

Buchsel, P.C., Leum, E.W., & Randolph, S.R. (1996). Delayed complications of bone marrow transplantation: An update. *Oncology Nursing Forum, 23,* 1267–1291.

Bush, W.W. (1999). Overview of transplantation immunology and the pharmacotherapy of adult solid organ transplant recipients: Focus on immunosuppression. *AACN Clinical Issues, 10*, 253–269.

Caccavelli, L., Field, A.C., Betin, V., Dreillard, L., Belair, M.F., Bloch, M.F., et al. (2001). Normal IgG protects against acute graft versus-host disease by targeting CD4+CD134+ donor alloreactive T cells. *European Journal of Immunology, 31*, 2781–2790.

Carlens, S., Remberger, M., Aschan, J., & Ringden, O. (2001). The role of disease stage in the response to donor lymphocyte infusions as treatment for leukemic relapse. *Biology of Blood and Marrow Transplantation, 7*, 31–38.

Carlens, S., Ringden, O., Remberger, M., Lonnqvist, B., Hagglund, H., Klaesson, S., et al. (1998). Risk factors for chronic graft versus host disease after bone marrow transplantation: A retrospective single center analysis. *Bone Marrow Transplantation, 22*, 755–761.

Carpenter, P.A., & Sanders, J.E. (2003). Steroid-refractory graft-vs.-host disease: Past, present and future. *Pediatric Transplantation, 7*(Suppl. 3), 19–31.

Cather, J.C. (2001). Cyclosporine and tacrolimus in dermatology. *Dermatology Clinics of North America, 19*, 119–137.

Cavazzana-Calvo, M., Andre-Schmutz, I., Hacein-Abina, S., Bensoussan, D., Le Deist, F., & Fischer, A. (2002). Improving immune reconstitution while preventing graft-versus-host disease in allogeneic stem cell transplantation. *Seminars in Hematology, 39*, 32–40.

Centers for Disease Control and Prevention, Infectious Diseases Society of America, & American Society of Blood and Marrow Transplantation. (2000). Guidelines for preventing opportunistic infections among hematopoietic stem cell transplant recipients. *Biology of Blood and Marrow Transplantation, 6*, 659–734.

Chakrabarti, S., Mautner, V., Osman, H., Collingham, K., Fegan, C., Klapper, P., et al. (2002). Adenovirus infection following allogeneic stem cell transplantation: Incidence and outcome in relation to graft manipulation, immunosuppression, and immune recovery. *Blood, 100*, 1619–1627.

Chakraverty, R., Peggs, K., Chopra, R., Milligan, D.W., Kottaridis, P.D., Verfuerth, S., et al. (2002). Limiting transplantation-related mortality following unrelated donor stem cell transplantation by using a nonmyeloablative conditioning regimen. *Blood, 99*, 1071–1078.

Champlin, R., Khouri, S., Kornblau, S., Marini, F., Anderlini, P., Ueno, N.T., et al. (1999). Allogeneic hematopoietic transplantation as adoptive immunotherapy: Induction of graft-versus-malignancy as the primary therapy. *Hematology/Oncology Clinics of North America, 13*, 1041–1057.

Chao, N.J. (1998). Graft-versus-host disease. In R.K. Burt, H.J. Deeg, S. Lothian, & G.W. Santos (Eds.), *Bone marrow transplantation* (pp. 478–497). Austin, TX: Landes Bioscience.

Chao, N.J. (1999a). *Graft-versus-host disease.* Austin, TX: Landes Company.

Chao, N.J. (1999b). Pharmacology and use of immunosuppressive agents after hematopoietic cell transplantation. In E.D. Thomas, K.G. Blume, & S.J. Forman (Eds.), *Hematopoietic cell transplantation* (2nd ed., pp. 176–185). Oxford, England: Blackwell Science.

Chao, N.J., Parker, P.M., & Niland, J. (1996). Paradoxical effect of thalidomide prophylaxis on chronic graft versus host disease. *Biology of Blood and Marrow Transplantation, 2*, 86–92.

Chao, N.J., Snyder, D., Jain, M., Wong, R., Niland, J., Negrin, R., et al. (2000). Equivalence of two effective graft versus host disease prophylaxis regimens: Results of a prospective double blind randomized trial. *Biology of Blood and Marrow Transplantation, 6*, 254–261.

Charuhas, P.M. (2000). Medical nutrition therapy in bone marrow transplantation. In P.D. McCallum & C.G. Polisena (Eds.), *The clinical guide to oncology nutrition* (pp. 90–98). Chicago: American Dietetic Association.

Chen, B., Cui, X., Liu, C., & Chao, N. (2002). Prevention of graft versus host disease while preserving graft versus leukemia effect after selective depletion of host reactive T-cells by photodynamic cell purging process. *Blood, 99*, 3083–3088.

Chen, B., Morris, R., & Chao, N. (2000). Graft versus host disease prevention by rapamycin: Cellular mechanisms. *Biology of Blood and Marrow Transplantation, 6*, 529–536.

Choi, C.J., & Nghiem, P. (2001). Tacrolimus ointment in the treatment of chronic cutaneous graft-versus-host disease. *Archives of Dermatology, 137*, 1202–1206.

Cohen, J.L., Trenado, A., Vasey, D., Klatzmann, D., & Salomon, B. (2002). CD 4+ CD 25+ immunoregulatory T cells: New therapeutics for graft versus host disease. *Journal of Experimental Medicine, 196*, 401–406.

Collins, R.H., Shpilberg, O., & Drobyski, W. (1997). Donor leukocyte infusions in 140 patients with relapsed malignancy after allogeneic bone marrow transplantation. *Journal of Clinical Immunology, 15*, 433–444.

Colombo, A.A., Alessandrino, E.P., Bernasconi, P., Arcese, G.W., Rabusin, M., Bacigalupo, A., et al. (1999). N-acetylcysteine in the treatment of steroid-resistant acute graft versus host disease: Preliminary results. *Transplantation, 58*, 1414–1416.

Couban, S., Simpson, D., Barnett, M., Bredeson, C., Hubesch, L., Howson-Jan, K., et al. (2002). A randomized multicenter comparison of bone marrow and peripheral blood in recipients of matched sibling allogeneic transplants for myeloid malignancies. *Blood, 100*, 1525–1531.

Couriel, D., Beguelin, G., Giralt, S., de Lima, M., Hosing, C., Kharfan-Dabaja, M., et al. (2002). Chronic graft versus host disease manifesting as polymyositis: An uncommon presentation. *Bone Marrow Transplantation, 30*, 543–546.

Couriel, D.R., Hicks, K., Giralt, S., & Champlin, R.E. (2000). Role of tumor necrosis factor-alpha inhibition with infliximAB in cancer therapy and hematopoietic stem cell transplantation. *Current Opinion in Oncology, 12*, 582–587.

Cronin, D.C., Faust, T.W., Brady, L., Conjeevaram, H., Jain, S., Gupta, P., et al. (2000). Modern immunosuppression. *Clinics in Liver Disease, 4*, 619–655.

Currie, D., Ludvigsdottir, G.K., Diaz, C., & Kamani, M. (2002). Topical treatment of graft versus host disease. *American Journal of Physical Medicine and Rehabilitation, 81*(2), 143–149.

Cutler, C., Giri, S., Jeyapalan, S., Paniagua, D., Viswanathan, A., & Antin, J. (2001). Acute and chronic graft-versus-host disease after allogeneic peripheral-blood stem cell and bone marrow transplantation: A meta-analysis. *Journal of Clinical Oncology, 19*, 3685–3691.

Daly, A., Hasegawa, W., Lipton, J., Messner, A., & Kiss, T. (2002). Transplantation-associated thrombotic microangiopathy is associated with transplantation from unrelated donors, acute graft versus host disease and venooclussive disease of the liver. *Transfusion and Apheresis Science, 27*, 3–12.

Darmstadt, G., Donnenberg, A.D., Vogelsang, G.B., Farmer, E.R., & Horn, T.D. (1992). Clinical, laboratory and histopathologic indicators of the development of progressive acute graft-versus-host disease. *Journal of Investigational Dermatology, 99*, 397–402.

Dazzi, F., Szydlo, R.M., Craddock, C., Cross, N.C., Kaeda, J., Chase, A., et al. (2000). Comparison of single dose and escalating-dose regimens of donor lymphocyte infusion for relapse after allografting for chronic myeloid leukemia. *Blood, 85*, 67–71.

Dazzi, F., Szydlo, R.M., & Goldman, J.M. (1999). Donor lymphocyte infusions for relapse of chronic myeloid leukemia after allogeneic stem cell transplant: Where we now stand. *Experimental Hematology, 27*, 1477–1486.

Deeg, H.J., & Henslee-Downey, P.J. (1990). Management of acute graft-versus-host disease. *Bone Marrow Transplantation, 6*, 1–8.

Deeg, H.J., Lin, D., Leisenring, W., Boeckh, M., Anasetti, C., Appelbaum, F., et al. (1997). Cyclosporine or cyclosporine plus methylprednisolone for prophylaxis of graft-versus host disease: A prospective randomized trial. *Blood, 89*, 3880–3887.

Dobbin, M., & Hartmuller, V.W. (2000). Suggested management of nutrition-related symptoms. In P.D. McCallum & C.G. Polisena (Eds.), *The clinical guide to oncology nutrition* (pp. 164–167). Chicago: American Dietetic Association.

Donnelly, L.J., & Morris, C.L. (1996). Acute graft versus host disease in children: Abdominal findings. *Radiology, 199*, 265–268.

Efremov, D.G., Georgievski, B., Cevreska, L., Pivkova, A., & Panovska, I. (2003). Lamivudine treatment for acute hepatitis B virus infection during allogeneic peripheral blood stem cell transplantation. *Bone Marrow Transplantation, 31*, 515–516.

Einsele, H., Ehninger, G., Hebart, H., Weber, P., Dette, S., Link, H., et al. (1994). Incidence of local CMV infection and acute intestinal GvHD in marrow transplant recipients with severe diarrhea. *Bone Marrow Transplantation, 14*, 955–963.

Elad, S., Garfunkel, A., Enk, C., Galili, D., & Or, R. (1999). Ultraviolet B irradiation: A new therapeutic concept for the management of oral manifestations of graft versus host disease. *Oral Surgery, Oral Medicine, Oral Pathology, 88*, 444–450.

Fefer, A. (1999). Graft versus tumor responses. In E.D. Thomas, K.G. Blume, & S.J. Forman (Eds.), *Hematopoietic cell transplantation* (2nd ed., pp. 316–326). Oxford, England: Blackwell Science.

Fehse, B., Frerk, O., Goldmann, M., Bulduk, M., & Zander, A.R. (2000). Efficient depletion of alloreactive donor T-lymphocytes based on expression of two activation-induced antigens (CD 25 and CD 69). *British Journal of Hematology, 109*, 644–651.

Fernandez-Aviles, F., Urbano-Ispizua, A., Aymerich, M., Colomer, D., Rovira, M., Martinez, C., et al. (2003). Serial quantification of lymphoid and myeloid mixed chimerism using multiplex PCR amplification of short tandem repeat-markers predicts graft rejection and relapse, respectively, after allogeneic transplantation of CD 34+ selected cells from peripheral blood. *Leukemia, 17*, 613–620.

Ferrara, J.L.M. (1995). Cytokine inhibitors and graft versus host disease. In R. Sackenstein, W. Janssen, & G. Elfenbein (Eds.), *Bone marrow transplantation: Foundations for the 21ˢᵗ century* (pp. 227–236). New York: New York Academy of Sciences.

Ferrara, J.L.M. (1998). The cytokine modulation of acute graft-versus-host disease. *Bone Marrow Transplantation, 21*(Suppl. 3), S13–S15.

Ferrara, J.L.M., & Antin, J.H. (1999). The pathophysiology of graft-versus-host disease. In E.D. Thomas, K.G. Blume, & S.J. Forman (Eds.), *Hematopoietic cell transplantation* (2nd ed., pp. 305–315). Oxford, England: Blackwell Science.

Ferrara, J.L.M., Levy, R., & Chao, N.J. (1999). Pathophysiologic mechanisms of acute graft-vs.-host disease. *Biology of Blood and Marrow Transplant, 5*, 347–356.

Filicko, J., Lazarus, H.M., & Flomenberg, N. (2003). Mucosal injury in patients undergoing hematopoietic progenitor cell transplantation: New approaches to prophylaxis and treatment. *Bone Marrow Transplantation, 31*, 1–10.

Fleming, D. (2002). Graft versus host disease: What is the evidence. *Evidence-Based Oncology, 3*, 2–6.

Flowers, M.E.D., Kansu, E., & Sullivan, K.M. (1999). Hematopoietic stem cell therapy: Pathophysiology and treatment of graft versus host disease. *Hematology/Oncology Clinics of North America, 13*, 1091–1112.

Flowers, M.E., Lee, S., & Vogelsang, G. (2003). An update on how to treat chronic GVHD. *Blood, 102*, 2312.

Foss, F.M., Gorgun, G., & Miller, K. (2002). Extracorporeal photopheresis in chronic graft versus host disease. *Bone Marrow Transplantation, 29*, 719–725.

French, L., & Rook, A. (2002). T-cell clonality and the effect of photopheresis in systemic sclerosis and graft versus host disease. *Transfusion and Apheresis Science, 26*, 191–196.

Furlong, T., Leisenring, W., Storb, R., Anasetti, C., Appelbaum, F., Carpenter, P., et al. (2002). Psoralen and ultraviolet A irradiation (PUVA) as therapy for steroid resistant cutaneous acute graft versus host disease. *Biology of Blood and Marrow Transplantation, 8*, 206–212.

Gavreau, J.M., Lenssen, P., Cheney, C.L., Aker, S.N., Hutchinson, M.L., & Barale, K.V. (1981). Nutritional management of patients with intestinal graft-versus-host disease. *Journal of the American Academy of Dietetics, 79*, 673–675.

Gaziev, D., Galimberti, M., Lucarelli, G., & Polchi, P. (2000). Chronic graft-versus-host disease: Is there an alternative to conventional treatment? *Bone Marrow Transplantation, 25*, 689–696.

Gillis, T., & Donovan, E.S. (2001). Rehabilitation following bone marrow transplantation. *Cancer, 92*, 998–1007.

Gilman, A., Beams, F., Tefft, M., & Mazumbder, A. (1996). The effect of hydroxychloroquine on alloreactivity and its potential use for graft-versus-host disease. *Bone Marrow Transplantation, 17*, 1069–1075.

Girardi, M. (2000). Cutaneous T-cell lymphoma and cutaneous graft versus host disease: Two indications for photopheresis in dermatology. *Dermatologic Clinics, 18*, 417–423.

Glucksberg, H., Storb, R., Fefer, A., Buckner, C.D., Neiman, P.E., Clift, R.A., et al. (1974). Clinical manifestations of graft-versus-host disease in human recipients of marrow from HLA-matched sibling donors. *Transplantation, 18*, 295–304.

Goerner, M., Gooley, T., Flowers, M.E., Sullivan, K.M., Kiem, H.P., Sanders, J.E., et al. (2002). Morbidity and mortality of chronic GvHD after hematopoietic stem cell transplantation from HLA-identical siblings for patients with aplastic or refractory anemias. *Biology of Blood and Marrow Transplantation, 8*, 47–56.

Goker, H., Haznedaroglu, I., & Chao, N. (2001). Acute graft-versus-host disease: Pathobiology and management. *Experimental Hematology, 29*, 259–277.

Gold, P., Flowers, M., & Sullivan, K. (1998). Outpatient management of marrow and blood stem cell transplant patients. In R.K. Burt, H.J. Deeg, S. Lothian, and G.W. Santos (Eds.), *Bone marrow transplantation* (pp. 524–531). Austin, TX: Landes Bioscience.

Goldberg, S., Cicogna, C., Rowley, S., & Pecora, A. (2003). Vaccinations against infectious diseases in hematopoietic stem cell transplant recipients. *Oncology, 17*, 539–554.

Goldman, D.A. (2001). Thalidomide use: Past history and current implications for practice. *Oncology Nursing Forum, 28*, 471–477.

Goldman, F., Gilman, A., Hollenback, C., Kato, R., Premack, B., & Rawlings, D. (2000). Hydroxychloroquine inhibits calcium signals in T-cells: A new mechanism to explain its immunomodulatory properties. *Blood, 95*, 3460–3466.

Gratama, J., Sinnige, L., & Weijers, T. (1987). Marrow donor immunity to herpes simplex virus: Association with acute graft versus host disease. *Experimental Hematology, 15*, 735–740.

Greinix, H.T., Volc-Platzer, B., Kalhs, P., Fischer, G., Rosenmayr, A., Keil, F., et al. (2000). Extracorporeal photochemotherapy in the treatment of severe steroid refractory acute graft versus host disease: A pilot study. *Blood, 96*, 2426–2431.

Grigg, A.P., Angus, P.W., Hoyt, R., & Szer, J. (2003). The incidence, pathogenesis, and natural history of steatorrhea after bone marrow transplantation. *Bone Marrow Transplantation, 31*, 701–703.

Grundmann-Kollmann, M., Behrens, S., Gruss, C., Gottlober, P., Peter, R.U., & Kersher, M. (2000). Chronic sclerodermic graft versus host disease refractory to immunosuppressive treatment response UVA1 phototherapy. *Journal of the American Academy of Dermatology, 42*(1), 134–136.

Haddad, J., Saade, N., & Safieh-Garabedian, B. (2003). Interleukin-10 and the regulation of mitogen-activated protein kinases: Are these signaling modules targets for the anti-inflammatory action of this cytokine? *Cellular Signaling, 15*, 255–267.

Hale, G., Zhang, M.J., & Bunjes, D. (1998). Improving the outcome of bone marrow transplantation by using CD 52 monoclonal antibodies to prevent graft versus host disease and graft rejection. *Blood, 92*, 4581–4590.

Harder, H., Cornelissen, J., Van Gool, A., Duivenvoorden, H.J., Eijkenboom, W.M.H., & van den Bent, M. (2002). Cognitive functioning and quality of life in long-term adult survivors of bone marrow transplantation. *Cancer, 95*, 183–192.

Hess, A.D. (1997). The immunobiology of syngeneic/autologous graft-versus-host disease. In J.L.M. Ferrara, H.J. Deeg, & S.J. Burakoff (Eds.), *Graft-vs.-host disease* (2nd ed., pp. 561–586). New York: Marcel Dekker.

Heymer, B. (2002). *Clinical and diagnostic pathology of graft-versus-host disease.* Berlin, Heidelberg: Springer-Verlag.

Hill, G.R., Crawford, J., Cooke, K., Brinson, Y., Pan, L., & Ferrara, J. (1997). Total body irradiation and acute graft-versus-host disease: the role of gastrointestinal damage and inflammatory cytokines. *Blood, 90,* 3204–3213.

Hill, G.R., & Ferrara, J.L. (2000). The primacy of the gastrointestinal tract as a target organ of acute graft versus host disease: Rationale for the use of cytokine shields in allogeneic bone marrow transplantation. *Blood, 95,* 2754–2759.

Hilton, D., Williams, L.C., & Nesbitt, L. (2000). Systemic glucocorticosteroid therapy in dermatology. *Dermatology Nursing, 12,* 258–265.

Hiraoka, A., Ohashi, Y., Okamoto, S., Moriyama, Y., Nagao, T., Kodera, Y., et al. (2001). Phase III study comparing tacrolimus with cyclosporine for graft versus host disease prophylaxis after allogeneic bone marrow transplantation. *Bone Marrow Transplantation, 28,* 181–185.

Ho, V., & Soiffer, R. (2001). The history and future of T-cell depletion as graft versus host disease prophylaxis for allogeneic hematopoietic stem cell transplantation. *Blood, 98,* 3192–3204.

Hsu, B., May, R., Carrum, G., Krance, R., & Przepiorka, D. (2001). Use of antithymocyte globulin for treatment of steroid-refractory acute graft versus host disease: An international practice survey. *Bone Marrow Transplantation, 28,* 945–950.

Iestra, J.A., Fibbe, W.E., Zwinderman, A.H., van Staveren, W.A., & Kromhout, D. (2002). Body weight recovery, eating difficulties and compliance with dietary advice in the first year after stem cell transplantation: A prospective study. *Bone Marrow Transplantation, 29,* 417–424.

Ippoliti, C., Champlin, R., Bugazia, N., Przepiorka, D., Neumann, J., Giralt, S., et al. (1997). Use of octreotide in the symptomatic management of diarrhea induced by graft versus host disease in patients with hematologic malignancies. *Journal of Clinical Oncology, 15,* 3350–3354.

Ippoliti, C., & Neumann, J. (1998). Octreotide in the management of diarrhea induced by graft versus host disease. *Oncology Nursing Forum, 25,* 873–878.

Ishii, T., Manabe, A., Ebihara, Y., Ueda, T., Yoshino, H., Mitsui, T., et al. (2000). Improvement in bronchiolitis obliterans organizing pneumonia in a child after allogeneic bone marrow transplantation by a combination of oral prenisolone and low dose erythromycin. *Bone Marrow Transplantation, 26,* 907–910.

Jacobsohn, D.A., Margolis, J., Doherty, J., Anders, V., & Vogelsang, G.B. (2002). Weight loss and malnutrition in patients with chronic graft versus host disease. *Bone Marrow Transplantation, 29,* 231–236.

Jacobsohn, D.A., Montross, S., Anders, V., & Vogelsang, G.B. (2001). Clinical importance of confirming or excluding the diagnosis of chronic graft-versus-host disease. *Bone Marrow Transplantation, 28,* 1047–1051.

Johnson, B.D., Becker, E.E., & Truitt, R.L. (1999). Graft versus host and graft versus leukemia reactions after delayed infusions of donor T-subsets. *Biology of Blood and Marrow Transplantation, 5*(3), 123–132.

Kanfer, E. (1995). Graft versus host disease. In J. Treleaven & P. Wiernik (Eds.), *Color atlas and text of bone marrow transplantation* (pp. 143–153). London: Mosby-Wolfe.

Kanold, J., Paillard, C., Halle, P., D'Incan, M., Bordigoni, P., & Demeocq, F. (2003). Extracorporeal photochemotherapy for graft versus host disease in pediatric patients. *Transfusion and Apheresis Science, 28,* 71–80.

Kaushik, S., Flagg, E., Wise, C., Hadfield, M., & McCarty, J. (2002). Granulomatous myositis: A manifestation of chronic graft versus host disease. *Skeletal Radiology, 31,* 226–229.

Kayaba, H., Hirokawa, M., Watanabe, A., Saitoh, N., Changhao, C., Yamada, Y., et al. (2000). Serum markers of graft versus host disease after bone marrow transplantation. *Journal of Allergy and Clinical Immunology, 106*(Suppl.), S40–S44.

Kharfan-Dabaja, M., Morgensztern, D., Santos, E., Goodman, M., & Fernandez, H. (2003). Acute graft versus host disease (aGVHD) presenting with an acquired lupus anticoagulant. *Bone Marrow Transplantation, 31,* 129–131.

Kiang, E., Tesavibul, N., Yee, R., Kellaway, J., & Przepiorka, D. (1998). The use of topical cyclosporin A in ocular graft versus host disease. *Bone Marrow Transplantation, 22,* 147–151.

Kim, R., Anderlini, P., Naderi, A., Rivera, P., Ahmadi, M.A., & Esmaeli, B. (2002). Scleritis as the initial clinical manifestation of graft versus host disease after allogeneic bone marrow transplantation. *American Journal of Ophthalmology, 133,* 843–845.

Kiss, T.L., Abdolell, M., Jamal, N., Minden, M., Lipton, J., & Messner, H.A. (2002). Long-term medical outcomes and quality of life assessment of patients with chronic myeloid leukemia followed at least 10 years after allogeneic bone marrow transplantation. *Journal of Clinical Oncology, 20,* 2334–2343.

Klein, S.A., Martin, H., Schreiber-Dietrich, D., Hermann, S., Caspary, W., Hoelzer, D., et al. (2001). A new approach to evaluating intestinal acute graft versus host disease by transabdominal sonography and colour Doppler imaging. *British Journal of Hematology, 115,* 929–934.

Klosner, G. (2001). Treatment of peripheral blood mononuclear cells with 8-methoxypsoralen plus ultraviolet A radiation induces a shift in cytokine expression from a Th1 to a Th2 response. *Journal of Investigational Dermatology, 116,* 459–462.

Kobbe, G., Schneider, P., Rohr, U., Fenk, R., Neumann, F., Aivado, M., et al. (2001). Treatment of severe steroid refractory acute graft-versus-host disease with infliximab, a chimeric human/mouse anti-TNFa antibody. *Bone Marrow Transplantation, 28,* 47–49.

Koc, S., Leisenring, W., Flowers, M.E., Anasetti, C., Deeg, H.J., Nash, R.A., et al. (2000). Thalidomide for treatment of patients with chronic graft versus host disease. *Blood, 95,* 3995–3996.

Koc, S., Leisenring, W., Flowers, M.E., Anasetti, C., Deeg, H.J., Nash, R.A., et al. (2002). Therapy for chronic graft versus host disease: A randomized trial comparing cyclosporine plus prednisone versus prednisone alone. *Blood, 100,* 48–51.

Kokalj, A., Greinix, H.T., Ciovica, M., Kittler, H., Kalhs, P., Knobler, R.M., et al. (2002). Effects of extracorporeal photo immunotherapy on soluble IL-2R alpha, TNF-R1, and CD8 in patients with steroid-resistant acute graft-versus-host disease. *Clinical Immunology, 104,* 248–255.

Kornblau, S., Benson, A.B., Catalano, R., Champlin, R.E., Engelking, C., Field, M., et al. (2000). Management of cancer treatment-related diarrhea. Issues and therapeutic strategies. *Journal of Pain and Symptom Management, 19*(2), 118–129.

Kottaridis, P., Milligan, D., Chopra, R., Chakraverty, R., Chakrabarti, S., Robinson, S., et al. (2000). In vivo CAMPATH-1H prevents graft-versus-host disease following non-myeloablative stem cell transplantation. *Blood, 96,* 2419–2425.

Kowdley, K.V. (2000). Ursodeoxycholic acid therapy in hepatobiliary disease. *American Journal of Medicine, 108,* 481–486.

Krijanovski, O.I., Hill, G.R., Cooke, K.R., Teshima, T., Crawford, J., Brinson, Y., et al. (1999). Keratinocyte growth factor separates graft-versus-leukemia effects from graft-versus-host disease. *Blood, 94,* 825–831.

Kumar, S., Wolf, R., Chen, M., Gastineau, D., Gertz, M., Inwards, D., et al. (2002). Omission of day +11 methotrexate after allogeneic bone marrow transplantation is associated with increased risk of severe acute graft versus host disease. *Bone Marrow Transplantation, 30,* 161–165.

LaDuca, J.R., & Gaspari, A.A. (2001). Targeting tumor necrosis factor alpha. New drugs used to modulate inflammatory disease. *Dermatology Clinics, 19,* 617–635.

Lanuza, D.M., & McCabe, M.A. (2001). Care before and after lung transplant and quality of life research. *AACN Clinical Issues, 12*(2), 186–201.

Lash, A.A. (2001). Sjogren's syndrome: Pathogenesis, diagnosis and treatment. *The Nurse Practitioner Journal, 26*(8), 50–58.

Lazarus, H.M., Vogelsang, G.B., & Rowe, J.M. (1997). Prevention and treatment of acute graft-versus-host disease: The old and the new. A report from the Eastern Cooperative Oncology Group (ECOG). *Bone Marrow Transplantation, 19*, 577–600.

Leano, A., Miller, K., & White, A. (2000). Chronic graft versus host disease-related polymyositis as a cause of respiratory failure following allogeneic bone marrow transplant. *Bone Marrow Transplantation, 26*, 1117–1120.

Lee, C.K., Gingrich, R.D., deMagalhaes-Silverman, M., Hohl, R., Joyce, J., Scott, S., et al. (1999). Prophylactic reinfusion of T cells for T cell-depleted allogeneic bone marrow transplantation. *Biology of Blood and Marrow Transplantation, 5*(1), 15–27.

Lee, S.J., Cook, E., Soiffer, R., & Antin, J. (2002). Development and validation of a scale to measure symptoms of chronic graft-versus host disease. *Biology of Blood and Marrow Transplantation, 8*, 444–452.

Lee, S.J., Vogelsang, G., & Flowers, M.E. (2003). Chronic graft versus host disease. *Biology of Blood and Marrow Transplantation, 9*, 215–233.

Lee, S.J., Vogelsang, G., Gilman, A., Weisdorf, D., Pavletic, S., Antin, J., et al. (2002). A survey of diagnosis, management and grading of chronic GvHD. *Biology of Blood and Marrow Transplantation, 8*, 32–39.

Lee, S.J., Wegner, S.A., McGarigle, C.J., Bierer, B.E., & Antin, J.H. (1997). Treatment of chronic graft versus host disease with clofazimine. *Blood, 89*, 2298–2302.

Lenssen, P., Bruemmer, B., Aker, S., & McDonald, G. (2001). Nutrient support in hematopoietic cell transplantation. *Journal of Parenteral and Enteral Nutrition, 25*, 219–228.

Lenssen, P., Sherry, M.E., Cheney, C.L., Nims, J.W., Sullivan, K.M., Stern, J.M., et al. (1990). Prevalence of nutrition-related problems among long-term survivors of allogeneic marrow transplantation. *Journal of the American Dietetic Association, 90*, 835–842.

Lewalle, P., Triffet, A., Delforge, A., Crombez, P., Selleslag, D., DeMuynck, H., et al. (2003). Donor lymphocyte infusions in adult haploidentical transplant: A dose finding study. *Bone Marrow Transplantation, 31*, 39–44.

Liesveld, J.L., Duerst, R.E., Rapoport, A.P., Constine, L.S., Abboud, C.N, Packman, C.H., et al. (1999). Continuous infusion cyclosporine and nifedipine to day +100 with short methotrexate and steroids as GvHD prophylaxis in unrelated donor transplants. *Bone Marrow Transplantation, 24*, 511–516.

Lindgren, C.G., Thompson, J.A., Robinson, N., Keeler, T., Gold, P.J., & Fefer, A. (1997). Interleukin-12 induced cytolytic activity in lymphocytes from recipients of autologous and allogeneic stem cell transplants. *Bone Marrow Transplant, 19*, 867–873.

Lister, J., Messner, H., Keystone, E., Miller, R., & Fritzler, M.J. (1987). Autoantibody analysis of patients with graft versus host disease. *Journal of Clinical and Laboratory Immunology, 24*, 19–23.

Litvinova, E., Maury, S., Boyer, O., Bruel, S., Benard, L., Boisserie, G., et al. (2002). Graft versus leukemia effect after suicide gene mediated control of graft versus host disease. *Blood, 100*, 2020–2025.

Locatelli, F., Bruno, B., Zecca, M., Van-Lint, M., McCann, S., Arcese, W., et al. (2000). Cyclosporin A and short-term methotrexate versus cyclosporin A as graft versus host disease prophylaxis in patients with severe aplastic anemia given allogeneic bone marrow transplantation from an HLA identical sibling: Results of a GITMO/EBMT randomized trial. *Blood, 96*, 1690–1697.

Loren, A.W., Porter, D., Stadtmauer, E., & Tsai, D. (2003). Posttransplant lymphoproliferative disorder: A review. *Bone Marrow Transplantation, 31*, 145–155.

Loughran, T.P., Sullivan, K.M., Morton, T., Beckham, C., Schubert, M., Witherspoon, R., et al. (1990). Value of Day 100 screening studies for predicting the development of chronic graft versus host disease after allogeneic bone marrow transplantation. *Blood, 76*, 228–234.

Mackinnon, S., Papadopoulos, E., Carabasi, M.H., Reich, L., Collins, N.H., Boulad, F., et al. (1995). Adoptive immunotherapy evaluating escalating doses of donor leukocytes for relapse of chronic myeloid leukemia after bone marrow transplantation: Separation of graft versus leukemia responses from graft versus host disease. *Blood, 86*, 1261–1268.

MacMillan, M.L., Weisdorf, D.J., Wagner, J.E., DeFor, T.E., Burns, L.J., Ramsay, N.K., et al. (2002). Response of 443 patients to steroids as primary therapy for acute graft versus host disease: Comparison of grading systems. *Biology of Blood and Marrow Transplantation, 8*, 387–394.

Marcellus, D., Altomonte, V., Farmer, E., Horn, T., Freemer, C., Grant, J., et al. (1999). Etretinate therapy for refractory sclerodermatous chronic graft versus host disease. *Blood, 93*, 66–70.

Marcellus, D.C., & Vogelsang, G.B. (2000). Chronic graft-versus-host disease. In E.D. Ball, J. Lister, & P. Law (Eds.), *Hematopoietic stem cell therapy* (pp. 614–624). New York: Churchill Livingstone.

Margolis, J.H., Phelps, M.L., & Chen, A. (2000). Pentostatin: A novel treatment for steroid refractory acute GvHD. *Blood, 96*, 400a.

Marks, D.I., Lush, R., Cavenagh, J., Milligan, D.W., Schey, S., Parker, A., et al. (2002). The toxicity and efficacy of donor lymphocyte infusions given after reduced-intensity conditioning allogeneic stem cell transplantation. *Blood, 100*, 3108–3114.

Martino, R., Caballero, M., Simon, J., Canals, C., Solano, C., Urbano-Ispizua, A., et al. (2002). Evidence for a graft versus leukemia effect after allogeneic peripheral blood stem cell transplantation with reduced-intensity conditioning in acute myelogenous leukemia and myelodysplastic syndromes. *Blood, 100*, 2243–2245.

Martino, R., Romero, P., Subira, M., Bellido, M., Altes, A., Sureda, A., et al. (1999). Comparison of the classic Glucksberg criteria and the IBMTR severity index for grading acute graft versus host disease following HLA-identical sibling stem cell transplantation. *Bone Marrow Transplantation, 24*, 283–287.

Matzinger, P. (1994). Tolerance, danger and the extended family. *Annual Review of Immunology, 12*, 991–1045.

Maury, S., Litvinova, E., Boyer, O., Benard, L., Bruel, S., Klatzmann, D., et al. (2002). Effect of combined cytostatic cyclosporin A and cytolytic suicide gene therapy on the prevention of experimental graft-versus-host disease. *Gene Therapy, 9*, 201–207.

Mavroudis, D.A. (1998). Graft-versus-leukemia effect of allogeneic BMT. In R.K. Burt, H.J. Deeg, S. Lothian, & G.W. Santos (Eds.), *Bone marrow transplantation* (pp. 499–502). Austin, TX: Landes Bioscience.

McCarthy, N.J., & Bishop, M.R. (2000). Non-myeloablative allogeneic stem cell transplantation: Early promises and limitations. *Oncologist, 5*, 487–496.

Michallet, M., Bilger, K., Garban, F., Attal, M., Huyn, A., Blaise, D., et al. (2001). Allogeneic hematopoietic stem cell transplantation after nonmyeloablative preparative regimens: Impact of pretransplantation and posttransplantation factors on outcome. *Journal of Clinical Oncology, 19*, 3340–3349.

Miura, Y., Thoburn, C., Bright, E.C., Sommer, M., Lefell, S., Ueda, M., et al. (2001). Characterization of the cell-cell repertoire in autologous graft-versus-host disease (GvHD): Evidence for the involvement of antigen drive T-cell response in the development of autologous GvHD. *Blood, 9*, 868–876.

Mookerjee, B., Altomonte, V., & Vogelsang, G. (1999). Salvage therapy for refractory chronic graft versus host disease with mycophenolate mofetil and tacrolimus. *Bone Marrow Transplantation, 24*, 517–520.

Morton, J., Hutchins, C., & Durant, S. (2001). Granulocyte-colony stimulating factor (G-CSF)-primed allogeneic bone marrow: Significantly less graft-versus-host disease and comparable engraftment to G-CSF-mobilized peripheral blood stem cells. *Blood, 98,* 3186–3191.

Murphy, B., & Krensky, A.M. (1999). HLA-derived peptides as novel immunomodulatory therapeutics. *Journal of the American Society of Nephrology, 10,* 1346–1355.

Muscaritoli, M., Grieco, G., Capria, S., Iori, A., & Fanelli, F. (2002). Nutritional and metabolic support in patients undergoing bone marrow transplantation. *American Journal of Clinical Nutrition, 75*(2), 183–190.

Nagler, R., & Nagler, A. (1999). Pilocarpine hydrochloride relieves xerostomia in chronic graft versus host disease: A sialometrical study. *Bone Marrow Transplantation, 23,* 1007–1011.

Nakamura, J. (2000). Serum levels of soluble IL-2 receptor, IL-12, IL-18, and IFN-gamma in patients with acute graft versus host disease after allogeneic bone marrow transplantation. *Journal of Allergy and Clinical Immunology, 106*(1 Pt. 2), S45–S50.

Nash, R.A., Antin, J.H., Karanes, C., Fay, J.W., Avalos, B.R., Yeager, A.M., et al. (2000). Phase 3 study comparing methotrexate and cyclosporine for prophylaxis of acute graft-versus-host disease after marrow transplantation from unrelated donors. *Blood, 96,* 2062–2068.

National Home Infusion Association. (2001). Infliximab therapy in patients with rheumatoid arthritis and Crohn's disease. *Infusion, 7*(6), 1–13.

Nestel, F.P., Greene, R.N., Kichian, K., Ponka, P., & Lapp, W. (2000). Activation of macrophage cytostatic effector mechanisms during acute graft-versus-host disease: Release of intracellular iron and nitric oxide-mediated cytostasis. *Blood, 96,* 1836–1843.

Noga, S.J., & O'Donnell, P.V. (1998). Manipulating the immunologic characteristics of both graft and host to improve transplant outcome. *Cancer Control, 5,* 385–393.

Norton, J. (1995). Graft versus host disease. In J. Treleaven & P. Wiernik (Eds.), *Color atlas and text of bone marrow transplantation* (pp. 185–192). London: Mosby-Wolfe.

Nunes, F., & Lucey, M. (1999). Gastrointestinal complications of immunosuppression. *Gastroenterology Clinics, 28,* 233–246.

Ogawa, H., Soma, T., Hosen, N., Tatekawa, T., Tsuboi, A., Oji, Y., et al. (2002). Combination of tacrolimus, methotrexate, and methylprednisolone prevents acute but not chronic graft versus host disease in unrelated bone marrow transplantation. *Transplantation, 74,* 236–243.

Okamoto, T., Takatsuka, H., Fujimori, Y., Wada, H., Iwasaki, T., & Kakishita, E. (2001). Increased hepatocyte growth factor in serum in acute graft versus host disease. *Bone Marrow Transplantation, 28,* 197–200.

Oliven, A., & Schechter, Y. (2001). Extracorporeal photopheresis: A review. *Blood Reviews, 15,* 103–108.

Ordemann, R., Hutchinson, R., Friedman, J., Burakoff, S.J., Reddy, P., Duffner, U., et al. (2002). Enhanced allostimulatory activity of host antigen-presenting cells in old mice intensifies acute graft-versus-host disease. *Journal of Clinical Investigation, 109,* 1249–1256.

Padovan, C., Gerbitz, A., Sostak, P., Holler, E., Ferrara, J., Bise, K., et al. (2001). Cerebral involvement in graft versus host disease after murine bone marrow transplantation. *Neurology, 56,* 1106–1108.

Palencia, S., Rodriguez-Peralto, J.L., Castano, E., Vanaclocha, F., & Iglesias, I. (2002). Lichenoid nail changes as the sole external manifestation of graft versus host disease. *International Journal of Dermatology, 41*(1), 44–45.

Panoskaltsis-Mortari, A., Lacey, D., Vallera, D., & Blazar, B. (1998). Keratinocyte growth factor administered before conditioning ameliorates graft-versus-host disease after allogeneic bone marrow transplantation in mice. *Blood, 92,* 3960–3967.

Parker, P.M., Chao, N., & Nademanee, A. (1995). Thalidomide as salvage therapy for chronic graft versus host disease. *Blood, 86,* 3604–3609.

Parkman, R., & Weinberg, K. (1999). Immunological reconstitution following hematopoietic stem cell transplantation. In E.D. Tho-

mas, K.G. Blume, & S.J. Forman (Eds.), *Hematopoietic cell transplantation* (2nd ed., pp. 704–711). Oxford: Blackwell Science.

Passweg, J.R., Rowlings, P.A., Atkinson, K.A., Barrett, A.J., Gale, R.P., Gratwohl, A., et al. (1998). Influence of protective isolation on outcome of allogeneic bone marrow transplantation for leukemia. *Bone Marrow Transplant, 21,* 1231–1238.

Patterson, A.E., & Korngold, R. (2001). Infusion of select leukemia-reactive TCR Vß+ T cells provides graft versus leukemia responses with minimization of graft versus host disease following murine hematopoietic stem cell transplantation. *Biology of Blood and Marrow Transplantation, 7,* 187–196.

Paumgartner, G., & Beuers, U. (2002). Ursodeoxycholic acid in cholestatic liver disease: Mechanisms of action and therapeutic use revisited. *Hepatology, 36,* 525–531.

Peggs, K.S., & Mackinnon, S. (2001). Exploiting graft versus tumor responses using donor leukocyte infusions. *Best Practice and Research Clinical Hematology, 14,* 723–739.

Penas, P.F., Jones-Caballero, M., Aragues, M., Fernandez-Herrera, J., Fraga, J., & Garcia-Diez, A. (2002). Sclerodermatous graft-versus-host disease: Clinical and pathological study of 17 patients. *Archives of Dermatology, 138,* 924–934.

Penn, E., & Kaz Soong, H. (2002). Cataract surgery in allogeneic bone marrow transplant recipients with graft versus host disease. *Journal of Cataract and Refractive Surgery, 28,* 417–420.

Picardi, M., Selleri, C., De Rosa, G., Raiola, A., Pezzullo, L., & Rotoli, B. (1998). Lamivudine treatment for chronic replicative hepatitis B virus infection after allogeneic bone marrow transplantation. *Bone Marrow Transplantation, 21,* 1267–1269.

Ponec, R.J. (1999). Endoscopic and histologic diagnosis of intestinal graft versus host disease after marrow transplantation. *Gastrointestinal Endoscopy, 49,* 612–621.

Porter, D.L., Collins, R.H., Shpilberg, O., Drobyski, W., Connors, J., Sproles, A., et al. (1999). Long-term follow-up of patients who achieved complete remission after donor leukocyte infusions. *Biology of Blood and Marrow Transplantation, 5,* 253–261.

Proujansky, R. (1999). Fixing the intestinal mucosa in the bone marrow transplant patient: Lessons from other intestinal immunodeficiencies and inflammatory disorders. *Pediatric Transplantation, 3*(Suppl. 1), 9–13.

Przepiorka, D. (2000). Prevention of acute graft-versus-host disease. In E.D. Ball, J. Lister, & P. Law (Eds.), *Hematopoietic stem cell therapy* (pp. 452–469). New York: Churchill Livingstone.

Przepiorka, D., Anderlini, P., Saliba, R., Cleary, K., Mehra, R., Khouri, I., et al. (2001). Chronic graft versus host disease after allogeneic blood stem cell transplantation. *Blood, 96,* 1695–1700.

Przepiorka, D., & Cleary, K. (2000). Therapy of acute graft-vs-host disease. In E.D. Ball, J. Lister, & P. Law (Eds.), *Hematopoietic stem cell therapy* (pp. 531–540). New York: Churchill Livingstone.

Przepiorka, D., Devine, S.M., Fay, J.W., Uberti, J.P., & Wingard, J.P. (1999). Practical considerations in the use of tacrolimus for allogeneic marrow transplantation. *Bone Marrow Transplantation, 24,* 1053–1056.

Przepiorka, D., Kernan, N.A., Ippoliti, C., Papadopoulos, E.B., Giralt, S., Khouri, I., et al. (2000). Daclizumab, a humanized anti-interleukin-2 receptor alpha chain antibody, for treatment of acute graft versus host disease. *Blood, 95,* 83–89.

Przepiorka, D., Nash, R., Wingar, J., Zhu, J., Maher, R., Fitzsimmons, W., et al. (1999). Relationship of tacrolimus whole blood levels to efficacy and safety outcomes after unrelated donor marrow transplantation. *Biology of Blood and Marrow Transplantation, 5*(2), 94–97.

Przepiorka, D., Smith, T., Folloder, J., Khouri, I., Ueno, N., Mehra, R., et al. (1999). Risk factors for acute graft-versus-host disease after allogeneic blood stem cell transplantation. *Blood, 94,* 1465–1470.

Rai, R.M., Hendrix, T.R., Moskaluk, C., Levine, D.S., & Pasricha, P.J. (1997). Treatment of idiopathic lymphocytic enterocolitis with oral beclomethasone diproprionate. *American Journal of Gastroenterology, 92*(1), 147–149.

Raiola, A.M., Van Lint, M.T., Valbonesi, M., Lamparelli, T., Gualandi, F., Occhini, D., et al. (2003). Factors predicting response and graft versus host disease after donor lymphocyte infusions: A study on 593 infusions. *Bone Marrow Transplantation, 31*, 6878–6893.

Ratanatharathorn, V., Ayash, L., Lazarus, H.M., Fu, J., & Uberti, J. (2001). Chronic graft versus host disease: Clinical manifestation and therapy. *Bone Marrow Transplantation, 28*, 121–129.

Ratanatharathorn, V., Nash, R.A., Przepiorka, D., Devine, S.M., Klein, J.L., Weisdorf, D., et al. (1998). Phase III study comparing methotrexate and tacrolimus (prograf, fk 506) with methotrexate and cyclosporine for graft versus host disease prophylaxis after HLA-identical sibling bone marrow transplantation. *Blood, 92*, 2303–2314.

Reddy, P., Teshima, T., Hildebrandt, G., Williams, D.L., Liu, C., Cooke, K.R., et al. (2003). Pretreatment of donors with interleukin-18 attenuates acute graft versus host disease via STAT 6 and preserves graft versus leukemia effects. *Blood, 101*, 2877–2885.

Remberger, M., Ringden, O., Blau, I., Ottinger, H., Kremens, B., Kiehl, M., et al. (2001). No difference in graft-versus host disease, relapse, and survival comparing peripheral stem cells to bone marrow using unrelated donors. *Blood, 98*, 1739–1745.

Richter, H.I., Stege, H., Ruzicka, T., Soehngen, D., Heyll, A., & Krutmann, J. (1997). Extracorporeal photopheresis in the treatment of acute graft versus host disease. *Journal of the American Academic of Dermatology, 36*(5 Pt. 1), 787–789.

Ringden, O. (1993). Management of graft versus host disease. *European Journal of Hematology, 51*, 1–12.

Ringden, O., & Deeg, H.J. (1997). Clinical spectrum of graft-versus-host disease. In J.L.M. Ferrara, H.J. Deeg, & S.J. Burakoff (Eds.), *Graft-vs-host disease* (2nd ed., pp. 525–559). New York: Marcel Dekker.

Rock, C.L. (2000). Nutritional issues and management in hematopoietic stem cell transplantation. In E.D. Ball, J. Lister, & P. Law (Eds.), *Hematopoietic stem cell therapy* (pp. 503–507). New York: Churchill Livingstone.

Rosenzweig, M.Q. (1998). Graft versus host disease. In C. Chernecky & B. Berger (Eds.), *Advanced and critical care oncology nursing: Managing primary complications* (pp. 172–188). Philadelphia: W.B. Saunders.

Ross, M., Schmidt, G., Niland, J., Amyulon, M., Dagis, A., Long, G., et al. (1999). Cyclosporine, ethotrexate, and prednisone compared with cyclosporine and prednisone for prevention of acute graft versus host disease: Effect on chronic graft versus host disease and survival. *Biology of Blood and Marrow Transplantation, 5*, 285–291.

Rossi, S., Blazar, B.R., Farrell, C.L., Danilenko, D.M., Lacey, D.L., Weinberg, K.I., et al. (2002). Keratinocyte growth factor preserves normal thymopoiesis and thymic microenvironment during experimental graft versus host disease. *Blood, 100*, 682–691.

Rovelli, A., Arrigo, C., Nesi, F., Balduzzi, A., Nicolini, B., Locasciulli, A., et al. (1998). The role of thalidomide in the treatment of refractory chronic graft versus host disease following bone marrow transplantation in children. *Bone Marrow Transplantation, 21*, 577–581.

Rowlings, P.A., Przepiorka, D., Klein, J.P., Gale, R.P., Passweg, J.R., Henslee-Downey, P.J., et al. (1997). IBMTR severity index for grading acute graft versus host disease: Retrospective comparison with Glucksberg grade. *British Journal of Hematology, 97*, 855–864.

Rudy, S.J., Pinto, C., & Townsend-Akpan, C. (2001). Caring for women of childbearing potential taking teratogenic dermatologic drugs. *American Journal for Nurse Practitioners, Spring*(Suppl.), 5–12.

Ruutu, T., Eriksson, B., Remes, K., Juvonen, E., Volin, L., Remberger, M., et al. (2002). Ursodeoxycholic acid for the prevention of hepatic complications of allogeneic stem cell transplantation. *Blood, 100*, 1977–1983.

Saito, T., Shinagawa, K., Takenaka, K., Matsuo, K., Yoshino, T., Kiura, K., et al. (2002). Ocular manifestation of acute graft versus host disease after peripheral blood stem cell transplantation. *International Journal of Hematology, 75*, 332–334.

Sanz, G.F., Saavedra, S., Jimenez, C., Senent, L., Cervera, J., Planelles, D., et al. (2001). Unrelated donor cord-blood transplantation in adults with chronic myelogenous leukemia: Results in nine patients from a single institution. *Bone Marrow Transplant, 27*, 693–701.

Sanz, M.A., & Sanz, G.F. (2002). Unrelated donor umbilical cord blood transplantation in adults. *Leukemia, 16*, 1984–1991.

Schetelig, J., Kroger, N., Held, T., Thiede, C., Krusch, A., Zabelina, T., et al. (2002). Allogeneic transplantation after reduced conditioning in high risk patients is complicated by a high incidence of acute and chronic graft versus host disease. *Haematologica, 87*, 299–305.

Schimmer, A., Minden, M., & Keating, A. (2000). Osteoporosis after blood and marrow transplantation: Clinical aspects. *Biology of Blood and Marrow Transplantation, 6*, 175–181.

Schlossberg, H., Klumpp, T., Sabol, P., Herman, J., & Mangan, K. (2001). Severe cutaneous ulceration following treatment with thalidomide for GvHD. *Bone Marrow Transplantation, 27*, 299–330.

Schmitz, N., & Barrett, J. (2002). Optimizing engraftment-source and dose of stem cells. *Seminars in Hematology, 39*(1), 3–14.

Schots, R., Kaufman, L., Van Riet, I., Lacor, P., Trullemans, F., De Waele, M., et al. (1998). Monitoring of c-reactive protein after allogeneic bone marrow transplantation identifies patients at risk of severe transplant related complications and mortality. *Bone Marrow Transplantation, 22*(1), 79–85.

Schubert, M., & Sullivan, K. (1990). Recognition, incidence, and management of oral graft versus host disease. *NCI Monographs, 9*, 135–143.

Seber, A., & Vogelsang, G. (1998). Chronic graft-versus-host disease. In J. Barrett & J. Treleaven (Eds.), *The clinical practice of stem cell transplantation* (pp. 620–634). Oxford, United Kingdom: ISIS Medical Media.

Seeley, K., & DeMeyer, E. (2002). Nursing care of patients receiving Campath. *Clinical Journal of Oncology Nursing, 6*, 138–143.

Sepkowitz, K.A. (2002). Antibiotic prophylaxis in patients receiving hematopoietic stem cell transplant. *Bone Marrow Transplantation, 29*, 367–371.

Seth, P., Alrajhi, A., Kagevi, I., Chaudhary, M., Colcol, E., Sahovic, E., et al. (2002). Hepatitis B virus reactivation with clinical flare in allogeneic stem cell transplants with chronic graft versus host disease. *Bone Marrow Transplantation, 30*, 189–194.

Sevilla, J., & Gonzalez-Vicent, M. (2001). Acute autoimmune hemolytic anemia following unrelated cord blood transplantation as an early manifestation of chronic graft versus host disease. *Bone Marrow Transplantation, 28*, 89–92.

Silberstein, L., Davies, A., Kelsey, S., Foran, J., Murrell, C., D'Cruz, D., et al. (2001). Myositis, polyserositis with a large pericardial effusion and constrictive pericarditis as manifestations of chronic graft-versus host disease after non-myeloablative peripheral stem cell transplantation, and subsequent donor lymphocyte infusion. *Bone Marrow Transplantation, 27*, 231–233.

Simpson, D. (2001). New developments in the prophylaxis and treatment of graft versus host disease. *Expert Opinion in Pharmacotherapy, 2*, 1109–1117.

Simpson, D. (2003). T-cell depleting antibodies: New hope for induction of allograft tolerance in bone marrow transplantation? *BioDrugs, 17*(3), 147–154.

Smith, E.P., Sniecinski, I., Dagis, A., Parker, P.M., Snyder, D.S., Stein, A., et al. (1998). Extracorporeal photochemotherapy for treatment of drug resistant graft versus host disease. *Biology of Blood and Marrow Transplantation, 4*(1), 27–37.

Socie, G., & Cahn, J.Y. (1998). Acute graft-versus-host disease. In J. Barrett & J. Treleaven (Eds.), *The clinical practice of stem cell transplantation* (pp. 596–618). Oxford, United Kingdom: ISIS Medical Media.

Socie, G., Devergie, A., & Cosset, J. (1990). Low dose total lymphoid irradiation for extensive, drug resistant chronic graft versus host disease. *Transplantation, 49*, 657–658.

Soiffer, R.J., Weller, E., Alyea, E.P., Mauch, P., Webb, I.L., Fisher, D.C., et al. (2001). CD 6+ donor marrow t-cell depletion as the sole form of graft versus host disease prophylaxis in patients undergoing allogeneic bone marrow transplant from unrelated donors. *Journal of Clinical Oncology, 19*, 1152–1159.

Sokos, D., Berger, M., & Lazarus, H.M. (2002). Intravenous immunoglobulin: Appropriate indications and uses in hematopoietic stem cell transplantation. *Biology of Blood and Marrow Transplantation, 8*, 117–130.

Solimando, D. (1998). Medications. In R.K. Burt, H.J. Deeg, S. Lothian, & G.W. Santos (Eds.), *Bone marrow transplantation* (pp. 544–566). Austin, TX: Landes Bioscience.

Stander, H., Schiller, M., & Schwarz, T. (2002). UVA1 therapy for sclerodermic graft versus host disease of the skin. *Journal of the American Academy of Dermatology, 46*, 799–800.

Strasser, S.I., & McDonald, G.B. (1999). Gastrointestinal and hepatic complications. In E.D. Thomas, K.G. Blume, & S.J. Forman (Eds.), *Hematopoietic cell transplantation* (2nd ed., pp. 627–658). Oxford, United Kingdom: Blackwell Science.

Strasser, S., Shulman, H., & McDonald, G. (1999). Cholestasis after hematopoietic cell transplantation. *Clinics in Liver Disease, 3*, 651–669.

Sudan, D., Grant, W., Iyer, K., Shaw, B., Horslen, S., & Langnas, A. (2002). Oral beclomethasone therapy for recurrent small bowel allograft rejection and intestinal graft versus host disease. *Transplantation Proceedings, 34*, 938–939.

Sullivan, K.M. (1999). Graft-versus-host disease. In E.D. Thomas, K.G. Blume, & S.J. Forman (Eds.), *Hematopoietic cell transplantation* (2nd ed., pp. 515–536). Oxford, United Kingdom: Blackwell Science.

Sullivan, K.M., Angura, E., Anasetti, C., Appelbaum, F., Badger, C., Bearman, S., et al. (1991). Chronic graft versus host disease and other late complications of bone marrow transplantation. *Seminars in Hematology, 28*, 250–259.

Sullivan, K.M., Kopecky, K.J., Jocom, J., Fisher, L., Buckner, C.D., Meyers, J.D., et al. (1990). Immunomodulatory and antimicrobial efficacy of intravenous immunoglobulin in bone marrow transplantation. *New England Journal of Medicine, 323*, 705–712.

Sullivan, K.M., & Siadak, M.F. (1997). Stem cell transplantation. In F.L. Johnson & K.S. Virgo (Eds.), *Cancer patient follow-up* (pp. 490–519). St. Louis, MO: Mosby

Sullivan, K.M., Storek, J., Kopecky, K.J., Jocom, J., Longton, G., Flowers, M., et al. (1996). A controlled trial of long-term administration of intravenous immunoglobulin to prevent late infection and chronic graft-versus-host disease after marrow transplantation: Clinical outcome and effect on subsequent immune recovery. *Biology of Blood and Marrow Transplantation, 2*, 44–53.

Sviland, L. (2000). The pathology of bone marrow transplantation. *Current Diagnostic Pathology, 6*, 242–250.

Sykes, M., & Strober, S. (1999). Mechanisms of tolerance. In E.D. Thomas, K.G. Blume, & S.J. Forman (Eds.), *Hematopoietic cell transplantation* (2nd ed., pp. 264–286). Oxford, United Kingdom: Blackwell Science.

Talmadge, J. (2003). Hematopoietic stem cell graft manipulation as a mechanism of immunotherapy. *International Immunopharmacology, 444*, 1–23.

Tauchmanova, L., De Rosa, G., Serio, B., Fazioli, F., Mainolfi, C., Lombardi, G., et al. (2003). Avascular necrosis in long-term survivors after allogeneic or autologous stem cell transplantation. *Cancer, 97*, 2453–2461.

Tauchmanova, L., Selleri, C., De Rosa, G., Pagano, L., Orlo, F., Lombardi, G., et al. (2002). High prevalence of endocrine dysfunction in long-term survivors after allogeneic bone marrow transplantation for hematologic diseases. *Cancer, 95*, 1076–1084.

Teshima, T., & Ferrara, J.L. (2002). Understanding the alloresponse: New approaches to graft-versus-host-disease prevention. *Seminars in Hematology, 39*, 15–22.

Teshima, T., Reddy, P., Liu, C., Williams, D., Cooke, K.R., & Ferrara, J.L. (2003). Impaired thymic negative selection causes autoimmune graft-versus-host disease. *Blood, 102*, 429–435.

Thompson, A., Couch, M., Zahurak, M., Johnson, C., & Vogelsang, G. (2002). Risk factors for post-transplant sinusitis. *Bone Marrow Transplantation, 29*, 257–261.

Treleaven, J. (1995). Late effects of bone marrow transplantation. In J. Treleaven & P. Wiernik (Eds.), *Color atlas and text of bone marrow transplantation* (pp. 193–200). London: Mosby-Wolfe.

Ustun, C., Arslan, O., Beksac, M., Koc, H., Gurman, G., Ozcelik, T., et al. (1999). A retrospective comparison of allogeneic peripheral blood stem cell and bone marrow transplantation results from a single center: A focus on the incidence of graft versus host disease and relapse. *Biology of Blood and Marrow Transplantation, 5*(1), 28–35.

Valcarcel, D., Martino, R., Caballero, D., Mateos, M., Perez-Simon, J., Canals, C., et al. (2003). Chimerism analysis following allogeneic peripheral blood stem cell transplantation with reduced-intensity conditioning. *Bone Marrow Transplantation, 31*, 387–392.

van Leeuwen, L., Guiffre, A., Atkinson, K., Rainer, S.P., & Sewell, W. (2002). A two phase pathogenesis of graft versus host disease in mice. *Bone Marrow Transplantation, 29*, 151–158.

Varadi, G., Or, R., Slavin, S., & Nagler, A. (1996). In vivo Campath-1 monoclonal antibodies: A novel mode of therapy for acute graft-versus-host disease. *American Journal of Hematology, 52*, 236–237.

Vickers, C.R. (1994). Gastrointestinal complications. In K. Atkinson (Ed.), *Clinical bone marrow transplantation: A reference textbook* (pp. 435–443). London: Cambridge University.

Vinayek, R., Demetris, J., & Rakela, J. (2000). Liver disease in hematopoietic stem cell transplant recipients. In E.D. Ball, J. Lister, & P. Law (Eds.), *Hematopoietic stem cell therapy* (pp. 541–556). New York: Churchill Livingstone.

Vivino, F., Al-Hashimi, I., Khan, Z., LeVeque, F., Salisbury, P., Ran-Johnson, T., et al. (1999). Pilocarpine tablets for the treatment of dry mouth and dry eye symptoms in patients with sjogren syndrome. *Archives of Internal Medicine, 159*, 174–181.

Vogelsang, G. (2000). Advances in the treatment of graft versus host disease. *Leukemia, 14*, 509–510.

Vogelsang, G. (2001). How I treat chronic graft-versus-host disease. *Blood, 97*, 1196–1201.

Vogelsang, G.B., Altomonte, V., & Farmer, E. (1993). Explosive graft versus host disease [Abstract]. *Blood, 82*(Suppl.), 422a.

Vogelsang, G.B., & Hess, A.D. (1994). Graft versus host disease: New directions for a persistent problem. *Blood, 84*, 2061–2067.

Vogelsang, G.B., Lee, L., & Bensen-Kennedy, D.J. (2003). Pathogenesis and treatment of graft-versus-host disease after bone marrow transplantation. *Annual Review of Medicine, 54*(1), 29–52.

Vogelsang, G.B., Wolff, D., Altomonte, V., Farmer, E., Morison, W.L., Corio, R., et al. (1996). Treatment of chronic graft versus host disease with ultraviolet irradiation and psoralen. *Bone Marrow Transplantation, 17*, 1061–1067.

Voltarelli, J., Ahmed, H., Paton, E., Stracieri, A., Holman, P., Bashey, A., et al. (2001). Beneficial effect of intravenous lidocaine in cutaneous chronic graft versus host disease secondary to donor lymphocyte infusion. *Bone Marrow Transplantation, 28*, 97–99.

Wada, H., Mori, A., Okada, M., Takatsuka, H., Tamura, A., Seto, Y., et al. (2001). Treatment of intestinal graft versus host disease using betamethasone enemas. *Transplantation, 72*, 1451–1463.

Wagner, J.L., Flowers, M.E.D., Longton, G., Storb, R., & Martin, P. (2001). Use of screening studies to predict survival among patients who do not have chronic graft-versus-host disease at Day 100 after bone marrow transplantation. *Biology of Blood and Marrow Transplantation, 7*, 239–240.

Wagner, J.L., Flowers, M.E.D., Longton, G., Storb, R., Schubert, M., & Sullivan, K.M. (1998). The development of chronic graft versus host disease: An analysis of screening studies and the impact of corticosteroids use at 100 days after transplant. *Bone Marrow Transplant, 22*, 139–146.

Weisdorf, S.S., & Schwarzenberg, S.J. (1999). Nutritional support of hematopoietic stem cell recipients. In E.D. Thomas, K.G. Blume, & S.J. Forman (Eds.), *Hematopoietic cell transplantation* (2nd ed., pp. 723–732). Oxford: Blackwell Science.

Wesorick, B. (1990). *Standards of nursing care: A model for clinical practice.* Philadelphia: J.B. Lippincott.

Wiesmann, A., Weller, A., Lischka, G., Klingebiel, T., Kanz, L., & Einsele, H. (1999). Treatment of acute graft versus host disease with PUVA (psoralen and ultraviolet irradiation): Results of a pilot study. *Bone Marrow Transplantation, 23*, 151–155.

Williams, M. (1999). Gastrointestinal manifestations of graft-versus-host disease: Diagnosis and management. *AACN Clinical Issues: Advanced Practice in Acute and Critical Care, 10*, 500–506.

Wingard, J., Nash, R., Przepiorka, D., Klein, J., Weisdorf, D., Fay, J., et al. (1998). Relationship of tacrolimus whole blood concentrations and efficacy and safety after HLA-identical sibling bone marrow transplantation. *Biology of Blood and Marrow Transplantation, 4*, 157–163.

Wolff, D., Reichenberger, F., Steiner, B., Kahl, C., Leithauser, M., Sibbe, T., et al. (2002). Progressive interstitial fibrosis of the lung in sclerodermoid chronic graft versus host disease. *Bone Marrow Transplantation, 29*, 357–360.

Wood, P.M., & Proctor, S.J. (1990). The potential use of thalidomide in the therapy of graft-versus-host disease—a review of clinical and laboratory information. *Leukemia Research, 14*, 395–399.

Zic, J.A., Miller, J.L., Stricklin, G.P., & King, L.E. (1999). The North American experience with photopheresis. *Therapeutic Apheresis, 3*(1), 50–62.

Zupan, I.P., Zver, S., & Pretnar, J. (2002). Immunosuppressive treatment of severe acute graft versus host disease after allogeneic hematopoietic stem cell transplantation. *Transplantation Proceedings, 34*, 2931–2933.

CHAPTER 7

Gail B. Johnson, MSN, RN, AOCN®
Kimberly Quiett, RN, MSN, AOCN®

Hematologic Effects

Introduction

The most common hematologic effects post-transplant include neutropenia, immunosuppression, thrombocytopenia, anemia, graft failure, and delayed engraftment. Although the most common cause of the complications is the transplant preparative regimen, other etiologic risk factors may occur. This chapter will discuss the pathophysiology, etiology, and management of each hematologic complication.

Neutropenia

Neutropenia and associated infections following transplant are the most common complications of hematopoietic stem cell transplant (HSCT). Many steps have been made toward limiting transplant-associated neutropenia and infections; however, infection remains the leading cause of post-transplant mortality and morbidity (Nichols & Boeckh, 2000). In addition, this complication has been found to add significant costs to the transplant procedure. In autologous transplantation, infection may add approximately $18,400, and for allogeneic transplantations, approximately $15,300 may be added to the cost of the procedure during the first 100 days post-transplant (Lee, Klar, Weeks, & Antin, 2000).

In caring for transplant recipients, it is vitally important to understand the neutropenic process and the diagnosis and treatment of infections often associated with neutropenia. The immune system of the transplant recipient is severely insulted by high-dose chemotherapy, with or without radiation, given prior to the transplant. Prolonged periods of neutropenia, combined with other complications of transplant, including impaired skin and mucosal integrity, graft versus host disease (GVHD), graft rejection, steroid therapy, malnutrition, and invasive venous catheters, increase HSCT recipients' risk for morbidity and mortality related to severe infections (Ellerhorst-Ryan, 1997; Walker & Burcat, 1997).

Infection Risk in Neutropenic Patients

The body has two basic lines of defense against invasion of infection-causing pathogens. The first line is the skin and mucosal linings, and the second is the white blood cell (WBC). The WBC community contains granulocytes, mono-cytes, macrophages, and lymphocytes. Neutrophils that seek out and kill microorganisms that enter the body comprise approximately 95% of the granulocyte population, making them a prominent component for an adequate immune system (Alcoser & Burchett, 1999). Chemotherapy and/or radiation therapies decrease the number of these infection-fighting cells, resulting in a condition known as neutropenia. See Table 7-1 for the National Cancer Institute's Common Toxicity Criteria (version 2.0) grading system for neutropenia for HSCT. Profound neutropenia with an absolute neutrophil count (ANC) < 100 cells per microliter is common to the HSCT population as a complication resulting from high-dose chemotherapy and/or radiation therapy (Phillips, 1999).

The point at which the neutrophil count is maintained at > 500/mm³ is considered neutrophil engraftment (Centers for Disease Control and Prevention [CDC], Infectious Diseases Society of America, and American Society of Blood and Marrow Transplantation, 2000). The duration of neutropenia for the HSCT recipient depends on several factors, including history of chemotherapy and radiation therapy, the type and number of cells used for the transplant, preparative regimen used, the use of growth factors post-transplant, and post-transplant complications.

Neutrophil Engraftment

Two of the most recognized and important factors in the fight against early infectious complications post-transplant are the use of colony-stimulating factors and mobilized peripheral blood progenitor cells. Transplants utilizing peripheral blood progenitor cells that have been mobilized with hematopoietic growth factors (specifically granulocyte–colony-stimulating factor [G-CSF]) improve hematologic recovery post-transplant for both autologous and allogeneic HSCT (Beyer et al., 1995; Pavletic et al., 1997). In the autologous transplant population, using mobilized peripheral blood stem cells (PBSCs) rather than bone marrow decreases the duration of neutropenia. Beyer et al. reported a randomized clinical trial that indicated that PBSCs mobilized with chemotherapy and G-CSF shortened the recovery time of engraftment to 10 days. Likewise, the use of PBSCs also has been evaluated in allogeneic transplant. Champlin et al. (2000) reported that the median time to engraftment was

Table 7-1. Grading of Neutropenia Using the National Cancer Institute's Common Toxicity Criteria

	Grade			
Subject	1	2	3	4
Neutrophils/granulocytes (absolute neutrophil count/absolute granulocyte count) for BMT studies	$1.0 - < 1.5 \times 10^9/l$ $1,000 - < 1,500/mm^3$	$0.5 - < 1.0 \times 10^9/l$ $500 - < 1,000/mm^3$	$0.5 - < 0.5 \times 10^9/l$ $100 - < 500/mm^3$	$< 0.1 \times 10^9/l$ $< 100/mm^3$

Note. Based on information from the National Cancer Institute, 1999.

shortened to 14 days, versus 19 days with traditional bone marrow. Pavletic et al. also reported a significantly shorter time to neutrophil engraftment using PBSCs compared to bone marrow (10 versus 14 days, respectively). PBSCs have been shown to shorten the interval between transplant and neutrophil engraftment.

In recent years, nonmyeloablative preparative regimens have been used for allogeneic stem cell transplant. With a shorter neutropenic phase and less mucosal tissue damage, incidence of bacterial infections may be decreased during the early phase of transplant (Junghanss & Marr, 2002). Patients undergoing nonmyeloablative transplant regimens have not had fewer infections in later phases of the transplant process.

The dose of cells given also has attributed to the duration of neutropenia. Cell dose is commonly calculated based on the number of CD34+ cells. CD34+ is a molecule on the surface of primitive progenitor cells. These earliest cells are most valuable in reestablishing hematopoiesis post-transplant. Therefore, the number of CD34+ cells to be transplanted has become a marker for engraftment potential. Kiss et al. (1997) and Shulman, Birch, Zhen, Pania, and Weaver (1999) both reported research indicating that faster neutrophil engraftment time was associated with CD34+ cell infusions $> 5.0 \times 10^6$ cells per kilogram in autologous transplant. Kiss et al. and Shulman et al. also reported the decrease of one day ($p = 0.004$, $p = 0.0001$, respectively) in the median days to neutrophil engraftment. Shulman et al. equated a CD34+ cell dose of $> 5.0 \times 10^6$ cells per kilogram with a reduction in patient resource utilization, including fewer platelet and red blood cell (RBC) infusions, decreased length of stay in the hospital, decreased use of intravenous antibiotics and antifungal agents, and decreased days of G-CSF administration.

CD34+ cell doses also have been shown to affect the duration of neutropenia. Bittencourt et al. (2002) reported that a CD34+ cell dose of at least 3×10^6 cells per kilogram significantly decreased the neutropenic duration ($p = 0.04$). In this study, neutrophil engraftment occurred prior to day +60 in 97.1% of patients, with a dose of at least 3×10^6 CD34+ cells per kilogram. Neutrophil engraftment occurred prior to day +60 in only 93.1% of patients when the cell dose was less than 3×10^6 cells per kilogram. Umbilical cord blood (UCB) has been used as a source of stem cells for allogeneic transplant. Although UCB has been noted as a rich source of stem cells, the quantity of cells available for transplant from a single umbilical cord is small, making the use of UCB limited for adults.

The use of colony-stimulating factors, such as G-CSF and granulocyte macrophage–colony-stimulating factor (GM-CSF), has decreased the duration of neutropenia following HSCT, both autologous and allogeneic. In autologous transplant, the use of growth factors may decrease the time from transplant to neutrophil engraftment by as much as 5.5 days (Klumpp, Goldberg, & Mangan, 1995). In allogeneic HSCT, neutrophil recovery may be decreased by an average of four days with the use of G-CSF post-transplant (Bishop et al., 2000). Decreasing the period of neutropenia may lead to decreased incidence and/or severity of infectious complications.

In a study reported by Bishop et al. (2000), the time to neutrophil engraftment was shortened from 15 to 11 days ($p = 0.0082$) for a sample of patients receiving allogeneic transplant followed by the administration of filgrastim starting on the day of transplantation. Currently, optimal timing for growth factor administration post-transplant remains controversial. Researchers have reported starting G-CSF on days 1, 3, 5, 6, and 7 post-autologous transplant (de Azevedo et al., 2002). In studies, the significant differences of neutrophil recovery were associated with patients who were given G-CSF versus those that were not, rather than the day on which G-CSF was started. Although specific groups may benefit from beginning the G-CSF nearer to the transplant, other patient groups may tolerate the delayed start of growth factors without clinical compromise. In a study reported by Ener et al. (2001), there was no statistically significant difference in autologous transplant recipients' days to neutrophil engraftment or days spent in the hospital for the transplant. It is known that the administration of growth factors following autologous and allogeneic transplant significantly lessens the duration of neutropenia. The American Society of Clinical Oncology (1996) guidelines for using colony-stimulating factors recognize that growth factors improve hematopoietic recovery, although a specific schedule for administration is not recommended. Doses of G-CSF and GM-CSF following HSCT range from 5–10 mg/kg/day and typically are given subcutaneously, although the doses may be administered intravenously when necessary.

Prolonged neutrophil recovery or delayed engraftment may occur following HSCT. Anderson et al. (2003) reported the patients receiving allogeneic PBSCs had neutrophil recovery by 17 days post-HSCT, and those receiving marrow had neutrophil recovery at an average of 24 days post-HSCT. In this same study, the incidence of bacteremia was higher in the marrow group (43%) versus the PBSC group (35%) at 100 days post-transplant.

The time from transplant to neutrophil engraftment is influenced by many factors. Studies have shown that the use of PBSCs versus bone marrow cells hastens the neutrophil recovery post-transplant. The use of colony-stimulating factors as well as nonmyeloablative preparative regimens has shortened this interval as well. Because prolonged neutropenia increases the potential for infection, decreasing the interval between transplant and neutrophil engraftment directly impacts the patient's outcome.

Infections During the Transplantation Process

The duration of neutropenia is directly related to the risk of infection in transplant recipients. Infection is the most common cause of morbidity and mortality in the transplant population. Infections typically are discussed in the context of the period of time post-transplant that they occur. Different risk factors and organisms are associated with different phases of the transplant process. For patients undergoing allogeneic transplant, infection is the primary cause (15%) or a contributory (35%) cause of death (Passweg et al., 1998). The most common infections, their prevention, and treatment throughout the transplant process will be discussed.

The transplant process may be defined in phases beginning with pretransplant, followed by the immediate post-transplant or pre-engraftment phase (0–30 days), the intermediate post-transplant or post-engraftment phase (30–100 days), and the late post-transplant phase (after day 100) (CDC et al., 2000; Phillips, 1999; van Burik & Weisdorf, 1999). Infectious complications common during each phase of the transplant process are described in Table 7-2.

Pre-Engraftment

During the pre-engraftment phase, transplant recipients are at risk for infection because of severe myelosuppression-causing neutropenia and gastrointestinal mucosal toxicity, which occur as expected side effects of the preparative regimen. An additional risk is the interruption of skin integrity due to central venous catheters. Previous exposure to infections such as herpes simplex virus and cytomegalovirus (CMV) poses an additional risk, as reactivation is possible during the neutropenic phase.

All of these factors contribute to the development of infectious complications. Bacteria are the most common cause of infection during this period. The incidence of bacterial infections in this population may be as high as 100% (Buchsel, 1997). Common bacterial infection-causing pathogens include gram-negative (*Escherichia coli*, *Klebsiella pneumoniae*, and *Pseudomonas aeruginosa*) and gram-positive (*Staphylococcus epidermitis*, *Staphylococcus aureus*, and *Streptococci*) species (Phillips, 1999; Walker & Burcat, 1997). The most common sites for infection include the oral mucosa and central venous catheters. Although prophylactic coverage is not recommended for the afebrile transplant patient (CDC et al., 2000), prophylaxis must be based on institutional-specific data. Common prophylactic interventions for the afebrile patient may include Pen-Vee K® (Wyeth Ayerst, Madison, NJ), Norfloxacin® (Merck, Whitehouse Station, NJ), and Bactrim® (Roche Pharmaceuticals, Nutley, NJ). With the first febrile episode, these medications should be discontinued, and coverage for gram-positive and gram-negative organisms should be instituted. Common antibiotic therapies include third and fourth generation cephalosporins (nafcillin, Primaxin® [Merck], Merrem® [AstraZeneca, Wilmington, DE]) quinolones (Levaquin® [Ortho-McNeil Pharmaceutical, Raritan, NJ]), aminoglycosides (tobramycin, gentamycin, amikacin), and vancomycin. Because of the emergence of vancomycin-resistant enterococcus, vancomycin should not be used as prophylaxis (CDC et al.) and should be discontinued if culture sensitivity is not documented. In conjunction with the change or implementation of antibiotic therapy, the nurse should expect other diagnostic tests, including blood cultures, chest x-ray, stool, and urine cultures.

Yeast and fungal infections also may be problematic during this pre-engraftment phase. The two species commonly identified are *Candida albicans*, primarily as stomatitis, and *Aspergillus*. More recently, infections caused by less common amphotericin-resistant molds have been described, including non-fumigatus *Aspergillus* species, *Fusarium* species, and *Scedosporium* species (Marr, 2001; Marr, Carter, Crippa, Wald, & Corey, 2002). Prophylaxis for fungal infection may include medications such as fluconazole, itraconazole, or voriconazole. Common treatment of invasive fungal infections, such as *Aspergillus*, includes amphotericin B, liposomal amphotericin preparations, or voriconazole. Oral treatments such as nystatin and clotrimazole troches may be used to treat mucosal candidiasis. Patients should be instructed to prevent exposure to yeasts and molds by avoiding construction sites, building renovation areas, and gardening (CDC et al., 2000). In hospitals with transplant units, it is very important to minimize immunocompromised patient exposure to fungal risk factors. It is recommended that hospitals provide high-efficiency particulate air filtration (HEPA), positive air pressure between the patient rooms and hallways, appropriately sealed doors, windows, and outlets, more than 12 air exchanges per hour in the patient room, and barriers that prevent dust from crossing into patient areas during periods of construction or renovation (CDC et al.).

Reactivation of viral infections, such as herpes simplex virus (HSV) I and II, HHV-6, and CMV, also may occur during the immediate post-transplant phase. Patients and donors should be evaluated for latent viral infections prior to beginning a transplant procedure. Herpes simplex most often manifests as stomatitis. Prophylaxis with acyclovir or famciclovir is common in the pre-engraftment phase. Allogeneic HSCT recipients have a much higher incidence of CMV antigenemia than autologous HSCT recipients. Of the allogeneic patients, those with acute GVHD beyond grade I have a higher incidence of CMV (Osarogiagbon, Defor, Weisdorf, Erice, & Weisdorf, 2000). The risk of CMV infec-

Table 7-2. Infectious Complications and Occurrence in Hematopoietic Stem Cell Transplantation Recipients

Organism	Common Sites	Treatment
First Month Post-Transplant		
Viral		
Herpes simplex virus (HSV)	Oral, esophageal, skin, gastrointestinal (GI) tract, genital	Acyclovir, famciclovir
Respiratory syncytial virus (RSV)	Sinopulmonary	Aerosolized ribavirin
Epstein-Barr virus (EBV)	Oral, esophageal, skin, GI tract	Treatment usually is not indicated.
Bacterial		
Gram + (*S. epidermidis, S. aureus, Streptococci*)	Skin, blood, sinopulmonary	Third and fourth generation cephalosporins,
Gram – (*E. coli, P. aeruginosa, Klebsiella*)	GI, blood, oral, perirectal	quinolones, aminoglycosides, vancomycin
Fungal		
Candida species (*C. albicans,* glabrata krusei	Oral, esophageal, skin	Fluconazole, voriconazole, itraconazole, amphotericin
Aspergillus (*fumagata,* flavum)	Sinopulmonary	B, liposomal amphotericin
One to Four Months Post-Transplant		
Viral		
Cytomegalovirus (CMV)	Pulmonary, hepatic, GI	Ganciclovir, foscarnet, valacyclovir, acyclovir
Enteric viruses (rotavirus, Coxsackie, adenovirus)	Pulmonary, urinary, GI, hepatic	No specific treatment
RSV	Sinopulmonary	Aerosolized ribavirin
Parainfluenza	Pulmonary	Possibly ribavirin, but no standard treatment
Bacterial		
Gram +	Sinopulmonary	Third and fourth generation cephalosporins, quinolones, aminoglycosides, vancomycin
Fungal		
Candida species	Oral, hepatosplenic, integument	Fluconazole, voriconazole, itraconazole, amphotericin B, liposomal amphotericin
Aspergillus species	Sinopulmonary, central nervous system (CNS)	
Mucormycosis	Sinopulmonary	
Coccidiomycosis	Sinopulmonary	
Cryptococcus neoformans	Pulmonary, CNS	
Protozoan		
Pneumocystis carinii	Pulmonary	Standard is trimethoprim-sulfamethoxazole (TMP-SMZ) Pentamidine, atovaquone may be used if allergic to sulfa
Toxoplasma gondii	Pulmonary, CNS	Pyrimethamine and sulfonamides may be combined with clindamycin and spiramycin, especially if sulfa allergy
4–12 Months Post-Transplant		
Viral		
CMV, echoviruses, RSV, Varicella zoster (VCV)	Integument, pulmonary, hepatic	CMV—ganciclovir, foscarnet, valacyclovir, acyclovir RSV—aerosolized ribavirin VCV—acyclovir, valacyclovir, famciclovir Echoviruses—no specific treatment, IVIG
Bacterial		
Gram + (*S. pneumoniae, H. influenza, Pneumococci*)	Sinopulmonary, blood	Third and fourth generation cephalosporins, quinolones, aminoglycosides, vancomycin
Fungal		
Aspergillus	Sinopulmonary	Fluconazole, voriconazole, itraconazole, amphotericin
Coccidiomycosis	Sinopulmonary	B, liposomal amphotericin

(Continued on next page)

Table 7-2. Infectious Complications and Occurrence in Hematopoietic Stem Cell Transplantation Recipients *(Continued)*

Organism	Common Sites	Treatment
4–12 Months Post-Transplant *(Continued)*		
Protozoan		
Pneumocystis carinii	Pulmonary	Standard is TMP-SMZ. Pentamidine, atovaquone may be used if allergic to sulfa.
Toxoplasma gondii	Pulmonary, CNS	Pyrimethamine and sulfonamides may be combined with clindamycin and spiramycin, especially if sulfa allergy.
Greater Than 12 Months Post-Transplant		
Viral		
VZV	Integument	Acyclovir, valacyclovir, famciclovir
Bacterial		
Gram + (*Streptococci, H. Influenza*, encapsulated bacteria)	Sinopulmonary, blood	Third and fourth generation cephalosporins, quinolones, aminoglycosides, vancomycin

Note. Based on information from Barnes 1998a, 1998b; Prentice et al., 1998; Riley, 1998; Shapiro et al., 1997; Westmoreland, 1998.

tion has been decreased to less than 3% in seronegative patients with the use of leukocyte filters for platelet and RBC transfusions. For seropositve patients, prophylaxis with ganciclovir, foscarnet, valacyclovir, or acyclovir is used in many HSCT centers (van Burik & Weisdorf, 1999). Ganciclovir is the standard treatment and prophylaxis for CMV; however, it may cause a decrease in WBC counts. Therefore, it is stopped just before transplant and restarted after engraftment. Screening for CMV should be performed for high-risk allogeneic patients at least one time per week from day 10 until day 100 post-transplant (CDC et al., 2000). Seropositive autologous patients who are being treated for hematologic malignancies should be tested for CMV reactivation weekly until 60 days post-transplant. Only autologous patients with CMV antigenemia or those who received a CD34+ selected transplant product should be treated with ganciclovir or foscarnet. Varicella zoster virus (VZV) and HSV are treated with acyclovir, valacyclovir, or famciclovir. Evaluating patients and donors for the presence of viruses prior to transplant provides a baseline for prophylaxis and treatment of the patient post-transplant. Testing for CMV is primarily performed through antigen detection techniques (Boeckh & Boivin, 1998), with the most common being the hybrid capture technique. Antigen detection techniques are less expensive and more specific in detecting early CMV.

In the allogeneic patient population, prophylactic treatment for *Pneumocystis carinii* pneumonia (PCP) with trimethoprim-sulfamethoxazole (TMP-SMZ) is recommended beginning pretransplant and continuing until the patient is no longer being treated for chronic GVHD (CDC et al., 2000). If the patient has an allergy to sulfa, pentamidine or atovaquone may be used. TMP-SMZ should be discontinued during the neutropenic period because a side effect of the medication is a decrease in WBC counts. Dur-

ing this time, pentamidine or atovaquone may be used as prophylaxis.

Other measures that are important to preventing early infections are the use of air filtration systems, such as HEPA or laminar airflow. Although these systems have been shown to be effective in significantly lowering the infection rates of allogeneic bone marrow transplant recipients (Passweg et al., 1998), this may not be necessary for all HSCT recipients. Russell et al. (2000) noted that strict isolation policies may not add significant protection against infection. As healthcare patterns have shifted and many patients are receiving treatment in the home or outpatient clinics, air filtration systems are not commonly used for autologous HSCT patients. Selected patients treated outside of filtered hospital rooms may not be at higher risk for infection during the pre-engraftment phase of transplant (Herrmann, Trent, Cooney, & Cannell, 1999). Likewise, carefully selected patients treated in the outpatient environment may use approximately the same amount of antibiotic treatment and develop fevers at approximately the same rate as those in inpatient settings (Meisenberg et al., 1998). Perhaps more important than air filtration systems is the patient's and family's understanding of appropriate hygiene, mouth care, care of indwelling central venous catheters, appropriate low bacterial diets, and avoidance of crowds, fresh flowers or plants, and other sources of bacterial contamination. Although the literature does not support one anti-infection regimen at this time, it is vitally important that patients with neutropenia and fever be treated immediately and proactively to prevent life-threatening complications (Phillips, 1999). Allowing treatment in the outpatient setting or sending patients out of the hospital prior to engraftment may improve the patient's emotional and social outlook without compromising safety. It is important that patients be carefully selected for programs allowing for this flexibility.

Postengraftment

In the postengraftment phase, differences between allogeneic and autologous transplants become more evident. For autologous patients, the risk of developing infectious complications decreases during the intermediate post-transplant or postengraftment phase, but infection occurs. However, for the allogeneic patient, risk factors such as GVHD, graft rejection, prolonged neutropenia, and continued immunosuppressive therapy cause a continued threat of infection (Phillips, 1999; Walker & Burcat, 1997). During this time, patients are especially at risk for nonbacterial infections, such as viral and fungal infections, although the threat of bacterial infection continues. Interstitial pneumonia (IP) that is often caused by a virus (CMV, HSV, parainfluenza, or respiratory syncytial virus) is more common between days 30 and 100 post-transplant (see chapter on cardiopulmonary effects for more discussion of IP) (Shapiro, Davison, & Rust, 1997). Localized or disseminated VZV infections also are seen during this phase. Treatment for zoster infections because of reactivation or a primary infection includes use of high-dose acyclovir. Fortunately, an often fatal infectious complication, *Pneumocystis carinii* pneumonia, has been essentially eliminated from the repertoire of postengraftment complications by the prophylactic administration of TMP-SMZ or pentamidine postengraftment (Walker & Burcat).

Nursing care of the patient during the postengraftment phase of HSCT includes frequent and thorough assessment, including central venous catheter sites, respiratory status, vital signs, and administration of antibiotics, antifungals, and antiviral medications. Only a few years ago, HSCT patients with infections in the intermediate post-transplant phase would be hospitalized. Currently, it is common for both allogeneic and autologous patients to be cared for in the home by homecare nurses and family members. Nursing care may revolve around education of the patient and caregivers. Teaching the patient and caregiver(s) the signs and symptoms of infection; accurate assessment of temperature, skin, and mucosal linings; and the use of interventions to minimize the risk of infection (e.g., hand washing, clean environment, medication administration) are often the most important nursing interventions during this phase of the HSCT process.

Late Post-Transplant

The final phase of the HSCT process is the late post-transplant phase. At this point, most patients will have engraftment of WBCs, healing of mucosal linings, and adequate skin integrity. Patients without ongoing complications of HSCT are not significantly at risk for major infectious complications. Patients with ongoing complications, such as GVHD, graft rejection or failure, or relapse or progression of disease, may continue to be more at risk for infectious complications. Common infections during this time are *Streptococcus pneumoniae*, *Haemophilus influenzae*, *Neisseria meningitidis*, sinusitis, and VZV (Buchsel, 1997; Phillips, 1999; van Burik & Weisdorf, 1999).

During the final phase of transplant, ongoing patient and caregiver education is imperative. These patients may be seen only on rare occasions, if at all, by the transplant team because of financial constraints, distance from the transplant center, or transportation limitations. It is necessary for nurses to provide education to the patient and caregivers regarding assessment and appropriate interventions for infectious complications, and it is also imperative that HSCT nurses share details of the patient's transplant course and information concerning appropriate monitoring and referral with the nurses and physicians who will resume care of the patient away from the transplant center. For patients still being seen by the transplant team, nursing care continues to include education, assessment, and administration of appropriate medications and interventions.

Thrombocytopenia

Thrombocytopenia is defined as an abnormal decrease in the number of circulating platelets (Whedon & Wujcik, 1997). Platelets are small fragments derived from megakaryocytes in the bone marrow. Under normal, healthy conditions, approximately 30,000 platelets/mm³ are formed each day. The production of platelets is regulated by a hormone-like substance called thrombopoietin, which is produced by the kidneys. Platelets are removed by the spleen if not used after approximately 10 days. Platelets are crucial for hemostasis and preventing hemorrhage or bleeding and also for maintaining vascular integrity in the absence of injury (Rutherford & Frenkel, 1994).

Thrombocytopenia commonly occurs in the post-transplant patient because of severe myelosuppression resulting from the preparative regimen of chemotherapy, immunotherapy, and/or radiation therapy (Whedon & Wujcik, 1997). Megakaryocytes are typically the last cell line to engraft following both autologous and allogeneic stem cell transplantation (Shapiro et al., 1997), although the engraftment period is shorter following PBSC transplantation (Ezzone, 1997). Normal platelet counts are not achieved for approximately one to three months following stem cell transplantation (Shapiro et al.). Persistent and chronic thrombocytopenia can indicate a poor prognosis for the patient (Dominietto et al., 2001). Thrombocytopenia may reoccur later in the post-transplant phase, after an initial recovery, because of viral infections, GVHD, delayed engraftment, and drug toxicity (Deeg, 1990; Shapiro et al.).

Although controversy exists about the platelet count threshold at which prophylactic transfusions are beneficial (Beutler, 1993; Labovich, 1997), most institutions use the criteria of petechiae, overt bleeding, increased bruising, and a platelet count less than 20,000 as a trigger for platelet transfusions. Severity of thrombocytopenia is graded using the National Cancer Institute Common Toxicity Criteria (see Table 7-3).

Thrombocytopenia can result from any mechanism that affects platelets: the use of prophylactic heparin for veno-occlusive disease (VOD), defective or suppressed production of platelets, abnormal distribution of platelets, or accelerated

Table 7-3. Grading of Thrombocytopenia Using the National Cancer Institute Common Toxicity Criteria

Grade	0	1	2	3	4
Platelets (X 10^9)		50–75	20–50	10–20	< 10

Note. Based on information from the National Cancer Institute, 1999.

platelet destruction or consumption (Belcher, 1993). The suppressed production of platelets is a common sequela of direct exposure to preparative regimens utilizing toxic antineoplastic agents and/or radiation therapy. There is a reduction in platelet count following exposure to antineoplastic therapies, a period of nadir followed by recovery. As the existing circulating platelets age and die, they are removed from the circulation through natural processes. They are not replaced because of the destructive impact of the therapy on cycling, differentiating precursor cells (Belcher). There is a lag between generations of hematopoietic cells that correspond to the period of lowest counts (the nadir) (Groenwald, Frogge, Goodman, & Yarbro, 1997).

Antineoplastic agents used in the preparative regimens of both allogeneic and autologous stem cell transplantation commonly cause myelosuppressive effects, such as thrombocytopenia. These agents include busulfan, carmustine, melphalan, cyclophosphamide, etoposide, thiotepa, carboplatin, cisplatin, cytarabine, and total body irradiation (Ezzone, 1997). Atrophy and fibrosis of bone marrow are late effects of chemotherapy and radiation therapy and may predispose transplant recipients to delayed and chronic thrombocytopenia (Deeg, 1990). In a study by Dominietto et al. (2001), thrombocytopenia correlated with poor transplant outcomes at 30-day, 60-day, and 180-day intervals in the allogeneic transplant setting.

In healthy individuals, approximately one-third of the total platelet volume is sequestered within the spleen (George & Rizvi, 2001). Thrombocytopenia that results from abnormal distribution is related to splenomegaly. An abnormally large number of platelets are sequestered in the spleen with this disorder. This disorder also may be seen in patients with various types of lymphomas and those with portal hypertension (Belcher, 1993).

Fever and systemic infection are processes that may cause thrombocytopenia through accelerated destruction and/or consumptive processes. Viral infections, including CMV, Epstein-Barr virus, HHV-6, Hantavirus, and HIV, commonly cause thrombocytopenia. Other infectious diseases that cause thrombocytopenia via these processes include mycoplasma and mycobacteria (George, Vesely, & Rizvi, 2001).

Drugs such as NSAIDs, aspirin, and aspirin-containing products cause disorders of platelet function. Other drugs such as Bactrim, heparin, quinine, and quinidine are thought to cause thrombocytopenia through an immune-mediated complex (George et al., 2001). Other drugs that may be implicated in thrombocytopenia in the transplant recipient include cyclosporine A, ganciclovir (Shapiro et al., 1997),

digoxin, furosemide, penicillin, vancomycin, and phenytoin (Shuey, 1996). These agents are commonly used in the allogeneic transplant setting (Shapiro et al.).

A complication of severe thrombocytopenia in the transplant recipient may be diffuse alveolar hemorrhage (DAH) (Armitage & Antman, 1992). *Aspergillus* pneumonia also may be a contributing factor resulting in alveolar hemorrhage. The onset of DAH correlates with the onset of WBC recovery. DAH is recognized on bronchoalveolar lavage when sequential instillation and aspiration of normal saline results in recovered fluid that becomes progressively bloodier with each recovered aliquot. Symptoms include dyspnea, diffuse consolidation on chest x-ray, high fevers, severe mucositis, and renal insufficiency. The majority of patients eventually require mechanical ventilation. DAH can proceed to death in more than 75% of patients. High-dose corticosteroids are commonly used for treatment (Armitage & Antman).

Another complication of thrombocytopenia is thrombotic thrombocytopenia purpura/hemolytic uremic syndrome (TTP/HUS). Initially described as a distinct disorder, TTP/HUS is more recently being recognized as a single clinical syndrome that can best be characterized as a spectrum of disorders (George et al., 2001). This syndrome has become more widely recognized in the post-transplant population during the last 15 years (Uderzo et al., 2000). Earlier descriptions of this syndrome included microangiopathic hemolytic anemia, thrombocytopenia, neurologic symptoms, renal function abnormalities, and fever. Currently, only the criteria of thrombocytopenia and microangiopathic hemolytic anemia, without other clinically apparent cause, are sufficient to establish this diagnosis (George et al.).

The pathophysiology of TTP/HUS is a vascular endothelial injury resulting in the release of von Willebrand factors and vascular micro-thrombi. Symptoms result from reversible platelet thrombus formation within the microvasculature, leading to transient ischemia of the brain, kidneys, and other organs (Moake & Byrnes, 1996). This disorder has been described as early as 2–3 months post-transplant and as late as 11 months post-HSCT. TTP/HUS may have multiple etiologies, including drug toxicity, infection, autoimmune processes, and bone marrow transplantation (George et al., 2001).

TTP/HUS has been problematic to recognize because the complications in the critically ill post-HSCT recipient can be similar (George et al., 2001). The factors that positively correlate with TTP/HUS include recipients of transplants from matched, unrelated donors and HLA-antigen mismatched donors, GVHD, total body irradiation as part of the preparative regimen, and infections. Nephrotoxicity and neurotoxicity associated with cyclosporine use also may be a complicated finding (George et al.).

Although the diagnosis of TTP/HUS should be suspected in the presence of microangiopathic hemolytic anemia and thrombocytopenia, most patients also present with renal and neurologic abnormalities. Symptoms may include aphasia, confusion, memory loss, paresis, and behavioral changes. Patients also may complain of abdominal symptoms: pain, nausea, vomiting, and diarrhea. The laboratory findings include thrombocytopenia, the appearance of shistocytes on peripheral blood smear, high serum LDH levels with isoenzymes reflecting hemolysis, and ischemic injury to multiple organs (George et al., 2001).

If not recognized and treated promptly, this syndrome can be fatal. The treatment for this disorder is plasma volume exchange and treating the underlying cause. Once the diagnosis is made, emergency plasma volume exchange is performed daily until the platelet count and LDH levels normalize and are stable for three days (BRT Laboratories, 2000). Unless there is severe, life-threatening bleeding, platelet transfusions are contraindicated, as they may contribute to the formation of microthrombi (Moake & Byrnes, 1996).

The apheresis process that healthy stem cell donors and autologous transplant recipients undergo may cause some transient thrombocytopenia. Studies have demonstrated a significant reduction in platelet counts during mobilization and collection of stem cells. These effects are transient, and donors' platelet counts returned to normal within a few days without transfusions. The mechanism for this phenomenon is not known (Wagner & Quinones, 1999; Walker, Roethke, & Martin, 1994).

Management of thrombocytopenia in the stem cell transplant recipient includes preventive measures, supportive care, and platelet transfusions. Prevention of bleeding is crucial. In the setting of thrombocytopenia, the most common sites of bleeding may be the mucous membranes, skin, gastrointestinal system, genitourinary system, respiratory tract, and intracranial compartment.

Preventive nursing management for transplant recipients during this time includes teaching patients to use very soft bristle toothbrushes or sponges when performing mouth care to prevent trauma and bleeding at the mucous membranes. Other measures to prevent trauma to mucous membranes include avoiding the use of rectal thermometers and rectal suppositories. Stool softeners may be used, and patients are encouraged to liberalize fluid intake to prevent constipation. Patients should be routinely monitored for nosebleeds, melanotic stools, and hematuria, as well as for occult bleeding in emesis, urine, and stool. Menstruating females are typically begun on hormone therapy to prevent vaginal bleeding of menstruation.

The U.S. Food and Drug Administration recently approved Neumega® (Wyeth), a thrombopoietic growth factor, for the prevention of severe thrombocytopenia following myelosuppressive chemotherapy in patients with nonmyeloid malignancies (Rust, Wood, & Battiato, 1999). This agent may have limited use in the transplant population because of the exclusion of its use in nonmyeloid malignancies. The side effects of this agent, including edema, dyspnea, and tachycardia, also may limit its usefulness. Although prophylactic platelet transfusions are controversial (Beutler, 1993), most transplant programs designate a minimum threshold as a trigger for platelet transfusion. Earlier studies indicated that hemorrhage was seen more frequently and with greater severity when the platelet counts were less than 10,000/mm^3. The same stud-

ies also indicated that gross visible hemorrhage rarely occurred with platelet counts greater than 20,000/mm^3 (Fuller, 1990). Thus, the 20,000/mm^3 threshold served as a trigger for initiating prophylactic platelet transfusion to prevent hemorrhage (Groenwald et al., 1997). Others suggested that prophylactic transfusions lead to sensitizing the patient to antigens found on platelets (alloimmunization), with subsequent inability to control hemorrhage when it occurred (Beutler; Fuller). Patients with thrombocytopenia who are actively bleeding require an aggressive approach to platelet transfusions and may be transfused for platelet counts less than 50,000/mm^3 (Fuller). Patients on heparin for VOD prophylaxis may be kept at a higher threshold, 30,000/mm^3, because of an increased incidence of bleeding.

Platelets for transfusion are obtained from one of two sources (Fuller, 1990; Triulzi, 2000): multiple, random donors or an HLA-matched single donor. Random donor platelets are pooled from the blood of several different donors. One unit of blood typically yields one unit of platelets. These are more readily available and less expensive. However, this source of platelets exposes the patient to several different donors, increasing the risk of developing transfusion transmitted disease and alloimmunization (Beutler, 1993; Fuller). Single-donor platelets are derived from an individual through apheresis. The donor platelets are harvested while the RBCs are returned during the apheresis procedure. This process yields 6–10 units of transfusable platelets (Fuller).

Alloimmunization is associated with multiple transfusions for which transplant recipients are at risk. When alloimunization occurs, platelet antibodies attack transfused platelets and may cause platelet levels to decrease after transfusions. There appears to be a dose response pattern for the development of alloimmunization. The more antigens the recipient is exposed to through multiple units of donor-derived blood and platelets, the more at risk the recipient is to develop alloimmunization (Labovich, 1997). For this reason, some would recommend that transplant recipients should only receive single-donor and/or HLA-matched platelets. Further, the discussion is raised that patients who are potential transplant candidates should *only* receive single-donor or HLA-matched platelet transfusions (Armitage & Antman, 1992; Fuller, 1990). Patients in whom alloimmunization is suspected should be tested by determining platelet count levels with serial blood draws after platelet transfusions. Blood tests are available to detect platelet refractory antiplatelet antibodies—cytotoxic anti-HLA antibodies. Alloimmunization risk can be minimized or delayed by the use of special filters that remove leukocytes from blood products before transfusion (Triulzi, 2001).

Anemia

Anemia is defined as a decrease in RBCs or the hemoglobin level that results in the reduction of oxygen-carrying capacity of blood (Erickson, 1996; Loney & Chernecky, 2000). Erythropoietin, an erythrocyte growth factor, is produced or suppressed based on a feedback mechanism involving oxygen tension. The kidneys produce more than 90% of the body's erythropoietin. When oxygen tension drops, interstitial renal cell and central vein hepatocyte receptors signal expression of an erythropoietin gene, resulting in erythropoietin production. As erythropoietin enters the systemic circulation, it quickly stimulates erythrocyte precursor cells in the bone marrow to accelerate RBC production and maturation (Loney & Chernecky). To keep the RBC mass stable, the bone marrow must produce and release approximately 2.5 billion RBCs per kg of body weight each day. The life span of the RBC is approximately 120 days.

Anemia may result from a decrease in RBC production, an increase in RBC destruction, or loss of RBCs through hemorrhage (see Table 7-4). Anemia also may be caused by the direct toxic effect of chemotherapy on the kidney resulting in an inability to respond to the stimulation of erythropoietin (Gillespie, 2002; Groopman & Itri, 1999; Rogers, 2002). Grading the severity of anemia may be described utilizing the National Cancer Institute and World Health Organization toxicity scales (see Table 7-5).

Anemia in the transplant recipient has several causative factors. These include hemolysis, malignancy type, blood loss due to bleeding, suppression of bone marrow function caused by antineoplastic agents and radiation therapy, nutritional deficiency, and kidney failure caused by antineoplastic agents as well as other drugs. For the transplant recipient, these factors may be complex and overlapping.

Chemotherapy agents used in the preparative regimens of transplant recipients suppress bone marrow function, including erythropoiesis, and can lead to poor dietary intake of iron and vitamins and cause RBC lysis and microangiopathic bleeding. All these mechanisms overlap to produce anemia in the transplant recipient.

The suppressive effects of intensive chemotherapy and radiation on the hematopoietic function of bone marrow are well documented. Radiation exposure results in a decrease in the production of RBCs when bone marrow–producing areas, such as the pelvis, sternum, and proximal ends of long bones, are included in the radiation field. Many of the drugs used in the transplant setting in addition to chemotherapeutic agents may be toxic to the kidneys, further compromising erythropoiesis (Franco & Gould, 1994; Groenwald et al., 1997; Whedon & Wujcik, 1997).

Immune hemolytic anemia is a complication of hematopoietic cell transplantation (Sniecinski & O'Donnell, 1999). The majority of these cases are due to ABO-RBC antigen incompatibilities between donor and recipient. The incidence may be as high as one-third of all allogeneic cell transplants. The incompatibilities can be minor or major. Donor-recipient ABO incompatibility is not a contraindication to successful transplantation, and there is no significant adverse impact on the incidence of graft rejection, GVHD, or survival. However, patients undergoing ABO-incompatible transplant are at risk for development of several complications (see Figure 7-1). Major ABO incompatibilities between donor and recipient have the potential for severe hemolytic reaction during marrow or peripheral blood infusion. At the least, incompatibilities could lead to delayed erythropoiesis and/or persistent hemolysis post-transplant (Sniecinski & O'Donnell).

Prevention strategies include removal of the incompatible RBCs from marrow aspirate before infusion. The RBC content in PBSC concentrate is less than in the marrow aspirate but may be sufficient to cause hemolysis at the time of the infusion (Sniecinski & O'Donnell, 1999).

Leukemias, lymphomas, multiple myelomas, and myelodysplastic syndromes are the cancers associated most frequently with anemia (Rogers, 2002). These also are among the most frequently transplanted malignant diseases (International Bone Marrow Transplant Registry/Autologous Blood and Marrow Transplant Registry, 2003). Some tumors possess factors that cause myelosuppression directly, which causes anemia (Rogers).

Prior myelosuppressive drug therapy, particularly platinum-derived agents, may have a cumulative impairment on

Table 7-4. Bleeding Complications and Etiologies That May Contribute to Anemia in the Transplant Recipient

Pathophysiology	Etiology	Signs/Symptoms	Management
• Myelosuppression induced by preparative regimen • Delayed platelet engraftment • Marrow suppressive medications • Coagulation abnormalities • Platelet autoantibodies • Graft rejection	• Graft versus host disease • Cyclosporine • Veno-occlusive disease • Altered mucosal barriers • Delayed/failed engraftment • Viral infection • ABO-incompatible bone marrow transplantation	Skin/mucosa: petechiae, ecchymoses, bruising, scleral hemorrhage Genitourinary: hematuria, menorrhagia Gastrointestinal: guaiac-positive stool/emesis, abdominal distension or discomfort Pulmonary: epistaxis, hemoptysis, change in breathing pattern Intracranial: headache, restlessness, change in pupil response, seizure, change in mental status/level of consciousness	Perform frequent assessment. Monitor hemoglobin/hematocrit, platelets, and coagulation studies. Minimize blood loss. Administer blood products. Avoid medications that inhibit platelet production and/or function. Avoid invasive procedures. Follow bleeding precautions.

Note. Based on information from Ezzone, 1997.

Table 7-5. Anemia Toxicity Scales

Grade	Severity	National Cancer Institute Scale	World Health Organization Scale
0	None	Normal limits*	> 11
1	Mild	10–normal	9.5–10
2	Moderate	8–10	8–9.4
3	Severe	6.5–7.9	6.5–7.9
4	Life threatening	< 6.5	< 6.5

*14–18 g/dl for men; 12–16 g/dl for women
Note. Based on information from Groopman & Itri, 1999.

erythropoiesis (Groopman & Itri, 1999). The intensive preparative conditioning regimens in the transplant setting create a hypoproliferative anemia because of the myelosuppressive effects on the bone marrow (Gillespie, 2002).

Transplant recipients commonly experience nausea and/or vomiting and mucositis as side effects of the preparative conditioning regimens. The intake of essential nutrients, including iron, folate, and vitamin B_{12}, for the normal differentiation and proliferation of erythroid progenitor cells is thus insufficient. The inability to take in adequate nutrients is compromised, adding another complicating factor for the development of anemia (Rogers, 2002).

Finally, acute hemolysis caused by cyclosporine A, Prograf® (Fujisawa, Chantilly, VA), ABO-incompatible graft, infection, or hemolytic uremic syndrome may cause bleeding, leading to anemia in the post-transplant recipient (Shapiro et. al., 1997).

The clinical features of anemia include fatigue, pallor and shortness of breath, headaches, dizziness and decreased cognition, sleep disorders, and sexual dysfunction (Gillespie, 2002). Hypotension and orthostasis may be present in the setting of an acute drop in hematocrit (Shapiro et. al., 1997).

The management of anemia in the transplant recipient includes anticipation of risk factors and initiating strategies to minimize risk to the patient. RBC transfusions should be anticipated to correct hemoglobin during the acute phases of transplant. Diagnostic studies include daily hemoglobin and hematocrit counts throughout the period of aplasia. These determinations are obtained more frequently if the patient is actively bleeding. Guaiac of emesis and stool and dipstick of urine for heme are important and appropriate nursing measures. The hemolysis workup includes urinalysis, complete blood count (CBC), haptoglobin, lactate dehydrogenase, direct and indirect Coombs' test, and fractionated bilirubin (Shapiro et al., 1997).

Tachycardia, tachypnea, hypotension, dyspnea at rest, and other symptoms of tissue hypoxia may occur as anemia becomes more severe (Erickson, 1996). The decision to transfuse RBCs is based upon hemoglobin concentration and the presence of signs or symptoms of anemia. Generally, when the hemoglobin is less than 8 g/dl and signs or symptoms of anemia may be present, transfusion is required. However, patients with underlying cardiopulmonary compromise and

older adults (Rogers, 2002) may require transfusions at higher hemoglobin thresholds (Rieger & Haeuber, 1995). One unit of packed RBCs (10–15 ml/kg in pediatric patients) can raise the hemoglobin increment by 1 g/dl (Shapiro et al., 1997).

An alternative or possible additive therapy made available in recent years has been recombinant erythropoietin alfa. Over a 12-week study, this agent was shown to increase hematocrit and decrease transfusion requirements and lead to the indication for its use in chemotherapy-induced anemia (Rieger & Haeuber, 1995). This agent may be given as a subcutaneous injection or intravenously weekly in the ambulatory treatment setting. Some side effects include hypertension and flu-like symptoms (Rieger & Haeuber).

Management Strategies for Anemia and Thrombocytopenia

Patients undergoing autologous or allogeneic stem cell transplantation will require multiple transfusions of platelets and packed RBCs during the period of aplasia following transplant, until stable recovery of hematopoiesis. Although component therapy is significantly safer now than in the past, there are still notable risks associated with transfusion therapy (Labovich, 1997). Three of those transfusion-related risks that will be discussed include infectious disease transmission, alloimmunization, and febrile nonhemolytic transfusion reactions.

The most notable transfusion-related risk is that of infectious disease transmission. Viruses with the potential for transmission include hepatitis A, B, and C, HIV, human T cell leukemia virus-1, parvovirus B19, Epstein-Barr virus, and CMV (Guertler, 2002). Bacterial and protozoal agents also have transmissible potential through the blood supply (Chamberland, 2002). However, leukofiltration and other measures have reduced the risk of disease transmission in recent years. With the current methods now employed, the estimated risk for infection by screened blood components

Figure 7-1. Complications of ABO-Incompatible Bone Marrow Transplantation

Major ABO incompatibility
- Immediate hemolysis of the red blood cells (RBCs) infused with donor marrow
- Delayed hemolysis of RBCs produced by engrafted marrow
- Delayed onset of erythropoiesis
- Pure red cell aplasia

Minor ABO incompatibility
- Immediate hemolysis of recipient RBCs by infused marrow
- Delayed hemolysis of recipient RBCs due to persistent production of marrow lymphocytes

Major and minor ABO incompatibility
- Immediate hemolysis caused by recipient and/or donor
- Delayed hemolysis caused by recipient and/or donor

Note. Based on information from Sniecinski & O'Donnell, 1999.

in Europe and the United States is 1 in 50,000—1.6 million transfused components (Vreilink & Reesink, 1998).

Another transfusion-related complication in the transplant recipient includes the risk of alloimmunization. Alloimmunization occurs when patients develop antibodies that destroy transfused blood components, most commonly platelets. This occurs as a consequence of being exposed to multiple transfusions over time (Labovich, 1997). The significant risk of alloimmunization is that it may lead to refractory thrombocytopenia, which is difficult to treat (Rowe et al., 1994). The use of leukofiltered platelets, single-donor platelets, and irradiated platelets minimizes this risk to the patient (Rowe et al.).

Febrile, nonhemolytic reactions are unexplained temperature increases of > 1°C or 2°F from baseline or the onset of chills or rigors in the patient who is receiving a transfusion. This may develop in patients within four to six hours of completing the transfusion. These reactions are the most common complication of platelet transfusions (Baldwin, 2002). Risk factors include previous transfusions, previous febrile reactions, and hematologic malignancy. Leukocyte reduction of all transfused blood products reduces the incidence of febrile nonhemolytic transfusions.

Commonly in the acute phases of transplantation, patients receive a transfusion of packed RBCs to correct hemoglobin deficits. A commonly used threshold for prophylactic transfusion of RBCs is ≤ or equal to 8 g/dl (Plaza, 2000). Pharmaceutical agents that may be useful for the management of chronic anemia include erythropoietin alfa and darbepoetin alfa. These agents are effective in increasing hemoglobin levels and decreasing the number of transfusions required. Erythropoietin alfa is dosed subcutaneously but can be administered intravenously. It is customarily dosed at 40,000 units as a weekly subcutaneous injection. The median time to response is 4 weeks, but 12 weeks may be needed to determine if the patient is responsive to therapy.

Darbepoetin alfa is a long-acting agent that stimulates erythropoiesis. The mean half-life is three times longer than epoetin alfa. This allows for less frequent dosing. A darbepoetin alfa dose of 3 mcg/kg given every two weeks produced similar hematopoietic responses to epoetin alfa dosed at 40,000–60,000 units weekly (Glaspy et al., 2002; Pirker & Smith, 2002).

Some transplant patients may need a higher threshold trigger for prophylactic platelet transfusion. This would include patients who are on chronic anticoagulation therapy and patients who are on mechanical ventilation and are frequently being suctioned.

Delayed Engraftment

Delayed engraftment and graft failure refer to the lack of functional hematopoiesis after marrow transplantation. Primary graft failure is the failure to establish hematopoiesis (Whedon & Wujcik, 1997). In autologous transplants, this may be because of inadequate volume, a defect in the quality of stem cells, cryopreservation, or damage during collec-

tion of cells (Shapiro et al., 1997; Whedon & Wujcik). In allogeneic transplants, graft failure is more commonly seen with HLA-mismatched donor marrow, cord blood transplant, or transplantation with T cell–depleted bone marrow (Lum, 1990).

Diagnostic studies include at least daily CBC with differential and platelets to follow engraftment trends and to evaluate transfusion needs. Bone marrow aspirate and biopsy and cytogenetics studies often are used to evaluate chimerism (Shapiro et al., 1997). Management of graft failure may include discontinuation of drugs known to be myelosuppressive (e.g., ganciclovir, Bactrim). Reinfusion of allogeneic marrow, back-up marrow with or without further conditioning, or attempted stimulation with colony-stimulating factors are all possible strategies (Shapiro et al.).

Conclusion

Hematologic and infectious complications are complex and all too common occurrences in the patient undergoing HSCT. Nurses traditionally have held key responsibility for symptom identification and management (Gillespie, 2002). Aggressive, proactive nursing care is critical in helping patients through these dangerous phases of the post-transplant period. A well-rounded grasp of current knowledge is essential to maintaining skills required to anticipate these complications and intervene early and effectively.

References

Alcoser, P.W., & Burchett, S. (1999). Bone marrow transplantation: Immune system suppression and reconstitution. *American Journal of Nursing, 99,* 26–32.

American Society of Clinical Oncology. (1996). Guidelines for use of CSFs as adjuncts to progenitor cell transplants. *Journal of Clinical Oncology, 14,* 1957–1960.

Anderson, D., DeFor, T., Burns, L., McGlave, P., Miller, J., Wagner, J., et al. (2003). A comparison of related donor peripheral blood and bone marrow transplants: Importance of late-onset chronic graft-versus-host disease and infections. *Biology of Blood and Marrow Transplantation, 9*(1), 52–59.

Armitage, J.O., & Antman, K.H. (Eds.). (1992). *High-dose cancer therapy. Pharmacology, hematopoietins, stem cells.* Baltimore: Lippincott Williams and Wilkins.

Baldwin, P.D. (2002). Febrile nonhemolytic transfusion reactions. *Clinical Journal of Oncology Nursing, 6,* 171–173.

Barnes, R.A. (1998a). Fungal infections. In J. Barrett & J.G. Treleaven (Eds.), *The clinical practice of stem cell transplantation, vol. 2* (pp. 723–740). St. Louis, MO: Mosby.

Barnes, R.A. (1998b). Other infections. In J. Barrett & J.G. Treleaven (Eds.), *The clinical practice of stem cell transplantation, vol. 2* (pp. 741–744). St. Louis, MO: Mosby.

Belcher, A.E. (1993). *Blood disorders.* St. Louis, MO: Mosby.

Beutler, E. (1993). Platelet transfusions: The 20,000/ul trigger. *Blood, 81,* 1411–1413.

Beyer, J., Schwella, N., Zingsem, J., Strohscheer, I., Schwanter, I., Oettle, H., et al. (1995). Hematopoietic rescue after high-dose chemotherapy using autologous peripheral-blood progenitor cells or bone marrow: A randomized comparison. *Journal of Clinical Oncology, 13,* 1328–1335.

Bishop, M.R., Tarantolo, S.R., Geller, R.B., Lynch, J.C., Bierman, P.J., Pavletic, Z.S., et al. (2000). A randomized, double-blind trial of filgrastim (granulocyte colony-stimulating factor) versus placebo following allogeneic blood stem cell transplantation. *Blood, 96,* 80–85.

Bittencourt, H., Rocha, V., Chevret, S., Socie, G., Esperou, H., Devergie, A., et al. (2002). Association of CD34 cell dose with hematopoietic recovery, infections, and other outcomes after HLA-identical sibling bone marrow transplantation. *Blood, 99,* 2726–2733.

Boeckh, M., & Boivin, G. (1998). Quantitation of cytomegalovirus: Methodologic aspects and clinical applications. *Clinical Microbiology Review, 11,* 533–554.

BRT Laboratories. (2000). *Thrombotic thrombocytopenia purpura.* Retrieved November 6, 2003, from http://www.rhlab.com/Winter2000.htm

Buchsel, P.C. (1997). Allogeneic bone marrow transplantation. In S.L. Groenwald, M.H. Frogge, M. Goodman, C.H. Yarbro, (Eds.), *Cancer nursing: Principles and practice* (pp. 459–506). Sudbury, MA: Jones and Bartlett.

Centers for Disease Control and Prevention, Infectious Diseases Society of America, and American Society of Blood and Marrow Transplantation. (2000). Guidelines for preventing opportunistic infections among hematopoietic stem cell transplant recipients. *Biology of Blood and Marrow Transplantation, 6,* 659–702.

Chamberland, M.E. (2002). Emerging infectious agents: Do they pose a risk to the safety of transfused blood and blood products? *Clinical Infectious Disease, 34,* 797–805.

Champlin, R.E., Schmitz, N., Horowitz, M.M., Chapuis, B., Chopra, R., Cornelissen, J.J., et al. (2000). Blood stem cells compared with bone marrow as a source of hematopoietic cells for allogeneic transplantation. *Blood, 95,* 3702–3709.

de Azevedo, A.M., Nucci, M., Maiolino, A., Vigorito, A.C., Simoes, B.P., Aranha, F.J.P., et al. (2002). A randomized multicenter study of G-CSF starting on day +1 versus day +5 after autologous peripheral blood progenitor cell transplantation. *Bone Marrow Transplantation, 29,* 745–751.

Deeg, H.J. (1990). Delayed complications and long term effects after bone marrow transplantation. *Hematology/Oncology Clinics of North America, 4,* 641–657.

Dominietto, A., Raiola, A.M., van Lint, M.T., Lamparelli, T., Gualandi, F., Berisso, G., et al. (2001). Factors influencing haematological recovery after allogeneic haemopoietic stem cell transplants: Graft-versus-host disease, donor type, cytomegalovirus infections and cell dose. *British Journal of Haematology, 112,* 219–227.

Ellerhorst-Ryan, J. (1997). Infection. In S.L. Groenwald, M.H. Frogge, M. Goodman, & C.H. Yarbro (Eds.), *Cancer nursing: Principles and practice* (pp. 585–603). Sudbury, MA: Jones and Bartlett.

Ener, R.A., Meglathery, S.B., Cuhaci, B., Topolsky, D., Styler, M.J., Crilley, P., et al. (2001). Use of granulocyte colony-stimulating factor after high-dose chemotherapy and autologous peripheral blood stem cell transplantation: What is the optimal timing? *American Journal of Clinical Oncology, 24,* 19–25.

Erickson, J.M. (1996). Anemia. *Seminars in Oncology Nursing, 12*(1), 2–14.

Ezzone, S. (Ed.). (1997). *Peripheral blood stem cell transplantation: Recommendations for nursing education and practice.* Pittsburgh, PA: Oncology Nursing Society.

Franco, T., & Gould, D.A. (1994). Allogeneic bone marrow transplant. *Seminars in Oncology Nursing, 10,* 3–11.

Fuller, A.K. (1990). Platelet transfusion therapy for thrombocytopenia. *Seminars in Oncology Nursing, 6,* 123–128.

George, J.N., & Rizvi, A.H. (2001). Diagnosis and management of thrombocytopenia. In R.W. Coman, J. Hirsh, V.J. Marder, A.W. Clowes, & J.N. George (Eds.), *Hemostasis and thrombosis: Basic principles and clinical practice* (pp. 1021–1031). Philadelphia: Lippincott Williams and Wilkins.

George, J.N., Vesely, S.K., & Rizvi, A.H. (2001). Thrombotic thrombocytopenia purpura-hemolytic uremic syndrome. In R.W.

Coman, J. Hirsh, V.J. Marder, A.W. Clowes, & J.N. George (Eds.), *Hemostasis and thrombosis: Basic principles and clinical practice* (pp. 1234–1242). Philadelphia: Lippincott Williams and Wilkins.

Gillespie, T.W. (2002). Effects of cancer-related anemia on clinical and quality of life outcomes. *Clinical Journal of Oncology Nursing, 6,* 206–211.

Glaspy, J.A., Jadeja, J.S., Justice, G., Kessler, J., Richards, D., Schwartzberg, L., et al. (2002). Darbepoetin alfa given every 1–2 weeks alleviates anemia associated with cancer therapy. *British Journal of Cancer, 87,* 268–276.

Groenwald, S.L., Frogge, M.H., Goodman, M., & Yarbro, C.H. (1997). *Cancer nursing: Principles and practice* (4th ed.). Sudbury, MA: Jones and Bartlett.

Groopman, J.F., & Itri, L.M. (1999). Chemotherapy-induced anemia in adults: Incidence and treatment. *Journal of the National Cancer Institute, 91,* 1616–1634.

Guertler, L. (2002). Virus safety of human blood, plasma, and derived products. *Thrombosis Research, 107*(Suppl. 1), S39.

Herrmann, R.P., Trent, M., Cooney, J., & Cannell, P.K. (1999). Infections in patients managed at home during autologous stem cell transplantation for lymphoma and multiple myeloma. *Bone Marrow Transplantation, 24,* 1213–1217.

International Bone Marrow Transplant Registry/Autologous Blood and Marrow Transplant Registry. (2003). Report on the state of the art in blood and marrow transplantation. *IBMTR/ABMTR Newsletter, 10,* 1.

Junghanss, C., & Marr, K.A. (2002). Infectious risks and outcomes after stem cell transplantation: Are nonmyeloablative transplants changing the picture? *Current Opinion in Infectious Diseases, 15,* 347–353.

Kiss, J.E., Rybka, W.B., Winkelstein, A., deMagalhaes-Silverman, M., Lister, J., Andrea, P.D., et al. (1997). Relationship of CD34+ cell dose to early and late hematopoiesis following autologous peripheral blood stem cell transplantation. *Bone Marrow Transplantation, 19,* 303–310.

Klumpp, T.R., Goldberg, S.L., & Mangan, K.F. (1995). Effect of granulocyte colony-stimulating factor on the rate of neutrophil engraftment following peripheral-blood stem-cell transplantation. *Journal of Clinical Oncology, 13,* 935–961.

Labovich, T.M. (1997). Transfusion therapy: nursing implications. *Clinical Journal of Oncology Nursing, 1,* 61–72.

Lee, S.J., Klar, N., Weeks, J.C., & Antin, J.H. (2000). Predicting costs of stem cell transplantation. *Journal of Clinical Oncology, 18,* 64–71.

Loney, M., & Chernecky, C. (2000). Anemia. *Oncology Nursing Forum, 27,* 951–964.

Lum, L.G. (1990). Immune recovery after bone marrow transplantation. *Hematology/Oncology Clinics of North America, 4,* 659–669.

Marr, K.A. (2001). Antifungal prophylaxis in hematopoietic stem cell transplant recipients. *Oncology, 15*(11 Suppl. 9), 15–19.

Marr, K.A., Carter, R.A., Crippa, F., Wald, A., & Corey, L. (2002). Epidemiology and outcomes of mold infections of hematopoietic stem cell transplant recipients. *Clinical Infectious Diseases, 34,* 909–917.

Meisenberg, B.R., Ferran, K., Hollenbach, K., Brehm, T., Jollon, J., & Piro, L.D. (1998). Reduced charges and costs associated with outpatient autologous stem cell transplantation. *Bone Marrow Transplantation, 21,* 927–932.

Moake, J.L., & Byrnes, J.J. (1996). Thrombotic microangiopathies associated with drugs and bone marrow transplantation. *Hematology/Oncology Clinics of North America, 10,* 485–497.

National Cancer Institute. (1999). *Common toxicity criteria* (version 2.0). Bethesda, MD: Author.

Nichols, W.G., & Boeckh, M. (2000). Conference report: 2nd international conference on transplant infectious disease. *Transplantation, 1,* 3.

Osarogiagbon, R.U., Defor, T.E., Weisdorg, M.A., Erice, A., & Weisdorf, D.J. (2000). CMV antigenemia following bone marrow transplantation: Risk factors and outcomes. *Biology of Blood and Marrow Transplantation, 6,* 280–288.

Passweg, J.R., Rowlings, P.A., Atkinson, K.A., Barrett, A.J., Gale, R.P., Gratwohl, A., et al. (1998). Red blood cell transfusions for anemia. *Seminars in Oncology Nursing, 6,* 117–122.

Pavletic, Z.S., Bishop, M.R., Tarantolo, S.R., Martin-Algarra, S., Bierman, P.J., Vose, J.M., et al. (1997). Hematopoietic recovery after allogeneic blood stem cell transplantation compared with bone marrow transplantation in patients with hematologic malignancies. *Journal of Clinical Oncology, 15,* 1608–1616.

Phillips, G.L. (1999). Management of infections. In H.J. Deeg, H.G. Klingemann, G.L. Phillips, & G. Van Zant (Eds.), *A guide to blood and marrow transplantation* (pp. 143–158). New York: Springer.

Pirker, R., & Smith, R. (2002). Darbepoetin alfa. Potential role in managing anemia in cancer patients. *Expert Review of Anticancer Therapy, 2,* 377.

Plaza, I.L. (2000, May). A practical approach to blood component transfusion therapy. *Transfusion Medicine Update.* Pittsburgh, PA: Institute for Transfusion Medicine.

Prentice, G., Grundy, J.E., & Kho, P. (1998). Cytomegalovirus. In J. Barrett & J.G. Treleaven (Eds.), *The clinical practice of stem cell transplantation, vol. 2* (pp. 697–707). St. Louis, MO: Mosby.

Rieger, P.T., & Haeuber, D. (1995). A new approach to managing chemotherapy-related anemia: Nursing implications of epoetin alfa. *Oncology Nursing Forum, 22,* 71–81.

Riley, U. (1998). Bacterial infections. In J. Barrett & J.G. Treleaven (Eds.), *The clinical practice of stem cell transplantation, vol. 2* (pp. 690–696). St. Louis, MO: Mosby.

Rogers, B. (2002). Management of anemia in the ambulatory patient with cancer. *Oncology Supportive Care Quarterly, 1*(1), 19–26.

Rowe, J.M., Ciobanu, N., Ascensao, J., Stadtmauer, E.A., Weiner, R.S., Schenkein, D.P., et al. (1994). Recommended guidelines for the management of autologous and allogeneic bone marrow transplantation. *Annals of Internal Medicine, 120,* 143–158.

Russell, J.A., Chaudhry, A., Booth, K., Brown, C., Woodman, R.C., Valentine, K., et al. (2000). Early outcomes after allogeneic stem cell transplantation for leukemia and myelodysplasia without protective isolation: A 10-year experience. *Biology of Blood and Marrow Transplantation, 6,* 109–114.

Rust, D.M., Wood, L.S., & Battiato, L.A. (1999). Oprelvekin. An alternative treatment for thrombocytopenia. *Clinical Journal of Oncology Nursing, 3,* 57–62.

Rutherford, C.J., & Frenkel, E.P. (1994). Thrombocytopenia. Issues in diagnosis and therapy. *Medical Clinics of North America, 78,* 555–575.

Shapiro, T.W., Davison, D.B., & Rust, D.M.A. (1997). *Clinical guide to stem cell and bone marrow transplantation.* Sudbury, MA: Jones and Bartlett.

Shuey, K.M. (1996). Platelet-associated bleeding disorders. *Seminars in Oncology Nursing, 12,* 15–27.

Shulman, K.A., Birch, R., Zhen, B., Pania, N., & Weaver, C.H. (1999). Effect of CD34+ cell dose on resource utilization in patients after high-dose chemotherapy with peripheral blood stem cell support. *Journal of Clinical Oncology, 17,* 1227–1233.

Sniecinski, I.J., & O'Donnell, M.R. (1999). Hemolytic complications of hematopoietic cell transplantation. In E.D. Thomas, K.G. Blume, & S.J. Forman (Eds.), *Hematopoietic cell transplantation* (2nd ed., pp. 674–682). Melbourne, Australia: Blackwell Science.

Triulzi, D.J. (2000). *Leuko reduction. Transfusion medicine update.* Retrieved January 13, 2004, from http://www.itxm.org/TMU200/TMU3_4-2000.htm

Uderzo, C., Fumagalli, M., DeLorenzo, P., Busca, A., Vassallo, E., Bonanomi, S., et al. (2000). Impact of thrombotic thrombocytopenic purpura on leukemic children undergoing bone marrow transplantation. *Bone Marrow Transplantation, 26,* 1005–1009.

van Burik, J.H., & Weisdorf, D.J. (1999). Infections in recipients of blood and marrow transplantation. *Hematology/Oncology Clinics of North America, 13,* 1065–1089.

Vreilink, H., & Reesink, H.W. (1998). Transfusion transmissible infections. *Current Opinion in Hematology, 6,* 396–405.

Wagner, N.D., & Quinones, V.W. (1999). Allogeneic peripheral blood stem cell transplantation: Clinical overview and nursing implications. *Oncology Nursing Forum, 25,* 1049–1055.

Walker, F., & Burcat, S. (1997). Hematologic effects of transplantation. In M.B. Whedon & D. Wujcik (Eds.), *Blood and marrow stem cell transplantation: Principles, practice, and nursing insights* (pp. 205–219). Sudbury, MA: Jones and Bartlett.

Walker, F., Roethke, S.K., & Martin, G. (1994). An overview of the rationale, process and nursing implications of peripheral blood stem cell transplantation. *Cancer Nursing, 17*(2), 141–148.

Westmoreland, D. (1998). Other viral infections. In J. Barrett & J.G. Treleaven (Eds.), *The clinical practice of stem cell transplantation, vol. 2* (pp. 709–721). St. Louis, MO: Mosby.

Whedon, M.B., & Wujcik, D. (Eds.). (1997). *Blood and marrow stem cell transplantation: Principles, practice, and nursing insights* (2nd ed.). Sudbury, MA: Jones and Bartlett.

CHAPTER **8**

Michelle M. Stevens, RN, BS, OCN®

Gastrointestinal Complications of Hematopoietic Stem Cell Transplantation

Introduction

The purpose of this chapter is to discuss the gastrointestinal (GI) complications of autologous and allogeneic pediatric and adult hematopoietic stem cell transplantation (HSCT), regardless of the source of stem cells. Topics include mucositis, salivary gland dysfunction and xerostomia, taste changes, nausea and vomiting, diarrhea, perineal-rectal skin alterations, and nutrition. Unless otherwise specified, the information provided in this chapter is applicable to all patients. Graft versus host disease (GVHD) is discussed fully in Chapter 6 and is only mentioned here when appropriate. Hematopoietic effects and general infection control practices are discussed in Chapter 7.

Mucositis

Mucositis is a major treatment-related toxicity that poses clinical problems to nearly all patients undergoing HSCT (see Figure 8-1). Mucositis occurs as a result of the direct and indirect effects of chemoradiotherapy, myelosuppression, and GVHD along the entire GI mucosa, including the oral mucosa, esophagus, pharynx, and the rest of the gut or GI tract (Wojtaszek, 2000). Oropharyngeal mucositis receives much attention because of its clinically obvious symptoms of ulceration and severe pain. However, it is important to identify and understand the effects of mucositis on the rest of the GI tract, which may include nausea and vomiting, abdominal cramping, and profuse watery diarrhea. The incidence and severity of mucositis of the gut is unknown but may pose a greater risk to patients because of its unique interactions with the immune system (Blijlevens, Donnelly, & DePauw, 2000). Mucositis complications may cause severe pain, fluid and electrolyte imbalances, dehydration, poor nutritional status, systemic infection, and hemorrhage and are associated with an increased morbidity and mortality.

Mucositis of the oropharynx and esophagus result in loss of the protective mucosal barrier, which serves as a portal for the spread of oropharyngeal pathogens, leading to systemic infections during periods of myelosuppression. More than 300 bacterial species make up the complex microflora of the oropharynx. Seventy percent are anaerobes, streptococci, and

gram-negative anaerobic rods. *Viridans streptococci*, normally found in the oral cavity, has been identified as a common cause of bacteremia in patients undergoing HSCT (Heimdahl, 1999). Systemic fungal infections, most commonly with the *Candida* species, usually follow colonization of the oral cavity and esophagus and are found in 15% of patients undergoing HSCT (Eisen, Essell, & Broun, 1997).

As with oropharyngeal mucositis, mucositis of the GI mucosa causes disruption of endogenous microflora and

---

Figure 8-1. Mucositis Risk Factors

Therapy-related risk factors
- Chemotherapeutic agents—antimetabolites, antitumor antibiotics, alkylating agents, vinca alkaloids, taxanes, epipodophyllotoxins
- Total body irradiation—depending on type, field, total cumulative dose, and treatment schedules
- Graft versus host reactions
- Medications—opiates, sedatives, antihistamines, antidepressants, phenothiazines, diuretics
- Prolonged hospitalization—microfloral shift to gram-negative organisms
- Use of broad-spectrum antibiotics—predisposes patients to resistant bacterial and fungal infections
- Prolonged myelosuppression—low absolute granulocyte and platelet counts
- Vomiting—irritation to oral mucosa, loss of proteins and water-soluble vitamins
- Transplanted cell dose < 3 x 10^8 nucleated cells/kg body weight

Patient-related risk factors
- Age—younger than 20 years, older than 65 years
- Oral health—poor oral hygiene, history of oral lesions, periodontal disease, dental-related sources of trauma (ill-fitting prosthesis, sharp teeth), preexisting oral/dental infections, inadequate dental restorations, impacted wisdom teeth
- Xerostomia
- Herpes simplex virus-positive serology—risk of reactivation is highest in patients with HSV IgG titer >10, 000 (ELISA)
- Hematologic malignancy
- Poor nutritional status
- Decreased renal function
- Tobacco use
- Alcohol consumption

Note. Based on information from Barker, 1999; Berger & Eilers, 1998; Heimdahl, 1999; Raber-Durlacher, 1999; Wojtaszek, 2000.

---

allows for the overgrowth of microbial pathogens. Although similar to the oral cavity, the gut harbors a much more complex endogenous microflora with a greater variety of aerobic and anaerobic bacteria (Blijlevens et al., 2000). Mucosal injury allows for bacterial translocation through the disrupted mucosal epithelium, allowing for the spread of microbial pathogens to extra-intestinal sites and the blood. The rate of translocation of pathogens, such as *Escherichia coli* and *Pseudomonas aeruginosa*, is strongly associated with the degree of neutropenia (Blijlevens et al.).

Pathophysiology

Oral mucositis has been described as occurring in four biologically successive phases: (1) an inflammatory phase followed by (2) an epithelial phase leading to (3) an ulcerative/microbiological phase and resolving in (4) the healing phase. Blijlevens et al. (2000) suggested this model could be applicable to the gut as well, even though the gut is a more complex organ with different functions and unique interactions with the immune system and luminal microflora. The direct result of chemoradiotherapy occurs at the cellular level approximately four to seven days following conditioning therapies and resolves with the engraftment of neutrophils, mirroring the course of neutropenia (Blijlevens et al.).

The initial phase of mucositis is the inflammatory phase. During this period, chemoradiotherapy induces the systemic release of cytokines, specifically interleukin- (IL-) 1, IL-6, and tumor necrosis factor-alpha, from activated macrophages and monocytes in the epithelial tissues causing local tissue damage. This causes an increased cellularity and vascularity of the epithelial tissues (Blijlevens et al., 2000; Wojtaszek, 2000).

During the second phase, the epithelial phase, chemoradiotherapy interferes with the mitosis of rapidly dividing cells, reducing epithelial cell renewal and thinning the basal epithelium. Mucosal atrophy, ulceration, and subsequent colonization with microbial pathogens occur from decreased cell renewal and cell death (Blijlevens et al., 2000; Wojtaszek, 2000).

The ulcerative/microbiological phase is the most symptomatic phase. The increased cellularity and vascularity of the inflammatory phase and the epithelial thinning of the epithelial phase culminates in erythema, edema, and erosions of the mucosal linings. Endogenous and nonendogenous microbial pathogens colonize oral submucosal tissues, which further stimulate cytokine release from the surrounding tissues and increases the risk of systemic infections. Local immune defenses of the oral cavity are impaired by a decrease in the quantity and quality of mucus and saliva, which contain host defense peptides (defensins), lactoferrin, lysozyme, and immunoglobulins (IgA, IgG, IgM) (Blijlevens et al., 2000). During this phase, GI permeability increases, allowing for the passage of microbial pathogens through the intestinal wall to extraintestinal sites and the blood (bacterial translocation) (Blijlevens et al.; Johansson & Ekman, 1997).

The healing phase occurs with neutrophil recovery. Epithelial proliferation and differentiation repair the tissues of the oral mucosa, usually within two to three weeks. In contrast, normal gut function takes several additional weeks to return to normal. Malabsorption and diminished enzyme activity continue to persist following structural repair (Blijlevens et al., 2000).

Assessment

Mucositis of the Mouth, Pharynx, and Esophagus

Nursing assessments of oral status are an integral part of mucositis management. The development and severity of mucositis is associated with many therapy-related and patient-related risk factors. Knowledge and recognition of these risk factors can alert nurses to those patients at highest risk and ensure the prompt initiation of preventative therapies (see Figure 8-1).

During assessments, nurses must be aware of common infections and their presenting signs and symptoms. Infections of the oropharyngeal and esophageal cavity may be bacterial, viral, or fungal in origin. Mucosal breakdown offers the perfect portal of entry for the systemic spread of oral pathogens, and, as such, all attempts at prevention should be employed. It is important to note that immunocompromised patients may not display the same signs and symptoms of inflammation and infection as immunocompetent patients. (Infection control guidelines and practices are discussed in Chapter 7.)

Reactivation of the herpes simplex virus (HSV) is the most common cause of early oropharyngeal and esophageal viral infections. Oral HSV infections appear mainly on the hard palate, gingiva, and lip as multiple painful vesicles or ulcers with raised, erythematous borders. Occasionally, HSV may present as a single painful lesion. Cytomegalovirus (CMV) infections of the esophagus may occur shortly after conditioning therapy and after engraftment when cell-mediated immunity is deficient and prophylactic therapy has been discontinued (Vargas & Silverman, 2000). CMV infection can be virulent and may be refractory to treatment in the HSCT population (Eisen et al., 1997).

Oral bacterial infections have been associated with systemic bacteremia in immunocompromised patients, so careful attention to the results of culture and sensitivity testing and biopsy are imperative. Bacterial infections may present as raised, ulcerative, yellow or yellow-white, painful lesions. Erythema may or may not be present. The most common pathogens include gram-positive Streptococci and Staphylococci and gram-negative *Pseudomonas, Klebsiella, Enterobacter, E. coli, Serratia,* and *Fusobacterium* (Majorana, Schubert, Porta, Ugazio, & Sapelli, 2000). Prophylaxis and treatment are dependent on institutional culture and sensitivity patterns and may include topical and systemic oral or IV therapy.

Oral fungal infections may develop from endogenous yeast flora (Van Burik & Weisdorf, 1999). Fungal infections may present as white patches or coatings on the tongue, hard palate, and gingiva that can be easily scraped away, revealing an ulcerated surface. Less commonly, leukoplakia-like plaques that do not rub off, patchy or diffuse erythema, and angular cheilitis may make up the clinical presentation (Eisen et al., 1997).

Patients and significant others should be taught how to assess the oral cavity to identify and accurately report early changes. A detailed oral assessment and history should be performed at the time of admission or presentation for transplant. Thereafter, a thorough oral assessment should be performed at least daily during myelosuppression and with any new complaints from the patient. Initial signs and symptoms include erythema, generalized tenderness, easy bleeding, dry/cracked lips, and difficulty and/or pain with swallowing and talking. As oral mucositis progresses, patients may exhibit ropy or absent saliva; ulcerations on the lips, tongue, gingiva, and mucus membranes of the mouth, pharynx, and esophagus; severe pain; difficulty or inability to talk and swallow; large areas of plaque and debris; and xerostomia (Wojtaszek, 2000).

The use of an oral assessment instrument is helpful in documenting baseline oral status and evaluating the changes and responses to interventions. In 1988, Eilers, Berger, and Petersen developed the Oral Assessment Guide (OAG) (see Figure 8-2) to provide clinicians with a concise, valid, and reliable tool to assess the oral cavity. The OAG assesses eight categories of the oral cavity: voice, swallow, lips, tongue, saliva, mucous membranes, gingiva, and teeth/dentures. A numeric value of 1 to 3 is assigned to each category. Normal findings are assigned a value of 1; mild alterations without severe compromise, a value of 2; severe compromise in integrity or system function, a value of 3 (Eilers et al.). Use of this instrument allows for evaluation of oral cavity changes and responses to therapy.

Mucositis of the Gastrointestinal Mucosa

As with oral mucositis, mucositis of the GI mucosa occurs as a result of the direct and indirect effects of chemoradiotherapy, myelosuppression, and GVHD. Symptoms may include nausea and vomiting, crampy abdominal pain, and profuse watery diarrhea. The differential diagnosis between infectious and noninfectious causes of GI complications, especially diarrhea, can be difficult. Careful attention to clinical symptoms, laboratory findings, and radiology testing must be employed. Diarrhea caused by mucosal damage or mucositis usually occurs following conditioning therapies and resolves around day 20 post-transplant (Cox et al., 1994). Diarrhea caused by infection, diarrhea-causing medications, or GVHD is most common between 20 and 100 days post-transplant (Cox et al.). Despite aggressive diagnostic practices, diarrhea of uncertain etiology occurs in approximately 40% of transplant patients (Cox et al.). Pathophysiology, assessment, and management of diarrhea is fully discussed later in this chapter.

To further complicate the issue, it is not uncommon for HSCT recipients to experience concomitant causes of GI symptoms. For example, patients with diarrhea associated with mucositis from their conditioning therapies may simultaneously experience diarrhea from an infections source, such as *Clostridium difficile*. Patients also may experience GI infection with more than one pathogen at a given time. Fungi, bacteria, protozoa, and viral pathogens all have been identified as a source of fever, sepsis, and gastroenteritis.

Adenovirus, rotavirus, and CMV are the most reported viral pathogens in cases of gastroenteritis in transplant recipients (Kingreen, Nitsche, Beyer, & Siegert, 1997; Van Kraaij et al., 2000). The incidence of adenoviral infections is reported between 4.9% and 20.9%, and an increased incidence has been attributed to the increased use of unrelated donor transplants (Hale et al., 1999). CMV infection has been found in half of the patients presenting with intestinal bleeding caused by acute GVHD (Kingreen et al.), and if left unchecked, intestinal obstruction, perforation, or life-threatening GI bleeding may occur (Vargas & Silverman, 2000). CMV infection also predisposes patients to infection with fungi and other opportunistic pathogens (Avery, Adal, Longworth, & Bolwell, 2000). HSV infection of the intestine is uncommon but has been reported as the cause of colitis in six allogeneic transplant patients (Kingreen et al.). HSV infection of the jejunum leading to diarrhea and death from uncontrolled GI bleeding has been reported in one allogeneic transplant recipient (Kingreen et al.).

Sporadic bacterial infections with *Giardia*, *Campylobacter*, *E. coli*, *Pseudomonas*, nondifficile *Clostridia*, and *Aeromonas* have been identified to cause GI infection among transplant patients. *Clostridium difficile* is the most common bacterial infection associated with GI symptoms, including diarrhea, in transplant recipients. Exposure to antimicrobial medications alters the normal microflora and allows for *Clostridium difficile* overgrowth and elaboration of toxins within the colon. *Clostridium difficile* may be present in the patient's endogenous microflora or acquired from an environmental source (Hanna et al., 2000).

Candida organisms are found in the normal microflora of the gut. During periods of GI mucositis and myelosuppression, translocation of yeasts such as *Candida albicans* can occur and cause systemic infections (Blijlevens et al., 2000). Diarrhea has been associated with *Candida* infections of the GI tract. Antimicrobial medications used for gut decontamination may increase GI yeast colonization and therefore increase the risk of invasive fungal infections with the *Candida* and *Aspergillus* species.

In the presence of severe neutropenia, patients may experience neutropenic enterocolitis, also called necrotizing enterocolitis or typhlitis. Neutropenic enterocolitis is a serious infection that occurs in the presence of severe neutropenia, with a reported mortality rate of 21%–48% (Kawai et al., 1998). The pathogenesis of neutropenic enterocolitis requires the simultaneous presence of mucositis, neutropenia, and invasion of the mucosa by microorganisms. Clinical symptoms include nausea, vomiting, abdominal pain, and fever and may progress to include signs of acute peritoneal inflammation (Vargas & Silverman, 2000). Aggressive medical management with antibiotics and supportive measures are required. Surgical resection may be necessary if perforation occurs or GI bleeding cannot be controlled. CMV, *Clostridium difficile*, *Pseudomonas aeruginosa*, and *Staphylococcus aureus* have been associated with neutropenic enterocoli-

Figure 8-2. Oral Assessment Guide

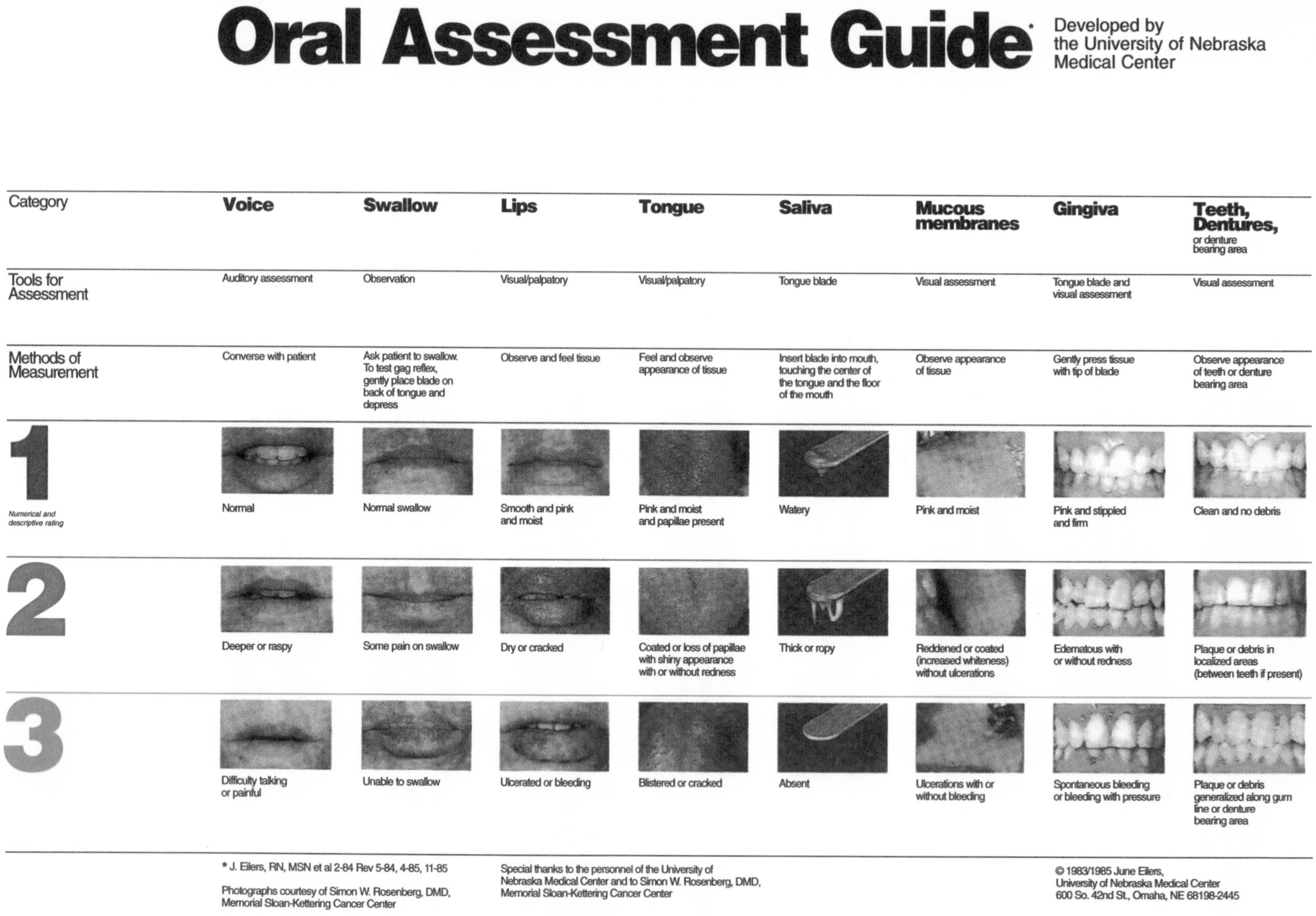

Oral Assessment Guide*

Developed by the University of Nebraska Medical Center

Category	Voice	Swallow	Lips	Tongue	Saliva	Mucous membranes	Gingiva	Teeth, Dentures, or denture bearing area
Tools for Assessment	Auditory assessment	Observation	Visual/palpatory	Visual/palpatory	Tongue blade	Visual assessment	Tongue blade and visual assessment	Visual assessment
Methods of Measurement	Converse with patient	Ask patient to swallow. To test gag reflex, gently place blade on back of tongue and depress	Observe and feel tissue	Feel and observe appearance of tissue	Insert blade into mouth, touching the center of the tongue and the floor of the mouth	Observe appearance of tissue	Gently press tissue with tip of blade	Observe appearance of teeth or denture bearing area
1 *Numerical and descriptive rating*	Normal	Normal swallow	Smooth and pink and moist	Pink and moist and papillae present	Watery	Pink and moist	Pink and stippled and firm	Clean and no debris
2	Deeper or raspy	Some pain on swallow	Dry or cracked	Coated or loss of papillae with shiny appearance with or without redness	Thick or ropy	Reddened or coated (increased whiteness) without ulcerations	Edematous with or without redness	Plaque or debris in localized areas (between teeth if present)
3	Difficulty talking or painful	Unable to swallow	Ulcerated or bleeding	Blistered or cracked	Absent	Ulcerations with or without bleeding	Spontaneous bleeding or bleeding with pressure	Plaque or debris generalized along gum line or denture bearing area

* J. Eilers, RN, MSN et al 2-84 Rev 5-84, 4-85, 11-85

Photographs courtesy of Simon W. Rosenberg, DMD, Memorial Sloan-Kettering Cancer Center

Special thanks to the personnel of the University of Nebraska Medical Center and to Simon W. Rosenberg, DMD, Memorial Sloan-Kettering Cancer Center

© 1983/1985 June Eilers, University of Nebraska Medical Center 600 So. 42nd St., Omaha, NE 68198-2445

Note. Photo courtesy of the University of Nebraska Medical Center. Used with permission.

tis, but *Clostridium septicum* and *Clostridium tertium* are most always found (Blijlevens et al., 2000; Kawai et al.; Vargas & Silverman).

Prevention and Management

There is no one scientifically proven intervention that can prevent or treat the numerous complications associated with mucositis. Detailed assessments and early multimodal interventions that prevent trauma and infection and control pain are the most important factors for the prevention and treatment of severe mucositis and infection (Barker, 1999). Oral lesions should be routinely cultured and sent for sensitivity studies. It may be necessary to biopsy lesions that do not respond to appropriate therapy. Evaluation of the esophagus with endoscopic exams and necessary biopsies and brushings should be performed as clinically warranted. Endoscopy and colonoscopy with biopsies, brushings, and cultures of lesions or erythematous areas may need to be performed in order to rapidly identify the causes of GI symptoms.

Decisions on antimicrobial medications used for prophylaxis and treatment should be made with knowledge of institutional sensitivity patterns. Routine gut decontamination is not recommended. The use of antibiotics for afebrile, asymptomatic, neutropenic patients has not been shown to reduce infection-related mortality and may predispose patients to infection with antibiotic-resistant organisms; therefore prophylactic use of antibiotics should be made with caution (Centers for Disease Control and Prevention [CDC], Infectious Diseases Society of America, & American Society of Blood and Marrow Transplantation, 2000).

Oral Hygiene

Oral hygiene should be performed after meals and at bedtime with increased intervals during periods of severe oral mucositis. Optimally, patients with severe mucositis should perform mouth care at least every one to two hours during the day and every two to four hours overnight, as tolerated. Practices and products used for oral hygiene management vary among transplant centers, and the use of many oral hygiene products is controversial and understudied.

Interventions for mechanical plaque removal, such as brushing, should be employed to reduce oral bacterial load and gingival inflammation (Raber-Durlacher, 1999). Patients should brush gently but thoroughly with a soft nylon bristle toothbrush and mild tartar-control fluorinated toothpaste more than two times daily, as tolerated. Toothpaste may need to be discontinued if burning or irritation develops. If patients are unable to tolerate a toothbrush, sponge toothettes may be used. They are less effective at mechanical plaque removal, but their efficacy is increased slightly when used with chlorhexidine solution (Peridex®, Proctor and Gamble, Cincinnati, OH) (Majorana et al., 2000). Majorana et al. reported effective plaque removal with the use of ultrasonic toothbrushes (Sonicare®, Philips Oral Healthcare, Snoqualmie, WA). However, the efficacy and safety of ultrasonic toothbrushes have not been evaluated in clinical tri-

als. Patients who are skilled at dental flossing should continue to floss daily to decrease interdental bacterial plaque. Flossing may need to be discontinued when platelet counts drop below 20,000/mm^3 (or per transplant center protocol) or when flossing causes trauma. Regular cleansing of dentures and changing of solutions in denture storage cups is recommended to avoid colonization with pathogens (Barker, 1999).

Mouthwashes and Rinses

Many different mouthwashes and rinses are used in transplant centers. Although the product(s) may be different, they share the same common goals of removing oral debris and microorganisms, providing mucosal hydration, decreasing inflammation, and decreasing pain (Wojtaszek, 2000).

Bland rinses of normal saline, sodium bicarbonate, or a combination of normal saline and sodium bicarbonate (salt and soda) are used to remove debris and moisturize the mucosal surface (Wojtaszek, 2000). They do not, however, have antimicrobial properties and are not effective at mechanical plaque removal.

Chlorhexidine mouthwash has the added benefits of plaque removal and antimicrobial properties; however, patients may experience burning or stinging of mucosal surfaces because of the alcohol content. Chlorhexidine may be most beneficial when mechanical plaque removal with brushing is not possible (Majorana et al., 2000). Biotène® Mouthwash (Laclede, Inc., Rancho Dominguez, CA) also has antimicrobial properties but does not contain alcohol and is therefore well tolerated by patients; however, its efficacy has not been determined in clinical trials involving HSCT recipients.

Half-strength hydrogen peroxide has been used for debridement and to loosen hemorrhagic accumulations. However, its use may inhibit fibroblast function and dry out and irritate mucosal surfaces (Barker, 1999; Majorana et al., 2000).

"Magic" mouthwashes use a variety of ingredients to provide pain relief, decrease inflammation, and coat inflamed mucosal surfaces. The most common ingredients are viscous lidocaine (Xylocaine®, Astra USA, Westborough, MA), Benadryl® (diphenhydramine hydrochloride, Warner-Lambert, Morris Plains, NJ), and Maalox® (magnesium aluminum hydroxide, Novartis, Summit, NJ) (Dodd et al., 2000). Some centers also include topical antifungal agents and corticosteroids in their mixtures.

Significant controversies exist in the literature with regard to the use of mouthwashes and rinses. A randomized, double-blind clinical trial was conducted by Dodd et al. (2000) to test the effectiveness of salt and soda, chlorhexidine, and "magic" mouthwashes to treat stomatitis in patients receiving stomatotoxic chemotherapy. Patients receiving radiation therapy to the head and neck and transplant recipients were excluded. No significant differences with time to cessation of symptoms were found between the three treatment groups. Unfortunately, there are no randomized, double-blind clinical trials that incorporate oral assessment, oral hygiene, and mouthwashes in the transplant population. Until clinical trials are performed, one must rely on anecdotal information and reports from clinical trials involving general patients with cancer.

Dental Evaluation and Management

The CDC, the Infectious Diseases Society of America, and the American Society of Blood and Marrow Transplantation published their guidelines for preventing opportunistic infections among stem cell transplant recipients in October 2000. Their recommendation stated that all patients undergoing HSCT should have a thorough dental consultation before conditioning therapy and all likely sources of dental infection and trauma should be vigorously eliminated.

Dental caries should be treated with permanent restoration whenever possible. Teeth with endodontic infections or abscesses need to be treated by endodontic therapy, when time permits, or extracted. Nonrestorable teeth also should be extracted (Majorana et al., 2000). Healing and resolution of infection must occur 10–14 days prior to conditioning therapy. Culture and sensitivity results of wound or abscess drainage should determine antibiotic use (Majorana et al.). Periodontal infections (gingivitis/periodontitis) are the cause of frequent dental infections in transplant recipients. Optimally, dental prophylaxis, scaling, and curettage should be performed when medically possible (Majorana et al.). To decrease the risk of mechanical trauma, secondary infection, and radiation backscatter, fixed orthodontic appliances (e.g., bands, brackets, arch wires) and space maintainers should not be worn from the start of conditioning until stomatitis resolves. Other sources of trauma, such as sharp teeth, should be eliminated prior to conditioning therapy.

Following transplantation, elective dental treatments should be postponed until full immune recovery has occurred. During dental procedures, aerosolization of bacteria can cause aspiration pneumonias. When dental procedures are required, prophylactic antibiotics and medical support with platelet transfusions may be necessary (Majorana et al., 2000).

Children transplanted under the age of 12 often develop changes in the size, shape, and eruption of teeth and overall growth of the jaw related to the effects of conditioning therapies (Majorana et al., 2000). There are no guidelines for the role and timing of orthodontic treatment for these complications, but children should be followed closely and seen at regular intervals by their dentist to optimally manage orthodontic complications.

Pain Management

Oropharyngeal mucositis is the principle etiology of pain in patients undergoing transplantation and often is described as the most traumatic experience of the transplant process. Pain occurs as a result of ulceration, edema, denuding of the epithelial lining, and the release of neurotransmitters (Wojtaszek, 2000). Mucositis pain varies in location, duration, and intensity from patient to patient but is generally described initially as a burning sensation that progresses over time to a continuous tender, sharp, aching feeling (Wojtaszek). The use of age-appropriate self-reports to assess pain intensity is the most reliable means because patients are best able to determine acceptable levels of pain intensity and distress. Instruments used for pain assessments vary among transplant centers because of institutional and protocol preference; however, all instruments should be simple, be easily understood by patients, be age appropriate, and have documented validity and reliability. Pain should be assessed as often as necessary to ensure optimal patient comfort and safety. Comprehensive nursing assessments are imperative for effective pain management, especially in nonverbal and critically ill children and adults.

More than three-fourths of transplant patients experience moderate to severe oral mucositis requiring IV opioid therapy by continuous infusion or patient-controlled analgesia (PCA) (Eisen et al., 1997). The efficacy of this therapy has been extensively documented in the literature. In a recent study, Pederson and Parran (1999) identified that children (age 5–17 years) and adults undergoing HSCT self-reported pain levels similarly, but children received 3 to 5.6 times more opioid medication than adults. Therefore, it is important for nurses to be prepared to give more opioids/kg to children in order to obtain comparable levels of comfort. Dosing of opioids should be individually based for all patients. Patients receiving opioid analgesics should be observed closely for signs and symptoms of overdose, including hypotension, bradycardia, decreased respirations, and oversedation. Opioid doses should be increased until comfort is achieved or until side effects prohibit further dose escalation.

HSCT recipients usually receive IV opioid therapy (continuous infusion or PCA) for more than one week and, as a result, are likely to develop physical dependence. Parran and Pederson (2000) developed the first opioid-taper algorithm for HSCT recipients. It is currently being studied and used in printed form with HSCT recipients five years of age and older. The tool is a systematic opioid taper plan that incorporates length of opioid taper, opioid doses at the beginning of taper, and patient responses. The tool allows for individualization by assessing patients' responses to taper by evaluation of withdrawal symptoms and self-reports of pain intensity. The algorithm is provided in Figure 8-3.

Other Interventions

Many studies have evaluated the effectiveness of other interventions on the prevention and treatment of oral mucositis in patients receiving chemoradiotherapy, but few have focused specifically on transplant recipients. One such study includes the helium-neon laser that has been reported to reduce the severity of oral lesions and time of wound healing. In 1997, Cowen et al. reported the results of a double blind randomized trial evaluating the efficiency of helium-neon laser for the prevention of stomatitis in transplant recipients. Laser treatments reduced severity, pain, time of onset, and duration of stomatitis. Improved wound healing occurred by increasing cell division, synthesis of myofibroblasts, and collagen production (Biron et al., 2000). Pain relief is thought to occur from modification of nerve conduction via

Figure 8-3. Opioid-Tapering Algorithm

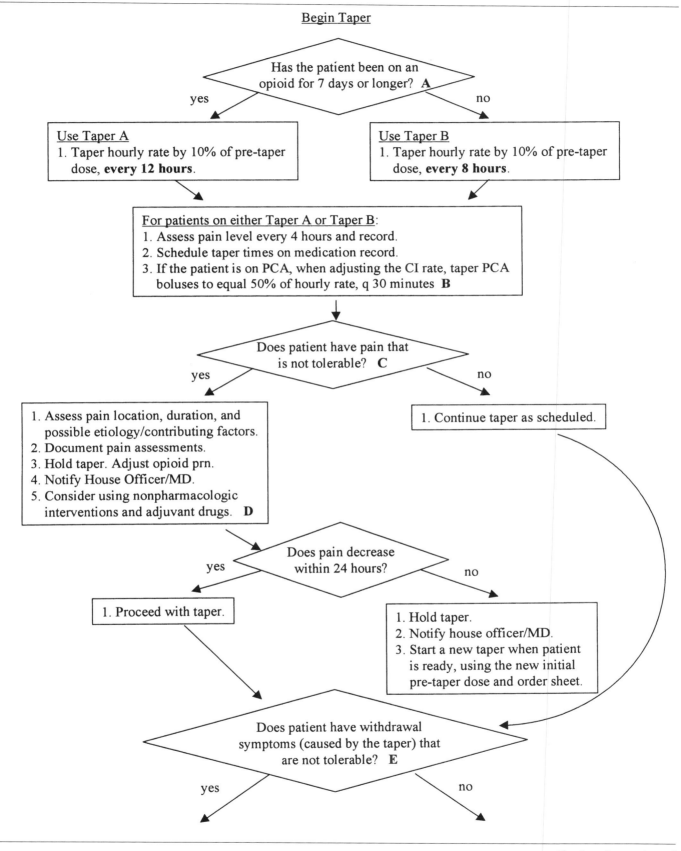

(Continued on next page)

Figure 8-3. Opioid-Tapering Algorithm *(Continued)*

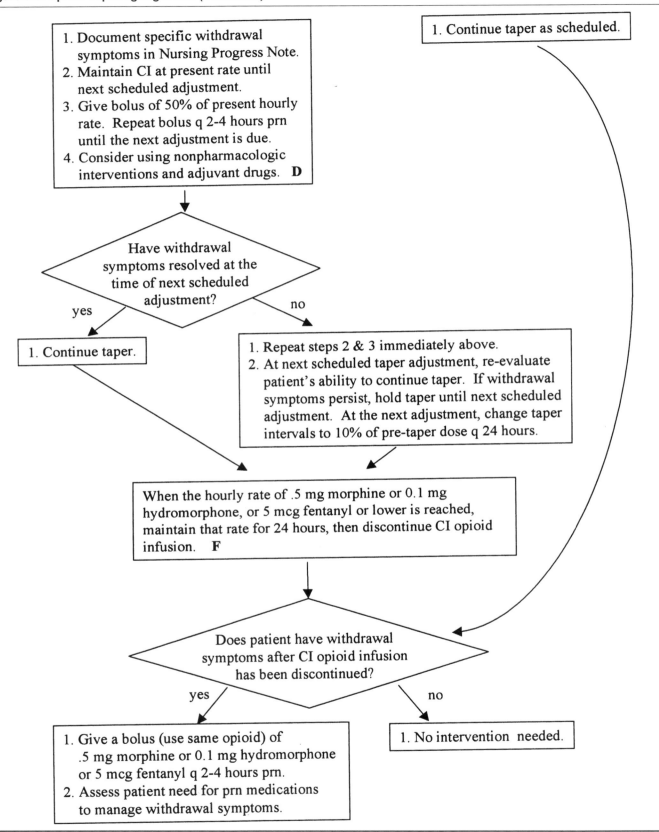

Note. From "Development of an Opioid-Taper Algorithm for Hematopoietic Cell Transplant Recipients," by L. Parran and C. Pederson, 2000, *Oncology Nursing Forum, 27,* p. 971. Copyright 2000 by the Oncology Nursing Society. Reprinted with permission.

the release of endorphins and enkephalins (Cowen et al.). Further studies are needed to identify the ideal timing and techniques of this application.

Growth factors, such as granulocyte–colony-stimulating factor (G-CSF) (Neupogen®, Amgen, Thousand Oaks, CA) and granulocyte macrophage–colony-stimulating factor (GM-CSF) (Leukine®, Immunex, Seattle, WA) may decrease the incidence of oral mucositis by shortening the duration of neutropenia. Recent studies have investigated the role of growth factors as topical oral agents to increase the restoration of normal oral epithelium. In a small (8 patients/32 cycles of chemotherapy) randomized placebo-controlled trial of high-grade lymphoma patients receiving stomatotoxic therapy, Karthaus et al. (1998) reported less frequent episodes of severe oral mucositis in the group that received oral G-CSF. They also found an earlier recovery from oral mucositis, reduction in the need for opioids, reduced hospital stay, and reduced incidence of fever. Bez et al. (1999) evaluated GM-CSF mouth rinses in a small group of transplant recipients (2 autologous/8 allogeneic). They found no significant difference in the mean mucositis score between the group receiving GM-CSF and the control group. However, the duration of severe stomatitis appeared to be reduced. Keratinocyte growth factor and transforming growth factor-beta 3 are additional growth factors currently under investigation (Peterson, 1999).

Misoprostol is a prostaglandin E1 analog that may exert a cytoprotective role on the oral mucosa. It has been evaluated in a double-blind, randomized trial with transplant recipients. When administered via oral rinse during myeloablative therapy, misoprostol was associated with a 43% reduction in stomatitis (Peterson, 1999). Large randomized clinical trials have not been completed.

These small studies demonstrate the need for new randomized clinical trials to evaluate the numerous factors involved in the treatment and prevention of oral mucositis in transplant recipients. Therapy-related oral mucositis continues to be a significant and unsolved problem. Many inconsistencies and controversies continue to exist. A multidisciplinary approach that includes detailed oral assessments and the promotion of early multimodal interventions that prevent trauma and infection and control pain are currently the mainstay of prevention and treatment.

Salivary Gland Dysfunction and Xerostomia

Pathophysiology

Xerostomia (dryness of the oral mucosa) and salivary gland dysfunction occur as a result of chemoradiotherapy toxicity. Mouth breathing, GVHD, and medications with anticholinergic effects may contribute to their severity (Eisen et al., 1997). Xerostomia occurs approximately 7–10 days after the conditioning regimen and may persist for several months. Saliva becomes thick and ropy with decreased flow rates leading to a sensation of oral dryness. Xerostomia oc-

curs along with a reduction in the immune components of saliva, specifically salivary amylase and immunoglobulins (IgA, IgG, and IgM). This reduction in immune components predisposes patients to infections with opportunistic pathogens and increases the risk of developing severe oral mucositis (Eisen et al.). Xerostomia increases the risk of *Candida* infections, and antifungal therapy should be instituted as clinically indicated (Majorana et al., 2000).

Management

Treatment usually focuses on symptomatic strategies. Suction should be available at the patient's bedside to deal with rope-like thick secretions. Bland mouth rinses, frequent sips of water, and artificial saliva can help to ease the sensation of severe dryness. Sodium bicarbonate rinses can reduce the viscosity of saliva and neutralize the acidic oral environment associated with xerostomia (Madeya, 1996b). Sialogogues can be effective in preventing and treating xerostomia by acting directly on the secretory cells of the salivary glands to increase saliva secretion (Madeya, 1996a). Aggressive oral hygiene practices that include topical fluorides, sealants, and a reduced dietary intake of refined carbohydrates can help to prevent dental decay.

Biotène products include toothpaste, gum, mouthwash, and gel developed to provide oral lubrication and protect the oral mucosa from irritation. These products may relieve dry mouth symptoms of burning, soreness, and swallowing difficulties. Biotène products have not been evaluated in randomized clinical trials involving HSCT recipients.

Taste Changes

Pathophysiology

Taste changes have been associated with radiation therapy, chemotherapy, stomatitis, xerostomia, and nutritional or immune deficiencies (Ripamonti & Fulfaro, 1998). Chemotherapeutic agents associated with taste changes are carboplatin, cisplatin, cyclophosphamide, doxorubicin, 5-fluorouracil, levamisole, and methotrexate. Toxicity to oropharyngeal taste receptors from conditioning regimens is a common cause of taste changes, including hypogeusia (loss of taste), dysgeusia (distorted taste), and ageusia (absence of taste) (Wickham et al., 1999). Nutritional deficiencies of zinc, nickel, niacin, and vitamin A also have been associated with decreased taste sensations (Madeya, 1996a). The loss of perception of sweet taste is most common. Less frequent are aversions to or reductions in the taste of sour, salt, and bitter.

Management

Strategies to improve taste changes include frequent oral hygiene, sucking on hard candy, and using artificial saliva. Patients may choose to improve the overall taste, smell, and appearance of food by increasing seasoning, eating small frequent portions, and avoiding fatty foods. Zinc supplements have been reported to be effective in improving taste changes following radiation therapy, although this has not been studied in transplant recipients (Majorana et al., 2000). Patients typically recover their sense of taste within one to three months following transplant (Majorana et al.).

Nausea and Vomiting

Preparative conditioning regimens that include high-dose chemotherapy with or without radiation therapy are highly emetogenic. Nausea and vomiting also may be caused by medications used for supportive care, organ damage, GI mucositis, infection, and GVHD. Nausea, vomiting, and retching are significant treatment-related side effects that are a source of enormous distress, discomfort, and anxiety and negatively impact quality of life of HSCT patients. Severe vomiting can lead to physical complications, such as fluid, electrolyte, and nutritional imbalances, decreased renal elimination of drugs, esophageal tears, and aspiration pneumonia (Ezzone, Baker, Rosselet, & Terepka, 1998). Nursing care involves accurate assessment, implementation of antiemetic therapies, evaluation of patient responses, and patient education.

Pathophysiology

Nausea is a subjective symptom usually described as a conscious recognition of the need to vomit. It is usually associated with symptoms of increased salivation, swallowing, and tachycardia (Hogan & Grant, 1997). Nausea associated with chemotherapy may be acute, occurring within minutes or hours of chemotherapy and lasting 24 to 48 hours; delayed, occurring 24 hours to several days after chemotherapy; or anticipatory, a conditioned response that begins prior to chemotherapy and develops from a prior experience with nausea and vomiting during chemotherapy (Hogan & Grant).

Acute nausea and vomiting occur as a result of numerous central and peripheral neurologic pathways capable of stimulating the vomiting center in the brainstem. These pathways include the vagal afferents, pharyngeal afferents, midbrain afferent, vestibular system, and chemoreceptor trigger zone (CTZ). 5-hydroxytryptamine$_3$ (5-HT$_3$), or serotonin, is a neurotransmitter that has been identified in the central and peripheral nervous systems and in the enterochromaffin cells that line the GI tract where 80% of the body's total serotonin is stored (Cunningham, 1997). Chemoradiotherapy causes damage to the GI mucosa, which causes the release of serotonin from the enterochromaffin cells of the duodenal mucosa. Serotonin binds to vagal afferent 5-HT$_3$ receptors at the GI site, which send impulses via vagal afferents to the vomiting center (Cunningham). In addition, the CTZ (located outside the blood-brain barrier in the area postrema to the fourth ventricle) detects the presence of nausea-mediating neurotransmitters (serotonin, dopamine, histamine, prostaglandins, and gamma-aminobutyric acid), which stimulate the vomiting center. In turn, the vomiting center signals cranial nerves VIII and X, causing the vomiting response to occur (Cunningham). 5-HT$_3$ is the most sensitive receptor in the first 24 hours following chemotherapy. 5-HT$_3$

receptor antagonist drugs are most effective during this time. During multiple-day or combination chemotherapy administration, the acute phase begins new with each new drug administration (Hogan & Grant, 1997).

The mechanisms involved in delayed and persistent nausea and vomiting are not well understood. Delayed nausea and vomiting are sensitive to prokinetic and steroid administration. Research is needed to better define this phenomenon and develop effective management strategies (Cunningham, 1997).

Assessment

Nursing assessments are critical to optimally manage nausea and vomiting in HSCT recipients. Initial patient assessments should include a thorough exploration of the patient's previous experiences with chemotherapy and nausea and vomiting, including the patient's previous experience with antiemetics and their effectiveness (Rhodes, 1997; Simpson, 2000). Nausea and vomiting should be assessed separately and include the duration, timing, and intensity of each episode as well as any precipitating factors (Rhodes). Patients' self-reports are the best way to evaluate the severity of symptoms because nurse and physician ratings often do not agree with the ratings of the patient (Wickham, 1996). Vomitus assessment should include quantity, color, smell, and the presence of food, blood, or medications. Vomitus from stomach contents may contain food and medications and have a greenish color. If blood is present, vomitus will have a coffee-grounds appearance. Vomitus from the distal ileum will be brown and have a fecal odor (Wickham).

Vomiting may cause fluid, electrolyte, and nutritional imbalances. Assessment of intake and output and monitoring for electrolyte imbalances such as potassium, chloride, and hydrogen are essential. Metabolic alkalosis may occur from the loss of electrolytes and large volumes of water with prolonged vomiting. Children are especially susceptible to fluid volume losses. Hourly intake and output measurements are necessary. Additional assessments should include weight loss, skin turgor, vital signs, and cardiac rhythm. Vomiting also may cause esophageal tears, aspiration pneumonia, and hemorrhage in thrombocytopenic patients (Ezzone et al., 1998).

Management

Antiemetic regimens should be individually prescribed, based upon the patient's previous experiences and the chemo-radiotherapy regimen to be used for conditioning therapy. Ongoing nursing assessments that include patients' responses to pharmacologic interventions are necessary for patient management. Patients younger than 45–55 years are more prone to nausea and vomiting and to the side effects of antiemetic medications than older patients (Wickham, 1996). Numerous antiemetic drugs are available, but no one drug has been found to be completely effective. Nearly all patients will require a combination of drug classes for effective management and support (see Table 8-1). However, despite the use of aggressive combination antiemetics, nausea and vomiting have been reported to occur in 75%–92% of patients receiving high-dose chemotherapy prior to HSCT (Ezzone et al., 1998).

Nonpharmacologic interventions have been used as an adjunct to antiemetic agents and have been found useful in minimizing nausea and vomiting (Ezzone et al., 1998). Most nonpharmacologic interventions involve acquiring new adaptive behavioral skills. These skills include relaxation, biofeedback, guided imagery, progressive muscle relaxation, and others. Additional nonpharmacologic interventions include acupuncture, acupressure, and music therapy (King, 1997). Behavioral interventions attempt to induce relaxation through learned responses. Behavioral interventions are particularly useful in children. They produce physiologic relaxation, serve as a distraction to divert the patient's attention away from a conditioned stimulus, and enhance feelings of control (King). Ezzone et al. tested the effect of music therapy as a diversional intervention in 39 patients undergoing high-dose chemotherapy prior to HSCT. The group of patients that received music therapy reported less nausea and fewer episodes of vomiting than the control group.

These interventions are useful in transplant patients because they have no side effects and can be self-administered easily. Nurses can positively influence their patients' experiences by teaching patients nonpharmacologic interventions.

Dietary modifications can be helpful in managing delayed nausea and vomiting. Antiemetics should be provided 30 minutes before meals. Patients should be instructed to eat a bland diet that does not include foods with heavy odors. Foods are best eaten cold or at room temperature. Foods high in fat content can delay gastric emptying and should be avoided. Some patients find sour-tasting foods ease nausea and vomiting. Patients should be instructed to elevate the head of the bed or sit up in a chair for 30–45 minutes following meals (Wickham, 1996).

Diarrhea

Pathophysiology

Diarrhea is a multifactorial process that results from an imbalance between absorption and secretion in the small bowel, although the mechanisms are not fully understood. Table 8-2 provides a description of the types of diarrhea and associated clinical syndromes that can be seen in transplant recipients. (GVHD of the GI tract, including the assessment and management of diarrhea, is discussed in Chapter 6.)

Chemotherapy agents associated with diarrhea include 5-FU, cytosine arabinoside, methotrexate, cisplatin, cyclophosphamide, and irinotecan. Radiation therapy and other agents, such as biologic-response modifiers (e.g., interferon,

Table 8-1. Commonly Used Antiemetic Agents

Drug	Mechanism of Action	Comments
5-HT$_3$ receptor antagonists Ondansetron (Zofran®, GlaxoSmithKline, Research Triangle Park, NC)	Blocks the stimulation of 5-HT$_3$ receptors peripherally on vagal afferent nerves and centrally in the chemoreceptor trigger zone (CTZ)	Most effective with acute nausea Headache, transient light-headedness during infusion, and constipation are common.
Granisetron (Anzemet®, Aventis Pharmaceuticals, Bridgewater, NJ)	Blocks the stimulation of 5-HT$_3$ receptors peripherally on vagal afferent nerves and centrally in the CTZ	
Phenothiazine Prochlorperazine	Binds to D$_2$ receptors to block vomiting impulse	Extrapyramidal side effects, especially in children; premedicate with diphenhydramine. May cause dry mouth, anxiety, hypotension.
Butyrophenone Droperidol	Pharmacokinetics are not fully understood, but dopaminergic blockade may be involved.	Major tranquilizer, akathisia, dystonic reactions, and extrapyramidal side effects; premedicate with diphenhydramine. Additive effects with other CNS depressants.
Substituted benzamide Metoclopramide	Blocks the stimulation of 5-HT$_3$ receptors in the gastrointestinal tract	Requires adequate plasma levels for best result. May cause extrapyramidal effects. Enhances gastric emptying, causing diarrhea. May cause headache and fatigue.
Benzodiazepine Lorazepam	Anxiolytic and amnesic	Particularly useful with highly anxious patients. Causes sedation and pleasant hallucinations. Use with caution in patients with hepatic or renal dysfunction.
Corticosteroid Dexamethasone	Pharmacokinetics not fully understood but may be inhibition of prostaglandins	Useful for acute and delayed nausea. Best used in conjunction with other antiemetics. May cause insomnia, anxiety, and euphoria.

Note. Based on information from Cunningham, 1997; Goodman, 1997; *Physicians' Desk Reference*, 2000.

Table 8-2. Types, Characteristics, and Causes of Diarrhea

Type of Diarrhea	Clinical Manifestations and Causes
Secretory	• Caused by an inhibition of mucosal absorption or the stimulation of secretion of fluid and electrolytes • Intestinal inflammation • Mucositis • Graft versus host disease
Exudative	• Caused from excessive blood, serum protein, and mucus in the intestine from inflammation, ulceration, and a loss of functional intestinal mucosa • Radiation therapy • Neutropenic enterocolitis • Infections
Osmotic	• Caused by the ingestion of nonabsorbable solutes, such as blood, that retard fluid absorption
Malabsorptive	• Caused by the malabsorption of solutes • Lactose insufficiency
Dysmotility	• Caused from dysfunctional intestinal motility resulting in an abnormally rapid transit time • Peristaltic stimulants • Fecal impaction or ileus

Note. Based on information from Engelking, 1998; Hogan, 1998; Ippoliti, 1998.

IL-2) contribute to the development of severe diarrhea (Hogan, 1998). Other drugs that cause diarrhea are laxatives, antacids, antibiotics, and nonsteroidal anti-inflammatory medications. Opioids used for the management of oral mucositis pain may cause patients to experience periods of constipation alternating with periods of diarrhea. Patients may experience massive fluid, protein, and electrolyte losses that can result in life-threatening hypotension, cardiac arrhythmias, and dehydration. Patients also are likely to experience a loss of skin turgor, perianal skin breakdown and ulceration, and malnutrition. Besides these clinical manifestations, uncontrolled or severe diarrhea has a profound impact on patients' quality of life and is a major cause of morbidity and mortality among patients undergoing HSCT (Kornblau et al., 2000).

Assessment

Accurate, detailed nursing assessments are critical to the effective management of diarrhea and should include history, physical examination, and evaluation of laboratory and diagnostic tests. History includes the onset, frequency, and duration of diarrhea, including any associated symptoms such as crampy or diffuse abdominal pain, flatus, and incontinence. Current dietary intake, including cause-and-effect relationships between consumption and diarrhea occurrence, as seen with dairy products, must be carefully assessed (Hogan, 1998). Assessment of intake and output and weight loss or gain is beneficial in determining fluid volume status.

Physical examination includes monitoring vital signs, skin turgor, and mucous membranes for signs of fluid volume losses, such as hypotension, postural hypotension, tachycardia, poor skin turgor, and dry mucous membranes. Elevated temperature may indicate the presence of infection. Abdominal assessments include the presence or absence of bowel sounds in all of the four quadrants and the presence of any pain or tenderness. Inspection of the stool should include quantity, color, consistency, frequency, and the presence of overt or occult blood (Hogan, 1998).

Analysis of laboratory and diagnostic testing is required in the assessment of diarrhea. Chemistry panels can detect electrolyte losses such as potassium, magnesium, sodium, and calcium and identify the presence of dehydration. Protein losses, especially albumin, may affect the blood levels of various medications and prompt the initiation of enteral or parenteral nutrition. Complete blood count with differential evaluates for the presence of neutropenia and thrombocytopenia. Analysis of the stool for electrolytes, microbial pathogens (bacteria, fungi, and viruses), and occult blood may be helpful in determining the etiology of diarrhea. X-rays and CT scans are used to diagnose the presence of perforation, obstruction, paralytic ileus, and neutropenic enterocolitis. Endoscopic examinations with biopsies, brushings, and cultures may be necessary in the evaluation and differential diagnosis of infection and GVHD (Hogan, 1998).

Scales for grading the severity of diarrhea are dependent on protocol and institutional preference; however, the National Cancer Institute (NCI) Common Toxicity Criteria for grading the severity of diarrhea is most often used. For transplant recipients, this scale only assesses the volume (ml/day) of diarrhea. Additional grading takes place with the separate grading of thrombocytopenia, hemorrhage/bleeding, pain, dehydration, and hypotension. Therefore, it lacks the ability to evaluate diarrhea comprehensively (Kornblau et al., 2000). If used inappropriately, clinicians may not adequately identify and evaluate diarrhea, which may lead to inadequate management and characterization of potential life-threatening sequelae (Hogan, 1998).

Management

Thorough assessments are critical for the management of diarrhea in the HSCT patient population. Interventions may include accurate recording of intake and output, including quantifying diarrhea amounts; replacement of fluids and electrolytes; monitoring for signs and symptoms of dehydration and electrolyte imbalances; monitoring for signs and symptoms of blood loss and hemorrhage (see Table 8-3); and monitoring the efficacy of pharmacologic interventions.

Dietary management may be beneficial in reducing the quantity and frequency of diarrhea for some patients, depending on the clinical situation. Patients should be advised to eat small, frequent, bland meals that are low in residue and include potassium-rich foods, such as in the BRAT diet (bananas, rice, applesauce, and toast). Dairy products that contain lactose should be avoided when lactose intolerance has been identified in the diarrhea assessment. Foods that

Table 8-3. Signs, Symptoms, and Interventions for Blood Loss and Hemorrhage, Dehydration, and Electrolyte Imbalances

Clinical Manifestation	Signs and Symptoms	Interventions
Blood loss and hemorrhage	• Hypotension • Postural hypotension • Tachycardia • Tachypnea • Pale mucous membranes	• Monitor results of complete blood count. • Monitor vital signs. • Assess mucous membranes for color and paleness. • Monitor stools for overt and occult blood. • Transfuse with packed red blood cells and platelets.
Dehydration	• Hypotension • Postural hypotension • Tachycardia • Dry mucous membranes • Decreased urinary output • Weight loss	• Monitor intake/output; quantify stool output. • Monitor vital signs. • Monitor for dizziness, weakness, and fatigue. • Assess mucous membranes for dryness. • Administer IV fluids. • Assess skin turgor. • Weigh patient (at least daily). • Encourage oral fluids.
Electrolyte imbalances Hypomagnesemia	• Symptoms rarely occur until serum mg < 1. • Confusion, seizures, vertigo, hyperactive deep tendon reflexes, muscle tremor/cramping, tachydysrhythmias	• Monitor results of chemistry testing. • Assess for signs and symptoms of electrolyte imbalances. • Replace electrolytes orally or parenterally.
Hypokalemia	• Weak irregular pulse, bradycardia, depressed T waves on ECG, hypotension, confusion, muscle cramps, nausea	
Hyponatremia	• Malaise, lethargy, weakness, muscle cramps, hyperreflexia, muscle twitching, seizures, vomiting, systolic BP < 90 mmHg	

Note. Based on information from Chernecky & Berger, 1998; Glynn-Tucker, 1998; Idemoto, 1998.

are too hot or cold and foods that cause gas (cabbage, onions) or irritation (caffeine, chocolate, dairy products) should be avoided (Hogan, 1998). Hyperosmotic supplements (Ensure® [Abbott Laboratories, Abbott Park, IL], Sustacal® [Bristol-Myers Squibb, Princeton, NJ]) also should be avoided. When possible, and not contraindicated, adult patients should be encouraged to drink approximately three liters of fluid daily to avoid dehydration. Fluids such as Pedialyte® (Abbott Laboratories) can replace fluid and electrolytes lost to diarrhea (Hogan). This amount of fluid intake is usually impossible, especially in the early transplant course, and requires fluids to be replaced intravenously.

Pharmacologic interventions are aimed at reducing fluid loss in the stool by inhibiting secretion, promoting absorption, and decreasing intestinal mobility, thereby promoting contact between intestinal fluids and epithelial cells where absorption of fluids and electrolytes takes place. However, in the presence of infectious diarrhea, inhibition of intestinal motility may compromise removal of infectious agents (Ippoliti, 1998). Infectious causes of diarrhea should be ruled out prior to initiating antidiarrheal medications, although this is controversial. Table 8-4 reviews current antidiarrheal medications, their mechanisms of action, and dosing schedules.

Perineal-Rectal Skin Alterations

Transplant recipients, especially children and infants in diapers, are at risk for alterations in perineal-rectal skin in-

tegrity from the effects of chemoradiotherapy, diarrhea, and GVHD. The skin is a primary barrier against infection, so close attention to perineal-rectal skin integrity is necessary during periods of myelosuppression.

Pathophysiology

The skin of the perineal-rectal area is susceptible to damage from chemoradiotherapy and diarrhea. Radiation and chemotherapy interfere with the mitosis of epithelial cells of the basal membrane, causing thinning of the epidermis, changes in pigmentation, hypersensitivity, and fibrosis of the dermis. Its anatomical structure and location hinder easy assessment and cleansing and increase the risk of bacterial growth. Mechanical or chemical trauma can occur from proteolytic enzymes in diarrhea or the frequent use of cleansing agents and result in perineal-rectal skin breakdown (Haisfield-Wolfe & Rund, 2000).

Assessment

Assessment of the perineal-rectal skin should be performed at least daily during myelosuppression and periods of diarrhea. Initially, erythema, increased skin temperature, and edema are seen. Symptoms may progress to dry and then moist desquamation, although patients may have several stages of skin reaction occurring simultaneously. Dry desquamation (dryness, flaking, and peeling of skin often accompanied by pruritus) that can occur as erythema is resolving (Maher, 2000).

Table 8-4. Antidiarrheal Medications

Antidiarrheal Medication	Mechanism of Action	Dosing Schedule
Diphenoxylate hydrochloride (Lomotil®, Searle & Co., Skokie, IL)	Opiate agonist[a] Intestinal transit inhibitor	• Not recommended for children younger than two years of age • Children: 0.3–0.4 mg/kg/day divided into four doses • Adult: 2.5–5.0 mg every six hours as needed (20 mg/day maximum dose)
Loperamide hydrochloride (Imodium®, McNeil Consumer Healthcare, Fort Washington, PA)	Opiate agonist[a] Intestinal transit inhibitor	• Not recommended for children younger than two years of age • Children: Recommended first day dosage schedule 2–5 years (13–20 kg) use liquid, 1 mg three times a day 6–8 years (20–30 kg) 2 mg two times a day 8–12 years (> 30 kg) 2 mg three times a day • Following initial treatment day, subsequent doses of 1 mg/10 kg should be given only after loose stool. • Total dose not to exceed recommended dosages for the first day. Adult: 4 mg by mouth followed by 2 mg by mouth after every loose stool (maximum dosing 16 mg/24 hrs)
Octreotide (Sandostatin® [injection], Sandostatin LAR® Depot [IV suspension], Novartis, Cambridge, MA)	Antisecretory drug	• Children: Octreotide has not been studied in children; there are no dosing recommendations. • Adults: maximal benefit seen when initiated early 100–150 mcg sq q8h for mild to moderate diarrhea • 500 mcg sq/IV q8h for severe diarrhea (has been given up to 2,000 mcg q8h; maximal dosing not yet established)

[a] Opiate agonists are contraindicated in the treatment of diarrhea with an infectious etiology.

Note. Based on information from Ippoliti, 1998; Ippoliti & Neumann, 1998; Kornblau et al., 2000; *Physicians' Desk Reference*, 2000.

Moist desquamation is seen with a total destruction of the epithelium, exposing nerve endings in the dermis and causing severe pain. Clinical manifestations of moist desquamation are bright red, sloughing skin with serous exudate oozing from the surface. The rate of skin regrowth following moist desquamation is dependent upon the severity of injury. Gradual thickening of skin will occur over time, but the skin will not regain its former thickness and will have fewer sweat and sebaceous glands, resulting in chronic dryness (Maher, 2000).

Management

Patients and their caregivers should be instructed in routine skin care and infection control practices. Routine and preventative skin care should be performed at least daily and following each bowel movement and urination. Haisfield-Wolfe and Rund (2000) developed a perineal-rectal skin management protocol for patients whose skin is at risk or altered from the side effects of chemotherapy or radiation therapy. The protocol (see Table 8-5) includes routine care and interventions for erythema, dry desquamation, and moist desquamation.

Transplant recipients are at risk for reactivation of HSV during periods of myelosuppression and following engraftment when prophylactic medications have been discontinued and cell-mediated immunity may be deficient. Perineal-rectal lesions should be routinely cultured for HSV and appropriate prophylaxis and treatment initiated.

Nutrition

Mucositis, pain, infection, diarrhea, xerostomia, taste changes, anorexia, nausea and vomiting, GVHD, and side effects of medications all have a profound impact on the nutritional status of HSCT recipients. During severe oropharyngeal and esophageal mucositis and severe diarrhea, patients may be unable to tolerate foods and fluids orally. Because mucositis resolves with neutrophil recovery, autologous transplant recipients can usually resume oral intake within one to two weeks post-transplant. However, allogeneic transplant patients may have a longer period of neutropenia, three to four weeks post-transplant, and may experience severe diarrhea from GI GVHD. Parenteral nutrition often is necessary in these circumstances. Whenever possible, the GI tract is the first choice for nutrition (Nitenberg & Raynard, 2000). Dietitians should be involved in the assessment of nutritional status and management and evaluation of nutritional support in HSCT recipients.

Assessment

Assessment parameters should include a thorough assessment of the patient's nutritional status prior to and during the transplant process. Daily or twice-daily weights, intake and output volumes, calorie counts, visceral protein measurements (albumin and prealbumin), transferrin levels, and nitrogen balance should be closely evaluated. Because weight can fluctuate with fluid balance, intake and output and weights should be evaluated together. An increase in weight may be related to fluid retention and mask the true loss of body mass. Visceral protein levels may decrease even though nutritional intake is adequate. Albumin levels may decrease from fever, stress, protein loss in diarrhea, and excessive IV hydration. Fever, stress, hepatic dysfunction, and renal dysfunction may affect prealbumin, transferrin, and nitrogen balance (Sigley, 1998). Calorie counts are useful

Table 8-5. Perineal-Rectal Skin Care Protocol

Routine Care

During morning care and after each episode of urination or defecation, the patient will receive the following care.
- Gently cleanse skin with tepid water or a mild cleansing agent followed by gently patting areas dry **or** cleanse with tepid to cool sitz baths.
- If open lesions are present, cleanse with a wound cleanser or normal saline solution and treat.
- Apply a moisturizing cream.
- Recommend cotton undergarments; avoid restrictive clothing.
- Perform a full assessment of the perineal-rectal skin.
- Perform a nutrition assessment followed by nutrition consult, if needed.
- Consult an enterostomal therapy or wound-care nurse as needed.

Assessment	Recommendations for Care
Erythema signs and symptoms Pink Tenderness	Gently cleanse using a mild cleansing agent (perineal skin cleansers). Apply a moisturizing, protective cream. If cleanser is not accessible and soap must be used, use a soap without perfumes and thoroughly rinse all soap residues from the skin. Avoid lotions or creams containing perfume and talc (if receiving radiation therapy to area, avoid products containing metals or ointments or cleanse prior to receiving radiation therapy). Frequency of skin care: Daily and after toileting.
Dry desquamation signs and symptoms Scaling Flaking Pruritus Pain	Cleanse with tepid water or a wound cleanser. Apply a protective cream. Assess for pruritus, if present. • Apply topical antihistamine creams. • Take a cool shower or bath. • Consider analgesics or antihistamines. Assess for fungal infection, if present. • Treat with topical antifungal or systemic antifungal agent. Frequency of skin care: Twice a day/as needed after toileting.
Moist desquamation signs and symptoms Pain Weeping Sloughing Abscess	Recommend sitz bath, shower or whirlpool as needed. Cleanse with a wound cleanser as needed. Apply a protective cream that will adhere to open skin. Apply an adhesive peripad or pantyliner without deodorant to the undergarments. Assess as needed for analgesics, pain medications. If desquamation worsens, apply a wound hydrogel. Frequency of skin care: Twice a day/as needed after toileting.
Possible complications of moist desquamation Vesicles Furuncle Carbuncles Abscess formation	Consult with physician or advanced practice nurse for treatment and systemic antibiotics. If vesicles are present, rule out herpes and treat appropriately.

Report to Physician	Documentation
Worsening of skin alteration Increase of inflammation Appearance of furuncle, carbuncles, abscess Appearance of vesicles Pain or increase in pain, change in character of pain	Anatomical area involved Size of involvement • Area may be difficult to measure because of the perineal-rectal anatomy. • Attempt to record in centimeters. • Measure from where the normal skin stops to where it begins again (use a disposable ruler). If open areas develop, measure width, length, and depth. • Record daily in acute care or weekly in home or long-term care. Changes in skin or wound conditions Colors of skin Drainage (i.e., amount, odor, color, consistency) Presence of sloughing or necrosis Presence and intensity of pain or pruritus Patient outcomes

Note. From "A Nursing Protocol for the Management of Perineal-Rectal Skin Alterations," by M.E. Haisfield-Wolfe and C. Rund, 2000, *Clinical Journal of Oncology Nursing, 4,* p. 19. Copyright 2000 by the Oncology Nursing Society. Reprinted with permission.

in determining if oral intake is adequate. Calorie requirements can be estimated by adding an activity factor to the calculated basal energy expenditure (BEE) results. The dietitian will evaluate and determine whether caloric needs are being met and recommend nutritional management strategies.

Management

A variety of recommendations exist for the nutritional management of autologous and allogeneic HSCT recipients. Some suggested nutritional strategies include the use of a neutropenic/low microbial diet, water safety practices, safe food handling, and parenteral and enteral nutrition. Differences in nutritional practices occur among transplant centers, and few research studies have been conducted that evaluate the impact of nutritional management on outcomes in transplantation.

Neutropenic/Low Microbial Diet

HSCT recipients' diets should be restricted to reduce the risk of food-related bacteria, yeasts, molds, viruses, and parasites. Patients should remain on restricted diets until immunosuppression resolves. It is recommended that this diet be continued for three months for autologous transplant recipients and until all immunosuppressive drugs are discontinued for allogeneic transplant recipients (CDC et al., 2000). Patients and caregivers should be instructed in dietary restrictions and appropriate food handling practices before the conditioning regimen begins (see Table 8-6 and Figure 8-4).

In addition, during periods of immunosuppression, HSCT recipients should avoid naturopathic medicines that may contain molds. Naturopathic medications should only be prescribed by licensed naturopathic physicians working in conjunction with transplant and infectious disease physicians (CDC et al., 2000).

Table 8-6. High-Risk Foods and Safer Substitutions

High-Risk Foods	Safer Substitutions
Raw or undercooked poultry, meats, fish, or shellfish (includes beef, pork, lamb, venison, or other wild game, or combination dishes containing raw or undercooked meats or sweetbread from these animals)	Well-done, cooked poultry, meats, and fish (a) Poultry cooked to internal temperature[a] of > 180°F (b) Meats and egg-containing casseroles and soufflés cooked to an internal temperature[a] of > 160°F (c) Hot foods kept to a temperature[a] of > 140°F
Deli meats, hot dogs, and processed meats	Should be avoided unless further cooked
Raw and undercooked eggs and foods that contain eggs (French toast, omelettes, Caesar and other salad dressings, puddings, hollandaise sauce, homemade mayonnaise, and egg nog)	Pasteurized or hard-boiled eggs
Unpasteurized dairy products, including milk, cheese, cheese-containing molds, cream, butter, and yogurt	Pasteurized dairy products
Fresh-squeezed or unpasteurized fruit or vegetable juices	Pasteurized juices
Raw fruits with rough texture (raspberries, strawberries)	Should be avoided
Smooth raw fruits	Washed under running water, peeled, or cooked
Raw vegetables	Washed under running water, peeled, or cooked
Undercooked or raw tofu	Cooked tofu (cut into 1-inch cubes and boiled for ≥ 5 minutes in water or broth before eating or using in recipes)
Unroasted raw nuts or roasted nuts in the shell	Cooked nuts, canned or bottled roasted nuts, or nuts baked in products
Raw or uncooked grain products	Cooked grain products, including bread, cooked and ready-to-eat cold cereal, pretzels, popcorn, potato chips, corn chips, tortilla chips, cooked pasta, rice
Raw or unpasteurized honey	Should be avoided
Raw, uncooked brewers yeast	Transplant recipients should avoid any contact with raw yeast; they should not make bread products themselves.
Unpasteurized beer (home-brewed and certain microbrewery beer)	Pasteurized beer (retail bottled or canned beer or draft beer that has been pasteurized after fermentation)
Mate tea	Should be avoided

[a] Internal temperature measured with a thermometer

Note. Based on information from CDC, Infectious Diseases Society of America, & American Society of Blood and Marrow Transplantation, 2000.

Figure 8-4. Food Safety Practices

- Raw poultry, meats, fish, and seafood should be handled on a separate surface (cutting board or countertop) from other food items. Separate cutting boards for poultry, meat, and vegetables should be used.
- All cutting or carving surfaces should be washed with warm water and soap between cutting different food items.
- Uncooked meats should not come in contact with other foods.
- After preparing raw poultry, meats, fish, and seafood and before preparing other foods, food handlers should wash their hands thoroughly in warm, soapy water.
- Cold foods should be stored at < 40°F; hot foods kept at > 140°F.
- Food handlers should
  - (a) Wash their hands in warm soapy water before handling leftovers.
  - (b) Use clean utensils and food-preparation surfaces.
  - (c) Divide leftovers into small amounts and store in shallow containers for quick cooling.
  - (d) Refrigerate leftovers within two hours after cooking and discard leftovers kept at room temperature for more than two hours.
  - (e) Reheat[a] leftovers or partially cooked foods to ≥ 165°F throughout before serving.
  - (f) Cook poultry to an internal temperature[a] of > 180°F; other meats and egg-containing casseroles and soufflés to an internal temperature[a] of > 160°F.
  - (g) Bring leftover soups, sauces, and gravies to a rolling boil before serving.
- Shelves, countertops, refrigerators, freezers, utensils, sponges, towels, and other kitchen items should be kept clean.
- All fresh produce should be washed thoroughly under running water before serving.

[a] Internal temperature measured with a thermometer

Note. Based on information from CDC, Infectious Diseases Society of America, & American Society of Blood and Marrow Transplantation, 2000.

Water Safety

To avoid possible exposure to *Cryptosporidium* and fecal or waterborne pathogens, HSCT patients should take precautions regarding water exposure and consumption. Patients should not walk, wade, swim, play in, or drink water from recreational sources such as ponds, rivers, or lakes that may be contaminated with sewage or animal or human wastes. Well water from private or public wells of small communities should not be consumed because tests for microbial pathogens are performed too infrequently. Water from municipal wells in highly populated areas is safe. In a boil-water advisory, all tap water used for drinking or brushing teeth should be boiled for > 1 minute(s) before it is used. Home water filters that remove particles > 1 μm in diameter or filter by reverse osmosis are only safe when used on municipal water sources (CDC et al., 2000). Patients should call the NSF International consumer line (800-673-8010) or contact them on the World Wide Web (www.nsf.org) for a list of filters certified under NSF Standard 053 for cyst removal. Home water filters are not appropriate or safe for use on private or small community public wells. Bottled water can be consumed if it has been processed to remove *Cryptosporidium* by reverse osmosis, distillation, or 1 μm particulate absolute filtration. Patients should contact the bottler directly. Contact information regarding water bottlers can be obtained by calling the International Bottled Water Association (703-683-5213) or by contacting them on the World Wide Web (www.bottledwater.org) (CDC et al.).

Parenteral Nutrition

Transplant centers have different criteria for the initiation of parenteral nutrition. Generally, when oral intake is less than 50% of minimal nutritional needs for four to seven days because of GI complications, such as mucositis; prolonged nausea, vomiting, and/or diarrhea; or GVHD, parenteral nutrition is recommended. In the allogeneic transplant setting, nutritional support with total parenteral nutrition is common and has been found to improve long-term survival (Lenssen, Bruemmer, Aker, & McDonald, 2001). In contrast, its use in the autologous transplant setting is rare, and its role has not been established (Lenssen et al.).

The quantity and components of parenteral nutrition should be titrated based on the patient's oral intake, weight, age, BEE (described previously), and clinical situation. Dextrose should provide 50%–60% of calories, lipids should provide no more than 25%–30% of calories, and protein should provide 15%–25% of calories (Sigley, 1998). Electrolytes, vitamins, and trace elements are also supplemented. Modifications in the components of parenteral nutrition may be made because of renal or hepatic insufficiency or dysfunction. Parenteral nutrition supplemented with glutamine, antioxidants, and lipids is being studied for its potential role in decreasing transplant-related toxicity, infections, and nutritional morbidity (Lenssen et al., 2001).

Enteral Nutrition

Enteral nutrition is only appropriate in patients without uncontrolled nausea, vomiting, and diarrhea and who have an intact digestive tract. As such, its utility in the transplant setting is limited. Some centers have successfully used enteral nutrition post-transplant (> 30 days) in patients who fail to maintain adequate nutritional status because of difficulties with oral intake and chronic GVHD (Nitenberg & Raynard, 2000).

Conclusion

The pathophysiology, assessment, and management of HSCT patients experiencing GI complications are complex. Patients usually have multiple GI complications occurring simultaneously, making the assessment and management of these patients even more difficult. In most cases, patients experiencing severe oral mucositis also will have fluid and electrolyte imbalances, infection, severe pain, and malnutrition. Concurrent mucositis of the GI mucosa usually occurs, causing diarrhea that predisposes patients to the development of perineal-rectal skin alterations and GI infection. Following the administration of myeloablative chemoradiotherapy, patients may experience xerostomia and taste alteration for several months, prolonging nutritional deficiencies. Specialized nursing care, assessments, and management can positively influence patient outcomes and experiences.

Nursing research regarding oral hygiene, skin care, nausea and vomiting, pain management, and diarrhea management are necessary to identify and implement standards of care that improve HSCT recipients' outcomes.

References

Avery, R.K., Adal, K.A., Longworth, D.L., & Bolwell, B.J. (2000). A survey of allogeneic bone marrow transplant programs in the United States regarding cytomegalovirus prophylaxis and preemptive therapy. *Bone Marrow Transplantation, 26,* 763–767.

Barker, G.J. (1999). Current practices in the oral management of the patients undergoing chemotherapy or bone marrow transplantation. *Supportive Care in Cancer, 7,* 17–20.

Berger, A.M., & Eilers, J. (1998). Factors influencing oral cavity status during high-dose antineoplastic therapy: A secondary data analysis. *Oncology Nursing Forum, 25,* 1623–1626.

Bez, C., Demarosi, F., Sardella, A., Lodi, G., Bertolli, V., Annaloro, C., et al. (1999). GM-CSF mouth rinses in the treatment of severe oral mucositis. *Oral Surgery, Oral Medicine, Oral Pathology, Oral Radiology and Endodontics, 88,* 311–315.

Biron, P., Sebban, C., Gourmet, R., Chvetzoff, G., Philip, I., & Blay, J.Y. (2000). Research controversies in management of oral mucositis. *Supportive Care in Cancer, 8,* 68–71.

Blijlevens, N.M.A., Donnelly, J.P., & DePauw, B.E. (2000). Mucosal barrier injury: Biology, pathology, clinical counterparts and consequences of intensive treatment for haematological malignancy: An overview. *Bone Marrow Transplantation, 25,* 1269–1278.

Centers for Disease Control and Prevention, Infectious Diseases Society of America, & American Society of Blood and Marrow Transplantation. (2000). Guidelines for preventing opportunistic infections among hematopoietic stem cell transplant recipients. *Morbidity and Mortality Weekly Report, 49*(RR–10).

Chernecky, C.C., & Berger, B.J. (1998). Hyponatremia. In C.C. Chernecky & B.J. Berger (Eds.), *Advanced and critical care oncology nursing: Managing primary complications* (pp. 355–370). Philadelphia: W.B. Saunders.

Cowen, D., Tardieu, C., Schubert, M., Peterson, D., Resbeut, M., Faucher, C., et al. (1997). Low energy helium-neon laser in the prevention of oral mucositis in patients undergoing bone marrow transplant: Results of a double blind randomized trial. *International Journal of Radiation Oncology, Biology, Physics, 38,* 697–703.

Cox, G.J., Matsui, S.M., Lo, R.S., Hinds, M., Bowden, R.A., Hackman, R.C., et al. (1994). Etiology and outcome of diarrhea after marrow transplantation: A prospective study. *Gastroenterology, 107,* 1398–1407.

Cunningham, R.S. (1997). 5-HT$_3$-receptor antagonists: A review of pharmacology and clinical efficacy. *Oncology Nursing Forum, 24*(Suppl. 7), 33–40.

Dodd, M.J., Dibble, S.L., Miaskowski, C., MacPhail, L., Greenspan, D., Paul, S.M., et al. (2000). Randomized clinical trial of the effectiveness of 3 commonly used mouthwashes to treat chemotherapy-induced stomatitis. *Oral Medicine, 90*(1), 39–47.

Eilers, J., Berger, A.M., & Petersen, M.C. (1988). Development, testing, and application of the Oral Assessment Guide. *Oncology Nursing Forum, 15,* 325–330.

Eisen, D., Essell, J., & Broun, E.R. (1997). Oral cavity complications of bone marrow transplantation. *Seminars in Cutaneous Medicine and Surgery, 16,* 265–272.

Engelking, C. (1998). Cancer-related diarrhea: A neglected cause of cancer-related symptom distress: Introduction. *Oncology Nursing Forum, 25,* 859–860.

Ezzone, S., Baker, C., Rosselet, R., & Terepka, E. (1998). Music as an adjunct to antiemetic therapy. *Oncology Nursing Forum, 25,* 1551–1556.

Glynn-Tucker, E.M. (1998). Hypomagnesemia. In C.C. Chernecky & B.J. Berger (Eds.), *Advanced and critical care oncology nursing: Manag-*

ing primary complications (pp. 342–354). Philadelphia: W.B. Saunders.

Goodman, M. (1997). Risk factors and antiemetic management of chemotherapy-induced nausea and vomiting. *Oncology Nursing Forum, 24*(Suppl. 7), 20–32.

Haisfield-Wolfe, M.E., & Rund, C. (2000). A nursing protocol for the management of perineal-rectal skin alterations. *Clinical Journal of Oncology Nursing, 4,* 15–21.

Hale, G.A., Heslop, H.E., Krance, R.A., Brenner, M.A., Jayawardene, D., Srivastava, D.K., et al. (1999). Adenovirus infection after pediatric bone marrow transplantation. *Bone Marrow Transplantation, 23,* 277–282.

Hanna, H., Raad, I., Gonzalez, V., Umphrey, J., Tarrand, J., Neumann, J., et al. (2000). Control of nosocomial *Clostridium difficile* transmission in bone marrow transplant patients. *Infection Control and Hospital Epidemiology, 21,* 226–228.

Heimdahl, A. (1999). Prevention and management of oral infections in cancer patients. *Supportive Care in Cancer, 7,* 224–228.

Hogan, C.M. (1998). The nurse's role in diarrhea management. *Oncology Nursing Forum, 25,* 879–886.

Hogan, C.M., & Grant, M. (1997). Physiologic mechanisms of nausea and vomiting in patients with cancer. *Oncology Nursing Forum, 24*(Suppl. 7), 8–12.

Idemoto, B.E. (1998). Hypokalemia. In C.C. Chernecky & B.J. Berger (Eds.), *Advanced and critical care oncology nursing: Managing primary complications* (pp. 327–341). Philadelphia: W.B. Saunders.

Ippoliti, C. (1998). Antidiarrheal agents for the management of treatment-related diarrhea in cancer patients. *American Journal of Health-System Pharmacy, 55,* 1573–1580.

Ippoliti, C., & Neumann, J. (1998). Octreotide in the management of diarrhea induced by graft versus host disease. *Oncology Nursing Forum, 25,* 873–878.

Johansson, J.E., & Ekman, T. (1997). Gastro-intestinal toxicity related to bone marrow transplantation: disruption of the intestinal barrier precedes clinical findings. *Bone Marrow Transplantation, 19,* 921–925.

Karthaus, M., Rosenthal, C., Huebner, G., Paul, H., Elser, C., Hertenstein, B., et al. (1998). Effect of topical oral G-CSF on oral mucositis: A randomized placebo-controlled trial. *Bone Marrow Transplantation, 22,* 781–785.

Kawai, K., Imada, S., Lida, K., Tsukamoto, S., Miyanaga, N., & Akaza, H. (1998). Neutropenic colitis as a complication of high-dose chemotherapy for refractory testicular cancer. *Japanese Journal of Clinical Oncology, 28,* 571–573.

King, C.R. (1997). Nonpharmacologic management of chemotherapy-induced nausea and vomiting. *Oncology Nursing Forum, 24*(Suppl. 7), 41–48.

Kingreen, D., Nitsche, A., Beyer, J., & Siegert, W. (1997). Herpes simplex infection of the jejunum occurring in the early post-transplantation period. *Bone Marrow Transplantation, 20,* 989–991.

Kornblau, S., Benson, A.B., Catalano, R., Champlin, R., Engelking, C., Field, M., et al. (2000). Management of cancer-treatment-related diarrhea: Issues and therapeutic strategies. *Journal of Pain and Symptom Management, 19*(2), 118–129.

Lenssen, P., Bruemmer, B., Aker, S.N., & McDonald, G.B. (2001). Nutrient support in hematopoietic cell transplantation. *Journal of Parenteral and Enteral Nutrition, 25,* 219–228.

Madeya, M.L. (1996a). Oral complications for cancer therapy: Part 1. Pathophysiology and secondary complications. *Oncology Nursing Forum, 23,* 801–807.

Madeya, M.L. (1996b). Oral complications for cancer therapy: Part 2. Nursing implications for assessment and treatment. *Oncology Nursing Forum, 23,* 808–821.

Maher, K.E. (2000). Radiation therapy: toxicities and management. In C.H. Yarbro, M.H. Frogge, M. Goodman, & S.L. Groenwald (Eds.), *Cancer nursing: Principles and practice* (5th ed., pp. 323–351). Sudbury, MA: Jones and Bartlett.

Majorana, A., Schubert, M.M., Porta, F., Ugazio, A.G., & Sapelli, P.L. (2000). Oral complications of pediatric hematopoietic cell transplantation: Diagnosis and management. *Supportive Care in Cancer, 8,* 353–365.

Nitenberg, G., & Raynard, B. (2000). Nutritional support of the cancer patient: Issues and dilemmas. *Critical Reviews in Oncology/Hematology, 34,* 137–168.

Parran, L., & Pederson, C. (2000). Development of an opioid-taper algorithm for hematopoietic cell transplant recipients. *Oncology Nursing Forum, 27,* 967–974.

Pederson, C., & Parran, C. (1999). Pain and distress in adults and children undergoing peripheral blood stem cell or bone marrow transplant. *Oncology Nursing Forum, 26,* 575–582.

Peterson, D.E. (1999). Oral infection. *Supportive Care in Cancer, 7,* 217–218.

Physicians' Desk Reference® (54th ed.). (2000). Montvale, NJ: Medical Economics Co.

Raber-Durlacher, J.E. (1999). Current practices for management of oral mucositis in cancer patients. *Supportive Care in Cancer, 7,* 71–74.

Rhodes, V.A. (1997). Criteria for assessment of nausea, vomiting, and retching. *Oncology Nursing Forum, 24,* 13–19.

Ripamonti, C., & Fulfaro, F. (1998). Taste alterations in cancer patients. *Journal of Pain and Symptom Management, 16,* 349–351.

Sigley, T. (1998). Nutrition support of the bone marrow transplant patient. *Clinical Nutrition, 13*(2), 35–50.

Simpson, J.K. (2000). Specialized nursing. In E.D. Ball, J. Lister, & P. Law (Eds.), *Hematopoietic stem cell therapy* (pp. 683–687). Philadelphia: Churchill Livingstone.

Van Burik, J.H., & Weisdorf, D.J. (1999). Infections in recipients of blood and marrow transplantation. *Hematology/Oncology Clinics of North America, 13,* 1065–1089.

Van Kraaij, M.G.J., Dekker, A.W., Verdonck, L.F., Van Loon, A.M., Vinje, J., Koopmans, M.P.G., et al. (2000). Infectious gastroenteritis: An uncommon cause of diarrhea in adult allogeneic and autologous stem cell transplant recipients. *Bone Marrow Transplantation, 26,* 299–303.

Vargas, H.E., & Silverman, W.B. (2000). Mucositis and other gastrointestinal complications. In E.D. Ball, J. Lister, & P. Law (Eds.), *Hematopoietic stem cell therapy* (pp. 557–561). Philadelphia: Churchill Livingstone.

Wickham, R.S. (1996). In S.L. Groenwald, M.H. Frogge, M. Goodman, & C.H. Yarbro (Eds.), *Cancer symptom management* (pp. 218–242). Sudbury, MA: Jones and Bartlett.

Wickham, R.S., Rehwaldt, M., Kefer, C., Shott, S., Glynn-Tucker, K.E., Potter, C., et al. (1999). Taste changes experienced by patient receiving chemotherapy. *Oncology Nursing Forum, 26,* 697–706.

Wojtaszek, C. (2000). Management of chemotherapy-induced stomatitis. *Clinical Journal of Oncology Nursing, 4,* 263–270.

Hepatorenal Complications of Hematopoietic Stem Cell Transplant

Introduction

Hepatorenal complications that are associated with hematopoietic stem cell transplant (HSCT) present a myriad of management challenges for all members of the transplant team. Management of this patient population is complex and requires constant vigilance by the transplant nurse. Transplant nurses with a sound knowledge base can facilitate prompt and accurate diagnoses of hepatorenal complications. The most common complications of the hepatic and renal systems will be reviewed, with focus on medical and nursing management strategies for these patients.

Liver Anatomy and Physiology

A normal liver weighs 1,000–1,500 grams, has a span of 6–12 centimeters, and is located in the right upper quadrant. The liver consists of two major lobes, which are divided into numerous functional units called lobules. Hepatic sinusoids are located throughout the lobules and are lined with endothelial and reticuloendothelial (Kupffer) cells (Ghany & Hoofnagle, 2001). The majority of cells making up the liver are hepatocytes, which are responsible for the major work of the liver. Blood enters the liver by way of the hepatic artery and the hepatic portal vein (Netter, 1997). The hepatic artery draws blood from the aorta, whereas the hepatic portal vein transports blood from the gastrointestinal (GI) tract and the spleen. The common bile duct follows the hepatic artery and hepatic portal vein pathway to form portal triads. These portal triads flow into the sinusoids, where white blood cells migrate through and around the Kupffer cells while red blood cells remain within the sinusoidal space. Blood then is drained from the liver via the hepatic vein into the inferior vena cava (Ghany & Hoofnagle).

The functional activities of the liver are numerous and vital to survival. The liver's functions include the metabolism of fats, carbohydrates, proteins, and drugs and their metabolites; the synthesis of clotting factors (I, II, V, VII, IX, X); the regulation of nutrients (fats, glucose, glycogen, and amino acids); the conjugation and excretion of bilirubin; and filtration of blood byproducts, bacteria, and products of coagulation (Ghany & Hoofnagle, 2001; Netter, 1997).

Hepatic Complications

Hepatic complications associated with HSCT are common; however, several factors have led to decreased incidence and severity of these complications. Strasser and McDonald (1999) reported that antiviral therapies, improved graft versus host disease (GVHD) prophylaxis, modified preparative regimens, and earlier recognition by practitioners have contributed to fewer and less severe hepatic complications. Figure 9-1 presents the most common hepatic complications associated with HSCT, with respect to expected time of onset.

Veno-Occlusive Disease

Hepatic veno-occlusive disease (VOD) is a clinical syndrome most commonly associated with the administration of high-dose chemotherapy and/or total body irradiation (TBI) in the transplant setting. The reported incidence of VOD is variable and ranges from 0%–70%, with mortality rates as high as 47% (Carreras et al., 1998). Carreras et al.

Figure 9-1. Hepatic Complications and Expected Time to Onset

Conditioning to Day +100
- Veno-occlusive disease
- Acute graft versus host disease (GVHD)
- Drug-induced cholestasis
- Total parenteral nutrition-induced injury
- Viral, bacterial, and fungal disease
- Cholecystitis

Day +100 and Beyond
- Chronic GVHD
- Chronic viral hepatitis
- Iron excess
- Metastatic disease
- Viral, bacterial, and fungal disease
- Cirrhosis
- Extrahepatic biliary obstruction
- Drug injury

Note. Based on information from Kim et al., 2000; Tomas et al., 2000.

---

reported a VOD incidence of 5.3% in 1,652 allogeneic and autologous transplant patients surveyed by the European Blood and Marrow Transplantation Group. Several factors place patients undergoing a myeloablative conditioning regimen at high risk for developing VOD in the immediate post-transplant period (see Figure 9-2).

The exact pathophysiology of VOD is not known. However, it appears that hepatic venular and sinusoidal endothelial injury are the key initiating events (Khoury et al., 2000; Williams & Vickers, 2000). Endothelial injury leads to cytokine and tumor necrosis factor activation, which stimulates coagulation and thrombosis within the hepatic venules and sinusoids. The resulting impairment of blood flow leads to the syndrome of hepatic VOD. These events are considered secondary to the hepatotoxic insult of conditioning therapy.

Jones et al. (1987) and McDonald, Sharma, Matthews, Shulman, and Thomas (1984) defined this clinical syndrome in seminal works. The syndrome is characterized by presentation of two or more of the following before transplant day 21: hyperbilirubinemia, hepatomegaly, right upper quadrant pain, and fluid retention. These cardinal clinical signs and symptoms remain the diagnostic criteria for VOD (Carreras et al., 1998; Zenz et al., 2001). The hepatic injury leads to various manifestations of liver disease, which are listed in Figure 9-3.

Further information can be gathered to support a diagnosis of VOD by obtaining a liver biopsy. Histopathology may reveal hepatic venular occlusion, sinusoidal fibrosis, phlebosclerosis, hepatocyte necrosis, and luminal narrowing of hepatic venules (Strasser & McDonald, 1999; Williams & Vickers, 2000). None of these changes is singularly diagnostic for VOD, but severity of disease is proportional to the amount of structural damage. Liver biopsies obtained via a transjugular approach allow for measurement of the hepatic venous pressure gradient. Gradients greater than 10 mm/Hg are 90% specific and 60% sensitive for a diagnosis of VOD (Strasser & McDonald). Transjugular biopsies are preferable to percutaneous needle biopsies because of the significant risks associated with thrombocytopenia and abnormal coagulopathies.

Doppler studies can be helpful in diagnoses of exclusion by evaluating for hepatic abscesses, gall bladder disease, and

Figure 9-3. Clinical Presentation of Veno-Occlusive Disease

1. Hyperbilirubinemia
2. Hepatomegaly
3. Right upper quadrant pain
4. Fluid retention/weight gain
5. Coagulopathies
6. Encephalopathy/hepatic coma
7. Increased platelet requirements
8. Ascites
9. Pulmonary edema/pleural effusion
10. Acute renal failure

Note. Based on information from Carreras et al., 1998; Zenz et al., 2001.

primary venous thromboses. The usefulness of Doppler in the early stages of VOD is limited; however, it may reveal a reversal of hepatic blood flow, which may be found in more advanced VOD (Williams & Vickers, 2000).

Treatment for VOD is primarily supportive in nature. To date, there are no proven effective therapies supported by reproducible prospective randomized trials for VOD (Williams & Vickers, 2000). Treatment studies have evaluated medical therapies, such as tissue plasminogen activator, defibrotide, high-dose methylprednisolone, and surgical interventions (e.g., transjugular intrahepatic portosystemic shunt, orthotopic liver transplantation) (Khoury et al., 2000; Ribaud & Gluckman, 2000; Rosen et al., 1996; Schriber et al., 1999; Zenz et al., 2001). Although some studies have shown positive results, no treatments are universally accepted. Once VOD has developed, the management of these patients focuses on treating the signs and symptoms of the disease (see Table 9-1).

Numerous earlier studies have examined prophylactic therapies for VOD with varying results. The focus of many studies has been the use of anticoagulants. Bearman et al. (1990) and Marsa-Vila et al. (1991) evaluated continuous infusion of low-dose heparin. Both groups found no positive effects from the experimental therapy. A similar study by Attal et al. (1992) found a 2.5% incidence of VOD for the experimental group receiving low-dose heparin compared to a 13.7% incidence for the control group. A more recent study evaluating ursodiol prophylaxis (Essell et al., 1998) found a 15% VOD incidence in the treatment group compared to a 40% VOD incidence in the placebo control group. Studies evaluating prophylactic therapies are as disappointing as those evaluating treatment therapies. Because 70% of patients diagnosed with VOD spontaneously resolve their disease, the current lack of treatment and prophylactic therapies support the importance of timely supportive management of these patients (Strasser & McDonald, 1999).

Nurses must provide much of the supportive care required by a patient with VOD. Close observation for subtle changes in patient status is imperative. The complications associated with VOD and possible multiorgan system failure require the nurse to have a broad knowledge base for physical care while remaining cognizant of patient and family education needs and psychosocial support (see Table 9-2).

Figure 9-2. Veno-Occlusive Disease Risk Factors

1. Pretransplant chemotherapy
2. Abdominal radiation
3. Pretransplant hepatotoxic drug therapy (e.g., amphotericin)
4. Elevated transaminases prior to conditioning regimen
5. HLA-mismatched or unrelated allogeneic donors
6. Vancomycin or acyclovir therapy (as markers of infection)
7. Viral hepatitis
8. Metastatic liver disease
9. Karnofsky score < 90%
10. Second transplant

Note. Based on information from Carreras et al., 1998; Williams & Vickers, 2000.

Table 9-1. Treating the Signs and Symptoms of Veno-Occlusive Disease

Factors	Management Practices
Strict fluid restriction/fluid management	Fluid restrictions minimize intravascular and extravascular fluid overload. Intravascular colloidal pressure should be maintained by hypertransfusion of packed red blood cells (hematocrit > 30%) or salt-poor albumin. Diuresis.
Renal function	Renal-dose dopamine may assist with renal artery dilatation and improve glomerular filtration. Minimize renal insult by dose adjusting nephrotoxic drugs.
Pain management	Severe hepatomegaly with concomitant right upper quadrant pain may require opioid analgesics. Pain also can exist from severe ascites and pleural effusions. Fentanyl is preferable because of limited hepatic metabolism.
Ascites/pleural effusion management	Paracentesis and thoracentesis can be performed to assist with abdominal pain/dyspnea; however, there is high risk of hypotension related to intravascular to extravascular fluid shifts following the procedure.
Bleeding risk	Coagulopathies and thrombocytopenia require frequent platelet transfusions and clotting factor replacement with cryoprecipitate or fresh frozen plasma.
Acute renal failure	Acute renal failure with resulting oliguria/anuria may require hemodialysis or continuous veno-venous hemodialysis for fluid management and filtration.
Safety risk	Severe hepatorenal disease can lead to encephalopathy and hepatic coma. Safety measures for confused and unstable ambulatory patients are required.

Note. Based on information from Bearman, 1995; Vinayek et al., 2000.

Hepatic Graft Versus Host Disease

GVHD of the liver is defined as either acute or chronic. Onset of acute GVHD of the liver most commonly occurs 2–4 weeks following transplant but can occur any time up to 100 days post-transplant. Chronic GVHD of the liver occurs any time after 100 days post-transplant (Crawford, 1997). Hepatic GVHD can occur independent of other organ involvement but frequently follows the presentation of cutaneous or GI GVHD.

The incidence of GVHD is dependent on several risk factors. The number of incidences rises with increased human leukocyte antigen (HLA) disparity, unrelated donors, age, sex-mismatched donor, donor parity, and increased radiation dose used in the conditioning regimen (Williams & Vickers, 2000). Risk of developing acute GVHD ranges from 35% for an HLA-identical sibling transplant to 70% for an unrelated donor transplant. The overall incidence of chronic GVHD is approximately 30% in long-term survivors (Williams & Vickers; Strasser & McDonald, 1999).

Clinical symptoms of hepatic GVHD are rarely evident. Elevated liver function tests are the first signs of hepatic GVHD. Direct and indirect bilirubin, serum alkaline phosphatase, and transaminases (AST, ALT) may reveal mild elevation or a significant rise to 10–20 times normal (Crawford, 1997). Progressive jaundice, hepatomegaly, and right upper quadrant pain are signs of severe GVHD of the liver. Patients who have signs of hepatic GVHD with concomitant cutaneous or GI GVHD rarely require further diagnostic evaluation of the liver. However, in situations where there is not biopsy-proven GVHD of other organs or when differential diagnoses cannot be ruled out by other means, a liver biopsy is required. Liver biopsy also is essential when there is evidence of improving cutaneous or GI GVHD in the face of worsening liver function tests.

Morphologic evaluation of the biopsy reveals changes throughout the disease course. Hepatocyte necrosis with lobular infiltrates is evident in early phases of the disease (Williams & Vickers, 2000). Later changes exhibit portal tract disease with biliary epithelial cell atypia and destruction of small bile ducts (Crawford, 1997; Williams & Vickers). Biopsies obtained in the chronic setting show lymphocytic infiltration of portal tracts along with periportal fibrosis and cholestasis (Strasser & McDonald, 1999).

Treatment of hepatic GVHD will vary based on the grade of disease, other organ involvement, and concurrent immunosuppressive therapy, such as tacrolimus, cyclosporine, or mycophenolate (see Table 9-3).

Grade I hepatic GVHD often is monitored without additional immunosuppressive therapy. The treatment of choice for grade II–IV hepatic GVHD is glucocorticoids at doses of 1–2 mg/kg/day. When there is no response to this treatment, further immunosuppressive therapy should be initiated. Additional agents, such as sirolimus (Rapamune®, Wyeth Pharmaceuticals, Madison, NJ), or more hepatic-specific steroids, such as beclomethasone, may be used. Liver function test abnormalities associated with GVHD may require months to normalize. More than 50% of cases of acute GVHD will progress to chronic GVHD of the liver, requiring use of immunosuppressive agents for extended periods of time. In addition to the increased risk of infection from immunosuppressants, hepatic GVHD is associated with significant immune defects (Williams & Vickers, 2000). This results in infection being the primary cause of death in patients diagnosed with hepatic GVHD.

The focus of nursing management once again spans far beyond the specific liver disease of hepatic GVHD. Specific management issues mirror much of that for VOD but also include close monitoring for signs and symptoms of infec-

Table 9-2. Nursing Management of Veno-Occlusive Disease

Factor	Management
Laboratory monitoring	Liver function tests, coagulation studies, platelet counts, renal functions, complete blood counts
Fluid management	Daily BID weights. Strict intake and output. Daily abdominal girth measurements. Restricting oral fluid intake. Maximally concentrating IV medications and hyperalimentation.
Administering medications/transfusions	Administer diuretics, colloids, blood product transfusions, and other medications as ordered. Continuously administer hepatotoxic medications, such as acetaminophen.
Renal function	Review medications and ensure dose adjustments are made for estimated creatinine clearance and hepatic function.
Pain management	Frequently assess pain level and assist with pain management strategies that are least harmful to the patient with VOD.
Patient safety	Evaluate mental status frequently, and provide an environment that is safe for the patient.
Patient/family education	Educate regarding VOD signs and symptoms, management strategies, and risks.
Identification of VOD risk	Review patient risk factors prior to initiation of conditioning regimen, past medical history, and liver function tests. Identify donor and HLA match.

Note. Based on information from Simpson, 2000.

tion and extensive education for patients and families regarding the importance of their specific immunosuppressive therapy.

Drug-Induced Cholestasis

The most frequent cause of post-transplant conjugated hyperbilirubinemia is cyclosporine (Williams & Vickers, 2000). Although extensive studies have not been performed with tacrolimus, similar clinical presentations can be seen with tacrolimus. Antifungal agents such as amphotericin, fluconazole, and itraconazole also are known to cause cholestasis (Vinayek, Demetris, & Rakela, 2000). Cyclosporine, and likely tacrolimus, inhibits canalicular bile transport and often causes mild elevations in bilirubin (Strasser & McDonald, 1999). Drug levels correspond directly with bilirubin elevation. Management of this condition involves decreasing drug doses or discontinuation of the drug, if possible.

Total Parenteral Nutrition-Induced Injury

Total parenteral nutrition (TPN)-induced hepatitis/cholestasis presents with mild elevations in bilirubin, alkaline phosphatase, and transaminases (Williams & Vickers, 2000). Clinical findings are rare but may include right upper quadrant tenderness or hepatomegaly. Liver biopsies are rarely diagnostic in drug-induced injury; however, obtaining biopsies may be helpful in the diagnosis of other liver processes (Williams & Vickers). Histologic evaluation of biopsies may reveal steatosis and cholestasis.

Abnormal liver function tests frequently normalize once the patient begins eating normally. Alteration of TPN composition or administration schedule also may resolve abnormal liver function tests.

Management goals in TPN-induced liver injury focus on returning the patient to a normal nutritional intake pattern. When this is not possible, steps should be taken to minimize the liver injury from TPN by cycling the administration or changing the TPN composition.

Hepatic Fungal Infections

Hepatic fungal infections are associated with disseminated fungal disease in 50% of cases (Vinayek et al., 2000). Patients who develop fungal infections are likely colonized with the fungus prior to experiencing prolonged neutropenia or undergoing immunosuppressive therapy. The most common pathogens causing hepatic disease are the *Candida* species (Vinayek et al.). The incidence of *Candida* hepatic infections has decreased with the common prophylactic use of fluconazole (Bowden, 1998). Other fungi such as *Aspergillus, Trichosporon,* and *Fusarium* also have been identified in fungal disease but are much less common pathogens.

The primary presenting sign is persistent fever, despite broad-spectrum antibacterial therapy, at the time of neutrophil recovery. Abdominal pain may be present in the absence of hepatomegaly. Liver function tests may reveal variable transaminases and bilirubin, with persistently elevated alkaline phosphatase. Liver function tests will worsen with disease progression.

Diagnostic workup should include computed tomography and ultrasonography; however, magnetic resonance imaging may be more sensitive in identifying microabscesses often seen in fungal liver disease (Vinayek et al., 2000). Negative radiologic examinations should not deter liver biopsy

Table 9-3. Hepatic Graft Versus Host Disease Grading System

Grade	Treatment
I	Total bilirubin 2–3 mg/dl or 35–52 mmol/l
II	Total bilirubin 3.1–6 mg/dl or 51–103 mmol/l
III	Total bilirubin 6.1–15 mg/dl or 104–256 mmol/l
IV	Total bilirubin > 15 mg/dl or > 256 mmol/l

Note. Based on information from Glucksberg, Storb, & Fefer, 1974.

as the diagnostic standard for fungal liver disease. Pathology results can confirm the presence of yeast or pseudohyphae seen with fungal growth. Fungal cultures may not result in growth and may take weeks to provide helpful information.

Antifungal therapy often is started empirically with suspected fungal infection. Drug therapy may include amphotericin B, liposomal amphotericin B, fluconazole, itraconazole, or voriconazole. Randomized controlled studies have not been performed to establish standard treatment protocols, so drug choice, dose, and duration of treatment remain questionable (Bowden, 1998). Granulocyte recovery and immunocompetency remain the most important factors in treatment of hepatic fungal disease.

Hepatic Viral Infections

The immunosuppressive therapy associated with HSCT places patients at risk for reactivation of latent viruses and acquisition of new viral infections. The degree of immunosuppression, toxicity of the conditioning regimen, presence of GVHD, and new viral exposure all contribute to the severity and timing of viral infections.

Viral infections that may involve the liver are herpes simplex virus (HSV), cytomegalovirus (CMV), varicella zoster virus (VZV), and adenovirus (Somervaille, Kirk, Dogan, Landon, & Mackinnon, 1999; Vinayek et al., 2000; Williams & Vickers, 2000). Hepatic viral infection from these pathogens tends to be low grade; however, infections can be severe and lead to fulminant liver failure and death (Williams & Vickers). Laboratory evaluation will commonly reveal isolated transaminitis, but with advanced disease, alkaline phosphatase and bilirubin levels also rise. Patients may have generalized symptoms, including fever, myalgias, and nausea and vomiting. Other clinical signs and symptoms are virtually nonexistent. Diagnostic tests may include evaluation by a polymerase chain reaction of serum for circulating viral DNA. The diagnostic standard, however, is liver biopsy with pathologic and microbiologic evaluation. Pathologic evaluation may reveal viral inclusion bodies within the hepatocytes and Kupffer cells as well as widespread hepatic necrosis (Vinayek et al.). Microbiologic evaluation includes special staining procedures to identify viral infections.

Antiviral therapies may include acyclovir, ganciclovir, valacyclovir, or foscarnet. HSV and VZV infections frequently respond to acyclovir therapy, whereas CMV infections require either ganciclovir, valacyclovir, or foscarnet (Vinayek et al., 2000). Many of these drugs carry significant side effects and require close monitoring (see Table 9-4). Immunoglobulin therapy may be added as a second agent if the disease is advanced or when the infection is not responding to single-agent therapy. No proven therapy has been found for adenovirus, but ribavirin and ganciclovir have been shown to have some activity against the virus (Vinayek et al.).

Hepatitis B and Hepatitis C

Patients who are hepatitis B antigen positive or whose donor is hepatitis B antigen positive are at risk for activation of the virus in the post-transplant period. Hepatitis B appears to become active once immune reconstitution occurs and when immunosuppression therapy is tapered (Williams & Vickers, 2000). Fulminant hepatitis with liver failure can occur; however, current antiviral therapies allow for a safe transplant course in the face of hepatitis B. Clinical presentation of active hepatitis B is the same for the disease outside of the transplant setting. The clinical picture may be clouded by the possibility of other hepatic complications, such as GVHD, VOD, and other infections. Laboratory evaluation will reveal isolated transaminitis with other liver function tests worsening with advanced disease. Antiviral therapies may include ganciclovir, lamivudine, or famciclovir (Williams & Vickers).

Patients who are infected with hepatitis C and have increased transaminases prior to transplant have increased risk of developing VOD in the immediate post-transplant period (Strasser et al., 1999). Strasser et al. found development of severe VOD in 48% of patients with hepatitis C when compared to 14% in those without. Despite this finding, the isolated infection of hepatitis C does not appear to increase risks for patients undergoing transplant (Strasser et al.). Acute activation of hepatitis C often is seen with the taper of immunosuppression and is frequently self-limited (Strasser & McDonald, 1999). The clinical presentation and natural course of the disease are not changed by transplant (Strasser et al.). Interferon has been used to reduce viral load but cannot be used while the patient is taking immunosuppressant agents. There is also risk of GVHD activation associated with interferon therapy (Williams & Vickers, 2000).

Renal Complications

Renal Anatomy and Physiology

The average adult kidney measures 10–12 centimeters and lies in the retroperitoneum between the parietal peritoneum and the posterior wall of the abdomen (Tortora, 1986). The renal artery, vein, and ureter enter the kidney at the hilus. The ureter drains urine from the centrally located renal pelvis. The vascular system enters the renal cortex and renal pyramids (striations of vessels and renal tubules), where blood filtrates through microscopic units called nephrons (Netter, 1997; Tortora). The nephron is the functional unit of the kidney and is responsible for filtration of blood, fluid balance, byproduct excretion, and pH balance. The ureter drains urine to the bladder, where urine is then passed through the urethra.

Renal Complications

Renal Insufficiency and Acute Renal Failure

Renal insufficiency (RI) and acute renal failure (ARF) are common complications of HSCT, with an incidence of 30%–80% in the first three months following transplant (Gruss et al., 1995; Noel, Hazzan, Noel-Walter, & Jouet, 1998; Savdie, 2000). Etiology of RI/ARF in the post-transplant period appears to be multifactorial in nature, with several major contributing insults. Nephrotoxic agents, including

Table 9-4. Management of Hepatic Infections

Infections	Therapies	Laboratory Tests	Management Issues

Fungal	Amphotericin B
	Liposomal
	  amphotericin
	Fluconazole
	Itraconazole
	Voriconazole
		Liver function tests (LFTs)
		Renal functions
		Electrolytes
		Fungal blood cultures
		Coagulation studies
			Monitoring of LFTs
			Electrolyte replacements
			Drug dose reductions for worsening
			  renal/liver functions
			Patient education

Viral	Acyclovir
	Ganciclovir
	Valacyclovir
	Foscarnet
	Ribavirin
	Immunoglobulin
		Liver functions
		Renal functions
		Electrolytes
		Serum for viral polymerase
		  chain reaction
			Monitoring of LFTs
			Electrolyte replacements
			Drug dose reductions for worsening
			  renal/liver functions
			Patient education

Hepatitis B and C	Ganciclovir
	Lamivudine
	Famciclovir
	Interferon
		Liver functions
		Renal functions
		Hepatitis B antigen and
		  DNA
		Hepatitis C viral counts
			Monitoring of LFTs
			Drug dose reductions for worsening
			  renal/liver functions
			GVHD monitoring
			Patient education

Note. Based on information from Bowden, 1998; Bzowej & Wright, 1998.

those in the conditioning regimen, and VOD are the most likely factors when determining the cause of RI/ARF. Less common toxic events include sepsis and tumor lysis syndrome (Savdie).

Nephrotoxic Agents

To review all nephrotoxic agents is not within the scope of this chapter. However, several drugs frequently used throughout the transplant process, such as cyclosporine, tacrolimus, amphotericin B, and aminoglycosides, have significant nephrotoxic qualities and will be discussed briefly (see Figure 9-4).

Cyclosporine and tacrolimus exhibit similar nephrotoxicity by decreasing renal blood flow and glomerular filtration rate by exerting powerful vasoconstriction (Savdie, 2000). Interstitial fibrosis, tubular atrophy, and vasculopathy result from this vasoconstriction (Kaplan & Mujais, 1996). These changes are more pronounced in patients who have received TBI and those receiving prolonged therapy with high trough levels. Although morbidity associated with cyclosporine and tacrolimus alone is low, the combined nephrotoxicity of other drugs and conditions can result in severe renal damage (Savdie). These drugs can lead to glomerular capillary thrombosis, hypertension, tubular abnormalities (with resulting hyperkalemia, hyperuricemia and hypomagnesemia), and impaired urinary concentration (Savdie). Volume depletion exacerbates renal insufficiency, and aggressive hydration is imperative.

Amphotericin B is a frequent cause of RI/ARF in the transplant setting. Lipid sterols of cell membranes are disrupted, and renal afferent arteriolar vasoconstriction diminishes blood flow, causing azotemia in 80% of patients who receive 2–3 grams of amphotericin B (Savdie, 2000). Renal insufficiency is dose dependent and is related to the degree of

concomitant nephrotoxins. Tubular abnormalities that lead to hypokalemia and hypomagnesemia also are seen with amphotericin B. Renal tubular acidosis and nephrogenic diabetes insipidus also can occur (Savdie). Adequate hydration is required to lessen the degree of renal insufficiency.

Aminoglycosides exert direct toxicity to the proximal tubules and can cause ARF that is nonoliguric. Factors that place patients at increased risk for ARF from aminoglycosides are liver disease, treatment course greater than five days, volume depletion, advanced age, and preexisting renal disease (Savdie, 2000). The most commonly used aminoglycosides are gentamicin and tobramycin. Drug levels should be monitored regularly and dose adjustments made accordingly to prevent excessive nephrotoxicity.

Hemorrhagic Cystitis

Hemorrhagic cystitis (HC) is a complication primarily affecting the lower urinary tract. Ifosfamide and cyclophos-

---

Figure 9-4. Nephrotoxic Agents

- Aminoglycosides
- Foscarnet
- Ifosfamide
- Melphalan
- Carboplatin
- Cisplatin
- Methotrexate
- Cyclosporine
- Tacrolimus
- Ganciclovir
- Acyclovir
- Amphotericin B

Note. Based on information from Noel et al., 1998; Savdie, 2000.

phamide are the leading causes of HC. Viral infection with CMV, BK virus, and adenovirus also are known to lead to HC later in the transplant process. Clinical manifestations include dysuria, frequency, urgency, and frank hematuria.

Acrolein is a metabolite of ifosfamide and cyclophosphamide that binds to the bladder wall, causing hemorrhage. Bleeding can be significant, and clot formation can cause further complications by occluding the ureters or urethra. The primary goal is to prevent HC. Hyperhydration, mesna, and bladder irrigation are the three prophylactic measures used to prevent HC. Mesna is a uroprotectant that binds to acrolein, forming an inactive compound that is then excreted in the urine. Mesna is well tolerated and is highly effective in preventing HC. Continuous bladder irrigation also is effective by rinsing the bladder free of acrolein on a continuous basis, disallowing the metabolite to bind to the bladder wall (Thomas & Grigg, 2000).

The most common viral infections that are known to cause HC are CMV, BK virus, and adenovirus. Clinical symptoms mirror those associated with ifosfamide- and cyclophosphamide-induced HC (see Table 9-5). There are no proven treatments for BK virus or adenovirus, but CMV can be treated with ganciclovir (Thomas & Grigg, 2000). There is a case report using cidofovir for treatment of BK virus with promising results (Held et al., 2000).

Hepatorenal Syndrome

The decreased intravascular volume and resultant low cardiac output that often is found in VOD can lead to renal hypoperfusion and RI/ARF. This condition is commonly known as the hepatorenal syndrome. Urine studies will indicate low sodium content (0–5 mmol), osmolality no greater than 400 mOsm/kg, and urinary sediment that is laden with granular and pigment (bile) casts (Savdie, 2000). Oliguria often develops with urinary output less than 400 ml/24 hours. Anuria will develop if renal perfusion is not increased and maintained by increasing intravascular volume and pressure.

The goal of therapy is to increase renal perfusion and increase sodium excretion. First-line therapy should include restriction of protein, sodium, and fluid intake. Intravascular volume expansion can be improved with colloids such as blood and salt-poor albumin. Renal dose dopamine (1.5–3 mcg/kg/min) may be assistive in dilating renal vasculature and increasing renal perfusion (Flancbaum, Dick, Choban, & Dasta, 1998). Powerful loop diuretics are contraindicated

Table 9-5. Recognition and Management of Hemorrhagic Cystitis

Factors	Early Onset	Late Onset
Risk	1. Cyclophosphamide (> 2 g/m²), ifosfamide (> 2 g/m²), or busulfan in conditioning regimen 2. Prior pelvic radiation 3. Previous busulfan therapy	1. Early onset hemorrhagic cystitis (HC) 2. Adenovirus infection 3. BK viral infection 4. Cytomegalovirus (CMV) viral infection 5. Graft versus host disease (GVHD)
Time of presentation	During or shortly after high-dose chemotherapy or chemo-radiotherapy	Weeks to months after conditioning therapy
Pathogenesis	1. Acrolein, a nonenzymatic metabolite of cyclophosphamide and ifosfamide, is excreted in the urine and is toxic to the bladder. 2. Busulfan is excreted in the urine and causes direct damage to the bladder mucosa from contact.	1. Not clearly understood 2. BK virus infects during childhood and persists in the kidney, reactivating in the immunocompromised host. 3. Adenovirus type II has an affinity for the bladder. 4. GVHD—role is not understood.
Diagnosis	Clinical diagnosis. Rule out urinary tract infection.	Send urine for urinalysis. Evaluate urine for BK virus by polymerase chain reaction (PCR), CMV PCR, and adenovirus culture.
Imaging	Not helpful. Ultrasound can evaluate for obstruction.	Not helpful. Ultrasound can evaluate for obstruction.
Medical/nursing management	1. Hyperhydration at 3 l/m²/day 2. Mesna; 100%–160% of cyclophosphamide or ifosfamide dose as a continuous infusion 3. Continuous bladder irrigation; 300–1,000 ml/hr 4. Hourly voids 5. Diuretics 6. Strict intake and output 7. Frequent evaluation of urine quality 8. Cystoscopy 9. Alum irrigation of the bladder for persistent bleeding 10. Phenazopyridine 100–200 mg TID for dysuria 11. Platelet transfusions	1. For persistent bleeding and risk of obstruction: hyperhydration, continuous bladder irrigation, or alum bladder irrigation 2. Hydration/irrigation is often less aggressive. 3. Cystoscopy 4. Phenazopyridine 100–200 mg TID for dysuria

Note. Based on information from Boyle, 2000; Long, 1996; Thomas & Grigg, 2000.

in the absence of other signs of fluid overload. The potential exists for depletion of intravascular volume, therefore worsening renal perfusion. Close observation of intake and output and signs of fluid overload, such as pulmonary edema, is integral to nursing care of these patients.

Conclusion

The hepatic and renal systems are complicated and intricate. The widespread effects of renal or hepatic dysfunction require extensive knowledge of all organ systems. The specialized team approach is imperative in the care of patients experiencing hepatorenal complications. It is important to remain vigilant throughout the transplant process as complications can arise at many points along the continuum. Continuing education and research are required to ensure quality and safe care.

References

Attal, M., Huguet, F., Rubie, H., Huynh, A., Charlet, J.P., Payen, J.L., et al. (1992). Prevention of hepatic veno-occlusive after bone marrow transplantation: Heparin or no heparin? *Blood, 79*, 2834–2840.

Bearman, S.I. (1995). The syndrome of hepatic veno-occlusive disease after marrow transplantation. *Blood, 85*, 3005–3020.

Bearman, S.I., Hinds, M.S., Wolford, J.L., Petersen, F.B., Nugent, D.L., Slichter, S.J., et al. (1990). A pilot study of continuous infusion heparin for the prevention of hepatic veno-occlusive disease after bone marrow transplantation. *Bone Marrow Transplantation, 5*, 407–411.

Bowden, R.A. (1998). Fungal infections after marrow transplantation. In R.A. Bowden, P. Ljungman, & C.V. Paya (Eds.), *Transplant infections* (pp. 325–338). Philadelphia: Lippincott Raven.

Boyle, D.M. (2000). Hematuria. In D. Camp-Sorrell & R.A. Hawkins (Eds.), *Clinical manual for the oncology advance practice nurse* (pp. 485–489). Pittsburgh, PA: Oncology Nursing Society.

Bzowej, N.H., & Wright, T.L. (1998). Viral hepatitis in the transplant patient. In R.A. Bowde, P. Ljungman, & C.V. Paya (Eds.), *Transplant infections* (pp. 309–324). Philadelphia: Lippincott Raven.

Carreras, E., Bertz, H., Arcese, W., Vernant, J.P., Tomas, J.F., Hagglund, H., et al. (1998). Incidence and outcome of hepatic veno-occlusive after blood or marrow transplantation: A prospective cohort study of the European group for blood and marrow transplantation. *Blood, 92*, 3599–3604.

Crawford, J.M. (1997). Graft-versus-host disease of the liver. In J.L. Ferrara, H.J. Deeg, & S.J. Burakoff (Eds.), *Graft-vs.-host disease* (2nd ed., pp. 315–336). New York: Marcel Dekker.

Essell, J.H., Schroeder, M.T., Harman, G.S., Halvorson, R., Lew, V., Callander, N., et al. (1998). Ursodiol prophylaxis against hepatic complications of allogeneic bone marrow transplantation. *Annals of Internal Medicine, 112*, 975–981.

Flancbaum, L., Dick, M., Choban, P.S., & Dasta, J.P. (1998). Effects of low-dose dopamine on urine output in oliguric, critically ill, renal transplant patients. *Clinical Transplantation, 12*, 256–259.

Ghany, M., & Hoofnagle, J.H. (2001). Liver and biliary tract disease. In E. Braunwald, A.S. Fauci, D.L. Kasper, S.L. Hauser, D.L. Longo, & J.L. Jameson (Eds.), *Harrison's principles of internal medicine* (15th ed., Vol. 2, pp. 1701–1711). New York: McGraw-Hill.

Glucksberg, H., Storb, R., & Fefer, A. (1974). Clinical manifestations of graft-versus-host disease in human recipients of marrow from HLA-matched sibling donors. *Transplantation, 18*, 295–304.

Gruss, E., Bernis, C., Tomas, J.F., Garcia-Canton, C., Figuera, A., Motellon, J.L., et al. (1995). Acute renal failure in patients following bone marrow transplantation: Prevalence, risk factors and outcomes. *American Journal of Nephrology, 15*, 473–479.

Held, T.K., Biel, S.S., Nitsche, A., Kurth, A., Chen, S., Gelderblom, H.R., et al. (2000). Treatment of BK virus-associated hemorrhagic cystitis and simultaneous CMV reactivation with cidofovir. *Bone Marrow Transplantation, 26*, 347–350.

Jones, R.J., Lee, K.S.K., Beschorner, W.E., Vogel, V.G., Grochow, L.B., Braine, H.G., et al. (1987). Venooclussive disease of the liver following bone marrow transplantation. *Transplantation, 44*, 778–783.

Kaplan, B., & Mujais, S. (1996). Disorders of renal function and electrolytes. In R.K. Burt, H.J. Deeg, S.T. Lothian, & G.W. Santos (Eds.), *On call in bone marrow transplantation* (pp. 408–422). Austin, TX: R.G. Landes.

Khoury, H., Adkins, D., Brown, R., Trinkaus, K., Vij, R., Miller, G., et al. (2000). Does early treatment with high-dose methylprednisolone alter the course of hepatic regimen-related toxicity? *Bone Marrow Transplantation, 25*, 737–743.

Kim, B.K., Chung, K.W., Sun, J.G., Min, W.S., Kang, C.S., Sim, S.I., et al. (2000). Liver disease during the first transplant year in bone marrow transplantation recipients: Retrospective study. *Bone Marrow Transplantation, 26*, 193–197.

Long, G.D. (1996). Regimen related toxicity—first 30 days early toxicity of high-dose therapy. In R.K. Burt, H.J. Deeg, S.T. Lothian, & G.W. Santos (Eds.), *On call in bone marrow transplantation* (pp. 504–522). Austin, TX: R.G. Landes.

McDonald, G.B., Sharma, P., Matthews, D.E., Shulman, H.M., & Thomas, E.D. (1984). Venocclusive disease of the liver after bone marrow transplantation: Diagnosis, incidence, and predisposing factors. *Hepatology, 4*, 116–122.

Marsa-Vila, L., Gorin, N.C., Laporte, J.P., Labopin, M., Dupuy-Montbrun, M.C., Fouillard, L., et al. (1991). Prophylactic heparin does not prevent liver veno-occlusive disease following autologous bone marrow transplantation. *European Journal of Haematology, 47*, 346–354.

Netter, F.H. (1997). *Atlas of human anatomy* (2nd ed.). East Hanover, NJ: Novartis.

Noel, C., Hazzan, M., Noel-Walter, M.P., & Jouet, J.P. (1998). Renal failure and bone marrow transplantation. *Nephrology Dialysis Transplant, 13*, 2464–2466.

Ribaud, P., & Gluckman, E. (2000). Hepatic veno-occlusive disease. In K. Atkinson (Ed.), *Clinical bone marrow and blood stem cell transplantation* (2nd ed., pp. 783–790). Boston: Cambridge University Press.

Rosen, H.R., Martin, P., Schiller, G.J., Territo, M., Lewin, D.N., Shackleton, C.R., et al. (1996). Orthotopic liver transplantation for bone-marrow transplant–associated veno-occlusive disease and graft-versus-host disease of the liver. *Liver Transplantation and Surgery, 2*(3), 225–232.

Savdie, E. (2000). Renal complications. In K. Atkinson (Ed.), *Clinical bone marrow and blood stem cell transplantation* (2nd ed., pp. 930–942). Boston: Cambridge University Press.

Schriber, J., Milk, B., Shaw, D., Christiansen, N., Baer, M., Slack, J., et al. (1999). Tissue plasminogen activator (tPA) as therapy for hepatotoxicity following bone marrow transplantation. *Bone Marrow Transplantation, 24*, 1311–1314.

Simpson, J.K. (2000). Specialized nursing. In E.D. Ball, J. Lister, P. Law (Eds.), *Hematopoietic stem cell therapy* (pp. 683–687). Philadelphia: Churchill Livingstone.

Somervaille, T.C.P., Kirk, S., Dogan, A., Landon, G.V., & Mackinnon, S. (1999). Fulminant hepatic failure caused by adenovirus infection following bone marrow transplantation for Hodgkin's disease. *Bone Marrow Transplantation, 24*, 99–101.

Strasser, S.I., & McDonald, G.B. (1999). Gastrointestinal and hepatic complications. In E.D. Thomas, K.G. Blume, & S.J. Forman (Eds.), *Hematopoietic cell transplantation* (2nd ed., pp. 627–658). Malden, MA: Blackwell Science.

Strasser, S.I., Myerson, D., Spurgeon, C.L., Sullivan, K.M., Storer, B., Schoch, H.G., et al. (1999). Hepatitis C virus infection and bone marrow transplantation: A cohort study with 10-year follow-up. *Hepatology, 29,* 1893–1899.

Thomas, D.M., & Grigg, A. (2000). Hemorrhagic cystitis. In K. Atkinson (Ed.), *Clinical bone marrow and blood stem cell transplantation* (2nd ed., pp. 806–811). Boston: Cambridge University Press.

Tomas, J.F., Pinilla, I., Garcia-Buey, M.L., Figuera, A., Gomez-Garcia de Soria, V., Moreno, R., et al. (2000). Long term liver dysfunction after allogeneic bone marrow transplantation: Clinical features and courses in 61 patients. *Bone Marrow Transplantation, 26,* 649–655.

Tortora, G.J. (1986). *Principles of human anatomy.* New York: Harper & Row.

Vinayek, R., Demetris, J., & Rakela, J. (2000). Liver disease in hematopoietic stem cell transplant recipients. In E.D. Ball, J. Lister, & P. Law (Eds.), *Hematopoietic stem cell therapy* (pp. 531–556). New York: Churchill Livingstone.

Williams, D.B., & Vickers, C.R. (2000). Hepatic complications. In K. Atkinson (Ed.), *Clinical bone marrow and blood stem cell transplantation* (2nd ed., pp. 912–924). Boston: Cambridge University Press.

Zenz, T., Rossle, M., Bertz, H., Siegerstetter, V., Ochs, A., & Finke, J. (2001). Severe veno-occlusive disease after allogeneic bone marrow of peripheral stem cell transplantation—role of transjugular intrahepatic portosystemic shunt (TIPS). *Liver, 21,* 31–36.

Cardiopulmonary Effects

Introduction

Cardiopulmonary complications are a significant cause of morbidity and mortality following hematopoietic stem cell transplantation (HSCT). It has been reported that 40%–60% of patients develop pulmonary complications at some point in the post-transplant period (Crawford, 1999a; Soubani, Miller, & Hassous, 1996). The incidence of cardiac complications in transplant recipients is approximately 25% (Shapiro, 1997).

Multiple factors contribute to pulmonary complications, including the preparative regimen, infection, underlying disease, human leukocyte antigen (HLA) disparity, and the development of graft versus host disease (GVHD) (Crawford, 1999a; Soubani et al., 1996). The lungs are susceptible to damage because of the sensitivity of the capillary bed to radiation and chemotherapy (Stover & Koner, 1997). Cardiac complications also are multifactorial and can result from the preparative regimen, previous treatment with anthracyclines, and an abnormal pretransplant ejection fraction (Brockstein, Smiley, Al-Sadir, & Williams 2000; Deeg, 1999) (see Figure 10-1). Cardiac tissue and the cardiac electrical conduction system are sensitive to damage from chemotherapy and radiation (Camp-Sorrell, 1999). Because cardiopulmonary complications are potentially life threatening or disabling, it is important for HSCT nurses to be aware of the potential for these complications (see Figure 10-2).

Pulmonary Complications

Idiopathic Pneumonia Syndrome

Idiopathic pneumonia syndrome (IPS) is defined as diffuse pneumonia in which no specific infectious pathogen has been identified (Crawford, 1999a; Kantrow, Hackman, Boeckh, Myerson, & Crawford, 1997; Soubani et al., 1996). The incidence of IPS has been reported to be 11%–17% following allogeneic transplant and 10% following autologous transplant (Kantrow et al.; Soubani et al.; Winer-Muram, Gurney, Bozeman, & Krance, 1996). IPS has a median onset of 39–52 days post-HSCT (Kantrow et al.; Winer-Muram et al.). The clinical presentation and cause of IPS varies; the only unifying defining factor is the lack of infectious cause

(Kantrow et al.; Winer-Muram et al.). Risk factors associated with IPS include total body irradiation (TBI)-containing preparative regimens, the presence of GVHD, methotrexate for GVHD prophylaxis, and a diagnosis of malignancy (Crawford, 1999a; Soubani et al.; Winer-Muram et al.).

The pathologic process in IPS is one of widespread alveolar injury. Histologically, there is an interstitial mononuclear infiltrate associated with diffuse alveolar damage (Soubani et al., 1996; Winer-Muram et al., 1996). The symptoms of IPS are tachypnea, fever, nonproductive cough, and hypoxemia. Radiographic studies conducted to evaluate or diagnose IPS include chest x-ray and computed tomography (CT). Chest x-ray reveals diffuse bilateral infiltrates, and chest CT scans demonstrate diffuse patchy opacities, thickened deep and superficial interlobular septa, and nodules of varying sizes (Crawford, 1999a; Winer-Muram et al.). CT scans are more sensitive than chest x-rays in early detection of IPS (Winer-Muram et al.).

The diagnosis of IPS can be difficult, as it cannot be readily differentiated from viral pneumonia or pulmonary edema (Crawford, 1999a). Diagnosis of IPS is usually made by excluding other possible causes, most frequently from a bronchoalveolar lavage (BAL) that shows no infectious pathogens (Soubani et al., 1996). IPS often progresses rapidly, leading to respiratory failure requiring mechanical ventilation. Mortality among intubated transplant recipients is high, approaching 80% (Price, Thall, Kish, Shannon, & Andersson, 1998; Rubenfeld & Crawford, 1996).

No proven effective treatment exists. Current treatment includes supportive care and mechanical ventilation when

---

Figure 10-1. Transplant Medications Potentially Toxic to the Lungs

- Amphotericin-B
- Busulfan
- Carmustine
- Cyclophosphamide
- Cytarabine
- Fludarabine
- Melphalan
- Methotrexate

Note. Based on information from Rossi et al., 2000.

Figure 10-2. Typical Onset of Pulmonary Complications Following Stem Cell Transplantation

Day 0 to Day 30
- Pulmonary edema
- Pleural effusion
- Leukoagglutinin reaction
- Idiopathic pneumonia syndrome
- Diffuse alveolar hemorrhage
- Aspergillosis
- Respiratory viruses—respiratory syncytial virus, parainfluenza, influenza
- Acute respiratory distress syndrome (ARDS)

Day > 30 to Day 100
- Pulmonary veno-occlusive disease
- Aspergillosis
- *Pneumocystis carinii* pneumonia
- Respiratory viruses—respiratory syncytial virus, parainfluenza, influenza
- ARDS
- Chemotherapy-associated pulmonary toxicity

Greater Than Day 100
- Aspergillosis
- Respiratory viruses—respiratory syncytial virus, parainfluenza, influenza
- Cytomegalovirus
- Pneumonia
- ARDS
- Bronchiolitis obliterans
- Bronchiolitis obliterans organizing pneumonia
- Chemotherapy-associated pulmonary toxicity

Note. Based on information from Bowden, 1999a, 1999b; Crawford, 1999a; Epler, 2001a, 2001b; Pai & Nahata, 2000; Shapiro, 1997; Shapiro et al., 1997; van Burik & Weisdorf, 1999; Zaia, 1999.

necessary (Crawford, 1999a). Corticosteroids have not been proven to be effective and may increase the risk of developing an infectious complication (Crawford, 1999a; Soubani et al., 1996). According to Crawford (1999a), survivors of IPS eventually will return to near normal pulmonary function. IPS is associated with a 60%–70% mortality rate.

Diffuse Alveolar Hemorrhage

Diffuse alveolar hemorrhage (DAH) occurs after both autologous and allogeneic transplantation, most commonly in the first few weeks (Crawford, 1999a; Soubani et al., 1996). An incidence of 21% in autologous transplant has been reported (Crawford, 1999a; Soubani et al.). Comparable numbers have been reported in allogeneic transplant recipients (Haselton, Klekamp, Christman, & Barr, 2000). DAH is associated with older age, solid malignancies, severe mucositis, renal failure, thrombocytopenia, and recovery of white blood cells (Crawford, 1999a; Lewis, DeFor, & Weisdorf, 2000; Soubani et al.). DAH usually occurs around the time of engraftment, typically around day +12 following transplant (Soubani et al.). Hemoptysis in DAH is rare (Crawford, 1999a; Soubani et al.). Onset is typically sudden with progressive dyspnea, nonproductive cough, fever, and hypoxemia. The chest x-ray findings show diffuse pulmonary infiltrates (Crawford, 1999a; Soubani et al.).

The pathology of DAH is one of diffuse alveolar damage with alveolar erythrocytes (Crawford, 1999a). The majority of patients with DAH have normal clotting factors (Crawford, 1999a; Soubani et al., 1996). Bronchoscopy fluid is grossly bloody, becomes increasingly bloodier with each instillation of saline, and contains hemosiderin-laden macrophages. There is no evidence of airway bleeding (Crawford, 1999a; Haselton et al., 2000). Mortality is high, although patients rarely die of the bleeding itself but rather because of the underlying injury to the lungs (Crawford, 1999a). The cause of DAH is unknown but may be the result of damage to the pulmonary vasculature secondary to the chemotherapy and radiation in the preparative regimen, which may be compounded by the return of inflammatory cells to the pulmonary vasculature at engraftment (Floreani et al., 1999).

Treatment of DAH includes correcting thrombocytopenia, treating renal failure, and providing supportive management, including mechanical ventilation (Crawford, 1999a). Corticosteroids have been used in the treatment of DAH with some success because of a belief that it may represent a nonspecific inflammatory response to an undefined initiating insult. However, mortality remains high, approaching 100% (Haselton et al., 2000; Lewis et al., 2000; Soubani et al., 1996).

Chemotherapy-Associated Pulmonary Toxicity

Chemotherapy can damage the lungs through a variety of mechanisms. Risk factors for chemotherapy-associated pulmonary toxicity include total cumulative dose, increased age, concurrent or previous radiation, oxygen therapy, other cytotoxic therapy, and preexisting pulmonary disease (Ben-Noun, 2000).

The pathology of chemotherapy-induced pulmonary toxicity is characterized by alveolar septal thickening with fibrosis, fibroblast proliferation, fibrin deposition, atypical type II pneumocytes, and pulmonary endothelial cell injury (McGaughey et al., 2001). Initially the endothelial and epithelial cells are damaged, resulting in fluid entering the interstitium and intra-alveolar spaces. This is followed by interstitial fibrosis (Rossi, Erasmus, McAdams, Sporn, & Goodman, 2000; Stover & Koner, 1997). The primary symptom of drug-induced pulmonary toxicity is dyspnea; other symptoms include nonproductive cough, fatigue, and malaise. The chest x-ray typically reveals a basilar or diffuse reticulonodular pattern (Stover & Koner). Pulmonary function tests typically reveal a reduced diffusing capacity for carbon monoxide (DLCO) and a restrictive ventilatory defect (Ben-Noun, 2000; Stover & Koner).

Agents used in transplant that most frequently cause chemotherapy-associated pulmonary toxicity include carmustine, busulfan, melphalan, and cytarabine (Stover & Koner, 1997). Chemotherapy-associated pulmonary toxicity is only definitively diagnosed by a biopsy of lung tissue, either with an open lung biopsy or fine needle aspirate; however, because this procedure often is not well tolerated by HSCT recipients, the diagnosis is typically made by exclusion of other possible causes.

The most sensitive noninvasive method of diagnosis is DLCO measurement on pulmonary function tests (PFTs). Diagnosis is made based on a drop in DLCO to less than 60% of predicted in the presence of dyspnea and a nonproductive cough with or without fever, or a drop in the DLCO of less than 50% of predicted without symptoms (Chap et al., 1997; McGaughey et al., 2001). Radiographic studies, including CT, have not been found to be specific or sensitive in diagnosing this condition (McGaughey et al.).

Onset of chemotherapy-associated pulmonary toxicity is two to eight months following transplant (Chap et al., 1997). Typical treatment involves administration of intravenous (IV) corticosteroids; however, the optimal dose and duration of treatment is not known. See Table 10-1 for an example of corticosteroid scheduling (Stover & Koner, 1997). Carmustine-containing regimens carry an incidence of 39%–64% of pulmonary toxicity (Bhalla et al., 2000). Pulmonary toxicity can be fatal if left untreated (Chap et al.; McGaughey et al., 2001). Initiating treatment promptly is imperative for a positive outcome. Nurses need to educate patients and families to notify the physician immediately if they develop dyspnea on exertion, a dry cough, or any change in respiratory status. In an effort to decrease the incidence of pulmonary toxicity, clinical trials have been performed using inhaled steroids as prophylaxis. The mechanism of action of inhaled steroids is not clear. They may reduce the amount of inflammatory cytokines present in the lungs following high-dose chemotherapy and help preserve pulmonary function. Inhaled steroids are easy to use and well tolerated; however, further study is needed before this treatment can be used as standard therapy (McGaughey et al.).

Radiation-Associated Pulmonary Toxicity

Radiation to the lungs can cause acute and chronic injury. Radiation pneumonitis typically occurs three to six weeks following completion of radiation. Radiation fibrosis presents six months to two years following radiation (McCoy-Adabody & Borger, 1996; Wesselius, 1999). The incidence of radiation-associated pulmonary toxicity has been reported to range from 7%–50% (Timmerman, 1998; Wesselius). The damage caused by radiation results from an inflammatory response to lung tissue damage. The damage occurs to the epithelial cells of the alveoli and the endothelium of the alveolar capillaries (Timmerman). The inflammation results in increased release of surfactant, causing alveolar wall thickening. Increased capillary permeability occurs, resulting in increased interstitial fluid (McCoy-Adabody & Borger). According to Crawford (1999b), there is a threshold dose under which no injury is detectable, followed by a steep dose-response curve at higher radiation levels. The lungs are the most radiation-sensitive structures in the body. The amount of damage to the lungs depends not only on dose of radia-

Table 10-1. Corticosteroid Administration Schedule for Chemotherapy-Associated Pulmonary Toxicity

Corticosteroid Dose	Length of Treatment
60 mg/day	5 days
50 mg/day	5 days
40 mg/day	5 days
30 mg/day	5 days
20 mg/day	5 days
10 mg/day	5 days
5 mg/day	5 days
2.5 mg/day	5 days
2.5 mg every other day	5 doses

Note. Based on information from Stover & Koner, 1997.

tion delivered but also on preexisting pulmonary impairment and concomitant and previous chemotherapy, such as bleomycin, carmustine, and cyclophosphamide (Crawford, 1999b; Timmerman).

Initially, patients with radiation pneumonitis may be asymptomatic; the first symptom is typically a dry nonproductive cough and diminished breath sounds. As it progresses, patients develop dyspnea, crackles on lung auscultation, fever, anorexia, tachypnea, and fatigue. Chest x-ray may be normal initially but will reveal interstitial and alveolar infiltrates as radiation pneumonitis progresses. A chest CT scan may reveal pulmonary infiltrates before the chest x-ray. Patients that progress to refractory hypoxemia may require mechanical ventilation. Treatment of radiation pneumonitis includes corticosteroids and oxygen. It may be necessary to continue steroids for several months. Antibiotics, antivirals, or antifungals should be instituted at the first sign of infection (McCoy-Adabody & Borger, 1996; Wesselius, 1999).

Radiation fibrosis is a more chronic reaction to radiation. Fibrosis may develop in patients who have had radiation pneumonitis, but it can develop in patients with no history of radiation pneumonitis (Wesselius, 1999). Fibrosis is a process in which the alveolar membrane is replaced with collagen, resulting in poor gas exchange and reduced compliance (McCoy-Adabody & Borger, 1996). The symptoms of fibrosis often are insidious. The patient may notice a gradual increase in dyspnea and/or a decrease in exercise tolerance (Wesselius). Late symptoms include cyanosis, clubbing of the nails, orthopnea, and cor pulmonale (Shapiro, 1997). Chest x-ray reveals "ground glass" appearance and hazy pulmonary markings (Shapiro). CT scan is more sensitive than chest x-ray (Wesselius). Pulmonary fibrosis typically is treated with corticosteroids; however, there is no evidence that the fibrosis is reversed by this treatment (Crawford, 1999b; Wesselius).

Pulmonary Embolism

Pulmonary embolism is defined as an occlusion of a portion of the vascular bed by an embolus, a thrombus (blood clot), a tissue fragment, a lipid, or an air bubble (Brashers & Davey, 1998). In the HSCT recipient, pulmonary embolism can be caused by the infusion of fat or bone spicules from poorly filtered marrow (Shapiro, Davison, & Rust, 1997). Other possible causes include deep vein thrombosis, coagulation disorder, congestive heart failure, and sickle cell disease (Brashers & Davey). Depending upon its severity, a pulmonary embolism can cause varying degrees of hypoxia, pulmonary edema, atelectasis, and hypotension (Brashers & Davey). The symptoms of pulmonary embolism are typically nonspecific and include tachypnea, tachycardia, dyspnea, and unexplained anxiety (Brashers & Davey). Chest x-ray is not a definitive test for pulmonary embolism. A perfusion scan reveals the venous circulation of the lungs and is the best diagnostic tool (Brashers & Davey). Treatment typically involves anticoagulants, although they can be difficult to manage in the HSCT population.

Pleural Effusion

Pleural effusion is defined as an accumulation of fluid in the pleural space. Pleural effusions can be the result of malignant or nonmalignant causes. In the HSCT recipient, pleural effusion most commonly occurs in the first few weeks following transplant and most often is associated with fluid retention (Crawford, 1999a). The pleural space is the gap between the visceral pleura that covers the lung and the parietal pleura, which covers the interior surface of the lung cavity (Collins, 1998). Typically, this space contains between 5 and 15 ml of fluid, but as much as 1–2 liters pass through this space every day. Pleural effusion results when more fluid enters the pleural space than can exit (Collins).

Pleural effusions in the HSCT patient can be caused by ascites secondary to veno-occlusive disease (VOD), vascular leak secondary to GVHD, hypoproteinemia, congestive heart failure, pulmonary emboli, pneumonia, lung infections, and pericardial effusion (Collins, 1998; Crawford, 1999a). Risk factors for pleural effusion include previous chest irradiation, methotrexate, cyclophosphamide, and malignancies such as lymphomas and leukemias (Collins). Symptoms of pleural effusion include shortness of breath, tachypnea, nonproductive cough, chest pain, and fever. Chest x-ray reveals blunting of the costophrenic angle and fluid accumulation (Collins). A thoracentesis often is necessary to determine the cause of the pleural effusion. The pleural fluid should be sent to the laboratory to be cultured and tested for cytology (Collins).

Treatment is aimed at eliminating the cause, removing the fluid, and obliterating the space so there is no space for the fluid to collect. Asymptomatic patients may be managed by diuresis or no treatment at all (Collins, 1998; Crawford, 1999a). The fluid can be removed by thoracentesis, although recurrent pleural effusion may require chest tube placement. Eliminating the pleural space is achieved through a procedure called pleurodesis. Pleurodesis results when chemicals are instilled into the pleural space resulting in fibrotic lesions that cause the visceral pleura and parietal pleura to stick together (Collins). The most common agents used in pleurodesis are talc, bleomycin, and doxycycline (Collins).

Chest tubes often are inserted at the bedside on the unit in stable patients. HSCT nurses may need an educational update on chest tube management, which includes positioning the patient to prevent the tubing from kinking, milking the tubing as ordered, avoiding dependent loops when positioning the chest drainage system, and increasing activity as tolerated. All of these measures are aimed at promoting chest tube drainage (Collins). Patients with pleural effusion often are most comfortable sitting upright and may require analgesia or sedation. Prognosis varies and often depends on the cause of the pleural effusion and if it can be managed effectively.

Leukoagglutinin Reaction

Leukoagglutinin reaction is a rare cause of febrile pneumonitis syndrome. This syndrome is characterized by abrupt onset of fever, rigors, tachypnea, nonproductive cough, and respiratory distress that occur within the first 24 hours following a blood product transfusion (Shapiro, 1997; Shapiro et al., 1997). The syndrome is believed to be the result of the interaction of preformed antibodies and antigens in the blood (Shapiro; Shapiro et al.). The antibodies are directed against the patient's leukocytes. The reaction is most commonly associated with granulocyte infusions. The reaction can be avoided by using blood products that are washed, packed, or frozen (Shapiro; Shapiro et al.).

Pulmonary Edema

Pulmonary edema is typically one of the earliest complications following HSCT. The onset is usually rapid and occurs in the first two or three weeks. Pulmonary edema is a relatively common complication of HSCT. The incidence has been reported in 11%–65% of patients (Winer-Muram et al., 1996). Risk factors include decreased cardiac function prior to transplant; underlying cardiac disease; previous chest irradiation; cyclophosphamide, cytarabine, or TBI in the preparative regimen; and previous cardiotoxic chemotherapy, such as doxorubicin. The exact mechanism of lung injury is unknown; however, the result is increased vascular permeability with leakage of fluid and protein into the alveolar spaces (Briasoulis & Pavlidis, 2001; Shapiro, 1997; Shapiro et al., 1997; Soubani et al., 1996). Granulocyte stimulating factor also has been implicated (Briasoulis & Pavlidis; Shapiro; Soubani et al.). Another factor that can contribute to pulmonary edema is the large volume of IV fluids that are typically part of the preparative regimen. Symptoms of pulmonary edema include severe dyspnea, cough, tachypnea, weight gain, hypoxemia, and fatigue (Briasoulis & Pavlidis). Chest x-ray reveals cardiac enlargement and confluent alveolar consolidations (Briasoulis & Pavlidis; Shapiro; Soubani et al.). Echocardiography typically reveals a dilated heart and poor left ventricular function (Soubani et al.).

Management of the patient with pulmonary edema includes fluid restriction, diuretic therapy, strict monitoring of intake and output, and supplemental oxygen (Briasoulis & Pavlidis, 2001; Shapiro, 1997; Shapiro et al., 1997; Soubani et al., 1996). Patients in true congestive heart failure may require digitalis. With careful management, patients can be successfully supported through this complication.

Pulmonary Veno-Occlusive Disease

Pulmonary veno-occlusive disease (PVOD) is a rare complication of HSCT. PVOD is characterized by narrowing or occlusion of the small pulmonary veins; this rapidly leads to pulmonary hypertension, which is typically fatal (Salzman, Adkins, Craig, Freytes, & LeMaistre, 1996). Onset of PVOD is typically three to four months following HSCT (Crawford, 1999a). Symptoms of PVOD include dyspnea on exertion, hypoxemia, and resting tachypnea (Crawford, 1999a; Holcomb, Loyd, Ely, Johnson, & Robbins, 2000; Salzman et al.). Chest x-ray reveals increased interstitial bronchovascular markings, enlarged proximal pulmonary arteries, and, in some cases, pleural effusions (Holcomb et al.; Salzman et al.). According to Crawford 1999a, the diagnostic procedure of choice is right heart catheterization with a pulmonary angiogram. Right heart catheterization reveals elevated pulmonary artery pressure with normal pulmonary artery wedge pressures. Angiography allows for thrombi to be excluded as the cause for pulmonary hypertension (Crawford, 1999a). Most often PVOD is diagnosed on autopsy, with evidence of grossly enlarged, congested, and occasionally hemorrhagic lungs (Salzman et al.). Histologically, PVOD consists of intimal fibrosis of the small post-capillary pulmonary veins. As the disease progresses, obliterative fibrosis and thrombosis with recanalization occur and, possibly, hypertrophy of the pulmonary arteries (Holcomb et al.; Salzman et al.).

The cause of PVOD is unknown; it is theorized that it occurs as a result of the toxic effects of chemotherapy and radiation on the blood vessels. Carmustine has been implicated as a possible causative agent in PVOD (Crawford, 1999a; Salzman et al., 1996). Alternatively it has been speculated that PVOD is caused by an underlying malignancy (Crawford, 1999a; Salzman). PVOD occurs in patients with coexisting hepatic VOD and interstitial pneumonitis, although the relationship is not well defined (Salzman et al.). Treatment of PVOD is difficult. Vasodilators, immunosuppressants, and anticoagulants have been used with occasional successes; however, the mortality rate remains high (Crawford, 1999a; Holcomb et al., 2000; Salzman et al.).

Bronchiolitis Obliterans Organizing Pneumonia

Bronchiolitis obliterans organizing pneumonia (BOOP) results from the formation of granulation tissue plugs within the lumens of the small airways, with scarring and occasional obstruction of these airways that extends into the alveolar ducts and alveoli (Epler, 2001a, 2001b; Thirman et al., 1992).

BOOP in the HSCT population is a rare pulmonary complication; only a handful of cases have been reported (Epler, 2001a, 2001b). BOOP has been associated with methotrexate and infections such as cytomegalovirus (CMV) and influenza, and there is speculation that it may represent chronic GVHD, although cases have been reported in patients without evidence of chronic GVHD (Epler, 2001a, 2001b). Symptoms of BOOP include dyspnea, inspiratory crackles, and nonproductive cough.

Pulmonary function testing reveals a restrictive ventilatory defect with a normal forced expiratory volume in one second (FEV_1) and a severely reduced DLCO (Floreani et al., 1999). Chest x-ray reveals patchy areas of consolidation or "ground glass" appearance and micronodular densities (Epler, 2001a; Floreani et al.; Thirman et al., 1992). CT findings are nonspecific and include air-space consolidation or a combination of air-space consolidation and "ground glass" attenuation. The consolidation is predominately subpleural and/or peribronchovascular. Nodules measuring 5–15 mm that are randomly distributed may be present (Winer-Muram et al., 1996).

BOOP can occur at any time in the transplant process, depending upon the suspected cause; though when it occurs concomitantly with chronic GVHD, the onset is typically after day +100 post-transplant (Epler, 2001a). Corticosteroids are the treatment of choice for BOOP. Treatment may need to continue for up to one year to prevent relapse (Baron et al., 1998; Epler, 2001a). Total recovery is seen in 65%–80% of patients treated (Epler, 2001a). Patients who have progressive BOOP while receiving corticosteroids have a poor prognosis (Epler, 2001a). Because BOOP typically occurs after day +100, patients and families need to be instructed to report shortness of breath or evidence of exacerbation of GVHD promptly; nurses' discharge teaching must emphasize the necessity of completing the full course of steroids prescribed.

Bronchiolitis Obliterans

Bronchiolitis obliterans (BO) is an obstructive airway disease defined as granulation tissue plugs within the lumens of the small airways, with scarring and occasional obstruction of these airways (Epler, 2001b; Thirman et al., 1992). The symptoms of BO include wheezing, nonproductive cough, and dyspnea on exertion. Pulmonary function testing reveals airflow obstruction as evidenced by severe decrease in FEV_1 and a normal DLCO (Floreani et al., 1999). Chest x-ray shows hyperinflation, diaphragmatic flattening, recurrent pneumothoraces, and occasional focal or diffuse opacities (Epler, 2001b; Thirman et al.; Winer-Muram et al., 1996). High-resolution CT reveals decreased lung density represented by lobular or segmental air trapping. The lung margins can be sharp or poorly defined. Other findings include centrilobular nodules and bronchiolectasis (Winer-Muram et al.).

The onset of BO can occur three months to two years post-transplant (Deeg, 1999). BO occurs in approximately

10% of allogeneic transplant recipients who have developed GVHD (Crawford, 1999a; Deeg; Randolph, Leum, & Buchsel, 1995; Soubani et al., 1996). Other risk factors include the use of cyclosporine and prednisone for GVHD prophylaxis, low serum IgG, and TBI-containing preparative regimens (Floreani et al., 1999). Diagnosis often is made based on clinical presentation and pulmonary function tests. BAL is useful in excluding an infectious cause. Transbronchial biopsies often provide insufficient tissue samples for diagnosis. Video-assisted thoracic surgery is the most effective means for obtaining sufficient tissue for diagnosis (Floreani et al.).

BO is typically treated with corticosteroids, initially at high doses, such as 1–1.5 mg/kg per day for four to six weeks. Bronchodilators have little effect but may help relieve some symptoms (Crawford, 1999a; Floreani et al., 1999; Soubani et al., 1996). BO carries a mortality rate of 65%–70% because the majority of patients respond poorly to treatment (Floreani et al.; Soubani et al.). See Table 10-2 for a comparison of the characteristics of BOOP and BO.

Acute Respiratory Distress Syndrome

Acute respiratory distress syndrome (ARDS) is defined as a clinical syndrome of acute lung injury that can occur in adults or children (Ware & Matthay, 2000). ARDS occurs as a result of injury to the lungs. In HSCT recipients, the most common causes are sepsis and pneumonia (Crawford, 1999a). ARDS typically has an acute onset that can rapidly lead to respiratory failure requiring mechanical ventilation (Ware & Matthay).

According to Ware and Matthay (2000), ARDS is characterized by three distinct stages. The acute or exudative phase is characterized by rapid onset of respiratory failure and hypoxemia that does not respond to supplemental oxygen. Chest x-ray reveals bilateral infiltrates that may be patchy or asymmetrical and may include pleural effusions. CT typically shows alveolar filling, consolidation, and atelectasis predominately in dependent areas of the lung. BAL reveals substantial inflammation throughout the lungs. Pathology reveals diffuse alveolar damage with neutrophils, macrophages, erythrocytes, hyaline membranes, and protein-rich edema fluid in the alveolar spaces, capillary injury, and disruption of the alveolar epithelium. Some patients have resolution of ARDS after the acute phase; others

progress to the second phase, which is typified by fibrosing alveolitis, persistent hypoxemia, increased alveolar dead space, and a further decrease in pulmonary compliance. The pulmonary capillary bed can be severely damaged, resulting in pulmonary hypertension that may lead to right ventricular failure. Chest x-ray shows linear opacities with evolving fibrosis. CT shows diffuse interstitial opacities and bullae. Pathology reveals fibrosis, acute and chronic inflammatory cells, and partial resolution of the pulmonary edema. The third phase, or the recovery phase, is characterized by gradual resolution of the hypoxemia and improved lung compliance. The chest x-ray will reveal complete resolution of the abnormalities. Pathology will typically be normal.

Treatment involves supportive care and treatment of the underlying cause of ARDS (Ware & Matthay, 2000). Appropriate treatment of any underlying infection is critical. Patients receiving prolonged mechanical ventilation may require enteral or parenteral feedings. It is important to maintain intravascular volume to maintain adequate systemic perfusion; however, excessive fluids will contribute to pulmonary edema, and vasopressors may be needed for adequate organ perfusion. Mechanical ventilation often is necessary. Typically, high tidal volumes have been employed; however, this approach may result in further lung injury. The use of lower tidal volumes is being investigated (Ware & Matthay).

Sepsis is associated with the highest risk of ARDS, approximately 40% (Ware & Matthay, 2000). The mortality from ARDS is 40%–60%; the majority of deaths are the result of sepsis or multiorgan failure rather than respiratory failure (Valta, Uusaro, Nunes, Ruokonen, & Takala, 1999; Ware & Matthay). In patients who survive, lung function can return to nearly normal within 6 to 12 months, although in severe cases and in those patients requiring prolonged mechanical ventilation, quality of life can be affected by permanent pulmonary damage (Ware & Matthay).

Pulmonary Infections

Viral

Cytomegalovirus Pneumonia

CMV is a member of the herpes virus family (Zaia, 1999). At least 50% of the population of the United States is seropositive for the IgG antibody to CMV, indicating a previous infection. As a result of the profound immunosup-

---

Table 10-2. Comparison Characteristics of Bronchiolitis Obliterans Organizing Pneumonia to Bronchiolitis Obliterans

Topic	Bronchiolitis Obliterans Organizing Pneumonia	Bronchiolitis Obliterans
Pathology	Granulation tissue plugs in small airway lumens; granulation tissue extends into alveolar ducts and alveoli.	Granulation tissue plugs in small airway lumens.
Chest x-ray	Patchy infiltrates	Normal or hyperinflation
Pulmonary function	Severely reduced DLCO, normal FEV$_1$	Normal DLCO, severely reduced FEV$_1$
Lung auscultation	Inspiratory crackles	Wheezing

Note. Based on information from Epler, 2001a, 2001b.

HEMATOPOIETIC STEM CELL TRANSPLANTATION: A MANUAL FOR NURSING PRACTICE

pression required for HSCT, there is a risk for CMV reactivation (Wilkin & Feinberg, 2000). The rate of CMV infection in CMV seronegative patients has been reduced from 40% to less than 3% with the use of seronegative or leukocyte filtered blood products (Adal & Avery, 2000; van Burik & Weisdorf, 1999). Antiviral prophylaxis has reduced the rate of CMV reactivation among CMV seropositive allogeneic patients from a high of 70% to between 20% and 40% (van Burik & Weisdorf). CMV infection is defined as isolation of the CMV virus in tissue culture; CMV disease is defined as a symptomatic CMV infection (Prentice & Kho, 1997; Zaia).

The risk factors for developing CMV pneumonia are older patient age, pretransplant seropositivity for CMV, HLA mismatch, and presence of GVHD (Zaia, 1999). The incidence of CMV pneumonia is less than 5% in CMV seropositive allogeneic patients that receive ganciclovir prophylaxis during the first 100 days post-transplant (van Burik & Weisdorf, 1999). CMV pneumonia is defined as progressive interstitial infiltrates on chest x-ray with concurrent evidence of CMV infection, such as a positive tissue culture (Zaia). CMV pneumonia typically is diagnosed by BAL (Zaia). Symptoms of CMV pneumonia include fever, nonproductive cough, dyspnea, hypoxemia, and diffuse interstitial infiltrates on chest x-ray (Soubani et al., 1996). Since the advent of CMV prophylaxis, CMV pneumonia most typically occurs after prophylaxis has been discontinued (van Burik & Weisdorf; Zaia).

CMV pneumonia is treated with IV ganciclovir and immune globulin (see Table 10-3 for dosing information). Ganciclovir may cause neutropenia; therefore, the patient's complete blood count should be monitored closely, and dosage adjustment may be necessary. In the event of severe neutropenia or resistance, foscarnet may be substituted for ganciclovir. Foscarnet is highly nephrotoxic and generally is not recommended for first-line treatment (Zaia, 1999). CMV-specific immune globulin is not recommended, as it has not been shown to provide a survival advantage over standard immune globulin (van Burik & Weisdorf, 1999). Early diagnosis and treatment of CMV pneumonia is imperative for patient survival. Survival rates of 31%–85% have been reported when CMV pneumonia is treated with this regimen (Zaia). This is a definite improvement: Prior to the advent of this treatment, CMV pneumonia carried an 85% mortality rate (Zaia).

Respiratory Viruses

There is increasing awareness of the importance of respiratory viruses as the cause of morbidity and mortality after HSCT. Respiratory viral infections may occur in as many as 20% of transplant recipients during the winter months (Bowden, 1999b). The respiratory viruses most commonly identified following transplant are respiratory syncytial virus (RSV), parainfluenza types 1, 2, and 3, and influenza types A and B (Bowden, 1999b). A respiratory virus infection can be acquired at any time during the transplant pro-

Table 10-3. Treatment of Cytomegalovirus Pneumonia

Induction Phase—21 days	Maintenance Phase (continue while on immunosuppression)
Ganciclovir 5 mg/kg IV every 12 hours	Ganciclovir 5 mg/kg IV 5 days per week
Immunoglobulin 500 mg/kg IV every other day	Immunoglobulin 500 mg/kg every week

Note. Based on information from Zaia, 1999.

cess. They most often are acquired from infected family members, healthcare workers, or the community. Respiratory viruses infect the epithelium of the respiratory tract, resulting in inflammation and necrosis. RSV is classified as a pneumovirus; the usual incubation period is one to four days. RSV is seasonal with infections, typically occurring in the winter and spring. Approximately 50% of transplant recipients infected with RSV will develop pneumonia (Bowden, 1999b; van Burik & Weisdorf, 1999). Symptoms of RSV infection include rhinorrhea, high fever, cough, and nasal congestion, which can rapidly lead to pneumonia in some patients (Bowden, 1999b). RSV pneumonia has a mortality rate of 80% in this population (van Burik & Weisdorf).

Parainfluenza virus has an incubation period of one to four days, and 22% of patients developing parainfluenza virus infection will go on to develop pneumonia (Bowden, 1999b). Symptoms of parainfluenza viral infection include rhinorrhea, high fever, cough, nasal congestion and sinusitis (Bowden, 1999b). Parainfluenza pneumonia has a mortality rate of 30%–35% (van Burik & Weisdorf, 1999).

Influenza is classified into three major types; type A is the most common, followed by type B. Type C is uncommon (Bowden, 1999b). The incubation period for influenza is two days. Symptoms include cough, rhinorrhea, and nasal congestion with or without high fever (Bowden, 1999b). Influenza type A rarely progresses to pneumonia; however, type B has a 25% chance of progressing to pneumonia in this population (Bowden, 1999b).

Standard treatment of respiratory viral pneumonia is supportive care. The use of aerosolized ribavirin has not been shown to be of benefit in clearing respiratory viruses or decreasing mortality (Bowden, 1999b). Patients who develop respiratory viral pneumonia prior to engraftment have poorer outcomes (van Burik & Weisdorf, 1999). During the respiratory virus season, all patients with respiratory symptoms should have nasopharyngeal washings tested for respiratory viruses (van Burik & Weisdorf). Transplantation in a patient with nasopharyngeal washings that are positive for one of the respiratory viruses should be delayed until the infection has resolved (Dykewicz, Jaffe, & Kaplan, 2000). Patient and family education are vital in preventing the spread of respiratory viruses. Families need to understand the potential implications of sick friends and relatives visiting HSCT recipients. Practicing good handwashing technique is the most effective measure for preventing the spread of respiratory viruses. Vaccinating family members and medical staff against influenza may help to control exposure (Dykewicz et al.; van Burik & Weisdorf).

Parasitic

Pneumocystis Carinii Pneumonia

Pneumocystis carinii is an opportunistic parasite capable of producing pneumonia in immunocompromised patients. Infection with *Pneumocystis carinii* is preventable with prophylaxis. The most effective prophylaxis is trimethoprim and sulfamethoxazole (TMP-SMZ). Dapsone-pyrimethamine can be used in patients that cannot take TMP-SMZ because of allergy or adverse effects. The most commonly reported side effects of TMP-SMZ are skin rash and bone marrow suppression. Another option for *Pneumocystis carinii* pneumonia (PCP) prophylaxis is aerosolized pentamidine. The primary advantage in using aerosolized pentamidine is that it only requires monthly administration and can be useful for patients that demonstrate poor compliance with oral TMP-SMZ or cannot take TMP-SMZ because of an allergy or side effects (Shapiro, 1997). However, according to the Centers for Disease Control and Prevention (CDC) and others, aerosolized pentamidine is associated with the lowest rate of preventing PCP and should only be used if the other agents cannot be tolerated (Dykewicz et al., 2000; Vasconelles, Bernardo, King, Weller, & Antin, 2000). Prophylaxis should be administered from engraftment until at least six months following transplant or for as long as the patient is receiving immunosuppressive therapy or has chronic GVHD (Dykewicz et al.). According to van Burik and Weisdorf (1999), *Pneumocystis carinii* infection usually results from an error in prophylaxis.

Pneumocystis carinii pneumonia presents with dyspnea, fever, and cough (van Burik & Weisdorf, 1999). Chest x-ray reveals a diffuse interstitial alveolar pneumonia that typically affects the lower lobes and is both bilateral and symmetrical (Shapiro, 1997). Median time of onset of PCP is two months post-transplant (Soubani et al., 1996). Definitive diagnosis is made by microbiologic identification of *Pneumocystis carinii* based on positive staining of induced sputum or BAL fluid or identification of *Pneumocystis carinii* cysts on transbronchial or open lung biopsy.

Treatment of choice for PCP is high-dose IV TMP-SMZ (van Burik & Weisdorf, 1999). For treatment of PCP, the dose of trimethoprim is 20 mg/kg per day, and the dose of sulfamethoxazole is 100 mg/kg per day in four divided doses given intravenously for 14 days (Shapiro, 1997). The response to treatment is good if it is started early, though a mortality rate of up to 30% has been reported (Shapiro; Soubani et al., 1996). Nurses are the vital link in teaching patients and families the importance of strict adherence to the prescribed PCP prophylaxis regimen. Because TMP-SMZ can cause neutropenia, the complete blood count should be monitored closely.

Fungal

Aspergillosis

Aspergillus is the most common fungal cause of pneumonia following HSCT (Soubani et al., 1996). The incidence of pulmonary aspergillosis ranges from 4%–12% (van Burik & Weisdorf, 1999). The incidence varies from center to center, and periodic outbreaks occur. The mortality rate from *Aspergillus* pneumonia is very high, approaching 85%–90% (Soubani et al.; van Burik & Weisdorf).

Aspergillosis is primarily contracted by inhalation of *Aspergillus* spores. Risk factors include prolonged granulocytopenia, the presence of GVHD, prolonged immunosuppression, construction in the vicinity of the hospital, HLA mismatch, and corticosteroid therapy (Mossad & Longworth, 2000; Soubani et al., 1996; van Burik & Weisdorf, 1999; Wilkin & Feinberg, 2000). Teaching should begin early in the transplant process and include ways to prevent possible exposure to *Aspergillus* (i.e., avoiding areas with high concentrations of dust, foods that contain molds, fresh plants, dried plants or moss) (Sanchez & Aberg, 2000).

The onset of aspergillosis typically occurs in a bimodal distribution either at a median of 16 days or 96 days post-transplant (Mossad & Longworth, 2000; van Burik & Weisdorf, 1999). The symptoms of *Aspergillus* pneumonia include fever, dyspnea, dry cough, wheezes, pleuritic chest pain, and occasionally hemoptysis (Soubani et al., 1996). Fungal infection should be suspected in patients who are persistently febrile despite receiving three to five days of broad-spectrum antibiotics (Soubani et al.).

The chest x-ray will vary from diffuse infiltrates, to local infiltrates, to cavitating lesions (Soubani et al., 1996). CT scan shows a halo surrounding the nodular lesions with focal aspergillosis. As the disease progresses, the lesions become larger consolidations or cavitary masses (Floreani et al., 1999). Aspergillosis is diagnosed by tissue culture; however, it may not always be possible to obtain tissue for evaluation. Fine needle aspiration or transbronchial biopsy may not provide enough tissue for diagnosis, and the patient's condition may preclude this approach. Sensitivity of BAL fluid cultures is less than 50% and has a negative predictive value of 90%. However, if acute angled fungal-like elements are isolated, *Aspergillus* should be suspected (Floreani et al.).

Suspected aspergillosis should be treated with amphotericin B, 1.0–1.5 mg/kg/day for a total dose of 3–4 grams (Bowden, 1999a; Soubani et al., 1996; van Burik & Weisdorf, 1999). Amphotericin B can cause fever, rigors, and nephrotoxicity. Patients may require premedication with acetaminophen, diphenhydramine, and meperidine. Serum creatinine and blood urea nitrogen should be monitored for signs of renal impairment. Lipid formulations of amphotericin have been developed with the hope that they will provide an efficacious and less toxic treatment option. According to Walsh et al. (1999), the toxicity of conventional amphotericin B results from the release of proinflammatory cytokines, whereas liposomal amphotericin is encapsulated in a liposomal structure that attenuates the release of these cytokines.

Studies have shown that although the efficacy of liposomal amphotericin is less than conventional amphotericin, the significant reduction in toxicity allows for much higher doses to be given (DeMarie, 2000). The dosage for liposomal amphotericin is 5 mg/kg/day (DeMarie).

Recommendations to decrease the risk of *Aspergillus* exposure include high-efficiency particulate air filtration, positive air pressure in patient rooms, properly sealed windows, high rates of air exchange, and barriers between patient care areas and construction (Dykewicz et al., 2000; Sanchez & Aberg, 2000). Growth factors have been used to decrease the neutropenic period following transplant, but they have not been proven to decrease the incidence of aspergillosis (Sanchez & Aberg). The use of low doses of amphotericin B to prevent *Aspergillus* infection has not been proven to be effective and remains controversial (Sanchez & Aberg).

Nursing Care

All patients undergoing HSCT are at risk for pulmonary complications. Nurses at the bedside are most likely to observe subtle changes in the patient's condition. Prompt reporting of changes can ensure proper and timely medical intervention and improved outcomes. Nursing care involves preventative interventions and frequent, careful assessment of the patient's pulmonary status. This includes rate and quality of respirations and lung auscultation, which should be performed at least every eight hours. Oxygen saturation should be obtained at the first sign of respiratory difficulty. Good pulmonary toilet should be encouraged. Coughing and deep breathing or use of the incentive spirometer every two to four hours are effective methods in preventing atelectasis. Nurses need to encourage patients to exercise. Activities such as riding a stationary bike, walking on a treadmill, or walking in the halls are effective. Consultation with the physical therapist to develop individual exercise plans can be helpful.

The likelihood that HSCT recipients will be admitted to the ICU varies, but admission rates ranging from 24%–40% have been reported (Jackson et al, 1998). The outcomes for these patients are poor, especially if they require mechanical ventilation (Jackson et al.; Price et al., 1998; Rubenfeld & Crawford, 1996). HSCT recipients with pulmonary complications should be monitored closely. Lungs should be auscultated at least every four hours. Antianxiety agents and oxygen therapy should help to relieve some of the anxiety associated with feeling short of breath. Both patients and families need to be educated about the specific condition and receive adequate psychosocial support. A patient's condition can deteriorate rapidly and result in the need for mechanical ventilation, so early transfer to the ICU should be considered. Some HSCT units provide intensive care, and transfer of patients is not necessary; however, this does not decrease the need for careful monitoring and early intervention.

Transfer to the ICU is a frightening experience for patients and families. Transfer frequently involves getting to know new nursing and medical staff. Ongoing involvement and support from the transplant team is critical. HSCT clinicians vary greatly in their opinions about what constitutes the appropriate level of care for these patients. However, it is not unusual for HSCT recipients to receive intensive care that includes measures such as mechanical ventilation, Swan-Ganz catheter placement, dialysis, and medications to support the blood pressure. Nurses play an important role in supporting and educating families during this difficult time. If withdrawal of life support is discussed, the nurse's role is vital. Some transplant physicians are advocating that guidelines based on the current grim mortality data be put in place to limit intensive care in cases that are felt to be futile (Rubenfeld & Crawford, 1996). Clearly, this is a complex controversy that has moral, ethical, and financial implications that will not be easily resolved.

Cardiac Complications

Arrhythmias

An arrhythmia is defined as an alteration in the rhythm or rate of the heart. The clinical significance of arrhythmias in HSCT recipients varies, and the degree of severity is typically based on the stability of the patients (Camp-Sorrell, 1999). Symptoms of less severe arrhythmias include stable heart rhythm, no chest pain, no dyspnea, and no change in vital signs or mental status. Severe arrhythmias are characterized by the presence of palpitations, anxiety, chest discomfort, dyspnea, mental status changes, a weak thready pulse, abnormal heart sounds, or hypotension (Camp-Sorrell). Arrhythmias are diagnosed by obtaining a 12-lead electrocardiogram (EKG). The EKG shows the rate, regularity, and pattern of the heart rhythm and defines the arrhythmia. Treatment is based on the specific arrhythmia diagnosed and the patient's tolerance to the treatment. Agents used in transplant that can cause arrhythmias include cisplatin, etoposide, ifosfamide, and cyclophosphamide (Camp-Sorrell; Nicolini, Rovelli, & Uderzo, 2000) (see Figure 10-3).

Cardiomyopathy

Cardiomyopathy is defined as damage to the myocardium; therefore, cardiomyopathy can cause a variety of conditions, depending upon the specific structures of the heart affected. Cyclophosphamide can cause an acute myocardial hemorrhage as a result of endothelial capillary damage (Steinherz & Yahalom, 1997). A pretransplant left ventricular ejection fraction of less than 50% increases the risk for cardiotoxicity (Steinherz & Yahalom). Radiation to the mediastinum is a well-known causative agent of cardiomyopathy. The pathology involves pericardial thickening that eventually leads to fibrosis (Steinherz & Yahalom).

Cardiac Infections

Cardiac infections in HSCT patients are rare. Among the most frequently reported causative organisms are *Candida albicans*, *Aspergillus*, *Pseudomonas*, *Clostridium*, *Streptococcus*, and *Staphylococcus* (Shapiro, 1997; Shapiro et al., 1997). Bacterial infections of the heart usually seed from the gastrointes-

Figure 10-3. Agents Potentially Toxic to the Heart

- Carmustine
- Cyclophosphamide
- Cytarabine
- Dacarbazine
- Etoposide
- Ifosfamide
- Cisplatin
- Busulfan
- Radiation

Note. Based on information from Pai & Nahata, 2000; Steinherz & Yahalom, 1997.

tinal tract. Bacteremia predisposes the HSCT recipient to valvular disease. Valvular vegetations can break off and become emboli. Bacterial infections of the heart also may result from central venous catheter infections (Shapiro et al.). *Aspergillus* is associated with endocarditis and pericarditis secondary to extrapulmonary spread (Shapiro et al.).

Diagnosing cardiac infections is difficult because the symptoms are nonspecific and include fever, chills, cough, malaise, and headache. Additional clinical findings that may indicate cardiac involvement include a change in heart sounds, EKG changes, or symptoms of congestive heart failure. Chest x-ray is nonspecific but may reveal increased heart size or pulmonary edema. Echocardiogram may reveal valvular vegetations and decreased ventricular function (Shapiro et al., 1997). Treatment should include broad-spectrum antibiotics. Amphotericin-B, 1–1.5 mg/kg/day should be started if the patient remains febrile after receiving three days of antibiotics. Fluids should be carefully managed, and administration of diuretics, digitalis, and nitroglycerin may be indicated (Shapiro et al.).

Cardiac Tamponade

Cardiac tamponade is caused when fluid in the pericardial space compresses the heart and decreases the cardiac output. The pericardial sac consists of two layers, the visceral pericardium that covers the outer surface of the heart and the parietal pericardium that is separated from the visceral pericardium by the pericardial space (Dragonette, 1998). The pericardial space normally contains no more than 50 ml of fluid. The fluid prevents friction between the two layers of the pericardium when the heart contracts and relaxes (Dragonette). As fluid accumulates in the pericardial space, right ventricular filling is impaired and may even result in the collapse of the right ventricle during diastole. This results in increased venous pressure, systemic venous congestion, and symptoms of right heart failure, such as distended jugular veins, edema, and hepatomegaly. As a result, less blood is delivered to the lungs, and left ventricle and cardiac output is reduced. Life-threatening circulatory collapse may occur. Compensatory mechanisms are initiated and may include an increased heart rate, constriction of peripheral blood vessels, and decreased blood flow to other organ systems. The end result of cardiac tamponade is arterial hypoten-

sion, venous hypertension, and hypoperfusion of all organ systems (Dragonette).

Cardiac tamponade can be caused by malignancy, radiation pericarditis, and viral or bacterial pericarditis. Doxorubicin, daunorubicin, and anticoagulants also have been implicated (Dragonette, 1998). Symptoms of cardiac tamponade include elevated central venous pressure, distant heart sounds, dyspnea, tachycardia, hypotension, and pulsus paradoxus. Pulsus paradoxus is present when the pulse is weaker or absent during inspiration or when the systolic blood pressure is more than 10 mmHg lower during inspiration than during expiration (Brashers, Haak, & Richardson, 1998; Dragonette).

Chest x-ray may reveal a "water-bottle" configuration of the cardiac silhouette. An echocardiogram is the most accurate and reliable method for detecting cardiac tamponade (Brashers et al., 1998). Treatment consists of pericardiocentesis, defined as the aspiration of the pericardial fluid. The fluid is analyzed to identify the cause, and the removal alone may provide dramatic symptom relief. Placement of a pericardial window may be indicated if cardiac tamponade persists after pericardiocentesis. A small section of the pericardium, a few centimeters square, is removed to allow the fluid to drain (Dragonette, 1998).

Cardiac tamponade is an emergency situation, and the patient typically will require transfer to the ICU. Nursing interventions include frequent monitoring of vital signs, close monitoring of intake and output, cardiac monitoring, oxygen administration, assessment for pulsus paradoxus, and administration of diuretics and corticosteroids (Dragonette, 1998). Prognosis often depends on the prompt recognition and treatment of the underlying cause and effective management of the symptoms. Malignant cardiac tamponade is typically fatal (Dragonette).

Nursing Care

The potential for cardiotoxicity should be recognized before the start of the preparative regimen. Nurses should know what chemotherapy and radiation the patients have received. Baseline EKG and ejection fraction should be obtained prior to HSCT. Nursing care requires careful assessment, auscultation of the heart, and monitoring of vital signs at least every eight hours. A 12-lead EKG should be performed prior to the administration of cyclophosphamide and 24–48 hours following the last dose. Any changes in the EKG should be reported to the physician promptly. Cardiac complications are rare following HSCT (see Table 10-4). Cardiology consultants can be very helpful in managing these patients.

Conclusion

Cardiopulmonary complications continue to be a significant source of morbidity and mortality following HSCT. It is important that nurses caring for these patients understand the potential for these complications to occur and are able to recognize the signs and symptoms. Ongoing assessment at all stages of the transplant process is imperative. Nurses

Table 10-4. Cardiotoxicity of Chemotherapy

Agent	Incidence	Dose	Onset	Risk Factors	Signs and Symptoms	Treatment	Monitoring and Prevention
Cyclophosphamide	25%	> 150 mg/kg over 2–4 days or > 1.5 g/m²/day	1–10 days after the first dose	Total dose/cycle, prior anthracycline or mitoxantrone therapy, mediastinal radiation	Congestive heart failure (CHF), chest pain, pleural and pericardial effusions, pericardial friction rub, cardiomegaly, loss of QRS voltage on EKG	CHF: diuretics, ACE inhibitors, digoxin Chest pain: supplemental oxygen, IV morphine, IV/sublingual nitroglycerin, evaluate for ongoing myocardial infarction (MI)	Identify and modify risk factors, serial measurements of 12-lead EKG, echocardiogram.
Ifosfamide	17%	Dose response trend, ≥ 12.5 g/m²	6–23 days after the first dose	Total dose	CHF, pleural effusion, re-entrant ventricular tachycardia, pulseless tachycardia, ST or T wave abnormalities, decreased QRS complex	CHF: diuretics, ACE inhibitors, digoxin Arrhythmias: Observe and treat based on seriousness of clinical signs and symptoms.	Identify and modify risk factors, serial measurements of 12-lead EKG, echocardiogram, fluid intake and output, weight, serum creatinine, electrolytes.
Cisplatin	Rare	Unrelated	Acute, within hours of infusion completion	Unknown	Palpitations, left-sided chest pain, nausea, vomiting, dyspnea, hypotension, arrhythmias, interventricular block, MI, ST-T wave changes, T wave inversion	Arrhythmias: Observe and treat based on seriousness of clinical signs and symptoms. Chest pain: supplemental oxygen, IV morphine, IV/sublingual nitroglycerin, evaluate for ongoing MI Hypotension: IV fluids, inotropes	12-lead EKG on symptoms, cardiac enzymes (CK-MB isozyme), electrolytes, especially magnesium
Carmustine	Rare	> 600 mg/m²	20–90 minutes after the start of infusion	Unknown	Chest pain, hypotension, sinus tachycardia, EKG changes	Hypotension: fluids, inotropes Chest pain: supplemental oxygen, IV morphine, IV/sublingual nitroglycerin, evaluate for ongoing MI Arrhythmias: Observe and treat based on seriousness of clinical signs and symptoms.	Blood pressure, continuous 12-lead EKG, cardiac enzymes if patient exhibits symptoms
Busulfan	Rare	≥ 7,200 mg cumulative dose (endocardial fibrosis)	3–9 years (endocardial fibrosis)	Unknown	CHF, palpitations, cardiac tamponade, pulmonary congestion, cardiomegaly, pericardial effusion, EKG changes	CHF: diuretics, ACE inhibitors, digoxin Arrhythmias: Observe and treat based on seriousness of clinical signs and symptoms.	Serial echocardiogram (LVEF, fractional shortening) if CHF suspected continuous 12-lead EKG
Cytarabine	Unknown	High dose ≥ 3 g/m²	3–28 days following infusion	Definitive information unknown, possibly cytarabine dose	Pericarditis with dyspnea, chest pain, pericardial friction rub, pulsus paradoxus, CHF, pleural and pericardial effusions	Chest pain: supplemental oxygen, IV morphine, IV/sublingual nitroglycerin, evaluate for ongoing MI	Serial echocardiogram (LVEF, fractional shortening) if CHF suspected continuous 12-lead EKG, cardiac enzymes if patient becomes symptomatic

(Continued on next page)

Table 10-4. Cardiotoxicity of Chemotherapy *(Continued)*						
Agent	**Incidence**	**Dose**	**Onset**	**Risk Factors**	**Signs and Symptoms**	**Treatment**	**Monitoring and Prevention**
Cytarabine (cont.)							Pericarditis: pericardiocentesis if required, prednisone, salsalate CHF: diuretics, ACE inhibitors, digoxin	
Etoposide	1%–2%	Unrelated	During the infusion	Definitive information unknown, possibly history of cardiac disease, mediastinal radiation, prior cardiotoxic chemotherapy	Hypotension, acute MI, EKG changes	Hypotension: discontinuation of infusion, IV fluids, slower rate of infusion, inotropes	Monitor blood pressure during and immediately after the infusion.
Dacarbazine	Unknown	High dose	During the infusion	Definitive information unknown, possibly history of cardiac disease, mediastinal radiation, prior cardiotoxic chemotherapy	Hypotension	Hypotension: discontinuation of infusion, IV fluids, slower rate of infusion, inotropes	Monitor blood pressure during and immediately after the infusion.

Note. Based on information from Pai & Nahata, 2000.

are most often the first to notice a change in the patient's condition. Understanding the significance of the change and facilitating early medical intervention can lead to better outcomes for these patients.

References

Adal, K.A., & Avery, R.K. (2000). Prevention of cytomegalovirus infection after allogeneic bone marrow transplantation. In B.J. Bolwell (Ed.), *Current controversies in bone marrow transplantation* (pp. 279–294). Totowa: NJ: Humana Press.

Baron, F.A., Hermanne, J.P., Dowlati, A., Weber, T., Thiry, A., Fassotte, M.F., et al. (1998). Bronchiolitis obliterans organizing pneumonia and ulcerative colitis after allogeneic bone marrow transplantation. *Bone Marrow Transplantation, 21,* 951–954.

Ben-Noun, L. (2000). Drug-induced respiratory disorders, incidence, prevention and management. *Drug Safety, 23*(2), 143–164.

Bhalla, K.S., Wilczynski, S.W., Abushamaa, A.M., Petros, W.P., McDonald, C.S., Loftis, J.S., et al. (2000). Pulmonary toxicity of induction chemotherapy prior to standard or high-dose chemotherapy with autologous hematopoietic support. *American Journal of Respiratory and Critical Care Medicine, 161,* 17–25.

Bowden, R.A. (1999a). Fungal infections after hematopoietic cell transplantation. In E.D. Thomas, K.G. Blume, & S.J. Forman (Eds.), *Hematopoietic cell transplantation* (pp. 550–559). Boston: Blackwell Science.

Bowden, R.A. (1999b). Other viruses after hematopoietic cell transplantation. In E.D. Thomas, K.G. Blume, & S.J. Forman (Eds.), *Hematopoietic cell transplantation* (pp. 618–626). Boston: Blackwell Science.

Brashers, V.L., & Davey, S.S. (1998). Alterations of pulmonary function. In K.L. McCance & S.E. Huether (Eds.), *Pathophysiology: The biologic basis for disease in adults and children* (pp. 1158–1200). St. Louis, MO: Mosby.

Brashers, V.L., Haak, S.W., & Richardson, S.J. (1998). Alterations of cardiovascular function. In K.L. McCance & S.E. Huether (Eds.), *Pathophysiology: The biologic basis for disease in adults and children* (pp. 1024–1092). St. Louis, MO: Mosby.

Briasoulis, E., & Pavlidis, N. (2001). Noncardiogenic pulmonary edema: An unusual and serious complication of anticancer therapy. *The Oncologist, 6,* 153–161.

Brockstein, B.E., Smiley, C., Al-Sadir, J., & Williams, S.F. (2000). Cardiac and pulmonary toxicity in patients undergoing high-dose chemotherapy for lymphomas and breast cancer: Prognostic factors. *Bone Marrow Transplantation, 25,* 885–894.

Camp-Sorrell, D. (1999). Surviving the cancer, surviving the treatment: Acute cardiac and pulmonary toxicity. *Oncology Nursing Forum, 26,* 983–990.

Chap, L., Shpiner, R., Levine, M., Norton, L., Lill, M., & Glaspy, J. (1997). Pulmonary toxicity of high-dose chemotherapy for breast cancer: A non-invasive approach to diagnosis and treatment. *Bone Marrow Transplantation, 20,* 1063–1067.

Collins, P.M. (1998). Malignant pleural effusions. In C.C. Chernecky & B.J. Berger (Eds.), *Advanced and critical care oncology nursing* (pp. 444–460). Philadelphia: W.B. Saunders.

Crawford, S.W. (1999a). Critical care and respiratory failure. In E.D. Thomas, K.G. Blume, & S.J. Forman (Eds.), *Hematopoietic cell transplantation* (pp. 712–722). Boston: Blackwell Science.

Crawford, S.W. (1999b). Noninfectious lung disease in the immunocompromised host. *Respiration, 66,* 385–395.

Deeg, H.J. (1999). Delayed complications after hematopoietic cell transplantation. In E.D. Thomas, K.G. Blume, & S.J. Forman (Eds.), *Hematopoietic cell transplantation* (pp. 776–788). Boston: Blackwell Science.

DeMarie, S. (2000). New developments in the diagnosis and management of invasive fungal infections. *Haematologica, 85,* 88–93.

Dragonette, P. (1998). Malignant pericardial effusion and cardiac tamponade. In C.C. Chernecky & B.J. Berger (Eds.), *Advanced and critical care oncology nursing* (pp. 425–443). Philadelphia: W.B. Saunders.

Dykewicz, C.A., Jaffe, H.W., & Kaplan, J.E. (2000). Guidelines for preventing opportunistic infections among hematopoietic stem cell transplant recipients. Recommendations of the CDC, Infectious Diseases Society of America, and the American Society of blood and Marrow Transplantation. *Biology of Blood and Marrow Transplantation, 6,* 659–727.

Epler, G.R. (2001a). *Bronchiolitis obliterans organizing pneumonia.* Retrieved December 23, 2003, from http://www.epler.com/boop1.html

Epler, G.R. (2001b). *Bronchiolar airway disorders and bronchiolitis obliterans.* Retrieved December 23, 2003, http://www.epler.com/boo1.html

Floreani, A.A., Sisson, J.H., Gurney, J., Romberger, D.J., Anderson, L.C., & Armitage, J.O. (1999). Thoracic complications related to bone marrow transplantation. *Chest Surgery Clinics of North America, 9,* 139–165.

Haselton, D.J., Klekamp, J.G., Christman, B.W., & Barr, F.E. (2000). Use of high-dose corticosteroids and high-frequency oscillatory ventilation of a child with diffuse alveolar hemorrhage after bone marrow transplantation: Case report and review of the literature. *Critical Care Medicine, 28,* 245–248.

Holcomb, B.W., Loyd, J.E., Ely, E.W., Johnson, J., & Robbins, I.M. (2000). Pulmonary veno-occlusive disease. *Chest, 118,* 1671–1679.

Jackson, S.R., Tweedale, M.G., Barnett, M.J., Spinelli, J.J., Sutherl, H.J., Reece, D.E., et al. (1998). Admission of bone marrow transplant recipients to the intensive care unit: Outcome, survival and prognostic factors. *Bone Marrow Transplantation, 21,* 697–704.

Kantrow, S.P., Hackman, R.C., Boeckh, M., Myerson, D., & Crawford, S.W. (1997). Idiopathic pneumonia syndrome. *Transplantation, 63,* 1079–1086.

Lewis, I.D., DeFor, T., & Weisdorf, D.J. (2000). Increasing incidence of diffuse alveolar hemorrhage following allogeneic bone marrow transplantation: cryptic etiology and uncertain therapy. *Bone Marrow Transplantation, 26,* 539–543.

McCoy-Adabody, A.M., & Borger, D.L. (1996). Selected critical care complications of cancer therapy. *AACN Clinical Issues, 7*(1), 26–36.

McGaughey, D.S., Nikevich, D.A., Long, G.D., Vredenburgh, J.F., Rizzieri, D., Smith, C.A., et al. (2001). Inhaled steroids as prophylaxis for delayed pulmonary toxicity syndrome in breast cancer patients undergoing high-dose chemotherapy and autologous stem cell transplantation. *Biology of Blood and Marrow Transplantation, 7,* 274–278.

Mossad, S.B., & Longworth, D.L. (2000). Can aspergillus infections be prevented in allogeneic bone marrow transplant recipients? In B.J. Bolwell (Ed.), *Current controversies in bone marrow transplantation* (pp. 279–294). Totowa: NJ: Humana Press.

Nicolini, B., Rovelli, A., & Uderzo, C. (2000). Cardiotoxicity in children after bone marrow transplantation. *Pediatric Hematology and Oncology, 17,* 203–209.

Pai, V.B., & Nahata, M.C. (2000). Cardiotoxicity of chemotherapeutic agents: Incidence, treatment, and prevention. *Drug Safety, 22,* 263–302.

Prentice, H.G., & Kho, P. (1997). Clinical strategies for the management of cytomegalovirus infection and disease in allogeneic bone marrow transplant. *Bone Marrow Transplantation, 19,* 135–142.

Price, K.J., Thall, P.F., Kish, S.K., Shannon, V.R., & Andersson, B.S. (1998). Prognostic indicators for blood and marrow transplant patients admitted to an intensive care unit. *American Journal of Respiratory and Critical Care Medicine, 158,* 876–884.

Randolph, S., Leum, E., & Buchsel, P. (1995). Long-term complications of BMT. In P.C. Buchsel & M.B. Whedon (Eds.), *Bone marrow transplantation* (pp. 323–350). Sudbury, MA: Jones and Bartlett.

Rossi, S.E., Erasmus, J.J., McAdams, P., Sporn, T.A., & Goodman, P.C. (2000). Pulmonary drug toxicity: Radiologic and pathologic manifestations. *RadioGraphics, 20,* 1245–1259.

Rubenfeld, G.D., & Crawford, S.W. (1996). Withdrawing life support from mechanically ventilated recipients of bone marrow transplants: A case for evidence based guidelines. *Annals of Internal Medicine, 125,* 625–633.

Salzman, D., Adkins, D.R., Craig, F., Freytes, C., & LeMaistre, C.F. (1996). Malignancy-associated pulmonary veno-occlusive disease: Report of a case following autologous bone marrow transplantation and review. *Bone Marrow Transplantation, 18,* 755–760.

Sanchez, J.L., & Aberg, J.A. (2000). The Wilkin/Feinberg article reviewed. *Oncology, 14,* 1708–1712.

Shapiro, T.W. (1997). Pulmonary and cardiac effects. In M.B. Whedon & D. Wujcik (Eds.), *Blood and marrow stem cell transplantation: Principles, practice, and nursing insights* (pp. 266–297). Sudbury, MA: Jones and Bartlett.

Shapiro, T.W., Davison, D.B., & Rust, D.M. (1997). *A clinical guide to stem cell and bone marrow transplantation.* Sudbury, MA: Jones and Bartlett.

Soubani, A.O., Miller, K.B., & Hassous, P.M. (1996). Pulmonary complications of bone marrow transplantation. *Chest, 109,* 1066–1077.

Steinherz, L.J., & Yahalom, J. (1997). Cardiac complications of cancer therapy. In V.T. DeVita, S. Hellman, & S.A. Rosenberg (Eds.), *Cancer: Principles and practice of oncology* (5th ed., pp. 2739–2756). Philadelphia: Lippincott-Raven.

Stover, D.E., & Koner, R.J. (1997). Pulmonary toxicity. In V.T. DeVita, S. Hellman, & S.A. Rosenberg (Eds.), *Cancer: Principles and practice of oncology* (5th ed., pp. 2729–2738). Philadelphia: Lippincott-Raven.

Thirman, M.J., Devine, S.M., O'Toole, K., Cizek, G., Jessurun, J., Hertz, M., et al. (1992). Bronchiolitis obliterans organizing pneumonia as a complication of allogeneic bone marrow transplantation. *Bone Marrow Transplantation, 10,* 307–311.

Timmerman, P. (1998). Pulmonary fibrosis. In C.C. Chernecky & B.J. Berger (Eds.), *Advanced and critical care oncology nursing* (pp. 512–535). Philadelphia: W.B. Saunders.

Valta, P., Uusaro, A., Nunes, S., Ruokonen, E., & Takala, J. (1999). Acute respiratory distress syndrome: Frequency, clinical course, and costs of care. *Critical Care Medicine, 27,* 2367–2372.

van Burik, J.H., & Weisdorf, D.J. (1999). Infections in recipients of blood and marrow transplantation. *Hematology/Oncology Clinics of North America, 13,* 1065–1089.

Vasconelles, M.J., Bernardo, M.V.P., King, C., Weller, E.A., & Antin, J.H. (2000). Aerosolized pentamidine as pneumocystis prophylaxis after bone marrow transplantation is inferior to other regimens and is associated with decreased survival and an increased risk of other infections. *Biology of Blood and Marrow Transplantation, 6,* 35–43.

Walsh, T.J., Finberg, R.W., Arndt, A., Hiemenz, J., Schwartz, C., Bodensteiner, D., et al. (1999). Lipsosomal amphotericin b for empirical therapy in patients with persistent fever and neutropenia. *New England Journal of Medicine, 340,* 764–771.

Ware, L.B., & Matthay, M.A. (2000). The acute respiratory distress syndrome. *New England Journal of Medicine, 342,* 1334–1348.

Wesselius, L.J. (1999). Pulmonary complications of cancer therapy. *Comprehensive Therapies, 25,* 272–277.

Wilkin, A., & Feinberg, J. (2000). Prophylaxis against fungal infections and cytomegalovirus disease after bone marrow transplantation. *Oncology, 14,* 1701–1708.

Winer-Muram, H.T., Gurney, J.W., Bozeman, P.M., & Krance, R.A. (1996). Pulmonary complications after bone marrow transplant. *Radiologic Clinics of North America, 34,* 97–118.

Zaia, J.A. (1999). Cytomegalovirus infections. In E.D. Thomas, K.G. Blume, & S.J. Forman (Eds.), *Hematopoietic cell transplantation* (pp. 560–583). Boston: Blackwell Science.

CHAPTER 11

Elizabeth (Beth) Warnick, RN, MSN, CRNP, BC

Neurologic Complications

Introduction

The impact that neurologic complications have on the stem cell recipient is not fully understood, as a majority of the literature has focused on autopsy results. More recently, research is evaluating the long-term impact that neurologic events have on individuals as survival rates improve. Most neurologic complications are associated with allogeneic stem cell transplantation and are limited in the autologous stem cell recipient. Although neurologic changes produce a great deal of stress on the immediate post-hematopoietic stem cell transplant (HSCT) phase, most are reversible with treatment. One study found that the development of neurologic complications had a negative impact on survival after day 90 (Antonini et al., 1998). Early identification and treatment of neurologic complications is crucial to recovery. Nurses with a basic knowledge of potential complications at each phase of the HSCT process are key in the early identification and treatment of neurologic toxicities. A detailed pretreatment neurologic assessment will not only enhance the nurse's ability to identify neurologic toxicities but also provide a more individualized post-transplant recovery. This chapter will focus on toxicities as related to the phases of HSCT and describe the more common neurologic complications.

Chemotherapy Agents

Chemotherapeutic agents used as part of conditioning regimens prior to HSCT use high drug dosages and can produce neurologic side effects. These side effects can be grouped as central nervous system (CNS) effects and peripheral nervous system effects. Patients often receive these drugs as part of initial treatment and may enter the HSCT process with preexisting neurologic abnormalities. Drugs commonly used in HSCT that may produce neurologic complications include busulfan, cyclophosphamide, ifosfamide, carmustine, methotrexate, cytarabine, cisplatin, etoposide, and paclitaxel (de Magalhaes-Silverman & Hammert, 2000).

Busulfan is a common component of many conditioning regimens and has been associated with seizure activity, although the exact mechanism of this toxicity is unclear. Busulfan is lipophilic and, thus, is able to cross the blood-brain barrier, accumulating sufficiently to produce seizures despite prophylaxis with phenytoin (Hassan, Ehrsson, & Ljungman, 1996). Typically, seizure activity is observed in adults after the second dose and after the last administered dose. Electroencephalograms (EEGs) may or may not be abnormal after seizure activity. In children, seizure activity has been found to be related to total dose of drug administered instead of timing, as with adults (Kobayashi et al., 1998). Seizure activity resolves without any long-term sequelae (Murphy, Harden, & Thompson, 1992).

Ifosfamide is a prodrug that requires activation in the liver by the cytochrome P450 enzymatic system; thus, concomitant use of drugs that inhibit this system may increase neurotoxicity. Renal insufficiency also can alter excretion of ifosfamide. It is thought that the accumulation of chloroacetaldehyde, a metabolite of ifosfamide, may be responsible because elevated levels have been found in patients who develop neurotoxicities. Other factors that may predispose one to develop neurotoxicity include age, female gender, cisplatin-induced renal insufficiency, hypoalbuminemia, and pelvic structural abnormalities (e.g., urinary obstruction). Acute neurotoxicity may develop within 96 hours after infusion has started and resolve between two and four days once discontinued. Toxicity is manifested by confusion, sleepiness, drowsiness, hallucinations, amnesia, clear dreams, epileptic episodes, and coma (Kerbusch et al., 2001). Irreversible mental status changes have been reported in children. Long-term sequelae, such as emotional instability, apathy, short-term memory problems, and mental focusing problems, have been reported (Cain & Bender, 1995; Kerbusch et al.).

Cytarabine is used in standard therapies to treat leukemia and lymphoma and also serves as a component of conditioning regimens used prior to HSCT. Documented neurotoxicities are associated with high dosages of cytarabine, increased age, renal insufficiency, rapid infusion, and repeated exposure (MacDonald, 1991; Schiller & Lee, 1997). Neurologic changes usually develop gradually and typically are observed several days after the initiation of therapy. They include confusion, somnolence, ataxia, dysarthria, and sometimes seizures and coma (MacDonald). These usually resolve within two weeks after therapy is stopped. Rapid infusion may cause an abrupt onset of these symptoms. Long-term neurologic effects include cerebellar toxicity, manifested by ataxia and slapping gait. Computerized tomography (CT) and magnetic resonance imaging (MRI) may reveal cerebellar atrophy (de Magalhaes-Silverman & Hammert, 2000; MacDonald; Schiller & Lee).

Carmustine crosses the blood-brain barrier and thus causes neurologic abnormalities at high doses. Vertigo, ataxia, and loss of equilibrium have been reported (Furlong, 1993). Confusion and seizures have been reported when used in high doses for HSCT (MacDonald, 1991). Headaches, facial flushing, and circumoral paresthesia have been reported when carmustine is used in the transplant setting (Woo, Ippoliti, et al., 1997).

Methotrexate is used in small doses post-transplant to prevent graft versus host disease (GVHD). Minimal neurotoxicity is associated with small doses; however, large doses can cause a stroke-like reaction. Symptoms include confusion, hemiparesis, seizures, and coma. These symptoms will resolve once the drug is discontinued. Delayed toxicity also can occur, manifested by personality changes, altered intellect, hemiparesis, and possibly seizures. Leukoencephalopathy may develop and is typically seen in children who have received cranial radiation in addition to methotrexate (Furlong, 1993; MacDonald, 1991).

Finally, a few drugs not commonly used in HSCT should be mentioned because of their neurotoxic side effects. Cisplatin is associated with sensorineural toxicity, causing high frequency hearing loss and peripheral neuropathy but rarely seizure activity. Cisplatin affects the large sensory fibers, causing disruption of position and vibratory sense, which leads to foot drop and gait disturbances. Etoposide also can cause peripheral neuropathy. The mechanism is felt to be a direct drug effect on small and large sensory fibers of the peripheral nervous system. Severity is associated with the total dose delivered. Etoposide and paclitaxel affect pain and temperature sensation, but this effect is reversible. Irreversible loss of deep tendon reflexes has been observed. Paclitaxel can cause reversible polyneuropathy of the distal extremities manifested by pain in the large muscle groups (Armstrong, Rust, & Kohtz, 1997; Furlong, 1993; MacDonald, 1991).

Worth mentioning are the neurologic toxicities associated with the use of prochlorperazine as an antiemetic. Its use has been associated with movement disorders such as akathisia and tardive dyskinesia, as well as Parkinson's neuroleptic malignant syndrome. Prochlorperazine works by blocking dopamine receptors, thus causing neurologic changes. Diphenhydramine can be used to prevent akathisia from developing but also causes sedation. Slowing the IV administration has been shown to decrease some degree of restlessness in patients treated for nausea, vomiting, or headache not related to chemotherapy treatments (Drotts & Vinson, 1999; Vinson & Drotts, 2001).

Total Body Irradiation

Acute side effects of total body irradiation (TBI) typically are associated with gastrointestinal and integumentary tox-

icities. However, there are acute complications as well as evidence suggesting long-term neurotoxicities associated with TBI. Prior treatment utilizing cranial radiation and intrathecal chemotherapy has been found to have an impact on neurologic status. An acute toxicity of TBI, somnolence syndrome, can develop six to eight weeks post-treatment. Symptoms include lethargy, headache, weakness, confusion, low-grade fever, EEG changes, and impaired cognition. The exact etiology is unclear but is felt to be related to cerebral edema that develops following TBI. Spontaneous recovery has been documented (Meriney & Grimm, 1997; Miyahara et al., 2000; Shank, 1999).

A case report describes radiation-induced myelitis in an HSCT survivor who received consolidative mediastinal radiation after TBI. The 38-year-old male developed right lateral truncal and abdominal hyperesthesia followed by right-sided distal weakness of the extremities and progressive impaired mobility 19 months following therapy. MRI demonstrated spinal cord edema between thoracic vertebra three and eight. These findings are consistent with radiation myelitis, and the authors concluded that TBI and intrathecal therapy, in addition to external consolidate radiation that included the spine in the treatment field, contributed to this patient's symptoms. This patient did recover (Schwartz, Schechter, Seltzer, & Chauncey, 2000).

Neuropsychological and cognitive effects secondary to TBI also have been studied in adult and pediatric populations, with conflicting results. A study evaluating the intelligence quotient (IQ) of a small sample of children (N = 73) who received TBI as part of their conditioning regimen found these children experienced a reduction in IQ during the first year following transplant. However, some improvement was observed at three years (Chou et al., 1996). Similar results have been observed when studying adult populations recovering from TBI. Wenz et al. (1999) found no changes in IQ when testing adults one hour before and one hour after TBI; however, this group (N = 22) scored lower than normal in pretreatment attention. This was felt to be a result of pretreatment anxiety (Wenz et al., 1999). A similar study evaluated patients (N = 21) at six months and 36 months after TBI. No changes were found in IQ or attention (Wenz et al., 2000). Extensive neuropsychological evaluations of 21 individuals over a 10-year period after TBI found performance to be comparable to pretreatment level (Peper et al., 2000). These studies used small patient populations. All authors suggested further studies, larger populations, and longer intervals of testing.

Cognitive dysfunction has been found to have an impact on HSCT survivors. In an early study, Andrykowski et al. (1990) found reduced cognitive function in 30 patients receiving TBI when tested between two and seven years after HSCT. They identified difficulty with problem solving, attention deficits, difficulty with concentration, and slowed reaction times. Another study evaluated a variety of HSCT recipients whose treatment may have included intrathecal chemotherapy, TBI, and/or high-dose chemotherapy (N = 42). Both cognitive and neuropsychiatric evaluations were performed. Twenty-eight percent experienced memory problems, whereas 17.5% demonstrated attention deficits. Impaired executive function and speed with which information was processed was found to be impaired after transplant. When quality of life and mood were evaluated, findings suggested that fatigue and physical limitations had an impact on the cognitive status of survivors. A majority of the participants received allogeneic HSCT (Harder et al., 2002).

Although data show conflicting results with regard to the long-term sequelae secondary to TBI, it would seem logical to evaluate HSCT survivors for any complaints regarding cognition and social functioning. Further studies are necessary to help delineate these treatment-related side effects.

Dimethyl Sulfoxide

Although it is generally felt that most treatment-associated toxicities often affect the outcome of the allogeneic recipient, the actual autologous stem cell infusion can carry a risk. Autologous stem cells are stored after mobilization and then reinfused after a conditioning regimen is administered. The stem cells are stored using dimethyl sulfoxide (DMSO) as a preservative. There have been reported cases of neurologic events occurring during the actual stem cell infusion, which are felt to be a direct effect of DMSO. It has been suggested that DMSO can cause cerebral ischemia resulting from acute vasospasm, thus impairing cerebral perfusion. Hypotension during stem cell infusion is common. Hoyt, Szer, and Gregg (2000) reported neurologic events in three of 179 patients receiving 10% DMSO with autologous stem cells. They reported transient global amnesia in one patient, a cerebral hemorrhagic infarct in a second, and a third who developed nystagmus, eye deviations, altered gag reflex, and bilateral positive Babinski reflex. A CT scan of the third patient demonstrated early infarct near the left cerebral artery. Although evidence is not clear as to the exact cause of these events, animal models suggest that cerebral vasospasm occurs, with infusion of DMSO as the causative agent. There also are reports of two cases of encephalopathy following autologous stem cell infusion that were thought to be a direct effect of DMSO (Dhodapkar, Goldberg, Terreri, & Gertz, 1994).

Immunosuppressant Agents

Cyclosporine (CSA) and tacrolimus (FK-506) are drugs that inhibit T cell production, thus preventing GVHD; however, they can have a profound effect on the CNS. HSCT recipients have a higher rate of neurologic events than those receiving solid organ transplant. This is felt to be related to drugs used prior to transplant, the effects of GVHD, and greater antibiotic use in the immediate post-transplant period (Koehler et al., 1995). Neurotoxicity secondary to immunosuppressants usually develops within one month of transplant (Garcia-Escrig, Martinez, Fernandez-Ponsati, Diaz, & Soto, 1994). Neurologic symptoms specific to CSA and FK-506 include tremor, confusion, agitation, headache, burning sensation of the palms and plantar regions, somnolence,

seizures, visual disturbances, and cortical blindness (de Brabander, Cornelissen, Sillervis-Smitt, Vecht, & van den Bent, 2000; Kahan, 1989; Steg, Kessinger, & Wszolek, 1999). In addition, CSA can induce a reversible extrapyramidal syndrome (Reece et al., 1991). FK-506 has been associated with problems of coordination, myoclonus, and psychosis (de Magalhaes-Silverman & Hammert, 2000). Both drugs have been associated with reversible leukoencephalopathy or changes in the white matter of the brain. Radiographic evaluation has documented this finding to occur one to eight days after the initiation of therapy (Bartynski et al., 2001). The incidence of drug-induced seizure activity can be as high as 25% (Gracia-Escrig et al., 1994). The exact mechanism of CSA/FK-506 neurotoxicity is unclear; however, some factors may predispose one to develop CNS changes. High circulating drug-blood levels, hypertension, renal dysfunction, hypomagnesemia, low cholesterol levels, and concurrent use of steroids have been factors identified as contributing to the development of seizures. Additionally, endothelial damage resulting in disruption of the blood-brain barrier and vasculopathy leading to brain hypoperfusion may cause seizures (Bartynski et al.; Trullemans, Grignard, Van Camp, & Schots, 2001; Woo, Przepiorka, et al., 1997). Sepsis also has been cited as another factor predisposing one to seizures (Woo, Przepiorka, et al.). Trullemans et al. reviewed the clinical records of 129 allogeneic HSCT recipients and found three who developed prodromal symptoms of headache, agitation, and confusion preceding seizure activity. When evaluating imaging studies of the brain in patients receiving CSA or FK-506, Bartynski et al. found that conditioning regimens had an impact on brain changes in patients who experienced abnormalities. Those who received cyclophosphamide with TBI had changes only in white matter, whereas those who received cyclophosphamide with thiotepa or busulfan developed additional cortical abnormalities, with cortical enhancement on radiographic evaluation. Edema was present at the lesion site. This suggests that CNS toxicity also may be affected by conditioning regimens. Discontinuation of the immunosuppressive agent will result in total reversal of symptoms, including brain abnormalities. CSA or FK-506 can be reintroduced at a lower dose or changed to the alternative drug (Bartynski et al.; Steg et al.).

Corticosteroids have a dual purpose in HSCT as antiemetics as well as in combination with other immunosuppressants to treat GVHD; prednisone, dexamethasone, and methylprednisolone are the most commonly used. Neuropsychiatric effects encompass a wide variety of symptoms ranging from mild mood disturbances to overt psychosis. Figure 11-1 lists some of the documented steroid-induced neuropsychiatric symptoms.

These symptoms are usually dose dependent and resolve once the drug has been withdrawn. Unfortunately, corticosteroids are used for an extended period of time to treat GVHD; thus, symptom management is often the preferred route to deal with side effects. Many times the addition of an antianxiety agent or neuroleptic medication may be helpful when attempting to control symptoms (de Magalhaes-

Figure 11-1. Neuropsychiatric Symptoms of Steroids

- Depression, anxiety, delirium
- Mania, euphoria, agitation
- Hallucinations, sleep disturbance, tremor
- Dysphoria, vivid dreams, nervousness
- Psychosis

Note. Based on information from de Magalhaes-Silverman & Hammert, 2000; Furlong, 1993; Meriney & Grimm, 1997.

Silverman & Hammert, 2000; MacDonald, 1991; Openshaw & Slatkin, 1999).

High-dose steroids administered for more than three weeks are associated with myopathy (Openshaw & Slatkin, 1999). Patients develop symmetrical changes of the proximal muscle groups resulting in weakness and decreased function with muscle atrophy. Symptoms include difficulty rising from a seated position, climbing stairs, or raising one's arms. Complaints of muscle tenderness and cramping also may accompany motor deficit. Neurologic examination shows extremity weakness. Electromyographic evaluation may be normal or show myopathic changes. Muscle biopsy typically shows type IIB fiber atrophy, which is a nonspecific finding. Treatment includes steroid taper, if possible, changing the type of steroid and physical therapy (de Magalhaes-Silverman & Hammert, 2000; Furlong, 1993; Meriney & Grimm, 1997; Openshaw & Slatkin). Fluorinated steroids, such as dexamethasone, are more myopathic than non-fluorinated agents, such as prednisone and methylprednisolone (Openshaw & Slatkin).

Anti-Infectives

Antibiotics and antivirals used to treat infection also have neurologic side effects. Certain factors appear to predispose one to develop CNS changes while undergoing drug therapy. Impaired renal function seems to play the most important role in the development of neurologic changes. Other risk factors include improper dosing, concurrent neurotoxic agents that decrease seizure threshold, concurrent nephrotoxic drugs, older age, and preexisting neurologic disorders. In most cases, removal of the agent will cause a gradual disappearance of the neurologic symptom. Adjusting the drug dosage for renal impairment is always suggested (Chatellier et al., 2002; Ernst & Franey, 1998; Snavely & Hodges, 1984).

Imipenem-cilastatin is associated with confusion, myoclonus, and seizures (Rivera, Crespo, Teruel, Marcen, & Ortuno, 1999). Seizures have been observed as early as 36 hours after initiation of therapy and as long as seven days after treatment was started. Carbapenem and meropenem also have been noted to have neurologic side effects (Wallace, 1997). Cephalosporins and other beta-lactamin antibiotics can cause headache, behavioral changes, confusion, hallucinations, nystagmus, seizures, and myoclonic jerks. Seizure activity is thought to be a result of the drug's direct effect at

the neurotransmitter gamma-aminobutyric acid. It is thought to act as a competitive antagonist at this site, inhibiting neurotransmission (Chatellier et al., 2002; Snavely & Hodges, 1984; Wong, Chan, Chan, & Li, 1999). Penicillin is thought to cause seizure activity by the same mechanism when high dosages are administered. Existing renal dysfunction is thought to play an important role in penicillin-induced seizure activity. Myoclonus and tonic clonic-type seizure activity also have been observed (Wallace).

Aminoglycosides can cause irreversible damage to the cochlea, resulting in unilateral or bilateral hearing loss. Initially, patients will complain of tinnitus or ear fullness with accompanying changes in hearing acuity. Actual hearing loss is the result of destruction to the sensory hair cells located in the inner ear. Concomitant use of loop diuretics may potentiate ototoxicity. These drugs also have caused vestibular damage, resulting in dizziness, gait disturbances, and nystagmus. One may develop compensatory adaptation to these neurologic effects. Neuromuscular blockade also has been documented. Incidentally, neurotoxicities from aminoglycosides may develop long after therapy has been discontinued. Vancomycin can cause hearing loss secondary to effects on the eighth cranial nerve. Finally, metronidazole can cause sensory peripheral neuropathy, gait disturbances, and seizures; however, these symptoms are associated with long-term drug administration (Snavely & Hodges, 1984; Wallace, 1997).

Cephalosporins have been found to cause nonconvulsive status epilepticus in patients with concurrent renal failure. Symptoms include decreased level of consciousness with disorientation and agitation. Myoclonic jerking has been documented. EEG demonstrates a pattern consistent with status epilepticus. Removal of the cephalosporin and treatment with an anticonvulsant produces improvement of symptoms (Martinez-Rodriguez et al., 2001).

Antiviral drugs also have induced neurologic toxicities that seem to be potentiated by concurrent renal impairment. Neurologic changes have been observed in those recipients with normal renal function, but less frequently. Discontinuation of the drug will reverse any effects, although there have been reports of ganciclovir re-challenge causing a return of the neurologic symptom(s) in patients with HIV. Acyclovir and ganciclovir are commonly used to treat varicella and cytomegalovirus (CMV) infections, respectively, in the transplant setting. Onset of neurologic symptoms is observed 24–72 hours after initiation of therapy and varies widely in presentation. Acyclovir has been documented to cause headache, vertigo, tremor, somnolence, depression, confusion, visual and motor impairment, paresthesias, aphasia, and epileptic seizures (Barkholt, Lewensohn-Fuchs, Ericzon, Tyden, & Andersson, 1999). Additional symptoms reported include myoclonus, agitation, hallucinations, dysarthria, asterixia, hemiparesthesia, and seizures (Ernst & Franey, 1998). Ganciclovir has caused confusion, headache, mental status changes, delirium, and agitation. Foscarnet, another antiviral agent used to treat CMV retinitis, has been reported to cause paresthesias and seizures (Barkholt et al.; Blohm,

Nurnberger, Aulich, Engelbrecht, & Burdach, 1997; Ernst & Franey; Openshaw & Slatkin, 1999).

Infections

Sources of CNS complications with an infectious etiology present during specific time periods during HSCT. Bacterial, fungal, and viral infections are seen during the period of neutropenia prior to engraftment, approximately 30 days after HSCT. Microbial prophylaxis has significantly decreased occurrence (de Magalhaes-Silverman & Hammert, 2000; Openshaw & Slatkin, 1999). After engraftment and during immunosuppressive therapy to treat GVHD, common pathogens include viruses, fungi, and parasites. Because autologous HSCT recipients do not require immunosuppressive therapy, CNS infection rates are low. Maschke et al. (1999) found CNS infections only in those patients (N = 571) who underwent allogeneic HSCT. A wide range of symptoms may be encountered if a CNS infection develops. Concomitant immunosuppressive therapy may alter specific presenting symptoms. Fever, headache, nucal rigidity, seizures (McLean & Douen, 2002), mental status changes, delirium, and depressed sensorium (Openshaw & Slatkin) may develop. Also, abnormalities found during neurologic examination will be specific to the area of the brain involved and will be verified radiographically. Factors influencing susceptibility include disruption of the blood-brain barrier, such as past treatment with TBI. CT, MRI, and cerebrospinal fluid evaluation should be included when any neurologic abnormality is found.

Bacterial etiologies are reported less frequently as causes of CNS infections. Bleggi-Torres et al. (2000) evaluated 180 autologous and allogeneic HSCT recipients at autopsy and found 27 (15%) to have CNS infections; however, only three cases were of bacterial origin. Bacterial pathogens included *Streptococcus epidermides* and *Staphylococcus aureus*. *Pseudomonas aerogenous*, *Hemophilus influenzae* and *Pneumococcus* were found by de Brabander et al. (2000) when studying neurologic complications of allogeneic HSCT recipients who received a graft from an alternative donor. *Nocardiosis* CNS infections also were found in HSCT recipients. They found *Nocardiosis* species to occur between one and six months post-HSCT exclusively in the allogeneic populations. Other bacterial offenders included *Klebsiella pneumoniae* and *Stenotrophomonas maltophilia*, but they did not delineate if these organisms were common to both solid organ and HSCT recipients or exclusive to one group.

Fungal infections of the CNS are found in allogeneic HSCT populations secondary to immunosuppression. *Aspergillus*, followed by *Candida*, is the most common infection and develops approximately 30 days after transplant. CNS invasion is the result of hematogenous spread or entrance via the nasal sinus, causing necrotic lesions with extension into surrounding vessels causing hemorrhage. Mortality rates are extremely high. Autopsy evaluation by Torres-Bleggi et al. (2000) found eight causes of death in 180 HSCT recipients to be caused by fungus. Likewise, of the 571 patients studied who were undergoing treatment of GVHD, 6 were found to have CNS fungal infections, and all 6 died (Maschke et al., 1999).

Viral infections of the CNS are uncommon and result from reactivation of a prior exposure. Human herpes virus 6 (HHV-6) is felt to pose the greatest threat to the CNS as opposed to other herpes viruses. After exposure during childhood, it lies dormant and reactivates during periods of immunosuppression, attacking CD4 lymphocytes, suggesting hematogenous spread. Infection has been documented to occur between two and four weeks and as long as 45 days after transplant. Specific symptoms include fever, abnormalities of speech, headache, seizures, mental status changes, and possibly coma (Singh & Husain, 2000). One report indicated amnesia as a presenting symptom (McLean & Douen, 2002). Cerebral spinal fluid samples may be positive. Radiographic examination may be unremarkable or indicate non-enhancing lesion of the white and gray matter. Foscarnet and ganciclovir have been effective in treatment, but some cases resolve spontaneously. When evaluating data on both organ and bone marrow transplant recipients, Singh and Husain found a mortality rate of 58% when patients developed HHV-6 infections. HHV-6 may predispose one to develop concurrent viral infections with CMV and Epstein-Barr virus. However, neurologic invasion by these viruses is not a common problem in the transplant setting, especially because CMV surveillance is a common practice. Varicella zoster virus (VZV) reactivation can occur; however, the disease is usually restricted to a specific dermatomal distribution or the viscera and responds well to antiviral therapy. Painful peripheral neuropathy has been associated with VZV. A case report describing an allogeneic bone marrow transplant recipient who developed meningoencephalitis after completing treatment for VZV rash was found in the literature (Tauro, Toh, Osman, & Mahendra, 2000).

A late complication of allogeneic HSCT is *Toxoplasmosis gondii*. This is a protozoan usually contracted from ingestion of oocysts found in infected food sources. A cyst will form in body tissues containing trophozoites. The CNS is a predominantly invaded organ. During immunosuppression, reactivation of the infection will occur. Specific neurologic symptoms include fever unresponsive to antibiotics (Zver, Cernelc, Mlakar, & Pretnar, 1999), mental status abnormalities, headache, seizures, and radiographic findings consistent with a cyst-like formation with ring enhancement in the periventricular region (Singh & Husain, 2000). Seropositive patients pretransplant or those with seropositive donors are at risk. Bactrim is felt to provide some protection against reactivation; however, infection is treated with clindamycin and pyrimethamine. Roemer et al. (2001) evaluated 301 matched alternative donors, allogeneic matched donors, and allogeneic mismatched recipients and found that six developed toxoplasmosis after Day 90. Interestingly, these six received either a matched alternative donor or allogeneic mismatched transplant, and no cases have been reported in autologous HSCT recipients (Singh & Husain). It has been suggested that extending Bactrim prophylaxis in high-risk HSCT recipients may help to prevent reactivation (Roemer et al.; Zver et al.).

Cerebrovascular

Intracranial hemorrhages, subdural hematomas, and ischemic strokes are three cerebrovascular complications of transplant. They are found in both allogeneic and autologous transplantation, with a slight increase in risk to patients with alternative donor transplants (de Brabander et al., 2000).

Intracranial hemorrhage occurs in approximately 2%–4% of both autologous and allogeneic patients (de Brabander et al., 2000; Graus et al., 1996; Pomeranz et al., 1994) and usually is related to refractory thrombocytopenia. In a review by Graus et al., both the diagnosis of acute myelogenous leukemia (AML) and platelet refractoriness were found to be risk factors for intracranial hemorrhages. This was thought to be because patients undergoing autologous transplant for AML experienced prolonged hematologic recovery and had higher platelet transfusion requirements.

In patients experiencing a CNS bleed, CT scan is preferable to MRI for evaluation. The clinical course can begin with the onset of hemiparesis or other localized neurologic defect, followed by depression of the sensorium, to other symptoms of brainstem herniation (Oppenshaw & Slatkin, 1999). Treatment involves aggressive platelet support and correction of any coagulopathies. Prophylactic platelet transfusions for platelet counts under 10,000–20,000/mm³ have decreased the incidence of life-threatening CNS bleeding.

Subdural hematomas are another cerebrovascular complication of transplant. They are frequently unrecognized because they present as a decrease in the patient's sensorium. These symptoms often are attributed to sedation or other metabolic etiologies. They have been reported in 5%–6% of patients after transplant (Staudinger et al., 1998). One study noted subdural hematomas to occur more frequently in patients undergoing autologous transplant, with this finding related to platelet refractoriness. An association also was noted between subdural hematomas and methotrexate-containing conditioning therapy, postlumbar puncture headache, prolonged thrombocytopenia, and coagulopathy (Colosimo et al., 2000). For subdural hematomas, CT scanning is preferable to MRI in evaluating patients. Treatment is directed at aggressive platelet support and correction of coagulopathies. Surgery usually is reserved for neurologic deterioration.

Subdural hygromas also have been noted post-transplant. A hygroma is a subdural fluid collection that appears hypodense on CT scan, ruling out hemorrhage as the underlying etiology of the defect. They usually present with the symptoms of nausea, vomiting, and headache. The cause is unclear. They are thought to be related to conditioning with high-dose chemotherapy and TBI. They occur within the first 30 days post-transplant with an incidence of 18%. Thrombocytopenia has not been found to be a risk factor. Hygromas are reversible and resolve within two to three months without surgical intervention, giving them a good overall prognosis (Staudinger et al., 1998).

The incidence of ischemic stroke in transplant recipients is low and ranges from 0.35%–3.3% (Antonini et al., 1998). The causes of stroke can be embolic from local thrombosis or from infectious causes.

A hypercoagulable state post-transplant has been identified as one cause of embolic stroke. Following autologous transplant, a decrease in the anticoagulants protein C and antithrombin with an increase in fibrinogen occurs. Following allogeneic transplant, this decrease in protein C levels also has been identified (de Magalhaes-Silverman & Hammert, 2000; Oppenshaw & Slatkin, 1999).

Stroke also can result from a local thrombosis or embolus from infectious or nonbacterial thrombotic endocarditis. These events usually occur in the early post-transplant period.

Infectious causes of stroke usually are related to fungal organisms, most commonly aspergillosis (Davis & Patchell, 1988; Oppenshaw & Slatkin, 1999). In a series evaluating stroke post-transplant, fungal infections were reported as a cause in 30.6% of patients. Unfortunately, 69% of patients experiencing stroke post-transplant do not survive. This percentage is likely higher, as many patients do not undergo autopsy (Coplin, Cochran, Levine, & Crawford, 2001).

Encephalopathy

Encephalopathies related to treatment include leukoencephalopathy and metabolic encephalopathy. Metabolic encephalopathy is one of the most common neurologic toxicities associated with transplant.

Leukoencephalopathy occurs in 7% of patients post-transplant and is a syndrome where the white matter of the brain is irreversibly damaged (Furlong, 1993). It may occur days to months post-transplant. Risk factors include extensive intrathecal methotrexate administration alone or in combination with cranial irradiation pre- and post-transplant (de Magalhaes-Silverman & Hammert, 2000; O'Connell, 2000).

The majority of patients with leukoencephalopathy are children with a diagnosis of acute lymphocytic leukemia (Johnson, Thomas, & Clark, 1981). Symptoms include dysarthria, ataxia, dysphagia, confusion, and decreased sensorium (de Magalhaes-Silverman & Hammert, 2000). In recent years, the risk has decreased because of careful use of cranial irradiation and intrathecal methotrexate (O'Connell, 2000). There is no known effective treatment.

Metabolic encephalopathy, the most common neurologic toxicity post-transplant, occurs in 9%–39% of patients. Patients receiving alternative donor transplants are at the highest risk (de Brabander et al., 2000; de Magalhaes-Silverman & Hammert, 2000). Causes of metabolic encephalopathy include gram-negative sepsis, sedative-hypnotic drugs, hypoxia/ischemia, hepatic dysfunction, renal dysfunction, electrolyte/acid-base disturbances, and GVHD.

The clinical presentation of metabolic encephalopathies includes depression of the CNS and altered sensorium, usually without focal neurologic findings (de Magalhaes-

Silverman & Hammert, 2000). In transplant recipients, the cause of metabolic encephalopathy can be multifactoral. Gram-negative sepsis and sedative-hypnotic drugs account for many of the cases. Other transplant-related etiologies include hypoxic encephalopathy occurring with pneumonias; GVHD or hepatic dysfunction from veno-occlusive disease, resulting in hepatic encephalopathy; uremic encephalopathy attributed to nephrotoxic drugs; radiation nephritis and hemolytic-uremic syndrome; and encephalopathy related to acid-base imbalances (Openshaw & Slatkin, 1999). Treatment is directed at managing the underlying cause.

Immune-Mediated Neurologic Toxicities

Immune-mediated neurologic complications are frequently a late effect of transplant. These complications include inflammatory demyelinating polyneuropathy, myasthenia gravis, and polymyositis. All are peripheral neuropathies. These complications are rare and have been associated with chronic GVHD. Most often, they are reported as case reports.

Inflammatory demyelinating polyneuropathy occurs in only 1% of allogeneic transplant recipients. It is associated with viral infections and disorders of reduced cellular immunity, although the exact mechanism is unknown. Many case reports have described an association with GVHD. It may occur acutely and lead to a rapid quadriplegic state, such as in Guillain-Barré syndrome. At other times, the onset of symptoms can occur two to three months after transplant, but cases have been reported to occur within one month (de Magalhaes-Silverman & Hammert, 2000; Openshaw & Slatkin, 1999; Wen et al., 1997).

Diagnosis is made using electromyography, nerve conduction studies, serologic testing for anticholinesterase antibody, and muscle biopsy. Treatment is usually with plasmapheresis, prednisone, and intravenous gamma globulin.

Myasthenia gravis is a rare complication occurring in allogeneic transplant recipients and often is associated with chronic GVHD (Mackey, Desai, Larratt, Cwik, & Nabholtz, 1997; Zaja et al., 1997). Openshaw and Slatkin (1999) described it as an immune-mediated disorder of the neuromuscular junction in which autoantibodies to the postsynaptic acetylcholine receptor produce a characteristic clinical syndrome of ptosis and extraocular muscle weakness, most often with proximal limb and facial muscle weakness. Myasthenia gravis usually responds to pyridostigmine treatment, immunosuppression, and plasmapheresis.

Polymyositis has been reported after both allogeneic and autologous transplant, with an incidence of 3%. In allogeneic transplant recipients, the disease has been associated with chronic GVHD. Patients present with proximal muscle weakness, muscle tenderness, dysphagia, and cardiac muscle involvement. In patients with GVHD, myositis has responded to CSA 5 and steroids (George, Danda, Chandy, Srivastava, & Mathews, 2001; Parker, Openshaw, & Forman, 1997).

Conclusions and Nursing Actions

Neurologic changes can be easily recognized during patient assessment or be so subtle that they are unnoticed until deleterious effects have taken place. Most patients will enter the HSCT process with preexisting neurologic changes, further complicating accurate and early identification during transplant. The initial nursing assessment is the most valuable tool, providing a detailed pretransplant neurologic status that can be used as a basis to identify new onset neurologic abnormalities. It will also identify those at risk for neurologic complications during the transplant process. Frequent assessment, especially at critical periods during treatment, such as the addition of new medications or altered laboratory values, is recommended. Global evaluation that includes changes in other organ systems also should be included, as altered renal and hepatic function have a significant impact on drug metabolism. Careful attention to transfusion requirements, specifically platelets, will help to prevent pathology of the brain, such as cerebral bleeds.

Familiarity with the neurologic side effects of chemotherapeutic agents used in conditioning regimens is an important step in maintaining patient safety and preventing complications of treatment. Immediately post-transplant, assessment should focus on factors affecting engraftment and medications such as antibiotic therapy. Proper administration of immunosuppressant agents and careful attention to drug levels are important steps to prevent CNS complications. Infectious offenders should be considered at any time during the HSCT process if CNS changes are identified. Preexisting neurologic defects identified at initial assessment may require care directed toward maximizing potential and play an important role once the patient has been stabilized post-HSCT. Physical and occupational therapy will play an important role in recovery.

HSCT has allowed survival to those who may not have lived because of their disease. Unfortunately, neurologic complications can develop and have a serious impact on survival. As nurses, we are at the best position to recognize early signs and symptoms so complications can be prevented.

References

Andrykowski, M., Altmaier, E., Burnett, R., Burish, T., Gingrich, R., & Henslee-Downey, P. (1990). Cognitive dysfunction in adult survivors of allogeneic marrow transplantation: Relationship to dose of total body irradiation. *Bone Marrow Transplantation, 6,* 269–276.

Antonini, G., Ceschin, V., Morino, S., Fiorellli, M., Gragnani, F., Mengarelli, A., et al. (1998). Early neurologic complications following allogeneic bone marrow transplant for leukemia: A prospective study. *Neurology, 50,* 1441–1445.

Armstrong, T., Rust, D., & Kohtz, J.R. (1997). Neurologic, pulmonary, and cutaneous toxicities of high-dose chemotherapy. *Oncology Nursing Forum, 24*(Suppl.1), 23–33.

Barkholt, L., Lewensohn-Fuchs, I., Ericzon, B.G., Tyden, G., & Andersson, J. (1999). High-dose acyclovir prophylaxis reduces cytomegalovirus disease in liver transplant patients. *Transplant Infectious Disease, 1,* 889–897.

Bartynski, W.S., Zeigler, Z., Spearman, M.P., Lin, L., Shadduck, R.K., & Lister, J. (2001). Etiology of cortical and white matter lesions in cyclosporin-A and FK-506 neurotoxicity. *American Journal of Neuroradiology, 22,* 1901–1914.

Bleggi-Torres, L.F., deMedeiros, B.C., Werner, B., Zanis, N.J., Loddo, G., Pasquini, R., et al. (2000). Neuropathological findings after bone marrow transplantation: An autopsy study of 180 cases. *Bone Marrow Transplantation, 25,* 301–307.

Blohm, M.E.G., Nurnberger, W., Aulich, A., Engelbrecht, V., & Burdach, S. (1997). Reversible brain MRI changes in acyclovir neurotoxicity. *Bone Marrow Transplantation, 19,* 1049–1051.

Cain, J., & Bender, C. (1995). Ifosfamide-induced neurotoxicity: Associated symptoms and nursing implications. *Oncology Nursing Forum, 22,* 659–666.

Chatellier, D., Jourdain, M., Mangalaboyi, J., Ader, F., Chopin, C., Derambure, P., et al. (2002). Cefepime-induced neurotoxicity: An underestimated complication of anti biotherapy in patients with acute renal failure. *Intensive Care Medicine, 23,* 214–217.

Chou, R.H., Wong, G.B., Kramer, J.H., Wara, D.W., Matthay, K.K., Crittenden, M.R., et al. (1996). Toxicities of total-body irradiation for pediatric bone marrow transplantation. *International Journal of Radiation Oncology, Biology, Physics, 34,* 834–851.

Colosimo, M., McCarthy, N., Jayasinghe, R., Morton, J., Taylor, K., & Durrant, S. (2000). Diagnosis and management of subdural haematoma complicating bone marrow transplantation. *Bone Marrow Transplantation, 25,* 549–552.

Coplin, W., Cochran, M., Levine, S., & Crawford, S. (2001). Stroke after bone marrow transplantation. *Brain: A Journal of Neurology, 124,* 1043–1051.

Davis, D., & Patchell, R. (1988). Neurologic complications of bone marrow transplantation. *Neurology Clinics of North America, 6,* 377–387.

de Brabander, C., Cornelissen, J., Sillervis-Smitt, P.A.E., Vecht, C.J., & van den Bent, M.J. (2000). Increased incidence of neurological complications in patients receiving an allogeneic bone marrow transplantation form alternative donors. *Journal of Neurology Neurosurgery and Psychiatry, 68,* 36–40.

de Magalhaes-Silverman, M., & Hammert, L. (2000). Neurologic complications. In E. Ball, J. Lister, & P. Law (Eds.), *Hematopoietic stem cell therapy* (pp. 578–588). New York: Churchill Livingstone.

Dhodapkar, M., Goldberg, S.L., Terreri, A., & Gertz, M.A. (1994). Reversible encephalopathy after cryopreserved peripheral blood stem cell infusion. *American Journal of Hematology, 45,* 187–188.

Drotts, D.L., & Vinson, D.R. (1999). Prochlorperazine induced akathisia in emergency patients. *Annals of Emergency Medicine, 34*(4 Pt. 1), 469–475.

Ernst, M.E., & Franey, R.J. (1998). Acyclovir and ganciclovir induced neurotoxicity. *Annals of Pharmacotherapy, 32,* 111–113.

Furlong, T.G. (1993). Neurologic complications of immunosuppressive cancer therapy. *Oncology Nursing Forum, 20,* 1337–1354.

Garcia-Escrig, M., Martinez, J., Fernandez-Ponsati, J., Diaz, J., & Soto, O. (1994). Severe central nervous system toxicity after chronic treatment with cyclosporine. *Clinical Neuropharmacology, 17,* 298–302.

George, B., Danda, D., Chandy, M., Srivastava, A., & Mathews, V. (2001). Polymyositis—An unusual manifestation of chronic graft-versus-host disease. *Rheumatology, 20,* 169–170.

Graus, F., Saiz, A., Sierra, J., Arbiaza, D., Rovira, M., Carreras, E., et al. (1996). Neurologic complications of autologous and allogeneic bone marrow transplantation in patients with leukemia: A comparative study. *Neurology, 46,* 1004–1009.

Harder, H., Cornelissen, J.J., Van Gool, A.R., Duvivenvoorden, H.J., Ejkenboom, W.M.H., & van den Bent, M.J. (2002). Cognitive functioning and quality of life in long-term adult survivors of bone marrow transplantation. *Cancer, 95,* 183–192.

Hassan, M., Ehrsson, H., & Ljungman, P. (1996). Aspects concerning busulfan pharmacokinetics and bioavailability. *Leukemia and Lymphoma, 22,* 395–407.

Hoyt, R., Szer, J., & Gregg, A. (2000). Neurological events associated with the infusion of cryopreserved bone marrow and/or peripheral blood progenitor cells. *Bone Marrow Transplantation, 25,* 1285–1287.

Johnson, F., Thomas, E., & Clark, B. (1981). A comparison of marrow transplantation with chemotherapy for children with ALL in second or subsequent remission. *New England Journal of Medicine, 305,* 846–851.

Kahan, B.D. (1989). Cyclosporine. *New England Journal of Medicine, 321,* 1725–1737.

Kerbusch, T., de Kraker, J., Keizer, H.J., van Putten, J.W.G., Groen, H.J.M., Jansen, R.L.H., et al. (2001). Clinical pharmacokinetics and pharmacodynamics of ifosfamide and its metabolites. *Clinical Pharmacokinetics, 40*(1), 41–62.

Kobayashi, R., Watanabe, N., Iguchi, A., Cho, Y., Yoshida, M., Arioka, H., et al. (1998). Electroencephalogram abnormality and high-dose busulfan in conditioning regimens for stem cell transplantation. *Bone Marrow Transplantation, 21,* 217–220.

Koehler, M.T., Howrie, D., Mirro, J., Neudorf, S., Blatt, J., Corey, S., et al. (1995). FK-506 (tacrolimus) in the treatment of steroid-resistant acute graft-versus-host disease in children undergoing bone marrow transplantation. *Bone Marrow Transplantation, 15,* 895–899.

MacDonald, D.R. (1991). Neurologic complications of chemotherapy. *Neurologic Complications of Systemic Cancer, 9,* 955–963.

Mackey, J., Desai, S., Larratt, L., Cwik, V., & Nabholtz, J. (1997). Myasthenia gravis in association with allogeneic bone marrow transplantation: Clinical observations, therapeutic implications and review of literature. *Bone Marrow Transplantation, 19,* 939–942.

Martinez-Rodriguez, J.E., Barriga, F.J., Santamaria, J., Iranzo, A., Pareja, J.A., Revilla, M., et al. (2001). Nonconvulsive status edioepticus associated with cephalosporins in patients with real failure. *American Journal of Medicine, 111,* 115–119.

Maschke, M., Dietrich, U., Prumbaum, M., Kastrup, O., Turowski, B., Schaefer, U.W., et al. (1999). Opportunistic CNS infection after bone marrow transplantation. *Bone Marrow Transplantation, 23,* 1167–1176.

McLean, H.J., & Douen, A.G. (2002). Severe amnesia associated with human herpes virus encephalitis after bone marrow transplantation. *Transplantation, 73,* 1086–1089.

Meriney, D.K., & Grimm, P. (1997). Neurological effects. In M.B. Whedon & D. Wujcik (Eds.), *Blood and marrow stem cell transplantation: Principles, practice, and nursing insights* (pp. 326–354). Sudbury, MA: Jones and Bartlett.

Miyahara, M., Azuma, E., Hirayama, M., Kobayashi, M., Hori, H., Komada, Y., et al. (2000). Somnolence syndrome in a child following 1200-cGy total body irradiation in an unrelated bone marrow transplant. *Pediatric Hematology and Oncology, 17,* 489–495.

Murphy, C.P., Harden, E.A., & Thompson, J.M. (1992). Generalized seizures secondary to high-dose busulfan therapy. *Annals of Pharmacotherapy, 26,* 30–31.

O'Connell, S. (2000). Complications of hematopoietic cell transplantation. In C.H. Yarbro, M. Frogge, M. Goodman, & S. Groenwald (Eds.), *Cancer nursing: Principles and practice* (pp. 528–535). Sudbury, MA: Jones and Bartlett.

Openshaw, H., & Slatkin, N.E. (1999). Neurological complications. In E.D. Thomas, K.G. Blume, & S.J. Forman (Eds.), *Hematopoietic cell transplantation* (pp. 659–673). Boston: Blackwell Science.

Parker, P., Openshaw, H., & Forman, S. (1997). Myositis associated with graft-versus-host disease. *Current Opinion in Rheumatology, 9,* 513–519.

Peper, M., Steinvorth, S., Schraube, P., Fruehauf, S., Haas, R., Kimmig, B.N., et al. (2000). Neurobehavioral toxicity of total body irradiation: A follow-up in long-term survivors. *International Journal of Radiation, Oncology, Biology, Physics, 46,* 303–311.

Pomeranz, S., Naparstek, E., Ashkenazi, E., Nagler, A., Lossos, A., Slavin, S., et al. (1994). Intracranial haematomas following bone marrow transplantation. *Journal of Neurology, 241,* 252–256.

Reece, D.E., Frei-Lahr, D.A., Shepherd, J.D., Dorovini-Zis, K., Gascovyne, R.D., Graeb, D.A., et al. (1991). Neurologic complications in allogeneic bone marrow transplant patients receiving cyclosporin. *Bone Marrow Transplantation, 8,* 393–401.

Rivera, M., Crespo, M., Teruel, J., Marcen, R., & Ortuno, J. (1999). Neurotoxicity due to imipenem/cilastatin in patients on continuous ambulatory peritoneal dialysis. *Nephrology Dialysis Transplant, 14,* 258–259.

Roemer, E., Nlau, I.W., Bassara, N., Kiehl, M.G., Bischoff, M., Gunzeimann, S., et al. (2001). Toxoplasmosis, a severe complication in allogeneic hematopoietic stem cell transplantation: Successful treatment strategies during a 5-year single-center experience. *Clinical Infectious Disease, 32,* E1–E8.

Schiller, G., & Lee, M. (1997). Long-term outcome of high-dose cytarabine-based consolidation chemotherapy for older patients with acute myelogenous leukemia. *Leukemia and Lymphoma, 25,* 1111–1119.

Schwartz, D.L., Schechter, G.P., Seltzer, S., & Chauncey, T.R. (2000). Radiation myelitis following allogeneic stem cell transplantation and consolidation radiotherapy for non-Hodgkin's lymphoma. *Bone Marrow Transplantation, 26,* 1355–1359.

Shank, B. (1999). Radiotherapeutic principles of hematopoietic cell transplantation. In E.D. Thomas, K.G. Blume, & S.J. Forman (Eds.), *Hematopoietic cell transplantation* (pp. 151–167). Boston: Blackwell Science.

Singh, N., & Husain, S. (2000). Infections of the central nervous system in transplant recipients. *Transplant Infectious Disease, 2,* 101–111.

Snavely, S.R., & Hodges, G.R. (1984). The neurotoxicity of antibacterial agents. *Annals of Internal Medicine, 101,* 92–104.

Staudinger, T., Heimberger, K., Rabitsch, W., Schneider, B., Greinix, H., Nowzad, S., et al. (1998). Subdural hygromas after bone marrow transplantation: results of a prospective study. *Transplantation, 65,* 1340–1344.

Steg, R.E., Kessinger, A., & Wszolek, Z.K. (1999). Cortical blindness and seizures in a patient receiving FK-506 after bone marrow transplantation. *Bone Marrow Transplantation, 23,* 959–962.

Tauro, S., Toh, V., Osman, H., & Mahendra, P. (2000). Varicella zoster meningoencephalitis following treatment for dermatomal zoster in an allo BMT patient. *Bone Marrow Transplantation, 26,* 795–796.

Torres-Bleggi, L.F., de Medeiros, B.C., Werner, B., Neto, Z., Loddo, G., & Pasquini, R. (2000). Neuro pathological findings after bone marrow transplantation: An autopsy study of 180 cases. *Bone Marrow Transplantation, 25,* 301–307.

Trullemans, F., Grignard, F., Van Camp, B., & Schots, R. (2001). Clinical findings and magnetic resonance imaging in severe cyclosporine-related neurotoxicity after allogeneic bone marrow transplantation. *European Journal of Hematology, 67,* 94–99.

Vinson, D.R., & Drotts, D.L. (2001). Diphenhydramine for the prevention of akathisia induced by prochlorperazine: A randomized, controlled trial. *Annals of Emergency Medicine, 37,* 125–131.

Wallace, K.L. (1997). Antibiotic induced convulsions. *Critical Care Clinics, 13,* 741–762.

Wen, P., Alyea, E., Simon, D., Herbst, R., Soiffer, R., & Antin, J. (1997). Guillain-Barré syndrome following allogeneic bone marrow transplantation. *Neurology, 49,* 1711–1714.

Wenz, F., Steinvorth, S., Lohr, F., Fruehauf, S., Hacke, W., & Wannenmacher, M. (1999). Acute central nervous system (CNS) toxicity of total body irradiation (TBI) measured using neuropsychological testing of attention functions. *International Journal of Radiation, Oncology, Biology, Physics, 44,* 891–894.

Wenz, F., Steinvorth, S., Lohr, F., Fruehauf, S., Wildermuth, S., van Kampen, M., et al. (2000). Prospective evaluation of delayed central nervous system (CNS) toxicity of hyperfractionated total body irradiation (TBI). *International Journal of Radiation, Oncology, Biology, Physics, 48,* 1497–1501.

Wong, K.M., Chan, W.K., Chan, Y.H., & Li, C. (1999). Cefepime-related neurotoxicity in a hemodialysis patient. *Nephrology Dialysis Transplantation, 14,* 2265–2266.

Woo, M.H., Ippoliti, C., Bruton, J., Mehra, R., Champlin, R., & Prezepiorka, D. (1997). Headache, circumoral paresthesia, and facial flushing associated with high-dose carmustine infusion. *Bone Marrow Transplantation, 19,* 845–847.

Woo, M.H., Przepiorka, D., Ippoliti, C., Warkentin, D., Khouri, I., Fritsche, H., et al. (1997). Toxicities of tacrolimus and cyclosporin A after allogeneic blood stem cell transplantation. *Bone Marrow Transplantation, 20,* 1095–1098.

Zaja, F., Barillari, G., Russo, D., Silvestri, F., Fanin, R., & Baccarani, M. (1997). Myasthenia gravis after allogeneic bone marrow transplantation. A case report and a review of the literature. *Acta Neurologica Scandinavia, 96,* 256–259.

Zver, S., Cernelc, P., Mlakar, U., & Pretnar, J. (1999). Cerebral toxoplasmosis—A late complication of allogeneic haematopoietic stem cell transplantation. *Bone Marrow Transplantation, 24,* 1363–1365.

CHAPTER 12

Relapse and Secondary Malignancies Following Hematopoietic Stem Cell Transplantation

Introduction

Hematopoietic stem cell transplantation (HSCT) has been proven to be a curative treatment modality in certain diseases, as presented in Table 12-1 (Whedon & Roach, 2000). Although the intent of HSCT is to cure disease, at times this is unsuccessful, and the disease relapses. On other occasions, years of remission and cure are followed by the diagnosis of a secondary malignancy, generally resulting from prior treatment modalities. This chapter will explore both of these results and the implications for nursing.

Relapse Following Autologous Transplantation

Relapse of the underlying malignancy is the major cause of treatment failure in 40%–75% of patients who receive autologous HSCT (Negrin, 1999). Relapse typically occurs within the first two years following autologous HSCT. The incidence of relapse is multifactorial and is related to the type of tumor involved and remission status at the time of transplantation (Sureda et al., 2001). Treatment options for patients who relapse following autologous HSCT are limited. New therapies, which use randomized clinical trials, should be used for patients who have been identified with a high risk of relapsing with traditional autologous HSCT (Nieto et al., 1999).

Several approaches have been proposed to reduce the rate of relapse and improve results following autologous HSCT. Identifying potential transplant candidates and completing autologous HSCT earlier in the course of the disease may decrease resistance to potential therapies and decrease exposure of stem cells to changes associated with prior therapies. Improved and intensified preparative regimens increase the likelihood that the high-dose chemotherapy will eradicate the malignancy. Manipulation of the stem cell graft through in vivo and ex vivo purging may decrease the likelihood the stem cell product is contaminated with tumor cells.

Purging autologous cells using pharmacologic agents include the use of certain chemotherapeutic agents, such as 4-hydroperoxycyclophosphamide. Immunologic agents include monoclonal antibodies such as alemtuzumab (Campath-1H®, Berlex Pharmaceuticals, Richmond, CA) and

rituximab (Rituxan®, IDEC Pharmaceuticals, San Diego, CA). Physical manipulation of the stem cell product may include the use of elutriation or cell selection methods. Effective methods to purge the stem cell product of malignant cells continue to be investigated (Cooper & Seropian, 2001).

More recently, the utilization of post-transplant immunotherapy is under investigation. Post-transplant immunotherapy strategies are aimed at reducing disease relapse, especially for patients with a high likelihood of microscopic relapse. Many approaches are being considered, including

Table 12-1. Estimated Five-Year Disease-Free Survival Following Transplantation

Disease	Stage	Five-Year Disease-Free Survival Allogeneic	Five-Year Disease-Free Survival Autologous
AML	1st CR	45%–70%	35%–45%
AML	2nd CR	20%–45%	15%–40%
ALL	1st CR	45%–60%	30%–60%
ALL	2nd CR	20%–40%	15%–40%
MDS	Combined	20%–45%	ND
CML	Chronic	60%–75%	50%
CML	Accelerated	30%–45%	25%
CML	Blast crisis	10%–20%	
NHL	1st relapse, 2nd CR	30%–50%	45%–60%
HD	1st relapse, 2nd CR	10%–30%	40%–60%
MM	Combined	30%–50%	30%
CLL		20%–55%	ND
Breast cancer	Stage IV	ND	15%–30%
Breast cancer	Stage III	ND	55%
Breast cancer	Stage II	ND	70%
Germ cell	Recurrent	ND	15%–20%
Brain tumors		ND	13%

ALL—acute lymphocytic leukemia; AML—acute myelogenous leukemia; CLL—chronic lymphocytic leukemia; CML—chronic myelogenous leukemia; CR—complete remission; HD—Hodgkin's disease; MDS—myelodysplastic syndrome; MM—multiple myeloma; ND—no data; NHL—non-Hodgkin's lymphoma

Note. From "Principles of Bone Marrow and Hematopoietic Cell Transplantation" (pp. 487–507) by M.B. Whedon and M. Roach in C.H. Yarbro, M. Goodman, M.H. Frogge, and S.L. Groenwald (Eds.), *Cancer Nursing*, 2000, Sudbury, MA: Jones and Bartlett. Copyright 2000 by Jones and Bartlett. Reprinted with permission.

the use of cytokines and interleukins (IL-2, IL-12; interferon); ex vivo activated cellular immunotherapy; immuno-modulating agents, such as cyclosporine and thalidomide; monoclonal and bispecific antibodies, such as rituximab (Rituxan) and trastuzumab (Herceptin®, Genentech Pharmaceuticals, San Francisco, CA); the induction of an autologous graft versus host reaction; and post-transplantation vaccination with tumor-specific proteins (Cooper & Seropian, 2001; Negrin, 1999). Clinical trials investigating post-transplant immunotherapy are ongoing.

Relapse Following Allogeneic Transplantation

High-dose chemoradiotherapy followed by allogeneic HSCT can be used successfully to cure hematologic malignancies and nonmalignant disorders in adults and children. The powerful immune reaction generated from donor cells reacting against residual tumor, known as graft versus tumor (GVT) effect, is unique to allogeneic transplantation. It is believed that because allogeneic stem cells have not been exposed to prior chemotherapy and/or radiation and are free of malignant disease, leukemogenesis and relapse are decreased (Deeg & Socié, 1998).

As more patients undergo allogeneic HSCT, longer survival data become available. Relapse of underlying leukemia has been identified in one study as the cause of death for 46% of patients who were disease-free two years after allogeneic transplantation (Socié et al., 1999). When relapse occurs, disease is still present in the host cells. This could be the result of an inadequate conditioning therapy that failed to eradicate tumor cells present in the marrow and other organs, graft failure, or the absence of graft versus host disease (GVHD), which may indicate inadequate GVT effect.

An allogeneic HSCT from a matched, related donor carries a lower risk of graft rejection and GVHD than one from a matched or partially mismatched unrelated donor. Although GVHD may be avoided by utilizing T cell depletion techniques, this carries a higher risk for graft rejection or graft failure and relapse than an unmanipulated stem cell product. GVHD is avoided with transplants between identical twins, but the incidence of relapse is higher in patients treated for leukemia because of the lack of graft versus leukemia effect (Fefer, 1999).

Relapse following allogeneic HSCT occurs in many forms. Systemic relapse of disease with rapid progression may occur. Extramedullary relapse can occur in so-called "sanctuary" sites or organs that are not usually penetrated by chemotherapy (Seo et al., 2000). Known sanctuary sites in acute lymphocytic leukemia include the testes, skin, eyes, and central nervous system (CNS). Most extramedullary relapses are followed by systemic relapses, and the patient's prognosis is usually dismal (Kolb, 1999). In other diseases, cytogenetic relapse may be detected before morphologic evidence of relapse occurs. Detection of disease earlier may lead to earlier treatment, which may prevent systemic relapses in the future.

Treatment of relapsed disease following allogeneic transplantation continues to evolve. No single treatment is effective for all patients. One successful approach is to withdraw immunosuppressive agents in an attempt to trigger a GVT effect. A disadvantage of this approach is the development of severe GVHD. Another approach is the use of cytokine injections to increase the number of tumor-fighting lymphocytes. Again, the disadvantage is the high risk of acute or chronic GVHD, which may be severe or life-threatening (Bishop et al., 2000; Giralt et al., 1993).

Donor leukocyte infusions are an option for certain disease relapses and have been studied extensively in the chronic myelogenous leukemia (CML) population (Dazzi, Szydlo, & Goldman, 1999). An effective therapeutic option for patients with CML in chronic phase with molecular relapse following allogeneic HSCT is withdrawal of immunosuppression followed by granulocyte–colony-stimulating factor primed T lymphocyte infusions from the original donor. Response rates vary from 57% (van Rhee et al., 1994) to 100% (Verdonck et al., 1998). This strategy has minimal effectiveness in relapsed acute myelogenous leukemia (AML) after allogeneic HSCT because adequate cellular responses are not able to develop in the presence of bulky, fast-growing disease (Levine et al., 2002).

Relapse following allogeneic transplantation presents a difficult situation for patients as well as the transplant team. Other strategies can be used in an attempt to re-induce a durable remission. Second myeloablative transplants following allogeneic HSCT are high risk, carry a significant risk of treatment-related mortality, and usually are not effective. For some diseases, experimental trials are being conducted using immunotherapy and monoclonal antibodies (Dazzi et al., 1999).

At times, the relapsed disease is no longer considered curable, and patients may elect not to receive any further therapy. In those cases, supportive and palliative care options should be discussed. Information should be provided to patients and their families so informed decisions regarding end-of-life care can be made. If the patient desires to receive no further treatment, nurses can facilitate their transition to hospice care (O'Connell, 2000).

Patients who survive HSCT should continue follow-up care with their oncologist to monitor for late toxicities of treatment. Blood tests and restaging scans and/or bone marrow biopsies are necessary to evaluate patients for engraftment, relapse, or secondary malignancies (Wingard, 2002). Transplant recipients also should receive routine health maintenance and health promotion education. Post-transplant follow-up is discussed in Chapter 13.

Secondary Malignancy

Secondary malignancy is a potential risk for patients receiving standard doses of chemotherapy and/or total body irradiation (TBI) for treatment of their underlying diseases. The use of certain chemotherapeutic agents (e.g., alkylating agents, such as busulfan, chlorambucil, CCNU, and cyclophosphamide; topoisomerase II inhibitors; anthracyclines) is commonly associated with deletion or loss of chromosomes 5 and 7 and can lead to the development of myelodysplastic syndrome (MDS) or AML following standard chemotherapy (Deeg & Socié, 1998; Leone, Mele, Pulsoni, Equitani, & Pagano, 1999; Yakoub-Agha et al., 2000).

Miller et al. (1994), in a retrospective review of 206 patients who received autologous HSCT for non-Hodgkin's lymphoma (NHL) and Hodgkin's disease, found a 14.5% ± 11.6% cumulative incidence of secondary acute leukemia or MDS at five years. Darrington et al. (1994), in a retrospective review of patients with lymphoma who received autologous HSCT, found there may be an increased risk of MDS after treatment with TBI-based regimens, which is independent of prior therapy. The risks and benefits of using TBI in preparative regimens for patients with lymphoma undergoing autologous HSCT still are being debated (Armitage, 2000; Berglund, Enblad, Carlson, Glimelius, & Hagberg, 2000).

It is known that the risk of secondary malignancy is high, but what is unknown is how that risk is compounded with transplantation. Many studies have been conducted exploring the incidence of secondary malignancies in the HSCT population. Results have been reported comparing HSCT recipients to the general population but one must remember that these patients should be compared to matched controls of patients who have undergone similar therapies without transplantation, so the actual incidence of secondary malignancies is unknown (Abruzzese et al., 1999; André et al., 1998; Bhatia et al., 2001; Deeg & Socié, 1998; Oddou et al., 1998; Pedersen-Bjergaard, Pedersen, Myhre, & Geisler, 1997; Socié et al., 2000; Traweek et al., 1996). Figure 12-1 depicts a scheme of the time and relative risk of the major categories of post-transplant malignancies.

The most common chemotherapy-related secondary malignant neoplasm is AML, following treatment with alkylating agents such as cyclophosphamide and melphalan. Epipodophyllotoxins or ionizing radiation also may contribute to the development of secondary malignancies (Darrington et al., 1994; Deeg & Socié, 1998; Leone et al., 1999; Micallef et al., 2000; Miller et al., 1994; Pedersen-Bjergaard et al., 1997; Stone et al., 1994; Sureda et al., 2001; Traweek et al., 1996).

Development of secondary malignancies is believed to result from damage to the DNA of hematopoietic stem cells and mainly occurs in autologous HSCT recipients. Deeg and Socié (1998) observed that MDS after autologous transplantation is related to pretransplant factors rather than the transplant itself. Cytogenetic studies of the bone marrow prior to autologous transplantation may identify patients at high risk for the development of secondary MDS/AML (Deeg & Socié; Stone et al., 1994).

Risk factors for the development of MDS/AML following autologous HSCT include age older than 40 years at the time of transplant, pretransplant irradiation, pretransplant therapy with alkylating agents, prior fludarabine therapy, mobilization of stem cells with etoposide, and low

Figure 12-1. Scheme of Time

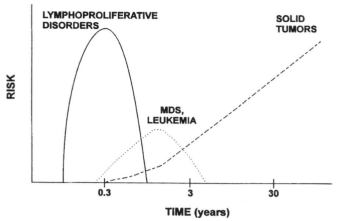

Scheme of time course and relative risk of the major categories of post-transplant malignancies. Whereas lymphoproliferative disorders occur almost exclusively in allogeneic transplant recipients, solid tumors are observed in both allogeneic and autologous patients. Myelodysplastic syndromes (MDS) and leukemia have been reported more frequently after autologous transplantation.

Note. From "Malignancies After Hematopoietic Stem Cell Transplantation: Many Questions, Some Answers," by H.J. Deeg and G. Socié, 1998, *Blood, 91,* p. 1840. Copyright 1998 by the American Society of Hematology. Reprinted with permission.

pretransplant platelet count (Childs, 2001; Leone et al., 1999; Mauch et al., 1996; Micallef et al., 2000; Riddell, 2001; Stone et al., 1994).

Micallef et al. (2000), in a retrospective review of 230 patients treated with cyclophosphamide therapy and TBI with autologous HSCT as remission consolidation for NHL at a median of six years follow-up, found a 12% incidence of treatment-related MDS or secondary AML. Micallef et al. further suggested that when researchers are developing new regimens for the treatment of NHL or other diseases, these findings and risk factors are taken into account because there are no effective treatments for secondary MDS/ AML.

Another secondary malignancy is a post-transplant lymphoproliferative disorder most commonly associated with B lymphocytes—B cell lymphoproliferative disorder (BLPD). BLPD is an aggressive and potentially fatal proliferation of B cell lymphoid cells of donor origin, which is associated with Epstein-Barr virus (EBV) infection (Deeg, 1999). BLPD generally occurs within the first six months following transplant and only affects allogeneic HSCT recipients (Bhatia et al., 1996; Riddell, 2001). The cumulative incidence of BLPD reported in the literature range from 0.6% to 10% (Bhatia et al., 1996).

Factors associated with increased risk of BLPD include matched, unrelated donor transplantation, T cell depletion of the graft, HLA-mismatched related donor, use of antithymocyte globulin or anti-CD3 monoclonal antibody for prophylaxis or treatment of acute GVHD, and an underlying diagnosis of primary immunodeficiency (Bhatia et al.,

1996; Curtis et al., 1999; Deeg & Socié, 1998). Patients may present with fever and progressive lymphadenopathy. Lesions may be extranodal and involve the spleen, liver, lungs, gastrointestinal tract, kidneys, and CNS.

Reducing immunosuppression and infusing unmanipulated donor leukocytes that contain cytotoxic T cells presensitized to EBV may successfully treat BLPD (Childs, 2001; Lucus, Pollok, & Emanuel, 1997). Other promising approaches used to treat a limited number of patients include the use of interferon-alpha, B cell–specific monoclonal antibodies, and cellular therapy (Deeg & Socié, 1998).

Secondary malignancies also may develop in the form of solid tumors. These occur following both autologous HSCT and allogeneic HSCT, with peak incidence occurring several years after transplant (Riddell, 2001). Major risk factors include the prior use of TBI in the preparative regimen; children younger than five years of age at the time of transplant; older patient age; patients with chronic GVHD who were treated with cyclosporine, thalidomide, azathioprine, or methotrexate; or patients with the diagnosis of Fanconi's anemia (Deeg, 2002; Deeg et al., 1996; Kolb et al., 1999; Socié et al., 2000).

Common secondary neoplasms may involve the skin, oral cavity, uterus, thyroid gland, breast, and glial tissue. Squamous cell carcinoma of the buccal cavity has been strongly linked with male gender and chronic GVHD (Curtis et al., 1997). Treatment of solid tumors is similar to that of nontransplant patients. The risk of secondary malignancies may be lowered with the use of nonmyeloablative regimens, which use little or no TBI.

Recipients of bone marrow transplants at a young age have an increased incidence of new solid neoplasms later in life. Transplant recipients should be followed indefinitely to detect early second cancers and precursor lesions (e.g., dysplastic nevi, actinic keratoses, oral leukoplakia) (Curtis et al., 1997). In addition, they should avoid exposure to carcinogenic agents and receive routine healthcare maintenance examinations annually.

Nursing implications for caring for patients at high risk for developing secondary malignancies include close monitoring and reporting of suspicious signs and symptoms. Patients should be educated on the early warning signs of cancer, the importance of routine cancer screening, and measures to prevent cancer development (Cohen & Ley, 2000).

Conclusion

Relapse and secondary malignancies can occur in any cancer survivor, not just those who have undergone HSCT. Transplant survivors are at a high risk for developing a second malignant neoplasm during their lifetime because of their previous chemoradiation and immunosuppression. Nurses must stress to their patients the importance of lifestyle changes, such as decreasing exposure to environmental carcinogens (tobacco and ultraviolet sunlight), which could lessen their chance of relapse or second malignancy in the future.

References

Abruzzese, E., Radford, J.E., Miller, J.S., Vredenburgh, J.J., Rao, P.N., Pettenati, M.J., et al. (1999). Detection of abnormal pretransplant clones in progenitor cells of patients who developed myelodysplasia after autologous transplantation. *Blood, 94*, 1814–1819.

André, M., Henry-Amar, M., Blaise, D., Colombat, P., Fleury, J., Milpied, N., et al. (1998). Treatment-related deaths and second cancer risk after autologous stem-cell transplantation for Hodgkin's disease. *Blood, 92*, 1933–1940.

Armitage, J. (2000). Myelodysplasia and acute leukemia after autologous bone marrow transplantation [Editorial]. *Journal of Clinical Oncology, 18*, 945–946.

Berglund, Å., Enblad, G., Carlson, K., Glimelius, B., & Hagberg, H. (2000). Long-term follow-up of autologous stem-cell transplantation for follicular and transformed follicular lymphoma. *European Journal of Haematology, 65*, 17–22.

Bhatia, S., Louie, A.D., Bhatia, R., O'Donnell, M.R., Fung, H., Kashyap, A., et al. (2001). Solid cancers after bone marrow transplant. *Journal of Clinical Oncology, 19*, 464–471.

Bhatia, S., Ramsay, N.K.C., Steinbuch, M., Dusenbery, K.E., Shapiro, R.S., Weisdorf, D.J., et al. (1996). Malignant neoplasms following bone marrow transplant. *Blood, 87*, 3633–3639.

Bishop, M.R., Tarantolo, S.R., Pavletic, Z.S., Lynch, J.C., Morris, M.E., Zacharias, D., et al. (2000). Filgrastim as an alternative to donor leukocyte infusion for relapse after allogenic stem cell transplantation. *Journal of Clinical Oncology, 18*, 2269–2272.

Childs, R.W. (2001). Allogeneic stem cell transplantation. In V.T. DeVita, Jr., S. Hellman, & S.A. Rosenberg (Eds.), *Cancer: Principles and practice of oncology* (pp. 2779–2797). Philadelphia: Lippincott Williams and Wilkins.

Cohen, M.Z., & Ley, C.D. (2000). Bone marrow transplantation: The battle for hope in the face of fear. *Oncology Nursing Forum, 27*, 473–480.

Cooper, D.L., & Seropian, S. (2001). Autologous stem cell transplantation. In V.T. DeVita, Jr., S. Hellman, & S.A. Rosenberg (Eds.), *Cancer: Principles and practice of oncology* (pp. 2767–2778). Philadelphia: Lippincott Williams and Wilkins.

Curtis, R.E., Rowlings, P.A., Deeg, H.J., Shriner, D.A., Socié, G., Travis, L.B., et al. (1997). Solid cancers after bone marrow transplantation. *New England Journal of Medicine, 336*, 897–904.

Curtis, R.E., Travis, L.B., Rowlings, P.A., Socié, G., Kingma, D.W., Banks, P.M., et al. (1999). Risk of lymphoproliferative disorders after bone marrow transplantation: A multi-institutional study. *Blood, 94*, 2208–2216.

Darrington, D.L., Vose, J.M., Anderson, J.R., Bierman, P.J., Bishop, M.R., Chan, W.C., et al. (1994). Incidence and characterization of secondary myelodysplastic syndrome and acute myelogenous leukemia following high-dose chemoradiotherapy and autologous stem-cell transplantation for lymphoid malignancies. *Journal of Clinical Oncology, 12*, 2527–2534.

Dazzi, F., Szydlo, R.M., & Goldman, J.M. (1999). Donor lymphocyte infusions for relapse of chronic myeloid leukemia after allogeneic stem cell transplant: Where we now stand. *Experimental Hematology, 27*, 1477–1486.

Deeg, H.J. (1999). Delayed complications after hematopoietic cell transplantation. In E.D. Thomas, K.G. Blume, & S.J. Forman (Eds.), *Hematopoietic cell transplantation* (pp. 776–788). Malden, MA: Blackwell Science.

Deeg, H.J. (2002). Malignancies after hematopoietic stem cell transplantation: Why do they occur? Can we prevent them? *American Society of Hematology Education Program Book*, pp. 433–444.

Deeg, H.J., & Socié, G. (1998). Malignancies after hematopoietic stem cell transplantation: Many questions, some answers. *Blood, 91*, 1833–1844.

Deeg, H.J., Socié, G., Schoch, M., Henry-Amar, M., Witherspoon, R.P., Devergie, A., et al. (1996). Malignancies after marrow transplantation for aplastic anemia and Fanconi anemia: A joint Seattle and Paris analysis of results in 700 patients. *Blood, 87,* 386–392.

Fefer, A. (1999). Graft-versus-tumor responses. In E.D. Thomas, K.G. Blume, & S.J. Forman (Eds.), *Hematopoietic cell transplantation* (pp. 316–326). Malden, MA: Blackwell Science.

Giralt, S., Escudier, S., Kantarjian, H., Deisseroth, A., Freireich, E.J., Andersson, B.S., et al. (1993). Preliminary results of treatment with filgrastim for relapse of leukemia and myelodysplasia after allergenic bone marrow transplantation. *New England Journal of Medicine, 329,* 757–761.

Kolb, H.J. (1999). Management of relapse after hematopoietic cell transplantation. In E.D. Thomas, K.G. Blume, & S.J. Forman (Eds.), *Hematopoietic cell transplantation* (pp. 929–936). Malden, MA: Blackwell Science.

Kolb, H.J., Socié, G., Duell, T., Van Lint, M.T., Tichelli, A., Apperley, J.F., et al. (1999). Malignant neoplasms in long-term survivors of bone marrow transplantation. *Annals of Internal Medicine, 131,* 738–744.

Leone, G., Mele, L., Pulsoni, A., Equitani, F., & Pagano, L. (1999). The incidence of secondary leukemias. *Haematologica, 84,* 937–945.

Levine, J.E., Braun, T., Penza, S.L., Beatty, P., Cornetta, K., Martino, R., et al. (2002). Prospective trial of chemotherapy and donor leukocyte infusions for relapse of advanced myeloid malignancies after allogeneic stem cell transplantation. *Journal of Clinical Oncology, 20,* 405–412.

Lucus, K.G., Pollok, K.E., & Emanuel, D.J. (1997). Post-transplant EBV induced lymphoproliferative disorders. *Leukemia and Lymphoma, 25,* 1–8.

Mauch, P.M., Kalish, L.A., Marcus, K.C., Coleman, N., Shulman, L.N., Krill, E., et al. (1996). Second malignancies after treatment for laprotomy staged IA-IIIB Hodgkin's disease: Long-term analysis of risk factors and outcome. *Blood, 87,* 3625–3632.

Micallef, I.N.M., Lillington, D.M., Apostolids, J., Amess, J.A.L., Neat, M., Matthews, J., et al. (2000). Therapy-related myelodysplasia and secondary acute myelogenous leukemia after high-dose therapy with autologous hematopoietic progenitor-cell support for lymphoid malignancies. *Journal of Clinical Oncology, 18,* 947–955.

Miller, J.S., Arthur, D.C., Litz, C.E., Neglia, J.P., Miller, W.J., & Weisdorf, D.J. (1994). Myelodysplastic syndrome after autologous bone marrow transplantation: An additional later complication of curative cancer therapy. *Blood, 83,* 3780–3786.

Negrin, R.S. (1999). Prevention and therapy of relapse after autologous hematopoietic cell transplantation. In E.D. Thomas, K.G. Blume, & S.J. Forman (Eds.), *Hematopoietic cell transplantation* (pp. 1123–1134). Malden, MA: Blackwell Science.

Nieto, Y., Cagnoni, P.J., Shpall, E.J., Xu, X., Murphy, J., Vredenburgh, J., et al. (1999). A predictive model for relapse in high-risk primary breast cancer patients treated with high-dose chemotherapy and autologous stem-cell transplant. *Clinical Cancer Research, 5,* 3425–3431.

O'Connell, S.A. (2000). Complications of hematopoietic cell transplantation. In C.H. Yarbro, M. Goodman, M.H. Frogge, & S.L. Groenwald (Eds.), *Cancer nursing: Principles and practice* (pp. 523–542). Sudbury, MA: Jones and Bartlett.

Oddou, S., Vey, N., Viens, P., Bardou, V.J., Faucher, C., Stoppa, A.M., et al. (1998). Second neoplasms following high-dose chemotherapy and autologous stem cell transplantation for malignant lymphomas: A report of six cases in a cohort of 171 patients from a single institution. *Leukemia and Lymphoma, 31,* 187–194.

Pedersen-Bjergaard, J., Pedersen, M., Myhre, J., & Geisler, C. (1997). High risk of therapy-related leukemia after BEAM chemotherapy and autologous stem cell transplantation for previously treated lymphomas is mainly related to primary chemotherapy and not to the BEAM-transplantation procedure. *Leukemia, 11,* 1654–1660.

Riddell, S.R. (2001). Transplantation-related malignancies. In V.T. DeVita, Jr., S. Hellman, & S.A. Rosenberg (Eds.), *Cancer: Principles and practice of oncology* (pp. 2597–2608). Philadelphia: Lippincott Williams and Wilkins.

Seo, S., Kami, M., Honda, H., Kashima, T., Matsumura, T., Moriya, A., et al. (2000). Extramedullary relapse in the so-called 'sanctuary' sites for chemotherapy after donor lymphocyte infusion. *Bone Marrow Transplantation, 25,* 226–227.

Socié, G., Curtis, R.E., Deeg, H.J., Sobocinski, K.A., Filipovich, A.H., Travis, L.B., et al. (2000). New malignant diseases after allogeneic marrow transplantation for childhood acute leukemia. *Journal of Clinical Oncology, 18,* 348–357.

Socié, G., Stone, J.V., Wingard, J.R., Weisdorf, D., Henslee-Downey, P.J., Bredeson, C., et al. (1999). Long-term survival and late deaths after allogeneic bone marrow transplantation. *New England Journal of Medicine, 341,* 14–21.

Stone, R.M., Neuberg, D., Soiffer, R., Takvorian, T., Whelan, M., Rabinowe, S.N., et al. (1994). Myelodysplastic syndrome as a late complication following autologous bone marrow transplant for non-Hodgkin's lymphoma. *Journal of Clinical Oncology, 12,* 2535–2542.

Sureda, A., Arranz, R., Iriondo, A., Carreras, E., Lahuerta, J.J., Garcia-Conde, J., et al. (2001). Autologous stem-cell transplantation for Hodgkin's disease: Results and prognostic factors in 494 patients from the Grupo Español de Linfomas/Transplante Autólogo de Médula Ósea Spanish cooperative group. *Journal of Clinical Oncology, 19,* 1395–1404.

Traweek, S.T., Slovak, M.L., Nademanee, A.P., Brynes, R.K., Niland, J.C., & Forman, S.J. (1996). Myelodysplasia and acute myeloid leukemia occurring after autologous bone marrow transplantation for lymphoma. *Leukemia and Lymphoma, 20,* 365–372.

van Rhee, R., Lin, F., Cullis, J.O., Spencer, A., Cross, N.C.P., Chase, A., et al. (1994). Relapse of chronic myeloid leukemia after allogeneic bone marrow transplant: The case for giving donor leukocyte transfusions before the onset of hematologic relapse. *Blood, 83,* 3377.

Verdonck, L.F., Petersen, E.J., Lokhorst, H.M., Nieuwenhuis, H.K., Dekker, A.W., Tilanus, M.G.J., et al. (1998). Donor leukocyte infusions for recurrent hematologic malignancies after allogeneic bone marrow transplantation: Impact of infused and residual donor T cells. *Bone Marrow Transplantation, 22,* 1057.

Whedon, M.B., & Roach, M. (2000). Principles of bone marrow and hematopoietic cell transplantation. In C.H. Yarbro, M. Goodman, M.H. Frogge, & S.L. Groenwald (Eds.), *Cancer nursing: Principles and practice* (pp. 487–507). Sudbury, MA: Jones and Bartlett.

Wingard, J.R. (2002). Overview of late complications. *American Society of Hematology Education Program Book,* pp. 422–441.

Yakoub-Agha, I., de La Salmonière, P., Ribaud, P., Sutton, L., Wattel, E., Kuentz, M., et al. (2000). Allogeneic bone marrow transplantation for therapy-related myelodysplastic syndrome and acute myeloid leukemia: A long-term study of 70 patients—Report of the French Society of Bone Marrow Transplantation. *Journal of Clinical Oncology, 18,* 963–971.

CHAPTER 13

Lori Williams, RN, MSN, OCN®, AOCN®

Post-Transplant Follow-Up

Introduction

Post-transplant follow-up traditionally begins with the patient's discharge from the inpatient transplant unit or from the care of the transplant center that performed the transplant. With the advent of early discharge and outpatient transplant, the start of this time period has become less clearly defined (Kelley, Randolph, & Leum, 2000). This chapter will consider post-transplant follow-up as beginning when the patient has engrafted, recovered from the acute toxicities of the transplant preparative regimen, and completed initial post-transplant care. Post-transplant follow-up continues until the patient's death.

Post-transplant follow-up has several purposes:
- Evaluation for and treatment of long-term physical and psychosocial side effects of the transplant
- Assessment, data collection, and reporting for research groups and registries to document recurrence of disease, overall survival, and quality of life
- Therapy administration to prophylax against late complications or to destroy any remaining traces of tumor and prevent recurrence
- Rehabilitation to ensure that the patient regains optimum functioning in as brief a time as possible (Deeg, 1994).

Care during this period of time may be accomplished in a variety of settings, depending on the needs of the patient and the resources available. Good communication between all facilities and healthcare providers is essential to meet the ongoing complex needs of these patients (Deeg, 1994; Kelley, McBride, Randolph, Leum, & Lonergan, 1998). Patient and family education is critical as patients are released from the intense oversight of the immediate post-transplant phase (Buchsel & Kapustay, 1999). Finally, extended follow-up to track the ultimate outcome of these patients is vital to the appropriate utilization of transplant therapy (Deeg).

Outpatient Care

Post-transplant follow-up care begins in the outpatient setting (Buchsel & Kapustay, 1999). It may start with the patient's first visit to an outpatient clinic after discharge from an inpatient unit; it may begin when the patient's care is transferred to a different outpatient clinic either in the same facility or a different facility; or it may be marked by a decrease in the frequency of visits to the same clinic. It often involves the shifting of care from one set of healthcare providers to another.

Communication

Whenever there is a transfer of some or all aspects of care, communication between the care teams is imperative. The new care providers must be aware that the patient is being assigned to their care, what the expectation of their role in the patient's care is, and when they are first expected to provide care to the patient. Ideally, written documents outlining the patient's current condition and needs are available at the time the patient is first seen and have been supplemented with one or more calls from the transferring facility (Kelley et al., 2000). Figure 13-1 lists information that may

---

Figure 13-1. Potential Information for Communication Between Care Providers After Hematopoietic Stem Cell Transplantation

Type of Information
- Patient name
- Allergies
- Patient date of birth
- Name of primary caregiver
- Primary diagnosis
- Type of transplant
- Date of transplant
- Current medications
- Other medical diagnoses
- Current history and physical
- Transplant course summary
- Current laboratory values
- Central venous catheter(s)
- Catheter care protocol
- Routine follow-up and testing needed
- Research studies in which patient is enrolled
- Documentation needs and follow-up schedule for research protocols
- Names and contact information for other providers participating in care
- Patient and family teaching that has been completed
- Additional patient and family education needs
- Other special needs and concerns

---

be useful to the new care provider. If the transplant center keeps detailed flow sheets or problem lists, it often is useful to send these to the new care provider. Actual copies of laboratory reports and diagnostic tests also may be useful. Careful thought should be given to the needs of each patient to ensure that needed information is communicated. Care also should be taken to guard the patient's privacy by not communicating information that is not needed by the new provider. The patient must be aware of information that is being communicated and consent to the communication (Dexter & Epstein, 2001). Carefully designed communication forms and checklists can help to ensure that items are not overlooked.

Routine Care

The care that is provided in this early post-transplant follow-up period usually involves complete blood counts several times a week to every two weeks to verify the stability of engraftment. Some patients will not yet have achieved platelet engraftment. These patients still may require platelet transfusions until platelet engraftment is established. Patients occasionally may require red blood cell transfusions during this time (Kapustay & Buchsel, 2000).

Patients, particularly allogeneic transplant recipients, may self-administer numerous medications during the early post-transplant follow-up period (Buchsel, 1999). If patients have been hospitalized prior to this period, they may require some help in organizing their medications so that they are taken correctly. A written list of medications with the generic and trade names of the medications, a description of the appearance of the medication, the strength of each unit of the medication, the total dose and number of units to be taken at each administration, the dosing schedule of the medication, space to write down the times of administration, the purpose of the medication, and any special instructions is helpful (Kelley et al., 1998). If this list can be computer-generated and printed in the clinic, a new list can be easily supplied to the patient when changes in medications, dosages, and schedules occur. An example of a patient medication list is in Table 13-1. It also is helpful to have patients bring their supply of medications to the clinic at each visit. The medications that the patient is taking can be verified and any changes in medication pointed out specifically to the patient. Some clinics provide patients with multidose, multiday pillboxes and even fill the boxes with the correct pills on a weekly basis. When the patient returns with the box each week, it can be determined if any dose of medication was skipped.

Infection Control

Although most patients are no longer neutropenic by the second and third months post-transplant, they still have increased susceptibility to infection. This susceptibility will be more severe and last longer in patients receiving corticosteroids or other immunosuppressants for transplant-related complications and patients with graft versus host disease (GVHD). Outpatient clinics need to protect patients from exposure to infectious diseases as long as they are immuno-suppressed (Foundation for the Accreditation of Cellular Therapy [FACT], 2002). Patients, caregivers, and all transplant clinic staff should practice good hand washing (Centers for Disease Control and Prevention [CDC], Infectious Disease Society of America, and the American Society of Blood and Marrow Transplantation, 2000). Patients should not wait in crowded waiting rooms or be exposed to other patients with known infectious diseases. Particular care should be taken during times when influenza, respiratory syncytial virus, and other community-acquired infections are prevalent. These patients also should be protected from contact with other patients who may have active herpes zoster, *Clostridium difficile*, or vancomycin-resistant enterococcus. Clinic staff, patients' families, and other caregivers should have up-to-date vaccinations, including influenza vaccinations, to decrease the risk of transmitting diseases to transplant recipients (CDC et al. ; Gaynes & Horan, 1999; Potter et al., 1997).

It has been documented that pretransplant antibody titers to routine vaccinations decline after autologous and allogeneic hematopoietic stem cell transplant (HSCT) (Ljungman et al., 1990, 1994; Pauksen et al., 1994). There are no research studies that describe the infectious history and outcome of revaccinated versus non-revaccinated transplant recipients. However, because transplant recipients may have increased susceptibility to infectious diseases, it is not unreasonable to consider revaccination as a precautionary measure. To be effective, revaccination should not be attempted until the patient's immune system has recovered to near normal (Avigan, Pirofski, & Lazarus, 2001). Transplant centers have developed numerous revaccination schedules (Henning, White, Sepkowitz, & Armstrong, 1997). Although limited data are available on the optimum revaccination schedule, the CDC has issued a suggested revaccination schedule in the "Guidelines for the Prevention of Opportunistic Infections Among Hematopoietic Stem Cell Transplant Recipients" (CDC et al., 2000). A brief summary of these recommendations is in Table 13-2. There are no specific recommendations for how long someone who has had a smallpox vaccination should avoid contact with someone who is immunosuppressed. The CDC recommendations are for reimmunization of HSCT recipients only.

As at other stages in the transplant process and with other patients with increased susceptibility to infectious diseases, good handwashing is the single most important factor in the prevention of infection. Patients and caregivers in the post-transplant period should be reminded to maintain their vigilance in washing their hands frequently, especially in the first six months post-transplant or if the patient remains on immunosuppressive agents (CDC et al., 2000). In addition, during this time period patients should avoid other people with upper respiratory infections and closed, crowded places. Influenza vaccination is strongly recommended for all healthcare workers caring for HSCT candidates and patients during each influenza season. Family members and other household contacts of HSCT recipients who still are immunocompromised should receive influenza vaccination

Table 13-1. Sample Post-Transplant Follow-Up Outpatient Clinic Patient Medication Instruction Sheet

Transplant Clinic Medication List

Patient name: _____   Date: _____

Each time that you come to the clinic, bring all of your medications with you. When you run out of medication, have your prescription refilled. Do not stop taking any medication until instructed to do so by your doctor or nurse. Do not take any medication not on this list, even a medication that you can buy at a drug store or health food store without a prescription, unless you check with your doctor or nurse.

Medication	Description	Strength	Dose	Schedule	Times	Reason	Comments
Diflucan®/ fluconazole	Pink, irregular-shaped tablet	200 mg	200 mg; 1 tablet	Every day	9 am	Prevent fungal infections	
Bactrim DS®/ sulfamethoxazole and trimethoprim/co-trimoxazole/TMP-SMX	Large white, oval tablet	Sulfamethoxazole 800 mg/Trimethoprim 160 mg	Sulfamethoxazole 800 mg/Trimethoprim 160 mg; 1 tablet	Twice a day on Monday and Thursday	9 am and 6 pm Monday and Thursday only	Prevent pneumonia	Take after eating.
Prilosec®/ omeprazole	Purple capsule	20 mg	20 mg; 1 capsule	Every day	8 am	Decrease stomach acid	
Prozac®/fluoxetine	Green and white capsule	20 mg	20 mg; 1 capsule	Every day	9 pm	Prevent depression	
Neoral®/cyclosporine	White, gelatin capsule	25 mg (small capsule) 100 mg (big capsule)	225 mg; 1 small capsule and 2 big capsules	Every 12 hours	10 am and 10 pm	Prevent graft versus host disease (GVHD)	Take at least 30 minutes before eating. When coming to clinic, do not take until after your blood work has been drawn.
Medrol®/methylprednisolone	White oval tablets	2 mg	4 mg; 2 tablets	Every day	9 am	Prevent GVHD	Take after eating.
Compazine®/ prochlorperazine	Yellow round tablets	10 mg	10 mg; 1 tablet	Every 4 hours as needed	As needed	Stop nausea and vomiting	Take if needed.
Ativan®/lorazepam	White, five-sided tablet	2 mg	2 mg; 1 tablet	Every 6 hours as needed	As needed	Stop anxiety; help with sleep	Take if needed.
Tylenol®/acetaminophen	White tablet	325 mg	325–650 mg; 1–2 tablets	Every 4 hours as needed	As needed	For mild pain	Take if needed.

Table 13-2. CDC Vaccination Recommendations for Autologous and Allogeneic Hematopoietic Stem Cell Transplant Recipients

Vaccine	Time Post-Transplant		
	12 Months	14 Months	24 Months
Tetanus-diphtheria toxoid (Td)[ab]	X	X	X
Haemophilus influenzae type b (Hib) conjugate	X	X	X
Hepatitis B (high-dose—40 mg/dose)	X	X	X[c]
23-valent pneumococcal polysaccharide	X		
Influenza	Starting six months after transplant, yearly at the start of influenza season		
Inactivated polio (IPV)	X	X	X
Measles-mumps-rubella (MMR)[d]			X[e]

[a] Only applies to people ≥ 7 years of age

[b] Should continue to be revaccinated every 10 years, as recommended for all adults

[c] Serum titer should be checked 1–2 months after third dose. If antibody not present, series of 3 vaccinations should be repeated.

[d] Live attenuated vaccine—administer only to patients assumed to be immunocompetent.

[e] A second dose is recommended 6–12 months later. If an outbreak of disease occurs, the second dose can be administered 4 weeks after the initial dose.

Note. Based on information from CDC et al., 2000.

each influenza season. Certain work sites, such as healthcare facilities, prisons, jails, and homeless shelters, increase the risk of exposure to tuberculosis and should be avoided (CDC et al., 2000).

To prevent a variety of opportunistic infections, patients in the first six months post-transplant, especially allogeneic transplant recipients and those on immunosuppressants, should avoid areas of construction, excavation, and other outdoor areas where the soil has been disturbed. They should be cautioned to avoid even passing through these areas when traveling from one place to another (Weems, Davis, Tablan, Kaufman, & Martone, 1987). Gardening and contact with soil or plants should be avoided. Patients also should avoid exposure to caves and areas where birds roost, smoking tobacco or other substances, and exposure to secondhand smoke. During this period, patients who are sexually active, even in long-term, monogamous relationships, should use latex condoms to reduce the risk of exposure to sexually transmitted viral diseases (CDC et al., 2000).

If patients have pets in the home during the first six months following transplant or while on immunosuppressives, care should be taken to ensure that the pets are healthy. Pets should be fed high-quality, fresh food. Raw pet

foods should be avoided. Patients and their household pets should not have contact with unfamiliar animals. Patients should not clean pet cages, fish tanks, or litter boxes or handle pet wastes. If these tasks cannot be avoided, patients should wear disposable gloves and wash their hands thoroughly immediately after disposing of the gloves. Cat litter boxes should be kept away from areas of food preparation. They should be cleaned daily by someone other than the patient and waste disposed of to prevent aerosolization. Certain animals, including reptiles, ducklings, chicks, and exotic animals, should be avoided completely (Angulo, Glaser, Juranek, Lappin, & Regnery, 1994; CDC et al., 2000; Elliot, Tolle, Goldberg, & Miller, 1985).

For the first six months following transplant and while immunosuppressed, patients should avoid wading, walking, swimming, or playing in lakes, rivers, and public swimming pools. They should not drink water from lakes, rivers, or wells that is not tested regularly for bacterial contamination (Kramer et al., 1998). Tap water may contain Cryptosporidium, so it should be boiled for at least one minute or filtered through a 1 mm filter prior to use. If bottled water is used, the label should be checked to be sure that it has been treated to remove Cryptosporidium. In restaurants and other public places, care should be taken to avoid water, ice, food, and drinks that may contain unboiled, unfiltered tap water (CDC et al., 2000).

Care should be taken in preparing food for transplant recipients. Family members and other caregivers should be educated on safe food preparation starting at the time of the patient's conditioning regimen. This will allow the family time to become familiar with the practices and to modify food preparation areas and equipment in the home before the patient becomes immunosuppressed. Raw meat, poultry, and seafood should be handled separately from other foods and cooked well before it is served to the transplant recipient. Fresh produce should be carefully washed under running water. Foods should be cooked to and stored at temperatures recommended by the U. S. Department of Agriculture (CDC et al., 2000).

The CDC recommends a low microbial diet for autologous transplant recipients for three months post-transplant and for allogeneic transplant recipients until all immunosuppressive medications are discontinued. In addition to avoiding undercooked meat, poultry, seafood, and dishes that may contain them, transplant recipients also should avoid raw or undercooked eggs and dishes that may contain them. Transplant recipients should use only pasteurized milk products and juices (Aker & Lenssen, 1999). Immunosuppressed transplant recipients should avoid naturopathic medicines because they may contain molds (CDC et al., 2000; Oliver, Van Voorhis, Boeckh, Mattson, & Bowden, 1996).

Finally, transplant recipients should be careful about traveling extensively, especially to developing countries, while they are immunosuppressed. Autologous transplant recipients should not travel to developing countries for three to six months post-transplant. Allogeneic transplant recipients should avoid such travel for six months to one year post-transplant, especially if they have or have had GVHD (CDC et al., 2000).

Toxicities and Complications

During post-transplant follow-up, patients are assessed to detect the development of any additional toxicities and to ensure that adequate progression to full recovery is occurring. Table 13-3 lists common late toxicities of HSCT along with recommendations for screening tests. Patients often receive prophylactic medications to prevent late complications, especially infections and GVHD. Although each transplant center decides which prophylactic medications will best meet the needs of each of their patients, Table 13-4 provides a list of some of the common medications used.

If toxicities occur after the initial recovery from HSCT, prompt identification and treatment offer the best chance for complete resolution (Vossen & Handgretinger, 2001). Awareness of the early signs and symptoms of late toxicities is critical for healthcare providers following patients at this time. If patients are returned to the care of primary care physicians or nontransplant specialists, information on identifying late toxicities should be provided to them. They should be aware of risk factors for particular late toxicities that specific patients may have. They should be advised when to contact the transplant team to assist in management of late toxicities and complications (Kapustay & Buchsel, 2000).

Engraftment syndrome has been reported to occur in 9%–55% of autologous transplant recipients following engraftment (Lee, Gingrich, Hohl, & Ajram, 1995; Moreb et al., 1997; Ravoet et al., 1996; Sica et al., 2000). Engraftment syndrome, sometimes referred to as autologous GVHD, appears to be an autoimmune reaction that is characterized by noninfectious fevers, skin rash, and occasionally diarrhea. Fluid retention, capillary leak, and pulmonary infiltrates may occur in severe cases (Edenfield, Moores, Goodwin, & Lee, 2000; Lee et al.; Moreb et al.; Ravoet et al.; Sica et al.). Engraftment syndrome is known to occur any time from engraftment until approximately 60 days post-transplant (Lee et al.; Moreb et al.; Sica et al.). Before the syndrome can be diagnosed, infectious causes and drug reactions must be ruled out. Treatment includes empiric antibiotics until infection is ruled out, antipyretics to control fever, careful review of current medications and continuation of only those that are absolutely necessary, topical, and/or systemic corticosteroids for the rash, and other supportive care as appropriate. The syndrome usually resolves spontaneously within two weeks to a month. Fatalities are reported infrequently in cases where capillary leak and pulmonary deterioration occur (Edenfield et al.; Lee et al.; Ravoet et al.; Sica et al.). The syndrome is most likely to occur in patients who receive a high dose of CD34+ cells/kg and experience early, rapid engraftment post-transplant (Edenfield et al.; Jillella, Helman, Larison, Litaker, & Cook, 2000; Ravoet et al.; Sica et al.). Engraftment syndrome is frustrating for patients and caregivers because the cause is never definitely identified, there is no treatment to resolve the syndrome, the fevers and rash cause significant discomfort, and the course of the syndrome is uncertain.

Following both allogeneic and autologous HSCT, some patients will develop multiple organ dysfunction syndrome (MODS). It has been suggested that MODS is a result of systemic inflammatory response syndrome (SIRS). Similar in presentation to engraftment syndrome, it is much more serious and often fatal (Haire, 2000). MODS is postulated to begin with tissue damage, most likely from the high-dose preparative regimen, infection, or GVHD. This damage induces cytokine production, which initiates coagulation and cytokine cascades in SIRS. The vascular endothelial damage eventually leads to major organ dysfunction, which may be one of the first signs of MODS (Haire; Takatsuka et al., 2000). The organs initially affected most often are lungs, central nervous system, or liver (Haire). Other symptoms related to SIRS include hyperthermia or hypothermia, tachycardia, tachypnea, and alteration in peripheral blood granulocyte count (Haire; Takatsuka et al.). Because of the cytokine cascade, there is a concern that colony-stimulating factors given to speed engraftment may play a role in SIRS and MODS. It has been suggested that patients be monitored daily during the engraftment period for signs of early organ dysfunction. Monitoring tests recommended are finger pulse oximetry, Mini-Mental Status Exam, serum bilirubin, and weight (Haire).

Post-Transplant Rehabilitation

In recent years, transplant programs have begun to use rehabilitation services to assist patients in recovery following transplantation (Dimeo et al., 1997). These services can assist patients in achieving a more rapid, complete recovery following transplant and improve patients' quality of life (Courneya, Keats, & Turner, 2000; Dimeo et al.). Patients can benefit from physical therapy to recover strength and stamina lost during the transplant process. Occupational therapy can assist patients in restructuring daily routines to achieve greater independence in self-care. Patients also can be taught strategies to cope with memory, concentration, and other executive function deficits that are known to occur after transplant (van Dam et al., 1998). Nutritional consultation can help patients to maintain adequate nutrition and eventually return to a normal diet while coping with taste changes, xerostomia, and temporary dietary restrictions. Seemingly minor gastrointestinal complications can lead to inadequate caloric intake, malnutrition, muscle wasting, and weight loss, if left untreated (Kelley et al., 1998). For patients at risk for nutritional compromise, a dietitian can be helpful in conducting nutritional assessments, providing dietary counseling, monitoring intake, and advising if oral supplements or parenteral nutrition are indicated (Kelley et al., 2000).

Home Care

Patients in the post-transplant follow-up period, who might otherwise require hospitalization, sometimes are able

Table 13-3. Long-Term Side Effects of Hematopoietic Stem Cell Transplantation

Side Effect	Expected Onset Post-HSCT	Evaluation Testing	Adult	Pediatric
Pulmonary				
Interstitial pneumonitis	80–150 days	O_2 sat; Chest x-ray; BAL; PFTs*[+]	X	X
Restrictive disease	Starting at 1 year	O_2 sat; Chest x-ray; PFTs*[+]	X	X
Obstructive disease	100–400 days	O_2 sat; Chest x-ray; PFTs*[+]	X	X
Bronchiolitis obliterans	90 days to 2 years	O_2 sat; Chest x-ray; PFTs*[+]	X	X
Infection	Up to 1 year or longer	O_2 sat; Chest x-ray; BAL; cultures*[+]	X	X
Central nervous system				
Leukoencephalopathy	30–150 days	Head CT scan or MRI	X	X
Cognitive dysfunction	90 days and longer	Cognitive function testing	X	X
Ocular				
Cataracts	1½–5 years	Ophthalmology exam; slit-lamp microscopy[+]	X	X
Sicca syndrome	1–5 years	Ophthalmology exam; Schirmer test[+]	X	X
Auditory				
Sensorineuronal deficit	180 days and longer	Auditory testing[+]		X
Dental				
Severe caries	90 days–1 year	Dental examination[+]	X	X
Tooth agenesis	Months to year	Dental examination[+]		X
Root abnormalities	Months to years	Dental examination[+]		X
Endocrine				
Hypothyroidism	Immediate to years	Thyroid function tests; thyroid scan[+]	X	X
Gonadal dysfunction	Immediate to years	Gonadotropin; sex steroid tests[+]	X	X
Infertility	Immediate to years	Gonadotropin; sex steroid tests[+]	X	X
Growth and development				
Decreased height growth	Immediate	Height measurement[+]		X
Insufficient weight gain	Immediate	Weight measurement[+]		X
Skeletal				
Avascular necrosis	90 days–1 year	Hip and shoulder x-rays	X	
Cardiac				
Decreased LVEF*	Up to 90–180 days	EKG; 2-D echocardiogram*[+]	X	X
Decreased LV wall size*	1 year or longer	EKG; 2-D echocardiogram*[+]		X
Liver				
Fibrosis	Several months to 1 year	LFTs; liver scan[+]	X	X
Functional liver disorder	1 month–1 year or longer	LFTs; liver scan[+]	X	X
Genitourinary				
Renal dysfunction	120 days–2 years	BUN, creatinine, urinalysis, B/P*[+]	X	X
Late hemorrhagic cystitis	More than 100 days	Urinalysis, cystoscopy[+]	X	
HUS*	30 days–2½ years	BUN, creatinine, platelet count[+]	X	X

(Continued on next page)

Side Effect	Expected Onset Post-HSCT	Evaluation Testing	Adult	Pediatric
Chronic GVHD	50 days to several years	Biopsy, x-rays, LFTs, PFTs*+	X	X
Infections	Up to 1 year or longer	Cultures	X	X
Impaired quality of life	Immediate to years	Validated quality-of-life assessment tool+	X	X
Disease relapse/recurrence	Immediate to years	Appropriate screening tests for disease+	X	X
Secondary malignancy				
Lymphoproliferative	Up to 1 year	CBC, bone marrow aspiration+	X	X
Leukemias	1–2 years	CBC, bone marrow aspiration+	X	X
Solid tumors	Many years	Biopsy, diagnostic scans	X	X

+ Italicized tests are standard screening tests that should be performed on a standard schedule of baseline pre-HSCT, 3 months, 6 months, and 12 months post-HSCT and then yearly for at-risk individuals.

* Abbreviations: BAL—broncho-alveolar lavage; B/P—blood pressure; EKG—electrocardiogram; HUS—hemolytic uremic syndrome; LFTs—liver function tests; LV—left ventricular; LVEF—left ventricular ejection fraction; O₂ sat—oxygen saturation by pulse oximeter; PFTs—pulmonary function tests

Note. Based on information from Buchsel, 1999; Deeg, 1994; Schwarze & Ranke, 2001.

to remain as outpatients with the support of home care. Although stable, patients may require long-term intravenous antimicrobials, immunosuppressives, or nutrition support (Kelley et al., 1998). Although some of this therapy can be provided in an outpatient clinic, the clinic may not be able to meet all of a patient's infusion needs. If home care can provide these services when clinic schedules and space do not permit, patients may be kept out of the hospital. Home care is less costly than hospitalization and is often more acceptable to patients (Buchsel & Kapustay, 1999; Kelley et al., 2000).

Homecare nurses can provide valuable insights into a patient's home environment and psychosocial status. Patients sometimes misunderstand instructions or have situations in their homes that they do not realize are dangerous to them. At other times, patients may have needs or problems that they are reluctant to share with healthcare providers. Patients often are more open in discussing concerns with healthcare providers in their own homes. Homecare nurses can counsel and educate patients about these issues. Homecare nurses can provide additional information to the primary healthcare team about the patient's needs. In addition, home healthcare nurses can continue and supplement patient and family education (Kelley et al., 1998, 2000).

Patients without a daytime caregiver may need home-health aide support for personal care and meal preparation. Because patients still are immunosuppressed, a regular thorough housecleaning schedule must be maintained (Kelley et al., 1998). If family members who must work are unable to do this, an aide to assist with the cleaning is invaluable.

For a homecare agency to provide optimum care to a transplant recipient, the staff must be aware of the patient's history, transplant course, current needs, and future treatment plans. Ideally, one or more members of the homecare agency staff will be part of the transplant program multidisciplinary team and attend regular transplant team meetings and patient reviews. When a patient is referred for home care, the homecare agency should receive written and verbal information about the patient (Kelley et al., 2000). Figure 13-1 contains information that may be useful to communicate when referral is made to a homecare agency. The homecare agency should provide prompt and complete records of all care provided to the patient's primary healthcare team. This information can be faxed to the physician's office or can be hand-carried by the patient to clinic visits. Care also must be taken to ensure that physician orders for care by the homecare agency are complete and that changes are communicated promptly (Kelley et al., 2000).

Personnel familiar with the process of transplant and the special needs of transplant recipients should provide home care. Personnel providing care in the home are an extension of the transplant program staff. Regardless of the level of expertise of agency staff, each transplant program should work with homecare and infusion agencies to provide education to all personnel that provide care in the home to their patients. Homecare and infusion agencies must see that their staff members are educated on general concepts of transplan-

Table 13-4. Common Prophylactic Medications Following Hematopoietic Stem Cell Transplantation

Medication	Purpose
Fluconazole/Diflucan® (Pfizer, New York, NY)	Prevent fungal infections
Sulfamethoxazole and trimethoprim/co-trimoxazole/Bactrim DS® (Women First HealthCare, San Diego, CA) or Septra DS® (Monarch, Fort Worth, TX)	Prevent *Pneumocystis carinii* pneumonia and bacterial infections
Penicillin V potassium/Pen-Vee K® (Wyeth, Philadelphia, PA)	Prevent bacterial infections
Acyclovir/Zovirax® (GlaxoSmithKline, London, UK) or Valacyclovir/Valtrex® (GlaxoSmithKline)	Prevent herpes simplex infections
Ganciclovir/Cytovene® (Roche, Nutley, NJ)	Prevent cytomegalovirus infection
Cyclosporine/Sandimmune® or Neoral® (Novartis, Cambridge, MA) or Tacrolimus/Prograf® (Fujisawa, Deerfield, IL)	Prevent graft versus host disease
Methylprednisolone/Medrol® (Pfizer)	Prevent graft versus host disease
Omeprazole/Prilosec® (AstraZeneca, Wilmington, DE)	Prevent gastric acid hypersecretion

Note. Based on information from Kapustay & Buchsel, 2000.

tation and specific practices of the individual transplant center (Kelley et al., 2000). Education efforts should cover the basic transplant information required of all staff in other areas of the transplant program as well as knowledge unique to the home setting, such as that listed in Figure 13-2. Ideally, the homecare agency will be able to assign a specific group of nurses and other personnel with special expertise and training in HSCT to rotate in providing all transplant patient home care (Kelley et al., 2000).

Post-Transplant Maintenance Therapy

Increasingly, transplant therapy is not considered the final or curative therapy for patients with malignancies but rather as another treatment modality in the total therapy of patients (Barlogie et al., 1999). The most common cause of death following transplant is relapse of disease. To significantly impact survival, effective methods to prevent relapse of the underlying malignancy are needed (Lazarus et al., 2001). In many patients, transplant renders a minimal residual disease state and provides an ideal setting for additional therapy to destroy the small numbers of remaining tumor cells (Guillaume, Rubinstein, & Symann, 1999).

In patients with lymphoma or breast cancer, radiation therapy frequently is given to areas of previous disease or with a high likelihood of recurrence following autologous transplantation (Marks et al., 1994; Schenkein et al., 1997). Radiation after transplant has been found to be less likely to induce toxicity in sensitive organs, such as the lungs, than radiation administered prior to high-dose therapy (van Besien et al., 1995). Care must be exercised not to irradiate the pelvis too soon after transplant, when the new stem cell graft is not well established. The decision to radiate the pelvis at a later time should take into consideration the robustness of the graft. Radiation therapy that does not involve the pelvis still can have hematologic consequences post-transplant. Marks et al. reported that patients with breast cancer, receiving chest wall and axillary radiation therapy following

high-dose chemotherapy and autologous bone marrow transplant, experienced more severe hematologic toxicity than did patients who had received only standard chemotherapy doses. The greater hematologic toxicity was due, in part, to the fact that the patients given high-dose chemotherapy began radiation therapy with lower white blood cell and platelet counts than patients receiving standard dose chemotherapy (Marks et al.). However, radiation therapy following transplant can significantly improve outcomes for select patients. In a large multivariate analysis, the use of involved field radiation following autologous transplant was shown to have a positive prognostic value for overall survival in patients with diffuse non-Hodgkin's lymphoma who never achieved a complete remission with standard dose chemotherapy (Vose et al., 2001).

Several other therapies are commonplace following transplant. Bisphosphonates are given to control bony disease or delay its onset and induce tumor cell apoptosis in multiple myeloma and metastatic breast cancer (Munshi, Barlogie, Desikan, & Wilson, 1999). Hormone-sensitive patients with breast cancer routinely receive selective estrogen receptor modulators post-transplant.

Despite concern for the immature stem cell graft, both Rahman et al. (1998) and Tallman et al. (1997) tested the feasibility of giving standard dose chemotherapy to patients with metastatic breast cancer following autologous stem cell transplantation. In both studies, patients were able to tolerate multiple courses of chemotherapy after transplant without unusual or significant toxicity. Because the number of patients in each study was small, it is not possible to comment on the efficacy of this approach. However, in both studies, the outcomes of the patients receiving the consolidation chemotherapy were encouraging (Rahman et al.; Tallman et al.). The feasibility of this approach following autologous transplantation in patients with hematologic malignancies and poorer stem cell reserves is uncertain.

Recently, post-transplant therapy to destroy minimal residual disease has focused on immune modulation. Manipulation of the immune system to destroy a minimal number of remaining tumor cells appears to be an encouraging strategy. Experience in allogeneic transplant with graft versus tumor effect has demonstrated that the immune system can be very effective post-transplant in eradicating remaining tumor cells and preventing recurrence of malignant disease. However, there has been some concern that slow immune reconstitution after transplant may interfere with attempts to boost the immune system against tumor cells (Guillaume et al., 1999).

Possibly the oldest and most widely used immune therapy post-transplant is the administration of interferon or dexamethasone maintenance therapy after autologous transplantation in patients with myeloma (Barlogie et al., 1999; Reece, Brockington, et al., 2000). The effect of interferon maintenance treatment on overall survival has been significant but limited (Ludwig, Meran, & Zojer, 1999). Besides interferon, the use of other cytokines, such as interleukin-2 (IL-2) and granulocyte macrophage–colony-stimulating factor, as maintenance therapy following transplantation has been proposed, and early studies are under way in patients with breast cancer and hematologic malignancies (Barlogie et al., 1998; Gravis et al., 2000; Meehan et al., 1996, 1999). These therapies are feasible and safe, especially if the dose of cytokine is kept relatively low (Gravis et al.; Meehan et al., 1999). Patients in some trials developed autologous GVHD during cytokine administration (Meehan et al., 1996, 1999). The efficacy of this approach remains to be seen.

Early studies describe the use of general and specific tumor vaccines in patients with breast cancer, ovarian cancer, and multiple myeloma following transplant (Holmberg et al., 2000; Reece, Foon, et al., 2000; Trudel et al., 2001). However, these studies are too early and the number of subjects too small to draw any conclusions about the efficacy of this approach. The therapy has been shown to be safe and feasible (Holmberg et al.; Reece, Foon, et al., 2000; Trudel et al.). Reichardt et al. (1999) reported the safe use of dendritic cells for idiotypic vaccination after autologous transplantation for multiple myeloma. The use of monoclonal antibodies as adjuvant immunotherapy post-transplant is being explored (Flinn & Lazarus, 2001).

Because of the donor immune system, allogeneic transplantation offers unique opportunities for immune manipulation post-transplant. Allogeneic transplant was one of the first areas where cytokine manipulation was used to treat post-transplant relapse. In 1993, Giralt et al. reported giving granulocyte–colony-stimulating factor (G-CSF) to patients with leukemia who were relapsing following allogeneic transplantation. The stimulation of residual donor marrow cells by the G-CSF reinduced remission in three of seven patients (Giralt et al.). Since this initial observation, a variety of strategies, including reduction in immunosuppression, infusion of additional donor lymphocytes with or without additional chemotherapy, and administration of various cytokines, has been used following allogeneic transplantation to treat relapsing and refractory disease or prevent relapse in high-risk patients with a variety of malignancies

(Badros et al., 2001; Collins et al., 1997; Shaffer, Giralt, Champlin, & Chan, 1995). Based on these early data, indolent hematologic and less advanced malignancies show better responses to this therapy than more aggressive, advanced disease (Collins et al.). These strategies must be used with extreme caution because they carry the risk of severe GVHD that can be extremely debilitating or fatal.

It is known that the bone marrow of patients with multiple myeloma has increased microvessel density compared to the bone marrow of people without multiple myeloma. This increased microvessel density does not disappear following autologous transplantation (Rajkumar, Fonseca, Witzig, Gertz, & Greipp, 1999). Therefore, the use of anti-angiogenesis agents post-transplant as maintenance therapy in multiple myeloma is a reasonable strategy. There have been a few reports of successful treatment of relapsed myeloma post-transplant with thalidomide (Tosi et al., 2001; Zomas, Anagnostopoulos, & Dimopoulos, 2000). The actual effectiveness of this approach as prophylactic maintenance therapy will need to be evaluated in large trials.

There is a relatively high rate of relapse following HSCT in children with certain hematologic malignancies and solid tumors. The use of IL-2, anti-CD 19 antibodies, activated cytotoxic T lymphocytes, or dendritic cells post-HSCT to improve immune function and prevent relapse in these children has been suggested (Vossen & Handgretinger, 2001). Early studies of immunologic manipulation as maintenance therapy post-HSCT in children with high-risk hematologic malignancies and solid tumors have found it a feasible treatment, but its efficacy has yet to be proven (Bonig et al., 2000; Dilloo et al., 1994; Messina et al., 1996; Pession et al., 1998; Robinson et al., 1996; Toren et al., 2000; Vivancos, Granena, Sarra, & Granena, 1999; Vlk et al., 2000).

Figure 13-2. Basic Educational Requirements for Nursing Staffs Caring for Hematopoietic Stem Cell Transplant Recipients

Areas of Knowledge
- Hematology/oncology patient care
- Usual transplant course
- HSCT patient assessment
- High-dose preparative regimens
- Prophylactic therapies
- Growth factor therapy
- Immunosuppressive agents
- Expected complications and toxicities
- Prevention and management of infectious complications in compromised hosts
- Nutritional needs of HSCT recipients
- Environmental assessment
- Psychosocial support of HSCT recipients and families
- HSCT patient and family education
- Blood component uses and administration
- Emergency care of the acutely ill patient
- Program-specific policies and procedures (e.g., central venous catheter care, patient and family education protocols, dietary restrictions)

Note. Based on information from FACT, 2002; Kelley et al., 1998.

Maintenance therapy following allogeneic or autologous transplant may begin anywhere from several days to several months post-transplant. Factors influencing the decision of when to start maintenance therapy include the consequences of delaying therapy, potential toxicities of the maintenance therapy, the vitality of the new graft, and the strength of the immune system that may be part of the maintenance strategy (Rahman et al., 1998). If patients are returned to the care of another physician or clinic while they are receiving maintenance therapy, the personnel assuming care of the patient must be aware of the therapy, its administration, its toxicities and side effects, and its goals. If the patient is receiving this therapy as part of a research protocol, he or she should be aware of all of the requirements of the protocol and who to contact if a problem arises. If the maintenance post-transplant involves an investigational drug or manipulation of the donor immune system, where GVHD could occur, it may be safer for the patient to remain at the transplant center until the maintenance therapy is complete.

Returning Care to the Referring Physician

The appropriate time to return the care of a transplant recipient to a referring physician can be a difficult decision. The expertise of the referring physician in the care of oncology and transplant patients will enter into the decision. If the referring physician is an experienced medical oncologist/hematologist and the patient has had an uncomplicated autologous transplant, the decision is easier, and the care can be transferred sooner after recovery from the transplant. Returning care for patients who have received allogeneic transplants who have had significant complications following autologous transplants or who have nononcologic/hematologic referring physicians is more problematic (Buchsel, 1999). These patients have increased assessment and follow-up care needs that the referring physician may be unprepared to provide. Patients also may feel strongly about returning to their referring physicians. If patients are anxious to return home, or if coming to the transplant center is inconvenient, they may be eager to return to the care of their referring physicians. Returning for follow-up to the referring physician may be an important step for a patient in the process of re-establishing a normal life post-transplant. However, patients sometimes become very attached to and dependent on transplant personnel. They may wish to remain under the care of the transplant physician team because they feel safe or have developed a good rapport (Buchsel). The transplant physician and staff should discuss with the patient and family early in the transplant process when the patient can expect to end care at the transplant center. When it is safe and appropriate, the patient should return to the referring physician. While under the care of the referring physician, the patient may occasionally return to the transplant center for long-term evaluations (Buchsel).

Transfer of the patient back to the referring physician is facilitated if the referring physician has been receiving regular reports every few weeks from the transplant center about the patient's progress through transplant. When care is actually transferred, the referring physician should receive a detailed summary of the patient's transplant course, current condition, and follow-up needs (Buchsel, 1999). Figure 13-1 lists potential information to be communicated to the referring physician when the patient is returned to his or her care. The referring physician and transplant physician also may be in contact regularly by telephone, fax, or e-mail for the first several weeks or months after the care of the patient has been transferred to ensure that the patient has no further transplant-specific needs. The referring physician and his or her staff can be extremely helpful to the transplant center staff in seeing that long-term post-transplant follow-up evaluations are performed appropriately and the results shared with the transplant center staff (Buchsel). If the staff in the referring physician's office is aware of the tests and assessments that the patient needs, understands the purpose and importance of the follow-up, and has ready access to staff at the transplant center for transmitting information and asking questions, they can be very helpful in facilitating the follow-up process. Tests and schedules that are commonly used to assess for common late side effects after HSCT are shown in Table 13-3.

Rehospitalization

Occasionally during the post-transplant period, patients will develop a late transplant-related complication or illness unrelated to transplant that requires hospitalization (Buchsel & Kapustay, 1999). If the patient is still being cared for in the same area as the transplant center, the hospitalization may be on the transplant unit. Some transplant centers do not admit transplant patients with late complications to the transplant unit because of space or other patient care considerations. If the patient has returned home away from the transplant center, rehospitalization may be to the transplant unit of a local transplant center, if available, or to a nontransplant unit. Once again, communication is the key to ensuring that the hospital staff caring for the transplant recipient is aware of the unique needs of the patient related to the transplant (Buchsel, 1999). It is advisable for the patient to wear a MedicAlert® identification bracelet or necklace to indicate that the patient has had a transplant. If the patient is unable to communicate when admitted to a hospital, the hospital staff will know to seek further information about the patient's current status. It also is advisable for the patient and family caregivers to have a copy of the patient's transplant summary, which includes contact information for the transplant center.

Rehospitalization can be a devastating emotional experience for the patient and family. The patient's and family's perception of the hospitalization will be dependent on their previous experiences with hospitalizations, their understanding of the patient's current medical condition, and other psychosocial factors (Buchsel, 1999). Whatever the reason for the hospitalization, the patient and family should be given honest, accurate information. If the hospitalization is planned for only a short time to stabilize a persistent or less serious problem, the patient and family should be offered reassurance that the hospitalization is precautionary and should be brief. If, however, the patient is admitted with a serious problem, the patient and family should be informed that the hospitalization could be lengthy and the outcome poor (Fallowfield, Jenkins, & Beveridge, 2002).

Long-Term Follow-Up

One of the most difficult tasks after HSCT is long-term follow-up of patients. As the time since transplant increases, it usually becomes more difficult to obtain accurate and complete information about patients. The process can be very time-consuming and frustrating for staff and may seem inconsequential compared to the needs of current patients. However, knowledge of the long-term effects and outcomes of transplantation are crucial in ultimately determining the use and value of transplantation as a treatment modality (FACT, 2002).

In an effort to maintain current, accurate records on all patients, some transplant centers are developing the role of long-term follow-up coordinator. This person may be a research nurse, data coordinator, or social worker. Depending on the number of patients in follow-up, this may be a full- or part-time position. A permanent follow-up phone number at the transplant center can facilitate reporting of information (R.M. Rifkin, personal communication, November 12, 1999).

Discussing the need for long-term follow-up with patients and families throughout the transplant process can help to make patients more active participants in the process. Patients and families who are willing to contact the transplant center if the patient's contact information changes or if a change in the patient's condition occurs can be a great help to the long-term follow-up coordinator. Soliciting help in follow-up from the staffs of referring physicians' offices also can improve the process. Spending time informing the referring physicians' staffs about how follow-up information is used and supplying them with reports that include information that they have provided gives them added incentive to aid in the follow-up process (White-Hershey & Nevidjon, 1990).

In general, the two most vital pieces of follow-up information are the patient's disease status and overall survival information. In addition, it is helpful to know if the patient has developed any further malignancies or hematologic disorders, if the patient has conceived a child, and if the patient has developed any significant medical problems that may be related to the transplant therapy. Information on any further therapy the patient has received and on the patient's performance status, employment status, and quality of life also is useful (FACT, 2002; International Bone Marrow Transplant Registry/Autologous Blood and Marrow Transplant Registry [IBMTR/ABMTR], 2002). A recommended minimum data set for post-HSCT follow-up is in Figure 13-3.

Figure 13-3. Suggested Minimum Data Set for Follow-Up of Hematopoietic Stem Cell Transplantation

Data Element
- Additional cell therapy or HSCT after first HSCT
  - Type of therapy
  - Date therapy began
- Date of white blood cell (WBC) engraftment (neutrophils ≥ 500 cells/μl)
  - Lack of engraftment or graft failure
  - Date of last WBC assessment
- ECOG/Karnofsky/Lansky performance status
- Maximum grade of acute graft versus host disease (GVHD)—allogeneic HSCT only
- Maximum extent of chronic GVHD—allogeneic HSCT only
  - Date of onset of chronic GVHD
- Disease status after HSCT
  - Type of assessment
  - Date of assessment
  - Date of progression or recurrence
- Best disease response to transplant
- Maintenance therapy post-HSCT
  - Type of therapy
- Development of second malignancy or lymphoproliferative disorder
  - Type of malignancy
  - Date of diagnosis
- Conception by patient or partner post-HSCT
- Employment/educational status
- Quality-of-life measurement
- Survival status
- Date of last contact or death
- Primary cause of death

Note. Based on information from FACT, 2002; IBMTR/ABMTR, 2002.

Dated documentation of all information in the patient's permanent medical record is vital (IBMTR/ABMTR, 2002). A written summary from the physician caring for the patient as well as copies of all relevant test results is ideal. If it is not possible to obtain these records, careful, detailed notation in the patient's medical record of conversations is acceptable. If possible, verbal information should be verified with a second source before it is documented as true. Names and contact numbers for all sources of verbal information should be included in the documentation (Weiss, 1998).

Conclusion

Care of the transplant recipient does not end with the engraftment of the stem cells. Patients and their families will continue to cope with the effects of transplantation for months and years after the transplant. Care of the patient over this extended period of time will take place in many settings. Systems to provide rapid, accurate, and complete information about the patient's past medical history and current condition are critical to ensuring that healthcare personnel can provide the best care to the patient. Patient and family education about the transplant process and post-transplant expectations and needs is essential. This process should not stop with the end of care at the transplant center. Without long-term follow-up, the ultimate impact of transplant therapy will never be known.

References

Aker, S.N., & Lenssen, P. (1999). Nutritional support of patients with hematological malignancies. In R. Hoffman, E.J. Benz, Jr., S.J. Shatill, B. Furie, H.J. Cohen, L.E. Silberstein, et al. (Eds.), *Hematology: Principles and practice* (3rd ed., pp. 1501–1514). New York: Churchill Livingstone.

Angulo, F.J., Glaser, C.A., Juranek, D.D., Lappin, M.R., & Regnery, R.L. (1994). Caring for pets of immunocompromised persons. *Journal of the American Veterinary Medicine Association, 205,* 1711–1718.

Avigan, D., Pirofski, L.A., & Lazarus, H. (2001). Vaccination against infectious disease following hematopoietic stem cell transplantation. *Biology of Blood and Marrow Transplant, 7,* 171–183.

Badros, A., Barlogie, B., Morris, C., Desikan, R., Martin, S.R., Munshi, N., et al. (2001). High response rate in refractory and poor-risk multiple myeloma after allotransplantation using a nonmyeloablative conditioning regimen and donor lymphocyte infusions. *Blood, 97,* 2574–2579.

Barlogie, B., Jagannath, S., Desikan, K.R., Mattox, S., Vesole, D., Siegel, D., et al. (1999). Total therapy with tandem transplants for newly diagnosed multiple myeloma. *Blood, 93,* 55–65.

Barlogie, B., Jagannath, S., Naucke, S., Mattox, S., Bracy, D., Crowley, J., et al. (1998). Long-term follow-up after high-dose therapy for high-risk multiple myeloma. *Bone Marrow Transplantation, 21,* 1101–1107.

Bonig, H., Laws, H.J., Wundes, A., Verheyen, J., Hannen, M., Kim, Y.M., et al. (2000). In vivo cytokine responses to interleukin-2 immunotherapy after autologous stem cell transplantation in children with solid tumors. *Bone Marrow Transplantation, 26,* 91–96.

Buchsel, P.C. (1999). Bone marrow transplantation. In C. Miaskowski & P. Buchsel (Eds.), *Oncology nursing: Assessment and clinical care* (pp. 143–186). St. Louis, MO: Mosby.

Buchsel, P.C., & Kapustay, P. (1999). Peripheral stem cell transplantation. In C. Miaskowski & P. Buchsel (Eds.), *Oncology nursing: Assessment and clinical care* (pp. 187–208). St. Louis, MO: Mosby.

Centers for Disease Control and Prevention. (2000). Guidelines for preventing opportunistic infections among hematopoietic stem cell transplant recipients: Recommendations of CDC, the Infectious Diseases Society of America and the American Society of Blood and Marrow Transplantation. *Biology of Blood and Marrow Transplant, 6,* 659–734.

Collins, R.H., Jr., Shpilberg, O., Drobyski, W.R., Porter, D.L., Giralt, S., Champlin, R., et al. (1997). Donor leukocyte infusions in 140 patients with relapsed malignancy after allogeneic bone marrow transplantation. *Journal of Clinical Oncology, 15,* 433–444.

Courneya, K.S., Keats, M.R., & Turner, A.R. (2000). Physical exercise and quality of life in cancer patients following high dose chemotherapy and autologous bone marrow transplantation. *Psychooncology, 9,* 127–136.

Deeg, H.J. (1994). Delayed complications after bone marrow transplantation. In S.J. Forman, K.G. Blume, & E.D. Thomas (Eds.), *Bone marrow transplantation* (pp. 538–544). Boston: Blackwell Scientific.

Dexter, F., & Epstein, R.H. (2001). Reducing family members' anxiety while waiting on the day of surgery: Systematic review of studies and implications of HIPAA health information privacy rules. *Journal of Clinical Anesthesia, 13,* 478–481.

Dilloo, D., Laws, H.J., Hanenberg, H., Korholz, D., Nurnberger, W., & Burdach, S.E. (1994). Induction of two distinct natural killer-cell populations, activated T cells and antineoplastic cytokines, by interleukin-2 therapy in children with solid tumors. *Experimental Hematology, 22,* 1081–1088.

Dimeo, F.C., Tilmann, M.H., Bertz, H., Kanz, L., Mertelsmann, R., & Keul, J. (1997). Aerobic exercise in the rehabilitation of cancer patients after high dose chemotherapy and autologous peripheral stem cell transplantation. *Cancer, 79,* 1717–1722.

Edenfield, W.J., Moores, L.K., Goodwin, G., & Lee, N. (2000). An engraftment syndrome in autologous stem cell transplantation related to mononuclear cell dose. *Bone Marrow Transplantation, 25,* 405–409.

Elliot, D.L., Tolle, S.W., Goldberg, L., & Miller, J.B. (1985). Pet-associated illness. *New England Journal of Medicine, 313,* 985–995.

Fallowfield, L.J., Jenkins, V.A., & Beveridge, H.A. (2002). Truth may hurt but deceit hurts more: Communication in palliative care. *Palliative Medicine, 16,* 297–303.

Flinn, I.W., & Lazarus, H.M. (2001). Monoclonal antibodies and autologous stem cell transplantation for lymphoma. *Bone Marrow Transplantation, 27,* 565–569.

Foundation for the Accreditation of Cellular Therapy. (2002). *FACT standards for hematopoietic progenitor cell collection, processing and transplantation* (2nd ed.). Omaha, NE: Author.

Gaynes, R.P., & Horan, T.C. (1999). Surveillance of nosocomial infections. In C.G. Mayhall (Ed.), *Hospital epidemiology and infection control* (2nd ed., pp. 1285–1317). Philadelphia: Lippincott Williams and Wilkins.

Giralt, S., Escudier, S., Kantarjian, H., Deisseroth, A., Freireich, E.J., Andersson, B.S., et al. (1993). Preliminary results of treatment with filgrastim for relapse of leukemia and myelodysplasia after allogeneic bone marrow transplantation. *New England Journal of Medicine, 329,* 757–761.

Gravis, G., Viens, P., Vey, N., Blaise, D., Stoppa, A.M., Olive, D., et al. (2000). Pilot study of immunotherapy with interleukin-2 after autologous stem cell transplantation in advanced breast cancers. *Anticancer Research, 20,* 3987–3991.

Guillaume, T., Rubinstein, D.B., & Symann, M. (1999). Immunological recovery and tumour-specific immunotherapeutic approaches to post-autologous haematopoietic stem cell transplantation. *Baillieres Best Practices in Research and Clinical Haematology, 12,* 293–306.

Haire, W.D. (2000). Multiple organ dysfunction syndrome. In J.O. Armitage & K.H. Antman (Eds.), *High-dose cancer therapy: Pharmacology, hematopoietins, stem cells* (3rd ed., pp. 609–624). Philadelphia: Lippincott Williams and Wilkins.

Henning, K.J., White, M.H., Sepkowitz, K.A., & Armstrong, D. (1997). National survey of immunization practices following allogeneic bone marrow transplantation. *JAMA, 277,* 1148–1151.

Holmberg, L.A., Oparin, D.V., Gooley, T., Lilleby, K., Bensinger, W., Reddish, M.A., et al. (2000). Clinical outcome of breast and ovarian cancer patients treated with high-dose chemotherapy, autologous stem cell rescue and theratope STn-KLH cancer vaccine. *Bone Marrow Transplantation, 25,* 1233–1241.

International Bone Marrow Transplant Registry/Autologous Blood and Marrow Transplant Registry. (2002, July). *Data collection.* Retrieved August 23, 2002, from http://www.ibmtr.org/datacollec/datacollec.research_dc.html

Jillella, A.P., Helman, S.W., Larison, J., Litaker, M.S., & Cook, L.O. (2000). High-dose chemotherapy followed by reinfusion of a high number of CD34+ progenitor cells is frequently associated with development of fever in the postengraftment period. *Journal of Hematotherapy and Stem Cell Research, 9,* 849–854.

Kapustay, P.M., & Buchsel, P.C. (2000). Process, complications, and management of peripheral stem cell transplant. In P.C. Buchsel & P.M. Kapustay (Eds.), *Stem cell transplantation: A clinical text book* (pp. 5.1–5.28). Pittsburgh, PA: Oncology Nursing Society.

Kelley, C.H., McBride, L.H., Randolph, S.R., Leum, E.W., & Lonergan, J.N. (1998). *Homecare management of the blood cell transplant patient* (3rd ed.). Sudbury, MA: Jones and Bartlett.

Kelley, C.H., Randolph, S.R., & Leum, E. (2000). Home care of peripheral stem cell transplantation recipients. In P.C. Buchsel & P.M. Kapustay (Eds.), *Stem cell transplantation: A clinical textbook* (pp. 13.1–13.16). Pittsburgh, PA: Oncology Nursing Society.

Kramer, M.H., Sorhage, F.E., Goldstein, S.T., Dalley, E., Wahlquist, S.P., & Herwaldt, B.L. (1998). First reported outbreak in the

United States of cryptosporidiosis associated with a recreational lake. *Clinical Infectious Diseases, 26,* 27–33.

Lazarus, H.M., Loberiza, F.R., Jr., Zhang, M.J., Armitage, J.O., Ballen, K.K., Bashey, A., et al. (2001). Autotransplants for Hodgkin's disease in first relapse or second remission: A report from the autologous blood and marrow transplant registry (ABMTR). *Bone Marrow Transplantation, 27,* 387–396.

Lee, C.K., Gingrich, R.D., Hohl, R.J., & Ajram, K.A. (1995). Engraftment syndrome in autologous bone marrow and peripheral stem cell transplantation. *Bone Marrow Transplantation, 16,* 175–182.

Ljungman, P., Lewensohn-Fuchs, I., Hammarström, V., Aschan, J., Brandt, L., Bolme, P., et al. (1994). Long-term immunity to measles, mumps, and rubella after allogeneic bone marrow transplantation. *Blood, 84,* 657–663.

Ljungman, P., Wiklund-Hammarsten, M., Duraj, V., Hammarström, L., Lonnqvist, B., Paulin, T., et al. (1990). Responses to tetanus toxoid immunization after allogeneic bone marrow transplantation. *Journal of Infectious Diseases, 162,* 496–500.

Ludwig, H., Meran, J., & Zojer, N. (1999). Multiple myeloma: An update on biology and treatment. *Annals of Oncology, 10*(Suppl. 6), 31–43.

Marks, L.B., Rosner, G.L., Prosnitz, L.R., Ross, M., Vredenburgh, J.J., & Peters, W.P. (1994). The impact of conventional plus high dose chemotherapy with autologous bone marrow transplantation on hematologic toxicity during subsequent local-regional radiotherapy for breast cancer. *Cancer, 74,* 2964–2971.

Meehan, K.R., Arun, B., Gehan, E.A., Berberian, B., Sulica, V., Areman, E.M., et al. (1999). Immunotherapy with interleukin-2 and alpha-interferon after IL-2-activated hematopoietic stem cell transplantation for breast cancer. *Bone Marrow Transplantation, 23,* 667–673.

Meehan, K.R., Verma, U.N., Rajogopal, C., Cahill, R., Frankel, S., & Mazumder, A. (1996). Stem cell transplantation with chemoradiotherapy myeloablation and interleukin-2. *Journal of Infusional Chemotherapy, 6,* 28–32.

Messina, C., Zambello, R., Rossetti, F., Gazzola, M.V., Varotto, S., Destro, R., et al. (1996). Interleukin-2 before and/or after autologous bone marrow transplantation for pediatric acute leukemia patients. *Bone Marrow Transplantation, 17,* 729–735.

Moreb, J.S., Kubilis, P.S., Mullins, D.L., Myers, L., Youngblood, M., & Hutcheson, C. (1997). Increased frequency of autoaggression syndrome associated with autologous stem cell transplantation in breast cancer patients. *Bone Marrow Transplantation, 19,* 101–106.

Munshi, N.C., Barlogie, B., Desikan, K.R., & Wilson, C. (1999). Novel approaches in myeloma therapy. *Seminars in Oncology, 2*(Suppl. 13), 28–34.

Oliver, M.R., Van Voorhis, W.C., Boeckh, M., Mattson, D., & Bowden, R.A. (1996). Hepatic mucormycosis in a bone marrow transplant recipient who ingested naturopathic medicine. *Clinical Infectious Diseases, 22,* 521–524.

Pauksen, K., Hammarström, V., Ljungman, P., Sjolin, J., Oberg, G., Lonnerholm, G., et al. (1994). Immunity to poliovirus and immunization with inactivated poliovirus vaccine after autologous bone marrow transplantation. *Clinical Infectious Diseases, 18,* 547–552.

Pession, A., Prete, A., Locatelli, F., Pierinelli, S., Pession, A.L., Maccario, R., et al. (1998). Immunotherapy with low-dose recombinant interleukin 2 after high-dose chemotherapy and autologous stem cell transplantation in neuroblastoma. *British Journal of Cancer, 78,* 528–533.

Potter, J., Stott, D.J., Roberts, M.A., Elder, A.G., O'Donnell, B., Knight, P.V., et al. (1997). Influenza vaccination of health care workers in long-term-care hospitals reduces the mortality of elderly patients. *Journal of Infectious Diseases, 175,* 1–6.

Rahman, Z., Kavanagh, J., Champlin, R., Giles, R., Hanania, E., Fu, S., et al. (1998). Chemotherapy immediately following autologous stem-cell transplantation in patients with advanced breast cancer. *Clinical Cancer Research, 4,* 2717–2721.

Rajkumar, S.V., Fonseca, R., Witzig, T.E., Gertz, M.A., & Greipp, P.R. (1999). Bone marrow angiogenesis in patients achieving complete response after stem cell transplantation for multiple myeloma. *Leukemia, 13,* 469–472.

Ravoet, C., Feremans, W., Husson, B., Majois, F., Kentos, A., Lambermont, M., et al. (1996). Clinical evidence for an engraftment syndrome associated with early and steep neutrophil recovery after autologous blood stem cell transplantation. *Bone Marrow Transplantation, 18,* 943–947.

Reece, D.E., Brockington, D.A., Phillips, G.L., Barnett, M.J., Klingemann, H.G., Nantel, S., et al. (2000). Prolonged survival after intensive therapy and purged ABMT in patients with multiple myeloma. *Bone Marrow Transplantation, 26,* 621–626.

Reece, D.E., Foon, K.A., Bhattacharya-Chatterjee, M., Hale, G.A., Howard, D.S., Munn, R.K., et al. (2000). Use of the anti-idiotype antibody vaccine TriAb after autologous stem cell transplantation in patients with metastatic breast cancer. *Bone Marrow Transplantation, 26,* 729–735.

Reichardt, V.L., Okada, C.Y., Liso, A., Benike, C.J., Stockerl-Goldstein, K.E., Engleman, E.G., et al. (1999). Idiotype vaccination using dendritic cells after autologous peripheral blood stem cell transplantation for multiple myeloma—a feasibility study. *Blood, 93,* 2411–2419.

Robinson, N., Sanders, J.E., Benyunes, M.C., Beach, K., Lindgren, C., Thompson, J.A., et al. (1996). Phase I trial of interleukin-2 after unmodified HLA-matched sibling bone marrow transplantation for children with acute leukemia. *Blood, 87,* 1249–1254.

Schenkein, D.P., Roitman, D., Miller, K.B., Morelli, J., Stadtmauer, E., Pecora, A.L., et al. (1997). A phase II multicenter trial of high-dose sequential chemotherapy and peripheral blood stem cell transplantation as initial therapy for patients with high-risk non-Hodgkin's lymphoma. *Biology of Blood and Marrow Transplant, 3,* 210–216.

Schwarze, C.P., & Ranke, M.B. (2001). Follow up and late effects. *Bone Marrow Transplantation, 28*(Suppl. 1), S6–S8.

Shaffer, L., Giralt, S., Champlin, R., & Chan, K.W. (1995). Treatment of leukemia relapse after bone marrow transplantation with interferon-alpha and interleukin 2. *Bone Marrow Transplantation, 15,* 317–319.

Sica, S., Chiusolo, P., Salutari, P., Piccirillo, N., Laurenti, L., Sora, F., et al. (2000). Autologous graft-versus-host disease after CD34+ purified autologous peripheral blood progenitor cell transplantation. *Journal of Hematotherapy and Stem Cell Research, 9,* 375–379.

Takatsuka, H., Takemoto, Y., Yamada, S., Wada, H., Tamura, S., Fujimori, Y., et al. (2000). Complications after bone marrow transplantation are manifestations of systemic inflammatory response syndrome. *Bone Marrow Transplantation, 26,* 419–426.

Tallman, M.S., Rademaker, A.W., Jahnke, L., Brown, S.G., Bauman, A., Mangan, C., et al. (1997). High-dose chemotherapy, autologous bone marrow or stem cell transplantation and post-transplant consolidation chemotherapy in patients with advanced breast cancer. *Bone Marrow Transplantation, 20,* 721–729.

Toren, A., Nagler, A., Rozenfeld-Granot, G., Levanon, M., Davidson, J., Bielorai, B., et al. (2000). Amplification of immunological functions by subcutaneous injection of intermediate-high dose interleukin-2 for 2 years after autologous stem cell transplantation in children with stage IV neuroblastoma. *Transplantation, 70,* 1100–1104.

Tosi, P., Ronconi, S., Zamagni, E., Cellini, C., Grafone, T., Cangini, D., et al. (2001). Salvage therapy with thalidomide in multiple myeloma patients relapsing after autologous peripheral blood stem cell transplantation. *Haematologica, 86,* 409–413.

Trudel, S., Li, Z., Dodgson, C., Nanji, S., Wan, Y., Voralia, M., et al. (2001). Adenovector engineered interleukin-2 expressing autologous plasma cell vaccination after high-dose chemotherapy for multiple myeloma—a phase 1 study. *Leukemia, 15*, 846–854.

van Besien, K., Tabocoff, J., Rodriguez, M., Andersson, B., Mehra, R., Przepiorka, D., et al. (1995). High-dose chemotherapy with BEAC regimen and autologous bone marrow transplantation to intermediate grade and immunoblastic lymphoma: Durable complete remissions, but a high rate of regimen-related toxicity. *Bone Marrow Transplantation, 15*, 549–555.

van Dam, F.S.A., Schagen, S.B., Muller, M.J., Boogerd, W., vd Wall, E., Fortuyn, M.E.D., et al. (1998). Impairment of cognitive function in women receiving adjuvant treatment for high-risk breast cancer: High-dose versus standard-dose chemotherapy. *Journal of the National Cancer Institute, 90*, 210–218.

Vivancos, P., Granena, Jr., A., Sarra, J., & Granena, A. (1999). Treatment with interleukin-2 (IL-2) and interferon (IFN) (alpha 2b) after autologous bone marrow or peripheral blood stem cell transplantation in onco-hematological malignancies with a high risk of relapse. *Bone Marrow Transplantation, 23*, 169–172.

Vlk, V., Eckschlager, T., Kavan, P., Kabickova, E., Koutecky, J., Sobota, V., et al. (2000). Clinical ineffectiveness of IL-2 and/or IFN alpha administration after autologous PBSC transplantation in pediatric oncological patients. *Pediatric Hematology Oncology, 17*, 31–44.

Vose, J.M., Zhang, M.J., Rowlings, P.A., Lazarus, H.M., Bolwell, B.J., Freytes, C.O., et al. (2001). Autologous transplantation for diffuse aggressive non-Hodgkin's lymphoma in patients never achieving remission: A report from the Autologous Blood and Marrow Transplant Registry. *Journal of Clinical Oncology, 19*, 406–413.

Vossen, J.M., & Handgretinger, R. (2001). Immune recovery and immunotherapy after stem cell transplantation in children. *Bone Marrow Transplantation, 28*(Suppl. 1), S14–S15.

Weems, J.J., Jr., Davis, B.J., Tablan, O.C., Kaufman, L., & Martone, W.J. (1987). Construction activity: An independent risk factor for invasive aspergillosis and zygomycosis in patients with hematologic malignancy. *Infection Control, 8*, 71–75.

Weiss, R.B. (1998). Systems of protocol review, quality assurance, and data audit. *Cancer Chemotherapy and Pharmacology, 42*(Suppl. 1), S88–S92.

White-Hershey, D., & Nevidjon, B. (1990). Fundamentals for oncology nurse/data managers—preparing for a new role. *Oncology Nursing Forum, 17*, 371–377.

Zomas, A., Anagnostopoulos, N., & Dimopoulos, M.A. (2000). Successful treatment of multiple myeloma relapsing after high-dose therapy and autologous transplantation with thalidomide as a single agent. *Bone Marrow Transplantation, 25*, 1319–1320.

CHAPTER 14

Ethical Considerations in Hematopoietic Stem Cell Transplantation Nursing

Introduction

Hematopoietic stem cell transplantation (HSCT) nurses, like oncology nurses in other settings, are confronted by a number of clinical situations that may challenge their technical skills and intellect as well as their beliefs, values, and principles. Nurses have a professional responsibility and obligation to advocate for patients during all phases of the transplantation experience. Nurses must come to terms with competing ethical principles presented by differences in resource allocation, religious beliefs, societal mores, and the research aspect of the treatment regimen. Hamric (2001) reflected on this nursing dilemma as "being in the middle." HSCT nursing is unique because the patients being seen present with a life-threatening illness for which standard therapy has failed or has a low probability of controlling the refractory disease. Uncertainty of outcomes might lead to difficulty in decision making. This chapter will focus on the ethical dilemmas related to treatment options, outcome of treatment, and end-of-life care that are challenging HSCT nurses and their patients.

In 1996, the American Nurses Association and Oncology Nursing Society published the *Statement on the Scope and Standards of Oncology Nursing Practice*. Included in this document is a standard on ethics, which states that the oncology nurse's decisions and actions on behalf of clients are determined in an ethical manner. It also encourages oncology nurses to examine their own philosophy; discuss ethical issues with other colleagues; address advance directives with patients and families; act as a patient advocate; maintain a sensitivity to patients' cultural diversity; protect patient autonomy, dignity, and rights; and seek resources to examine issues and formulate ethical decisions.

Figures 14-1 and 14-2 provide a brief review of ethical principles relevant in today's society that may influence decision making related to clinical situations. It is important to remember that these ethical principles do not stand alone. Different clinicians will have varied opinions; therefore, policies and politics are necessary.

HSCT as a Treatment Option

Many factors must be considered when cancer treatment decisions are made. Offering treatments to patients when there is little or no chance of cure or control of disease can contradict the ethical principles of beneficence and nonmaleficence. Some centers have espoused a 5% or 10% rule (i.e., therapies will not be offered if there is less than a 10% chance of a positive outcome). Yet other clinicians might say that as long as the patient knows the survival outcome data, all treatment options should be offered and administered, if the patient chooses. When clinicians take this position universally, it may conflict with what may be considered best medical practice. Additionally, consideration must be given to resource allocation and cultural differences of international patients who are seeking state-of-the-art care at major cancer centers.

Resource allocation was the major factor in the landmark case of Colby Howard of Oregon in the mid-1980s. Colby was a seven-year-old boy with leukemia who needed a bone marrow transplant. Initially, Oregon Medicaid had agreed to fund the procedure, which was to be performed in the neighboring state of Washington. Before the transplant process was started, the Oregon legislature voted to discontinue funding of solid organ and bone marrow transplantation, which was expected to benefit only 34 people over a two-year period. The $2.8 million savings were to be used to fund prenatal and pediatric care for 1,500 low-income mothers and children. Colby died waiting for the funds needed for the transplant (Pentz, 1999). The competing ethical principles or considerations that lawmakers were faced with in

---

Figure 14-1. Bioethical Principles

1. Beneficence: To benefit or help persons
2. Nonmaleficence: To prevent or avoid harm to persons; "do no harm"
3. Sanctity of Life: Human life is held in high regard and respect.
4. Justice: Professionals have a duty to act with fairness, giving every individual what is owed them.
5. Personal Autonomy: Competent individuals or their surrogate have a right to decide for or against treatment.
6. Benefit-Burden: Only medical treatments that provide more benefit than burden are ethically mandated (Beauchamp & Childress, 2001).

Note. Figure courtesy of Rebecca Pentz, PhD, clinical ethicist, University of Texas M.D. Anderson Cancer Center, Houston, TX. Used with permission.

making their decision were justice (Colby was entitled to what was promised) and benefit versus burden (the greater good for the most people).

When considering aggressive therapies such as HSCT as a treatment option, clinicians know that many factors will have an impact on outcomes. The aftercare of the patient requires compliance with medications, clinic visits to monitor blood counts and perform physical exams, and compliance with guidelines for self-care activities (see Figure 14-3). A requirement of many HSCT programs is availability of a caregiver 24 hours a day, 7 days a week. Some centers have developed an algorithm (see Figure 14-4) for patients who meet the medical eligibility for transplant but have special needs or situations that may put them at risk for harm (nonmaleficence) with the prescribed therapy (Neumann, 2001). Ideally, these issues should be addressed and resolved before the patient begins therapy, whether inpatient or outpatient. The goal is to provide a means of success in the cure or control of the patient's cancer diagnosis. As providers of health care, clinicians have a responsibility to be good stewards of available resources and create criteria with guidelines for judicious use of therapies, especially new therapies that tend to be extremely costly.

Frequently, the research or clinical nurse is the one who validates the patient's understanding of the experimental nature of this therapy. Patients need to understand the fact that alternative treatment options exist and that their physician also may be the principal investigator of the study and, therefore, may have a vested interest concerning the study in which they are being asked to participate. The media have reported on legal actions taken against institutions in which alleged breaches in the informal consent process have surfaced (Marshall, 2001). Recently, knowledge of alternate therapies and potential conflicts of interest have been added to most informed consent documents (Daniels & Sabin, 2000). Because of the research aspect of this treatment option, members of the nursing staff may have difficulty accepting the aggressive nature of the therapy. New transplant nursing staff members need to have an understanding of the goals of a research program and acknowledge that the patient accepts the experimental nature of treatment with unknown outcomes. Nurses may have the perception of being caught in the middle of competing goals of the medical team and the patient and family (Hamric, 2001). It may take skill and diplomacy on the nurse's part to ensure that mutual goals are understood.

In addition, HSCT team members, including physicians, need to agree with basic assumptions and ethical considerations that may include the following.

- We have an obligation to provide potential life-saving treatment (beneficence).
- Numerous factors, in addition to medical eligibility, will influence outcomes and patient safety (nonmaleficence).
- Success is dependent on a team of professionals who are empowered to make decisions.
- A patient's verbal commitment should be demonstrated with actions (e.g., compliance with appointments, tests, treatments).
- People (patients) do not change coping styles during a crisis, such as during HSCT. Team members need to provide other tools and conditions to decrease dependence on coping skills that may have negative outcomes; refusals of psychosocial assessment and intervention can be just as serious as refusals of cardiac medications or insulin.

Other variables that may influence a clinician's decisions related to treatment include the patient's age, toxicities, and cost. Elderly patients frequently receive less aggressive therapy because of regimen-related toxicity or clinician biases (Clarke, 2001; Hutchins, Unger, Crowley, Coltman, & Albain, 1999). In the past, HSCT has been a treatment modality for younger patients, but nonmyeloablative stem cell transplantation therapy can include patients from all age groups. Although nonmyeloablative transplantation is associated with less toxicity than conventional transplantation, complications related to comorbid conditions of the older patient can make management equally as complex. In addition, the post-transplant complications such as graft versus host disease also require careful monitoring.

Informed Consent

Truth telling regarding the treatment and prognosis can pose the greatest concern. Frequently, families, in an attempt to "protect" the patient, will request the alteration of truth so that their loved ones will not give up hope or decide to stop treatment. If the patient is very young or old or of an ethnic background that follows a paternalistic philosophy, a patient surrogate may serve as the decision maker or spokesperson. Unless the healthcare practitioner is fluent in the language spoken by the patient, the use of an interpreter is recommended. The interpreter also may assist in the acquisition of culturally sensitive information that could influence the decision-making process. The clinician, either the nurse or the physician, is faced with the challenge of ensuring that the patient's wishes or interests are met and protected.

The goal and requirements of HSCT must be that which best meet the patient's physical and psychosocial condition.

Self-Care as a Patient in the Blood and Marrow Transplant Program

This information describes how you and your health care team will contribute to your care while you are in the Blood and Marrow Transplant program. Please read this information carefully and ask a member of your health care team if there is anything you do not understand. You will be asked to sign a patient acknowledgement form, once you understand your role in your care. The signed form will be kept with your medical record and you will receive a copy.

The Blood and Marrow Transplant Center approaches your care as a team. You and your caregiver are important members of this team, just like your doctors, nurses, pharmacists and other health care professionals. You will do better physically and emotionally when you take an active role in your treatment and recovery. It is very important that you be involved in your care at the hospital and when you are discharged.

It is important that you remain as active as possible, even if you feel very tired. The more independent you are the better you may feel. If you are unable to do certain self-care activities, your doctors and nurses will make sure that you have someone to help you.

Self-Care Activities

Your nurse or doctor will explain your self-care activities in detail. It is important for you to participate in these activities as much as possible.

If you are an **inpatient**, your self-care activities will include:

1. Keeping a record of fluid intake.
2. Showering once a day, preferably in the morning before the doctor examines you. If you are taking certain chemotherapy drugs, you may need to shower at least 3 times a day.
3. Walking for 10 minutes, at least 3 times per day. You must have permission from the nurse or doctor to leave the inpatient unit.
4. Performing mouth care every 2 hours while you are awake.
5. Keeping a record of the amount of food you eat when instructed by your doctor, nurse or dietitian.
6. Breathing exercises, at least 4 times a day, ~~using an incentive spirometer.~~ *deep breathing exercises*
7. Learning how to give yourself injections of growth factor. If you are unable to inject yourself, your caregiver will need to learn how to give the injections.
8. Attending 2 classes that will teach you how to flush your central venous catheter (CVC) and change your dressing, if needed.
9. Using a collection "hat" container each time you urinate or have a bowel movement.
10. Ordering your meals every day by filling out menus or calling room service.

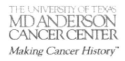
THE UNIVERSITY OF TEXAS
MD ANDERSON
CANCER CENTER
Making Cancer History

(Continued on next page)

11. **Not eating** fresh fruit or vegetables, even if family or friends bring these foods for you to eat.

If you are an **outpatient**, your self-care activities will include:

1. Keeping a record of fluid intake.
2. Showering once a day.
3. Walking for 10 minutes, at least 3 times per day.
4. Performing mouth care every 2 hours while you are awake.
5. Keeping a record of the amount of food you eat when instructed by your doctor, nurse or dietitian.
6. Breathing exercises, at least 4 times a day, using an incentive spirometer.
7. Learning how to give yourself injections of growth factor. If you are unable to inject yourself, your caregiver will need to learn how to give the injections.
8. Attending 2 classes that will teach you how to flush your central venous catheter (CVC) and change your dressing, if needed.
9. Learning how to give yourself intravenous antibiotics or fluid, if needed.
10. **Not eating** fresh fruit or vegetables, even if family or friends bring these foods for you to eat.

Your Caregiver

You **must** choose a caregiver before you are admitted to the hospital for your transplant. Your caregiver will provide essential support to you, both physically and emotionally. Your caregiver must stay with you at all times after you are discharged from the hospital. He or she will help you in your recovery, and will ensure that you come to the hospital or clinic for appointments or emergencies, and will make sure you follow your health care team's instructions and remain safe during recovery. Your caregiver may also help arrange blood or platelet donations for you if you need them.

Your Health Care Team

Your health care team will keep you and your caregiver informed about your care. They will also:

1. Perform a physical exam, including exam of your mouth and perineum (bottom), to check for infection and bleeding. This will be done at every hospital shift or at each clinic visit.
2. Evaluate your condition closely and discuss your progress. They will:
   a. Check your vital signs at least every 4 hours or at each clinic visit.
   b. Record your weight daily or at each clinic visit.
   c. Measure and record urine, stool, and vomit output, when in the hospital.
   d. Perform tests (blood draws and X-rays) and activities (physical therapy) when instructed by the health care team.
3. Explain procedures and tests.

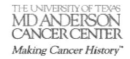
THE UNIVERSITY OF TEXAS
MD ANDERSON
CANCER CENTER
Making Cancer History™

(Continued on next page)

4. Review your medication schedule
5. Review and discuss blood counts, trends and whether blood or platelets are needed.
6. Administer blood products, as needed.
7. Review your treatment plan.
8. Teach you how to do your self-care activities.
9. Provide resources to assist you with your emotions and concerns.
10. Consult with specialist from other departments (i.e. pain service, pulmonary, cardiology) as needed.
11. Provide support and encouragement.
12. Answer questions or refer you to a person or department who can answer your questions.

While you are an **inpatient**, you will also receive:

1. Medications and treatment supplies from hospital stock.
2. Consistency in staff assigned to care for you whenever possible.
3. Clean bed linens daily.
4. Extended periods of rest whenever possible.
5. Quick response to your call light by intercom or in person.

Symptoms to Report

 If you are experiencing problems or having symptoms, such as nausea, vomiting, shortness of breath, diarrhea, sore areas or pain, please tell your health care team or caregiver.

Medications

Do not take any prescription or over-the-counter medications, vitamins, herbs, or herbal supplements from your own supply while in the hospital or after you are discharged unless your doctor, nurse or pharmacist approves it.

Coping With Your Situation

To help you through your treatment, your health care team will include staff from the Psychiatry and Social Work department. Patients going through this procedure experience many emotions and may need additional support. Sharing your fears and worries with your team will help you better cope with treatment and daily activities. At times, your team may request assistance from the psychiatry department in determining which medications will be most helpful with anxiety or depression.

Preventing Infection

It is important that you protect yourself from germs. Always wear a mask when you leave your room and while you are out in public. It is very important that you wash your hands before removing your mask, after using the bathroom, before handling food, and if you have been out of

© 2003 The University of Texas M. D. Anderson Cancer Center, 02/18/03
Patient Education Office

THE UNIVERSITY OF TEXAS
MD ANDERSON
CANCER CENTER
Making Cancer History™

(Continued on next page)

your room.

Leaving the Hospital

If you have been admitted to the hospital for transplant, you will be discharged from the hospital when you have sufficiently recovered. At the time of discharge, you and your caregiver will attend a discharge class and will be given an instruction sheet to follow.

Follow Up

It is important that you keep all follow up appointments as scheduled. If you are unable to make an appointment or will be late to an appointment, you must call your assigned clinic as soon as possible.

 If you have **any** signs or symptoms that are listed on the instruction sheet given to you when you were discharged from the hospital, come to the M.D. Anderson Emergency Center immediately.

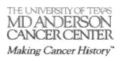

THE UNIVERSITY OF TEXAS
MD ANDERSON
CANCER CENTER
Making Cancer History

Note. Figure courtesy of the University of Texas M.D. Anderson Cancer Center. Used with permission.

Figure 14-4. Algorithm for Hematopoietic Stem Cell Transplant Recipients With Special Needs

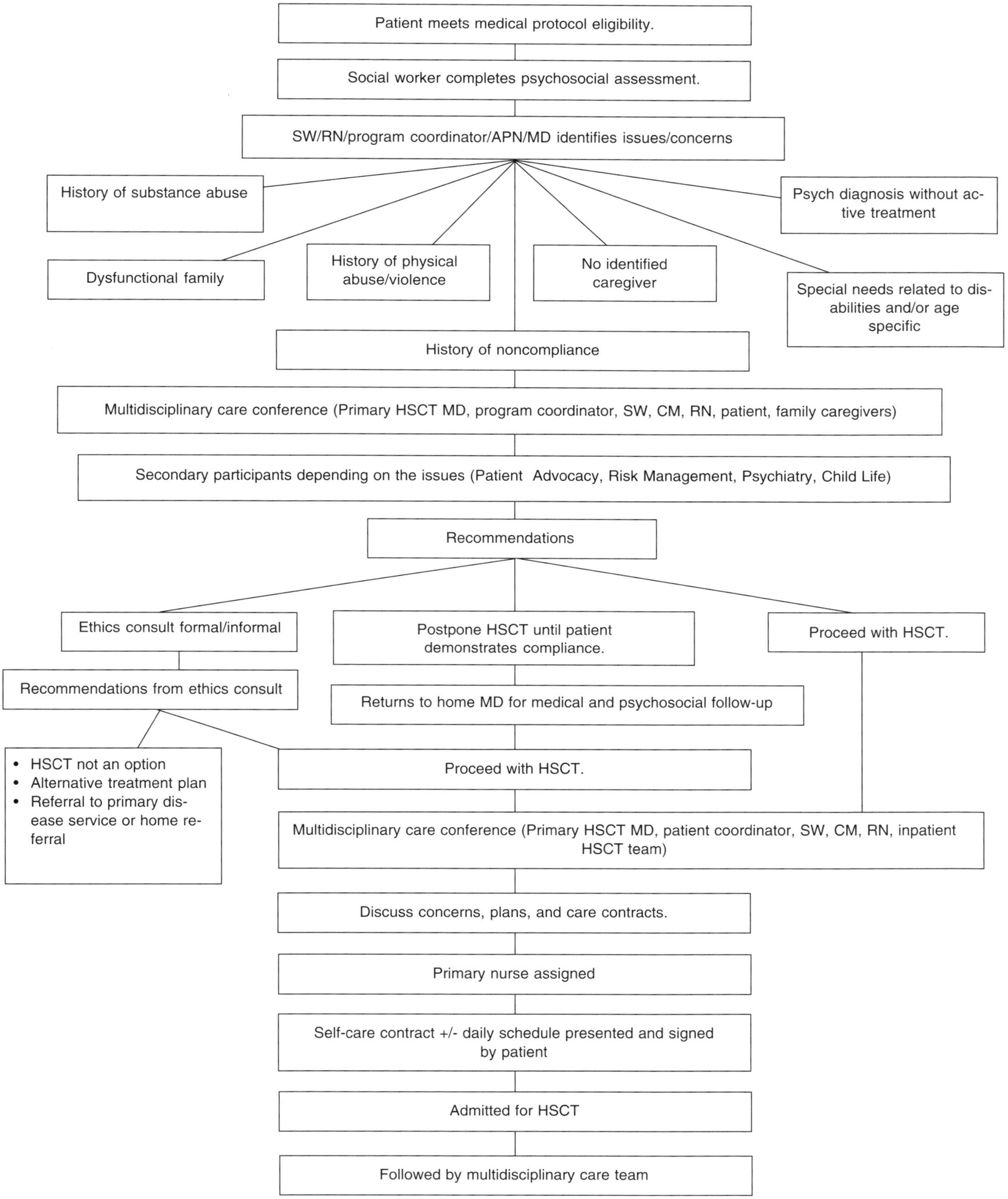

Patient meets medical protocol eligibility.

Social worker completes psychosocial assessment.

SW/RN/program coordinator/APN/MD identifies issues/concerns

History of substance abuse

Psych diagnosis without active treatment

Dysfunctional family

History of physical abuse/violence

No identified caregiver

Special needs related to disabilities and/or age specific

History of noncompliance

Multidisciplinary care conference (Primary HSCT MD, program coordinator, SW, CM, RN, patient, family caregivers)

Secondary participants depending on the issues (Patient Advocacy, Risk Management, Psychiatry, Child Life)

Recommendations

Ethics consult formal/informal

Postpone HSCT until patient demonstrates compliance.

Proceed with HSCT.

Recommendations from ethics consult

Returns to home MD for medical and psychosocial follow-up

- HSCT not an option
- Alternative treatment plan
- Referral to primary disease service or home referral

Proceed with HSCT.

Multidisciplinary care conference (Primary HSCT MD, patient coordinator, SW, CM, RN, inpatient HSCT team)

Discuss concerns, plans, and care contracts.

Primary nurse assigned

Self-care contract +/- daily schedule presented and signed by patient

Admitted for HSCT

Followed by multidisciplinary care team

The concepts of informed consent and informed decision making are important issues at this point. The purpose of informed consent is to give the care recipient or patient surrogate information related to the treatment plan, medications to be given, side effects, complications, risks, cost, benefits, and rights (Jacoby et al., 1999). The recipient or surrogate can then make the appropriate decision for the recipient's specific situation. The patient must be aware of all potential side effects. Clinicians often have differing opinions on whether to tell patients about side effects that may occur infrequently. Many believe that patients only should be informed of side effects or complications that have a 5% or greater chance of occurring. As healthcare professionals, it is important to present an unbiased impression informing the patient of side effects that are most likely to occur with additional detail when requested.

In research protocols, a written informed consent document is used to provide information and obtain the patient's permission to receive treatment. The patient receives a copy of the signed document. It also serves to document and register the patient on the protocol. Providing and having patients sign an informed consent for standard of care therapies is a suggested practice but not one that is uniformly practiced. By signing a consent, even for what would be considered standard of care treatment, one assumes an increased sense of responsibility by both the practitioner and patient to understand the treatment planned (Jacoby et al., 1999). In the case of a minor undergoing HSCT, most institutions have a policy in place and an assent clause in the informed consent document. This generally is obtained in minors who are under the chronological age of 18 years and above the age of 7 years with regard to mental comprehension (American Academy of Pediatrics, 1995).

Patient Education

Patient information should be provided to give a more detailed explanation of what the patient might expect during the therapy. Some HSCT centers also provide a care contract or agreement, a document that specifically outlines what is expected of the patient or caregiver and what they can expect of the healthcare facility and providers of care (see Figure 14-5). This is especially helpful if there is concern about the patient's and caregiver's level of understanding or commitment (see Figure 14-6). Ensuring that patients know that some care requirements are non-negotiable at certain times also helps with limit setting that may be required later. Patients also need to know that systems are not perfect. One method used might be to request that the patient identify his or her most important concern or issue and communicate this to all providers via the Kardex® (Kardex Systems, Inc., Marietta, OH) or care plan. This will help to eliminate misunderstandings, to individualize care, and to inform the patient that the team is willing to meet his or her personal needs. For some patients, receiving information about their blood counts daily is most important. For others, it is knowing that certain premedications

will be given before blood products or that every effort will be made to ensure that the patient gets four uninterrupted hours of sleep in the hospital. Communicating the patient's individual requests to all care providers will help to lessen distress, potential maladaptive behavior, and potential ethical dilemmas.

Occasionally, a patient wants to know little or nothing of the details of the treatment, whereas others may request that only positive information be given. These types of patient preferences present some ethical challenges, as it is the healthcare provider's *responsibility to inform the patient*. One suggested way to deal with these issues is to have the patient identify a family member who can act as a surrogate.

To increase the patient's knowledge of planned therapy, the HSCT nurse may assist the patient to formulate questions and provide additional information concerning the long-term consequences of the planned therapy. When discussing the treatment plan, the patient may have questions or concerns regarding fertility issues, plans to return to work or "normal" life, the plan if complications occur, and end-of-life care. Ideally, these questions and concerns should be addressed before treatment begins.

When conducting *phase I clinical trials*, the clinician must ensure that patients understand that there may be little or no direct benefit to them and that the goal of the trial is to define the maximum tolerated dose of therapy (Jenkins, 1991). Studies suggest that even after being informed that the protocol in which they have been enrolled is a phase I study, patients often believe they will personally gain a clinical benefit from their participation (Daugherty et al., 1995). With the advent of the Internet, savvy consumers have many opportunities to explore treatment options, both standard therapies and unproven treatment options. Practitioners need to be able to explain these options to patients in such a way that they understand not all options are suitable or appropriate for their condition.

Donor Issues

Healthcare professionals have an ethical responsibility to inform the normal donor of the risks associated with the donation of stem cells through bone marrow harvest or collection through apheresis procedure. The risks to a young normal, healthy donor are minimal for either procedure. However, in nonmyeloablative therapy, the donor may be of older age and have multiple comorbid conditions; these factors may increase the risks for donors. Special consideration also is required when the donor is a child or minor (Schaison, 1992). If the treatment has a low chance of success, the risks to the normal donor may be the primary factor in the decision not to proceed, although this was not the case in a study examining the use of pediatric donors, as reported by Chan et al. (1996). In this study of 56 North American BMT centers, there was general consensus about using BMT with experimental protocol. In addition, the projected outcome of treatment did not influence the decision to use the minor donor. Patients and families may become

Figure 14-5. Hematopoietic Stem Cell Transplant Patient Care Agreement

Patient and Caregiver Acknowledgement Form

THE UNIVERSITY OF TEXAS
MD ANDERSON
CANCER CENTER

Patient and Caregiver Acknowledgement

Blood and Marrow Transplantation

Page 1 of 1

Patient Acknowledgement

I have received a copy of the **Blood and Marrow Transplantation (BMT) Patient Education Manual** and **Role of the Caregiver in the BMT Process**, which outlines information about my care, my caregiver's responsibilities, and the transplant process.

I have also read **Self-Care as a Patient in the Blood and Marrow Transplant Program** and understand my responsibilities as a BMT patient. I agree to actively participate in my care, to follow my self-care instructions and to work with my health care team in providing the best care possible.

A copy of the **Self-Care as a Patient in the Blood and Marrow Transplant Program** document and the **Patient & Caregiver Acknowledgement Form** will be given to me. I understand that these documents are to help prepare me for my transplant, but should not take the place of any discussion with my health care team.

_____   _____
Patient Signature   Date

_____   _____
Health Care Provider Signature   Date

Caregiver Acknowledgement

I have received a copy of the **Blood and Marrow Transplantation (BMT) Patient Education Manual** and **Self-Care as a Patient in the Blood and Marrow Transplant Program**, which outlines information about the patient's care and the transplant process.

I have read **Role of the Caregiver in the BMT Process** and understand my responsibilities as caregiver of a BMT patient. I agree to perform these responsibilities during treatment and during the recovery phase.

A copy of the **Role of the Caregiver in the BMT Process** document and the **Patient & Caregiver Acknowledgement Form** will be given to me.

_____   _____
Patient Signature   Date

_____   _____
Health Care Provider Signature   Date

Patient and Caregiver Acknowledgement

File Under: Consent   BMT462003 04/03

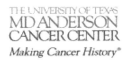

THE UNIVERSITY OF TEXAS
MD ANDERSON
CANCER CENTER
Making Cancer History®

Note. Figure courtesy of the University of Texas M.D. Anderson Cancer Center. Used with permission.

Role of the Caregiver in the Blood and Marrow Transplant Program

A BMT caregiver provides essential physical and emotional support to the patient. Caregivers assist patients in their recovery, ensure that they come to the hospital for appointments or emergencies, make sure they eat, drink, sleep, and take their medications as instructed, and help them remain safe during recovery.

This information describes how you will contribute to the care of your patient while they are in the Blood and Marrow Transplant program. Please read this information carefully and ask a member of the patient's health care team if there is anything you do not understand. You will be asked to sign a caregiver acknowledgement form, once you understand your role as a caregiver. The signed form will be kept with the patient's medical record and you will receive a copy.

Various members of the health care team will work with you and educate you about your role during inpatient and outpatient care. If you are employed, you will need to take time off from work. Some caregivers use vacation time from work, while others take leave under the FMLA (Family Medical Leave Act). If you need a letter or a form completed for an employer, you may contact the patient's assigned social worker. The social worker will help you to complete the paperwork.

The health care team must have your name and phone numbers of where you can be reached. If there is more than one caregiver, the health care team will also need their information as well. Also, the health care team needs a schedule showing when you and the other caregivers will be caring for the patient.

Caregiver Duties

Throughout the transplant period, you will have many different roles, including that of driver, cook, cleaner, bather/dresser, entertainer, advocate, and friend.

You will:
- Care for the patient's Central Venous Catheter (CVC). Before the patient is discharged from the hospital, the caregiver must learn how to care for his or her CVC. Classes are held regularly.
- Attend the Transplant Discharge Teaching class with the patient before he or she leaves the hospital.
- Assist the patient, once he or she has been discharged from the hospital, in getting to the Ambulatory Treatment Center (ATC) or Fast-Track Clinic as scheduled.
- Shop for and prepare nutritious meals and snacks for the patient. Also, encourage the patient to eat adequate amounts of food daily.

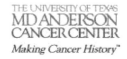

(Continued on next page)

- Help the patient comply with a no fresh fruits and vegetables diet and practice safe food handling.
- Help the patient take his or her medications on time
- Help the patient contact social workers, chaplains, and community resources if needed.

In some cases, patients may not recognize problems that develop. They may be unaware of the problems, or may fear going back into the hospital. However, the health care team **must be notified** of any changes in the patient's condition, such as fever, chills, vomiting, diarrhea, eating or drinking difficulties, depression, or changes in mental status. **Failure to notify the health care team may seriously affect the outcome of the treatment and safety of the patient.**

You may be asked to keep a daily record of patient activities and to provide the record to the health care team. You must remember to encourage the patient to perform as much of his/her care as he/she can do safely, and to resume normal activities as soon as he/she is able to do so. If safety is an issue and/or the patient needs help with appropriate exercise, or if the patient cannot do activities of daily living because of fatigue, discuss the possibility of starting physical therapy and/or occupational therapy with the health care team.

It is important to keep family and friends informed of the patient's condition, but that is not always easy. Since many medical concepts and terms are difficult to comprehend, repeatedly explaining them can be frustrating. Some patients have found it helpful to share an informational newsletter or email with family and friends. Others have found it easier to designate someone close to them to provide information, and some patients use church bulletins, etc. to keep people informed. The health care team can help you, the patient, or another designated person explain the information in layman's terms.

Taking Care of Yourself

Fatigue, weakness and difficulty eating are challenges not only for the patient, but for the caregiver as well. It is important that you communicate concerns to the health care team. Remember, your role is valued and important.

Your duties are like a full-time job. You should not be afraid to ask for help if needed. Family members and friends are often willing to assist caregivers and may be willing to assume responsibilities like child-care, paying bills, housework and yardwork. Family and friends can also help arrange blood donors if needed. This often will help them to feel that they are helping, so caregivers should tell them what is needed.

The multiple responsibilities and tasks require that you be physically and mentally fit. If you have a medical condition that requires follow-up and/or monitoring by a physician, you should ask your physician the best way to accomplish this. There are hospitals and clinics in the Houston area that you can contact directly if medical needs arise.

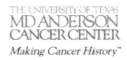

(Continued on next page)

It is important that you keep in good health. Without you, the patient cannot make progress and succeed in their treatment. You must take time to exercise, walk, and eat right. Exercise can help motivate the patient as well as yourself.

The Place … of wellness offers support for those who care for someone with cancer. Caregivers: I've Got Feelings Too! meets on Thursdays, 11 a.m. to noon. For more information, you can contact the Place… of wellness at 713-794-4700.

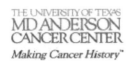

THE UNIVERSITY OF TEXAS
MD ANDERSON
CANCER CENTER
Making Cancer History™

Note. Figure courtesy of the University of Texas M.D. Anderson Cancer Center. Used with permission.

desperate to find treatment options. Normal donors' rights must be protected through program or institutional policies that provide a mechanism to ensure voluntary, confidential, and safe practices when harvesting stem cells, whether through apheresis or bone marrow procurement.

When the donor is a minor, extensive psychosocial and developmental assessment by experts in child psychology is recommended. The emotional dilemmas may be profound because of the age of both the patient and donor as well as the need for immediacy of decision making in some clinical situations. In the case of a child donating to a parent, a separate healthcare team usually is assigned for the patient and donor to eliminate the possibility of competing interests. When obtaining informed consent for a minor donor, most centers will obtain consents or assents from the donor as well as the parent(s), if possible (Massimo, 1996). In the case of a very young or incompetent minor donor, a formal ethics consult may be standard practice during the consenting process. In the extreme but infrequent case of dissension between a minor donor's joint-custody parents, the legal system may have to get involved to resolve the issue. If any concerns develop about donor rights or interests, regardless of age, a formal ethics consult should be initiated by any member of the healthcare team.

Caring for international patients coming from countries where systems and ethics are different from those in the United States may pose other problems. Solicitation of a donor by unauthorized review of hospital records or offering incentives are two situations that an institution's ethical committee or administrative review board may encounter (Pentz, Chan, Neumann, Champlin, & Korbling, in press).

In the case of an unrelated donor, the national and international bone marrow registries have set up strict guidelines to protect the normal donor's and patient's rights and confidentiality. Assessment of the donor for possible increased risk factors related to general anesthesia in the case of bone marrow harvest or increased fluid and electrolyte shifts during an apheresis procedure are evaluated. Donor center personnel deal with concerns about potential withdrawal of consent by the donor after the patient's conditioning regimen has been started by validating the level of commitment of the donor and the donor's signature on a letter of intent. Selection of a date for the donation may be somewhat complicated and sometimes is inflexible once set. Specific information (i.e., donor's name and address) is provided to the patient and donor after a year only if both parties agree.

The Outcome of Disease/Treatment

Most cancer therapies are aimed at cure, but with advanced disease, the goal of therapy may be control of disease or palliation. Ethical issues that may be present during the treatment or aftercare of HSCT recipients include advance directives, "Do Not Resuscitate" (DNR) orders, and discontinuation of medically inappropriate care (futility). Individual states and institutions may have differing regulations related to each of these issues.

Advance Directives

In 1991, the U.S. Congress enacted the Patient Self-Determination Act, which mandates that patients must be informed of their rights to accept or refuse treatments, including resuscitative measures, in accordance with their state laws or statutes (Jezewski & Finnell, 1998). The term *advance directives* usually refers to three separate documents: the living will, medical power of attorney, and out-of-hospital DNR. The social work or clinical ethics department usually assists patients and families in completing the advance directive forms and answers questions. Historically, people who do not wish to be kept alive by artificial means if their medical condition is considered irreversible have written a living will. An irreversible condition may be defined as

a condition, injury, or illness: that may be treated, but is never cured or eliminated; that leaves a person unable to care for or make decisions for the person's own self; and that, without life-sustaining treatment provided in accordance with the prevailing standard of medical care, is fatal. (Advance Directives Act, 1999)

Recently, an additional statement was added to the living will. In some states, with support from the "Right to Life" coalition, the individual can indicate that they want all life support measures to be maintained. The additional statement reads, "I request that I be kept alive in this terminal condition using available life-sustaining treatment, and I request that I be kept alive in this irreversible condition using available life-sustaining treatment (this does not apply to hospice care)" (Advance Directives Act, 1999; Texas Department of Human Services, 2000). Although this may give more choices to the individual completing the document, it is more restrictive to the healthcare provider. This reflects the principle of self-autonomy to the extreme and has the potential to create a barrier to clinicians exercising what would be viewed as sound medical practice; for example, CPR is not indicated in a terminally ill HSCT patient with multisystem failure. This also does not include the choice of assisted suicide for those people whose wishes may include ending their lives if their condition is intolerable to them.

These documents need to be reviewed and ideally will become a forum for preemptive discussions, especially when the patient is about to undergo treatment regimens that have a high risk for complications, which may necessitate transfer to an intensive-care unit (ICU) and intubation. The communication skills of clinicians are very important when presenting the information related to diagnosis and treatment options to patients and families. Improved communication skills with compassionate and clear messages naturally will lead to decreased conflict and fewer ethical dilemmas.

Do Not Resuscitate Order

The DNR order is a medical decision based upon the judgment of the patient's physician that the use of extraordinary measures (e.g., CPR, defibrillation, emergency medications, intubation) in conditions that are irreversible will not change the outcome for the patient who has no reasonable hope for recovery. The physician, however, should not do this unilaterally, nor should the physician put the burden of the DNR decision on the patient or family exclusively. Frequently, there is disparity in definitions and the meaning of DNR among patients, providers, and families, which can lead to conflict in the consent process (Olver, Eliott, & Blake-Mortimer, 2002). Patients and families may assume that they need to sign a document before the DNR order can be written. This is the case in some institutions or states. In some states, a statute exists that mandates that adult patients (or designee) give verbal or written consent before a physician writes the order to withhold resuscitation. Physicians or patients/families may have the perception that the quality of nursing care will be less in the setting of a DNR order. Some may believe that a DNR order represents a death sentence or that the patient will lose all hope and give up if a DNR order is written.

Some institutions have created a preprinted order sheet on which the physician has various treatment options to choose from (including cardiac defibrillation, vasoactive drugs, antiarrhythmic drugs, cardiac pacemaker, tracheostomy, chemotherapy, antibiotics, dialysis, blood products, hyperalimentation, tube feeding, IV fluids, oxygen, and tests) and specifies that patient comfort always takes priority. Establishing the specific goal of care is paramount to decide which of these measures to withhold. Knowledge of HSCT patient trends also is critical in making sound judgments about which conditions may be considered irreversible. In studies published by Hinds et al. (2001) and Groeger et al. (1998), the authors identified variables that influence the mortality of patients with cancer admitted to the ICU. They included CPR within 24 hours prior to admission, intubation, intracranial mass, allogeneic HSCT, recurrence of disease, poor baseline performance status, prothrombin time longer than 15 seconds, albumin less than 2.5 g/dl, bilirubin greater than 2 mg/dl, BUN greater than 50 mg/dl, and number of hospital days prior to ICU admission. For example, allogeneic HSCT recipients who are intubated and have an infection or a gastrointestinal bleed have a 4% chance of survival (Price, Thall, Kish, Shannon, & Andersson, 1998).

Discontinuation of Medically Inappropriate Care (Futility)

At times, measures are instituted when it is not clear if the patient's condition is reversible. When it becomes apparent that the patient has little or no chance for recovery, the decision may be made to discontinue those measures that are life sustaining and switch to measures with the goal of a peaceful death with dignity. This may be difficult for families, and they may liken it to euthanasia. Many factors must be considered when having this discussion, such as individual preferences, religious beliefs, and cultural traditions. For example, individuals of the Muslim faith may believe withholding or withdrawing life-sustaining measures would be totally unacceptable under any circumstances. Institutions

and hospitals, especially those with religious affiliations, may hold the ethical principle of the sanctity of life in highest regard. This may lead to conflict with what practitioners might consider an appropriate medical decision regarding termination of care. With the exception of aggressive relapsed disease, the transplant medical team frequently has difficulty discontinuing aggressive therapy for complications of transplantation. Perry, Rivlin, and Goldstone (1999) conducted a review of the literature on decision making and practices related to stopping treatment for HSCT recipients with life-threatening organ failure. They concluded that greater attention should be paid to these topics during pretransplant counseling, including the identification of treatment limits.

When families and clinicians disagree on medical care, an ethics consult may be called, and the institutional medical futility (inappropriate medical care) policy may need to be enacted. This usually involves a review process that includes clinical experts not directly involved in the case, members of the ethics committee, the patient's family, the medical team, and a representative from the hospital administration. If the decision is made to terminate life support, a designated waiting period will be established so the patient and family can find another care facility that will continue to provide the level of care requested. During this process, provisions usually are in place to maintain the same level of life-sustaining care, and an agreement (within the institution's physician group) is made that no other physician will take over the case, thereby changing the goal and plan of care as decided by the committee. If the family does not choose to move the patient to another facility, life-sustaining measures will be discontinued and comfort measures will be continued until the patient dies (M.D. Anderson Cancer Center, 2001).

Summary

Transplant nurses encounter many ethical issues in their role as patient advocates. Initial studies are being done to try to quantify the issues nurses face in their practice (Fry & Duffy, 2001). Nurses working in research centers where phase I trials are being performed may have additional issues because of the unknown results of these studies and the possibility of severe side effects and complications as new therapies are being developed. Nurses are encouraged to become involved in their institution's ethics committee and in writing policies that can help to define practice and lessen potential conflicts. Measures to support the nurse in the role of caregiver and patient advocate also should be examined. At the University of Texas M.D. Anderson Cancer Center, monthly ethics rounds on the inpatient bone marrow transplant unit were initiated. Results of a staff survey after one year of ethics rounds indicated that the nurses had an increased knowledge of ethical principles and that the nursing staff felt more comfortable discussing ethical issues with physician colleagues (Neumann, Pentz, & Flamm, 2001).

Nurses also have a responsibility to know their states' current regulations, as well as the policies of their institutions, related to the issues presented here. Finally, to truly advocate for patients, it is imperative to know the goal of care and challenge inconsistencies if they arise between the patient's understanding of that goal and the medical plan of care.

References

Advance Directives Act, Tex. Health & Safety Code Ann. §§166.001 et seq. (1999). Retrieved September 16, 2003, from http://www.capitol.state.tx.us/statutes/he/he0016600.html

American Academy of Pediatrics. (1995). Policy statement RE9510: Informed consent, parental permission, and assent in pediatric practice. *Pediatrics, 95,* 314–317.

American Nurses Association & Oncology Nursing Society. (1996). *Statement on the scope and standards of oncology nursing practice.* Washington, DC: American Nurses Publishing.

Beauchamp, T.L., & Childress, J.F. (2001). *Principles of biomedical ethics* (5th ed.). New York: Oxford University Press.

Chan, K.W., Gajewski, J., Supkis, D., Pentz, R., Champlin, R., & Bleyer, W. (1996). Use of minors as bone marrow donors: Current attitude and management. A survey of 56 pediatric transplantation centers. *Journal of Pediatrics, 128,* 644–648.

Clarke, C.M. (2001). Rationing scarce life-sustaining resources on the basis of age. *Journal of Advanced Nursing, 35,* 799–804.

Daniels, N., & Sabin, J.E. (2000). Last-chance therapies and managed care: Pluralism, fair procedures, and legitimacy. In J.H. Howell & W.F. Sale (Eds.), *Life choices: A Hastings Center introduction to bioethics* (2nd ed., pp. 89–108). Washington, DC: Georgetown University Press.

Daugherty, C., Ratain, M.J., Grochowski E., Stocking, C., Kodish, E., Mick, R., et al. (1995). Perceptions of cancer patients and their physicians involved in phase I trials. *Journal of Clinical Oncology, 13,* 1062–1072.

Fletcher, J. (Ed.). (1993). *Introduction to clinical ethics.* Charlottesville, VA: Center for Biomedical Ethics, University of Virginia.

Fry, S., & Duffy, M. (2001). The development and psychometric evaluation of the ethical issues scale. *Journal of Nursing Scholarship, 33,* 273–277.

Groeger, J., Lemshow, S., Price, K., Nierman, D.M., White, P., Jr., Klar, J., et al. (1998). Multicenter outcome study of cancer patients admitted to the intensive care unit: A probability of mortality model. *Journal of Clinical Oncology, 16,* 761–770.

Hamric, A. (2001). Reflections on being in the middle. *Nursing Outlook, 49,* 254–257.

Hinds, P., Oakes, L., Furman, W., Quargnenti, A., Olson, M.S., Fopiano, P., et al. (2001). End-of-life decision making by adolescents, parents, and healthcare providers in pediatric oncology: Research to evidence-based practice guidelines. *Cancer Nursing, 24,* 122–135.

Hutchins, L., Unger, J., Crowley, J., Coltman, C., & Albain, K. (1999). Underrepresentation of patients 65 years of age or older in cancer-treatment trials. *New England Journal of Medicine, 341,* 2061–2067.

Jacoby, L.H., Maloy, B., Cirenza, E., Shelton, W., Goggins, T., & Balint, J. (1999). The basis of informed consent for BMT patients. *Bone Marrow Transplantation, 23,* 711–717.

Jenkins, J. (1991). Oncology nursing practice: The role of the nurse in support of progress in cancer treatment. In M.B. Burke, K. Ingwersen, G.M. Wilkes, D. Berg, & C.K. Bean (Eds.), *Cancer chemotherapy: A nursing process approach* (pp. 3–20). Sudbury, MA: Jones and Bartlett.

Jezewski, M., & Finnell, D. (1998). The meaning of DNR status: Oncology nurses' experiences with patients and families. *Cancer Nursing, 21,* 212–221.

M.D. Anderson Cancer Center. (2001). *The determination of medically inappropriate interventions.* Policy VII.A.1.064. Houston, TX: Author.

Marshall, E. (2001). Fred Hutchinson Center under fire. *Science, 292*(6), 25.

Massimo, L. (1996). Ethical problems in bone marrow transplantation in children. *Bone Marrow Transplantation, 18,* 8–12.

Neumann, J. (2001). Ethical issues confronting oncology nurses. *Nursing Clinics of North America, 36,* 827–841.

Neumann, J., Pentz, R., & Flamm, A. (2001). Evaluating the impact of ethics rounds on nurses' roles as caregiver and patient advocate [Abstract 206]. *Oncology Nursing Forum, 28,* 362.

Olver, I., Eliott, J., & Blake-Mortimer, J. (2002). Cancer patients' perceptions of do not resuscitate orders. *Psycho-Oncology, 11,* 181–187.

Pentz, R. (1999). *Case presentation: Core curriculum. Fellows ethics course.* Houston, TX: University of Texas M.D. Anderson Cancer Center.

Pentz, R., Chan, K.W., Neumann, J.L., Champlin, R.E., & Korbling, M. (in press). Designing an ethical policy for bone marrow donation by minors and others lacking capacity. *Cambridge Quarterly of Healthcare Ethics, 13*(2).

Perry, A., Rivlin M., & Goldstone, A. (1999). Bone marrow transplant patients with life-threatening organ failure: When should treatment stop? *Journal of Clinical Oncology, 17,* 298–312.

Price, K., Thall, P., Kish, S., Shannon, V.R., & Andersson, B.S. (1998). Prognostic indicators for blood and marrow transplant patients admitted to an intensive care unit. *American Journal of Respiratory Critical Care Medicine, 158,* 876–884.

Schaison, G.S. (1992). The child conceived to give life. The point of view of the hematologist. *Bone Marrow Transplantation, 9,* 93–94.

Texas Department of Human Services. (2000). *Directive to physicians and family or surrogates (living will).* Retrieved September 18, 2003, from http://www.dhs.state.tx.us/providers/ltc-policy/AdvanceDirectives/LivingWill-English.pdf

Quality-of-Life Issues in Hematopoietic Stem Cell Transplantation

Introduction

Over a period of more than 25 years, hematopoietic stem cell transplantation (HSCT) has emerged from being an experimental procedure to frontline therapy for a number of malignant and nonmalignant diseases. Advances in technology and supportive care and the increasing numbers of transplants performed annually have resulted in an expanded number of people who are survivors 10–20 years post-transplant. Early research in transplantation focused on identification of those medical outcomes, with the greatest impact on relapse rates and disease-free survival. In the early days of bone marrow transplantation (BMT), issues related to physical recovery and management of complications during the acute phase of the transplant process took priority in both research and clinical practice arenas with less attention being given to the impact of transplant on survival and quality-of-life (QOL) issues. Currently there is an ongoing and growing consensus that these traditional outcome variables are inadequate when used alone to measure the effectiveness of transplantation. Information on psychosocial adaptation, social reintegration, and QOL provide a more comprehensive picture of patient outcomes than survival and relapse-free intervals alone. As such, there is an increased interest in researching these QOL issues from a more multidimensional view (Andrykowski, 1994).

Defining Quality of Life

The concept of QOL is not a new one; in fact, concerns with the constituents of human happiness and satisfaction have been topics of discussion for centuries. Despite this long history, no consensus has been reached on a single definition of QOL. Recent research has acknowledged QOL as multidimensional and subjective, with most definitions focusing on the ability to live a normal life, happiness or satisfaction with life, achievement of personal goals, or social utility (Ferrans, 1990). From the social science literature, definitions of QOL incorporate the subjective nature of the construct with recognition that QOL can only be fully understood from the perspective of the individual (Caplan, 1984). Satisfaction with one's life is determined by the dif-

ference between one's perceived needs or expectations with what is actually possessed or achieved. In addition, although QOL can be defined in terms of global happiness or satisfaction, this global perception is influenced by numerous domains or dimensions of life (Anderson & Burckhardt, 1999). Caplan also stated that QOL is an assessment for the potential for growth. It is the difference, at a particular point in time, between hopes and expectations. QOL therefore depends on individual experiences and life expectations (Molassiotis, 1997). Ferrans defined QOL as "the person's sense of well-being that stems from satisfaction or dissatisfaction with the areas of life that are important to him/her" (p. 15).

Conceptual Model of Quality of Life

Searching for a theoretical framework within the QOL research literature remains elusive. King et al. (1997), in a review of QOL research, identified theories of uncertainty, discrepancy, hope, and meaning as guiding several studies. In the BMT literature, theories of hope (Ersek, 1992) and finding meaning (Steeves, 1992) have been explored. Reasons for the lack of theoretical frameworks are attributed to a focus on content to define and describe QOL in various populations and the development of reliable instruments to measure the concept (King et al.).

A conceptual model that can be used to guide research and understand QOL in transplant recipients comes from the work of Ferrell et al. (1992a, 1992b). This model views QOL from a multidimensional, subjective perspective. The assumptions underlying the model are based on individualistic ideologies and view individuals as complex beings, health as a multidimensional construct, and QOL as dependent on the unique experiences of each individual (Vallwrand, Breckenridge, & Hodgson, 1998). Ferrell et al. (1992a, 1992b) pioneered the exploration of QOL in BMT survivors using a qualitative approach resulting in the development of a model consisting of four domains (see Figure 15-1). A qualitative study consisting of a one-time interview with 119 BMT recipients was conducted to explore the specific impact of transplantation on QOL. The researchers developed six open-ended questions and collected data via a written sur-

Figure 15-1. Quality-of-Life Domains in Bone Marrow Transplantation

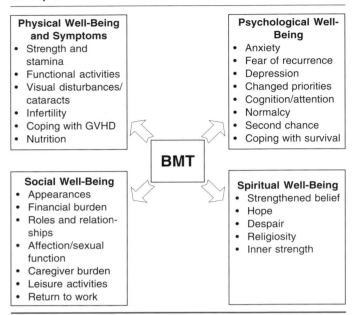

Physical Well-Being and Symptoms	Psychological Well-Being
• Strength and stamina • Functional activities • Visual disturbances/cataracts • Infertility • Coping with GVHD • Nutrition	• Anxiety • Fear of recurrence • Depression • Changed priorities • Cognition/attention • Normalcy • Second chance • Coping with survival
Social Well-Being	**Spiritual Well-Being**
• Appearances • Financial burden • Roles and relationships • Affection/sexual function • Caregiver burden • Leisure activities • Return to work	• Strengthened belief • Hope • Despair • Religiosity • Inner strength

Note. From "The Meaning of Quality of Life for Bone Marrow Transplant Survivors: Part 1. The Impact of Bone Marrow Transplant on Quality of Life," by B. Ferrell, M. Grant, G. Schmidt, M. Rhiner, C. Whitehead, P. Fonbuena, et al., 1992, *Cancer Nursing, 15,* p. 159. Copyright 1992 by Lippincott Williams and Wilkins. Reprinted with permission.

vey. Questions were derived to capture the meaning of QOL, what impact did BMT have on QOL, what were the positive and negative influences on QOL, and how physicians and nurses could improve QOL. The researchers performed content analysis verbatim on the written responses to the questions and conducted thematic coding. A summary of the responses showed that BMT survivors value health as the major factor of QOL and describe their perceptions of QOL in the same dimensions of physical, psychological, social, and spiritual well-being as other populations (Ferrell et al., 1992a). The data then were reconstructed to reflect a multidimensional model of QOL (see Figure 15-1) consisting of four domains: physical well-being and symptoms, psychological well-being, social well-being, and spiritual well-being. The physical well-being domain is defined as "the control or relief of symptoms and the maintenance of function and independence" (Ferrell, 1996, p. 911). From the transplant data, this domain is characterized by strength and stamina, functional activities, visual disturbances/cataracts, recurrent infections, infertility, chronic graft versus host disease, and nutrition (Whedon & Ferrell, 1994). Psychological well-being is "seeking a sense of control in the face of a life-threatening illness characterized by emotional distress, altered life priorities, and fears of the unknown, as well as positive life changes" (Ferrell, p. 912). Psychological well-being for the BMT survivor encompasses the areas of regaining normalcy, anxiety, depression, fear of recurrence, and coping with survival (Whedon & Ferrell). Social well-being

is "providing a way to view not only the cancer or its symptoms but also the person surrounding the tumor. It is the means by which we recognize people with cancer, their roles, and relationships" (Ferrell, p. 913). Social well-being for the BMT survivor encompasses issues of intimacy, relationships, family, employment, and social reintegration (Whedon & Ferrell). Spiritual well-being is "the ability to maintain hope and derive meaning from the cancer experience that is characterized by uncertainty. Spiritual well-being involves issues of transcendence and is enhanced by one's religion and other sources of spiritual support" (Ferrell, p. 913). For BMT survivors, issues of spirituality include survivorship, hope, finding meaning, inner strength, and religion (Cohen, Headley, & Sherwood, 2000; Whedon & Ferrell).

Reflections of the lived experience from BMT survivors reveal a concern for the physical sequelae of the transplant, a realization of the impact of the experience on ability to adjust and cope with the uncertainty of the future, a need for transition with intimate and social relationships, and a transcendence to find meaning and reconciliation. These responses imply interrelationships between domains and that the construct of QOL is a process involving multiple dimensions, changes over time, and can be profoundly influenced by illness and survival from life-threatening events.

Review of the Literature

Recovery from HSCT requires a prolonged period of time and often is accompanied by acute morbidity. A review of the current literature identifies areas of post-transplant recovery that are most vulnerable to both positive and negative changes (see Table 15-1).

When addressing the physical outcomes, symptom inventories in long-term BMT survivors commonly are reported. Wolcott, Wellisch, Fawzy, and Landsverk (1986) studied 26 allogeneic BMT recipients, with 75% reporting an overall good QOL. Twenty-five percent of the participants, however, reported ongoing medical symptoms. Self-reports of current physical health were positively related to time since transplant. Additional studies (Bush, Donaldson, Haberman, Dacanay, & Sullivan, 2000; Chiodi et al., 2000; Duell et al., 1997; Molassiotis, Boughton, Burgoyne, & van den Akker, 1995; Wingard, 1994) are consistent with the findings that, although the majority of transplant survivors do quite well, subsets of individuals report moderate to severe problems with physical health and functional status. Two studies identified older age at the time of transplant (Andrykowski, Bruehl, Brady, & Henslee-Downee, 1995) and presence of chronic graft versus host disease (Wolcott et al.) as contributing to ongoing physical problems in the post-transplant period. Among the symptoms reported, fatigue appears to be a significant problem. Whedon and Ferrell (1994) indicated that among 29 patients, fatigue was the most commonly reported symptom, with 50% indicating moderate to severe levels as many as three years post-transplant. These reports were confirmed by Andrykowski, Bruehl, et al., in a multicenter study of 200

Table 15-1. Quality-of-Life Dimensions in Hematopoietic Stem Cell Transplantation

Author	Sample Size	Sample Characteristics	Design	Time of Measurement	Instruments	Results
Physical Well-Being/Symptoms						
Andrykowski, Greiner, et al. (1995)	N = 200 • 46% allogeneic • 54% autologous	60% male 40% female Mean age = 38.5 years Range = 19–70 years	Quantitative Retrospective	Single time point Mean time since BMT = 41 months Range = 12–127 months	• Profile of Mood States (POMS) • Psychosocial Adjustment to Illness Scale (PAIS)—Sexual Relationship Subscale • Sickness Impact Profile (SIP) subscale • Recovery of Function Scale—BMT	• BMT recipients perceived physical health as poorer than normal population. • Most frequently reported symptoms were feeling tired, sleep problems, stiff joints, headaches. • Ability to engage in vigorous physical activity and sexual activity were compromised.
Andrykowski et al. (1997)	N = 172 • 45% allogeneic • 55% autologous	62% male 38% female Mean age = 39 years	Quantitative Retrospective	12 months and 18 months Mean time since BMT = 43.5 months	• POMS • Functional Living Cancer Index • Symptom Experience Report • Pittsburgh Sleep Quality Index	• 65% experienced problems with energy level. • 51% reported sleep difficulty. • No significant difference in energy level or sleep between the two time points
Bush et al. (1995)	N = 125 • 87% allogeneic • 11% syngeneic • 2% autologous	51% male 49% female Mean age = 38 years Range = 26–62 years	Quantitative Retrospective	Single time point Mean time since BMT = 10.1 years Range = 6–18 years	• EORTC QLQ-C30 • Late Complications of BMT Module • Demands of BMT Recovery Inventory • POMS • Ware Health Perceptions Questionnaire • Long-Term BMT Recovery	• 74% reported quality of life (QOL) same or better than pre-BMT. • 5% rated QOL as poor. • 80% rated health as good to excellent. • Ongoing symptoms included sexual dysfunction, fatigue, eye problems, sleep disturbances, and cognitive dysfunction.
Bush et al. (2000)	N = 415 • 67% allogeneic • 33% autologous	Mean age = 41.8 years Range = 19–65 years	Quantitative Prospective Longitudinal	N = 415 year 1 N = 217 year 2 N = 117 year 3 N = 35 year 4 N = 6 year 5	• EORTC QLQ-C30 • Late Complications of BMT Module • Demands of BMT Recovery Inventory • POMS • Ware Health Perceptions Questionnaire • Long-Term BMT Recovery	• All reported at least one BMT-related symptom at each annual assessment, and most were rated mild. • 17%–27% reported dissatisfaction with sexual appeal, ability to share warmth and intimacy, or sexual interest. • When compared to general population, BMT recipients perceived significantly poorer prior health, were more worried about their health, and were more susceptible to illness. • Patients had greater focus on big picture and overall value and life priorities.
Chiodi et al. (2000)	N = 244 Allogeneic	54% male 46% female	Quantitative Retrospective	Good QOL • < 60 months (n = 22) • > 60 months (n = 122)	• PAIS	• 31% reported poor QOL. Factors associated with poor QOL were older age, presence of long-term sequelae, and chronic graft versus host disease (GVHD). • QOL improves greatly at > 5 years. • Females had greater difficulty with sexual function and psychological distress.

(Continued on next page)

Table 15-1. Quality-of-Life Dimensions in Hematopoietic Stem Cell Transplantation *(Continued)*

Author	Sample Size	Sample Characteristics	Design	Time of Measurement	Instruments	Results
Physical Well-Being/Symptoms (Continued)						
Duell et al. (1997)	N = 798 Allogeneic	56% male 44% female	Quantitative Retrospective	Single time point Mean time since BMT = 8.4 years Range = 5–19 years	• Karnofsky Performance Status score • Survival	• 93% have Karnofsky scores of 90%–100%. • 89% returned to work or school.
Heinomen et al. (2001)	N = 109 Allogeneic	48% male 56% female Age range = 21–59 years	Quantitative Retrospective	Single time point Range = 4–171 months post-BMT • 4–12 months (n = 18) • 13–36 months (n = 29) • 36–60 months (n = 25) • 60 months (n = 37)	• POMS • FACT-BMT • Activities of Daily Living (ADL) scale • Medical Outcomes Study (MOS)—Survey of Social Support • Brief Measure of Social Support	• Physical well-being, educational level, age at BMT, and social support have an impact on perceived QOL. • Greatest impact on physical well-being were lack of energy, side effects, and sleeping. • Mean scores and functional well-being improved over time.
Lee et al. (2001)	N = 320 • 114 autologous • 201 allogeneic • 5 syngeneic	66% male 48% female Age range 19–66 years Hematologic malignancy	Quantitative Longitudinal	6, 12, and 24 months	• Survey developed for study. • Data include survival, general health, frequency and severity of post-transplant symptoms, and return to work.	• Both groups reported recovery just beginning at 6 month. • At 12 months and 24 months, 40% of both groups perceived their lives as not having returned to normal. • Overall, patients were most bothered by fatigue and sexual difficulties. • These symptoms reached a plateau at 12 months and did not improve significantly at 24 months.
Marks et al. (1999)	N = 20 Allogeneic unrelated donors	55% male 45% female Median age at transplant = 26 years Range = 17–48 years	Quantitative Retrospective	Single time point Median time since BMT = 42 months Range = 23–95 months	• MOS • Satisfaction With Life Domains Scale (SLDS)-Cancer • Significant Others Scale • Employment Questionnaire	• Overall satisfaction with life was above average. • Patients expressed dissatisfaction with physical strength and appearance. • 30% fewer were in full-time employment as compared to pre-BMT. • GVHD correlated on health, daily activities, and overall QOL.
Prieto et al. (1996)	N = 117 60% allogeneic 37% autologous 3% syngeneic	56% male 44% female Mean age = 33 Range = 15–54 years	Quantitative Retrospective	Single time point Mean time since BMT = 55 months Range = 6–156 months	• Nottingham Health Profile • General Health Status	• Patients exhibited high and varied physical morbidity ranging from 4%–30%. • Physical symptoms, sexual dysfunction, educational level, age at BMT, and time since transplant were significant predictors of global QOL. • Women had greater physical and psychological recovery.

(Continued on next page)

Table 15-1. Quality-of-Life Dimensions in Hematopoietic Stem Cell Transplantation *(Continued)*

Author	Sample Size	Sample Characteristics	Design	Time of Measurement	Instruments	Results
Physical Well-Being/Symptoms *(Continued)*						
Somerfield et al. (1996)	N = 156 • 75% allogeneic • 25% autologous	55% male 45% female	Quantitative Retrospective	Single time point Mean time since BMT = 55 months Range = 9–181 months	• BMT Problem Checklist • COPE Inventory	• 54% reported physical problems. • Feelings of increased vulnerability and uncertain future • Reduced energy • Concerns about infertility
Sutherland et al. (1997)	N = 231	54% male 46% female Age range = 19–57 years	Quantitative Retrospective	Single time point Median time = 40 months Range = 1–253 months	• MOS • SLDS • Symptom Experience Report	• When compared to general population, BMT recipients had significantly diminished QOL in areas of performing physical activities, problems with work, and interference with normal social activities.
Whedon et al. (1995)	N = 29 Autologous	45% male 55% female Mean age = 38.5 years Range = 20–54 years	Qualitative/ Quantitative Retrospective	Single time point Mean time since BMT = 37 months Range = 14–76 months	• City of Hope QOL—BMT Instrument • Open-ended interview questionnaire	• Overall QOL was good. • Most common physical problems were fatigue, sexual problems, and vision problems. • 93% reported distress over the illness's effect on the family. • Lowest scores on social domain were sexual pleasure and intimacy. • 66% were able to return to work or school. • Spiritual well-being was defined in terms of hope and having a sense of purpose.
Psychological Well-Being						
Andrykowski, Brady, et al. (1995)	N = 172 • 45% allogeneic • 55% autologous	62% male 38% female Mean age = 39 Range = 19–70	Quantitative/ Qualitative Retrospective	Single time point Mean time since BMT = 43.5 months Range = 12–124 months	• Semistructured Interview • POMS • PAIS—Psychological Distress Subscale • Rosenberg Self-Esteem Scale • Positive and Negative Affect Schedule (PANAS)	• 52% reported having not returned to normal post-BMT in regard to working outside the home, engaging in sexual activity, and engaging in vigorous physical activity.
Broers et al. (2000)	N = 123 • 51% allogeneic • 49% autologous	60% male 40% female	Quantitative Prospective	Pre-BMT = 123 • 1 month = 90 • 6 months = 59 • 1 year = 55 • 3 years = 38	• Functional Limitations Battery • General Health Questionnaire • Symptom Checklist-90 • Rosenberg Self Esteem Scale	• At three years, 25% were limited in several functional areas. • 90% reported good QOL despite functional and somatic problems. • Changes in QOL could be explained entirely by changes in functional limitations and somatic problems. • Changes in psychological distress related to baseline status and functional and somatic issues.

(Continued on next page)

Author	Sample Size	Sample Characteristics	Design	Time of Measurement	Instruments	Results
				Psychological Well-Being (Continued)		
Fromm et al. (1996)	N = 90 • 51% allogeneic • 49% autologous	58% male 42% female Mean age = 39 years	Quantitative Retrospective	Single time point Mean time since BMT = 49.5 months	• Semistructured Interview • Functional Living Index—Cancer • Sickness Impact Profile • PAIS—Psychological Distress and Sexual Relationship Subscales • POMS • PANAS • Rosenberg Self-Esteem Scale • Cantril Global QOL Ladder	• Positive changes most reported were - New philosophy of life (59%) - Change in personal attributes (54%) - Improved family relationships (52%) - Family more supportive (51%) - Greater appreciation of life (47%) • Negative changes most reported were - Increased uncertainty about future (59%) - Emotionally taxing on family (52%) - Depression (43%) - Family uncertainty about future (40%)
Molassiotis (1997)	N = 91 • 42% allogeneic • 58% autologous	67% male 33% female Mean age = 36 years Range = 18–61 years	Quantitative/ Qualitative Retrospective	Single time point Mean time since BMT = 39.8 months Range = 6–122 months	• PAIS • Hospital Anxiety and Depression Scale (HADS) • Rotterdam Symptom Checklist • Family Environmental Scale	• Five meaningful transition times - 6 months–2 years (psychological dysfunction, sexual concerns, adjustment with social environment) - 3 years (sexual concerns, loss of control, grieving followed by life re-evaluation) - 4 years (sexual concerns, adjustment with social environment, loss of control, occupational adjustment) - 5 years (sexual concerns, despair, health concerns - 6 years (sexual concerns, occupational adjustment, moving on with life or stuck phase)
Vickberg et al. (2001)	N = 85 Allogeneic	49% male 51% female Mean age = 40 years Range = 17–59 years	Quantitative Retrospective	Single time point Mean time since BMT = 4 years Range = 6 months–11 years	• Personal Meaning Index • Brief Symptom Inventory • PTSD Checklist • MOS—Short Form 36 (MOS—SF-36)	• Global meaning (purpose in life and psychological adjustment) was inversely related to anxiety and depression. • Global meaning was positively related to emotional role functioning, mental functioning, and vitality.
				Social Well-Being/Sexuality		
Altmaier et al. (1991)	BMT group: N = 12 Chemo group: N = 10	BMT group: 58% male 42% female Chemo group: 50% male 50% female	Retrospective	BMT group: 24–41 months post Mean = 33 months Chemo group: actively getting treatment	• Semistructured interview • Interviewer rating of Karnofsky status • Interviewer rating of psychological distress	• 33% of overall BMT group reported worsening of relationship, in contrast to 10% of chemo group. • 42% reported diminished sexual desire (4 males, 1 female). • 17% reported diminished sexual function (2 males). • 25% reported inability to perform (3 males). • 33% reported difficulties with partner over sex (3 males, 1 female).

(Continued on next page)

Table 15-1. Quality-of-Life Dimensions in Hematopoietic Stem Cell Transplantation (Continued)

Author	Sample Size	Sample Characteristics	Design	Time of Measurement	Instruments	Results
				Social Well-Being/Sexuality (Continued)		
Andrykowski, Greiner, et al. (1995)	N = 200	60% male 40% female	Retrospective	12–127 months post-BMT Mean = 41 months	• POMS • PAIS—Sexual Relationship Subscale • SIP • Recovery of Function Scale • Perceived Health Questionnaire • Perceived Quality of Life Questionnaire • Symptom Experience Report	• 37% reported compromised sexual activity on Recovery of Function scale. • Subjects with chronic GVHD had significantly lower scores on PAIS sex subscale ($p < 0.01$). • 12% of BMT group experienced serious sexual relationship dysfunction relative to other patients with cancer.
Andrykowski, Bruehl, et al. (1995)	N = 28	57% male 43% female	Prospective	Pre-BMT and 12–16 months post-BMT Mean = 14 months	• POMS • Functional Living Index—Cancer • PAIS • SIP • Symptom Experience Report • Sleep, Energy, and Appetite Scale	• Significant differences were seen from pre-BMT to one year post-BMT, with poorer sexual relationship at one year.
Curbow et al. (1993)	N = 135	61% male 39% female	Retrospective	6–149 months post-BMT Mean = 47 months	• 9 open-ended questions in fixed order	• Loss themes expressed most often were interruption in life plans, inability to have children, difficulties with sexual functioning, physical disability, and psychological loss. • Women were more likely than men to report children/sexuality themes (52.8% versus 30.5%).
Molassiotis, Boughton, et al. (1995)	N = 50	64% male 36% female	Retrospective	6–97 months post-BMT Mean = 42 months	• PAIS • HADS • RSCL	• No significant difference was seen between allogeneic and autologous groups with regard to psychological or physical dysfunction. • 20% of allogeneic patients reported decreased sexual interest. • 33% of autologous patients reported decreased sexual interest. • 25% of both groups had failed to return to full-time work/school.

(Continued on next page)

Table 15-1. Quality-of-Life Dimensions in Hematopoietic Stem Cell Transplantation *(Continued)*

Author	Sample Size	Sample Characteristics	Design	Time of Measurement	Instruments	Results
				Social Well-Being/Sexuality *(Continued)*		
Molassiotis et al. (1997)	N = 91	67% male 33% female	Retrospective	16–122 months post-BMT Mean = 40 months	• PAIS • HADS • RSCL • FES	• Sexual function concerns were present throughout all time points post-BMT.
Prieto et al. (1996)	N = 117	56% male 44% female	Retrospective	6–156 months post-BMT Median = 55 months	• Nottingham Health Profile • General Health Status (GHQ-28)	• Women had overall higher Nottingham Health Profile scores (p = 0.001) and higher GHQ-28 scores (p = 0.03) than men, indicating higher levels of perceived health problems, impact on life, and psychiatric morbidity. • Women had sex life affected more than men. • Overall QOL (total Nottingham Health Profile score) correlated with psychosocial distress: correlation with total GHQ-28 score and all categories of Nottingham Health Profile. Strongest association was with sex life. • 31% of subjects reported disturbances in sex life.
Somerfield et al. (1996)	N = 156	55% male 45% female	Cross-sectional survey	9–81 months post-BMT Mean = 55 months	• BMT Problem Checklist • Cope Inventory-52	• Single patients indicated greater concern over infertility and greater concern over physical appearance. • Younger patients indicated greater concern over infertility, whereas older patients were more likely to have difficulty with sexual intercourse.
Sutherland et al. (1997)	N = 231	54% male 46% female	Cross-sectional	1–253 months post-BMT Median = 40 months	• MOS—SF-36 • SLDS-BMT • Symptom Experience Checklist	• The two areas with the least satisfaction on the SLDS-BMT were physical strength (28%) and sexual satisfaction (28%), followed by decreased satisfaction with body (17%) and appearance (17%). • Health-related QOL (MOS-SF) was significantly lower in BMT recipients than normal.
Zittoun et al. (1997)	N = 98	Allogeneic BMT: N = 35 Female = 15 Male = 20	Retrospective Cross-sectional	12–89 months from achieving remission Mean = 53 months	• Sexual Functioning and Fertility questionnaire addressing interest, satisfaction, level of activity, ability to have intercourse, and infertility problems	• Sexual functioning impaired in one-third of all subjects: 68% allo BMT, 30% auto BMT, 22% chemo. Significant differences were seen between groups: Decreased interest: - Allo BMT: 60%

(Continued on next page)

Table 15-1. Quality-of-Life Dimensions in Hematopoietic Stem Cell Transplantation *(Continued)*

Author	Sample Size	Sample Characteristics	Design	Time of Measurement	Instruments	Results
Social Well-Being/Sexuality *(Continued)*						
Zittoun et al. (1997) (cont.)		Autologous BMT: N = 29 Female = 7 Male = 22 Chemo: N = 34 Female = 15 Male = 19			• Disease Related Modification Module • Symptom Checklist • Functional Scale	- Auto BMT: 21% - Chemo: 15% Decreased sexual activity: - Allo BMT: 68% - Auto BMT: 30% - Chemo: 22% Decreased satisfaction: - Allo BMT: 47% - Auto BMT: 18% - Chemo: 22% Decreased ability to engage in sex: - Allo BMT: 53% - Auto BMT: 29% - Chemo: 21% Sexual problems were more frequently reported by females versus males (46% versus 25%) and older people (46 years and older) versus younger (70% versus 25%).

BMT survivors who averaged 41 months post-transplant. Fatigue was perceived as the most common symptom, with 78% of the sample feeling consistently tired.

This population also identified issues related to fertility and sexual functioning as a major concern in this population. Loss of reproductive capability following transplantation is influenced by the type of preparative regimen and age at transplant, with those receiving total body irradiation and those post-pubertal at the time of transplant at higher risk (Saunders et al., 1988). Issues of intimacy and sexual functioning are, however, not necessarily related to issues of sterility. Baruch et al. (1991) studied sexual functioning in male BMT recipients (6–154 months post-BMT) and found that 26% of the participants reported moderate to severe sexual problems. Mumma, Mashberg, and Lesko (1992) examined long-term psychosexual adjustment in 21 adult BMT survivors with comparison made to adult leukemia survivors who had received conventional chemotherapy treatment. No differences were seen between the two groups. When compared to physically healthy individuals, female BMT survivors reported less sexual satisfaction, and both male and female survivors reported poorer body image. Wingard, Curbow, Baker, Zabora, and Piantadosi (1992) assessed sexual satisfaction in 126 adult BMT recipients (6–149 months post-BMT) and found that 22% reported dissatisfaction. Syrjala et al. (1998) reported significant sexual problems in survivors of transplantation. In a prospective study from pretransplant through three years post-transplant, type and severity of sexual problems were measured. Women reported a more significant number of problems than men across all time periods. These problems did not improve over time but rather seemed to influence all aspects of sexual function. Hormone replacement therapy improved sexual function but did not ensure QOL.

Several studies have examined indicators of psychological distress as outcomes of BMT including inability to assume social roles (Molassiotis, 1997), worries about the future (Bush et al., 2000; Fromm, Andrykowski, & Hunt, 1996), work problems (Duell et al., 1997; Marks, Gale, Vedhara, & Bird, 1999), and life satisfaction (Vickberg et al., 2001). As with the physical domain of QOL, the majority of individuals adjust quite well psychologically and socially following BMT with a subset of individuals, somewhere between 15%–25%, who exhibit ongoing problems (Molassiotis, Boughton, et al., 1995; Neitzert, Dancey, Murray, & Avery, 1998). One study (Andrykowski, Brady, et al., 1995) reported that less than half of the BMT recipients felt "back to normal" 12–24 months following transplant. Two studies (Haberman, Bush, Young, & Sullivan, 1993; Syrjala, Chapko, Vitaliano, Cummings, & Sullivan, 1993) evaluated individuals at 4–18 years post-transplant and reported a 5%–10% incidence of continued psychological and social difficulties.

Family relationships influence recovery of BMT recipients in both positive and negative ways. Belec (1992) found the subset family had the greatest impact on QOL, and Syrjala et al. (1993) reported that high levels of family conflict pre-BMT were a predictor of post-BMT difficulties. Molassiotis (1997) found similar results in long-term BMT survivors, for whom social support and strong family relationships were associated with better adjustment and decreased psychological distress.

Few studies examined the spiritual or existential domain of QOL post-transplantation. Belec (1992) reported that the BMT experience results in the patient reassessing priorities and values and the development of inner strength and hope for the future, all of which are seen as positive outcomes from the perspective of the individual. Haberman et al. (1993) supported these findings in a study of long-term survivors in which participants reported a new valuing of life and a changed perspective. Life was considered precious, with each day being seen as important.

Family/Caregiver Quality of Life

The impact of transplant on the family is significant as disruptions occur in roles, communication, future goals, and QOL. Little research has examined family needs throughout the transplant process. These studies identified the family as critical for adaptation and recovery after transplantation; the burden of care is intense and often unexpected, and there are often feelings of being ill-prepared to provide the necessary care (Compton, McDonald, & Stetz, 1996; Molassiotis, 1997; Rivera, 1997; Stetz, McDonald, & Compton, 1996; Wochna, 1997). Using focus group interviews, Stetz et al. evaluated the informational needs of the 19 adult family members of transplant recipients. The informational themes that emerged from the data included preparation for the caregiver role, provision of the physical care, anticipation of the stress and barriers to care, developing supportive strategies, and discovering unanticipated rewards such as personal growth and family cohesion. Results suggest a unique set of informational needs and demands on caregivers as well as patients. However, demands and better QOL could be mitigated through education strategies and support from healthcare providers.

In a qualitative study, Foxall and Gaston-Johansson (1996) described the burden of care and health outcomes (anxiety, depression, symptom distress, and fatigue) in family caregivers to BMT recipients. Disruptions in daily life, energy expenditure, financial concerns, fear about the future, interpersonal relationships, and whether the caregiver felt useful all were correlated with caregiver outcomes. In a study of QOL after autologous transplantation, Boyle et al. (2000) reported that caregivers regain normalcy and satisfaction with life one to six years after transplant. However, care responsibilities and demands to assume new roles were ongoing.

Pediatric Quality-of-Life Issues

The impact of BMT on the QOL in children has been addressed in few studies. A study assessing the psychological adjustment of 26 pediatric recipients of stem cell transplantation revealed high levels of anxiety (35%), increased sense of vulnerability and sensitivity (62%), and unfulfilled needs in their love lives. There were no differences in self-esteem, family and peer relationships, and school performance as compared to similar populations (Felder-Puig et al., 1999).

QOL also was evaluated in a sample of 36 children and adolescents who underwent BMT (Nespoli, Verri, Locatelli, & Bertuggia, 1995). Parents reported that most of the children did not seem to think back to the BMT experience because they did not discuss it with family and friends. Anxiety levels were slightly higher in preschool children than in older children, and 16% reported some physical problems resulting from the transplant.

In another study (Matthes-Martin et al., 1999), researchers evaluated the QOL of 155 pediatric BMT recipients. The physical and psychosocial aspects of QOL most affected in this group included restricted peer relationships (8%), restricted "normal activities" (4%), and severe physical handicap (3%). Most patients (75%) reported no physical or psychosocial impairment.

In a longitudinal study, the impact of family cohesion on adjustment of children post-transplant was addressed (Phipps & Mulhern, 1995). Significant declines were observed in post-BMT social competence and overall self-esteem. Additionally, perceptions of family variables were highly predictive of post-BMT adjustment. Perceived family cohesion and expressiveness promoted resilience to the stresses of BMT, thereby promoting adjustment, whereas perceived family conflict adversely affected adjustment regardless of stress level.

Conclusion and Recommendations for Further Research

In general, most survivors of HSCT rate their life satisfaction as favorable. Life satisfaction correlates with physical health, age, and ability to retain work and social roles (Baker, Curbow, & Wingard 1991; Syrjala et al., 1993). Despite ongoing medical problems and physical symptoms, most individuals retain an overall positive view on life satisfaction. Researchers need to continue to design prospective studies with long-term follow-up periods and to focus on subgroups of HSCT survivors who continue to have difficulties with both the physical and psychosocial domains of QOL. Research can continue to define and evaluate the interrelationships among the domains of QOL, to develop comparison studies between HSCT groups and other cancer survivors, and to develop intervention studies that, perhaps, can identify those at highest risk for problems post-transplant and offer effective strategies to promote healthy outcomes.

It is apparent that the concept of QOL is not an easy one to understand, nor are there single definitions or tools for measurement. A need exists for continued investigation of QOL in subjective ways, for the use of theoretical models to guide research, and for expanding the boundaries to include cultural diversities. Patients and families need information that will prepare them for the impact of transplant on their everyday lives and ongoing support to deal with the physical, psychological, social, and spiritual changes in life perception and satisfaction.

References

Altmaier, E.M., Gingrich, R.D., & Fyfe, M.A. (1991). Two-year adjustment of bone marrow transplant survivors. *Bone Marrow Transplantation, 7*, 311–316.

Anderson, K.L., & Burckhardt, C.S. (1999). Conceptualization and measurement of quality of life as an outcome variable for health care intervention and research. *Journal of Advanced Nursing, 29*, 298–306.

Andrykowski, M. (1994). Psychosocial factors in bone marrow transplantation: A review and recommendations for research. *Bone Marrow Transplantation, 13*, 357–375.

Andrykowski, M.A., Brady, M.J., Greiner, C.B., Altmaier, E.M., Burish, T.G., Antin, J.A., et al. (1995). 'Returning to normal' following bone marrow transplantation: Outcomes, expectations and informed consent. *Bone Marrow Transplantation, 15*, 573–581.

Andrykowski, M.A., Bruehl, S., Brady, M.J., & Henslee-Downee, P.J. (1995). Physical and psychosocial status of adults one-year after bone marrow transplantation: A prospective study. *Bone Marrow Transplantation, 15*, 837–844.

Andrykowski, M., Carpenter, J., Greiner, C., Altmaier, E., Burish, T., Antin, J., et al. (1997). Energy level and sleep quality following bone marrow transplantation. *Bone Marrow Transplantation, 20*, 669–679.

Andrykowski, M., Greiner, C., Altmaier, E., Burish, T., Antin, J., Gingrich, R., et al. (1995). Quality of life following bone marrow transplantation: findings from a multicentre study. *British Journal of Cancer, 71*, 1322–1329.

Baker, F., Curbow, B., & Wingard, J.R. (1991). Role retention and quality of life of bone marrow transplant survivors. *Social Science and Medicine, 32*, 697–704.

Baruch, J., Benjamin, S., Treleaven, J., Wilcox, A., Barron, J., & Powles, R. (1991). Male sexual dysfunction following bone marrow transplantation. *Bone Marrow Transplantation, 7*(Suppl. 2), 52.

Belec, R.H. (1992). Quality of life: Perceptions of long-term survivors of bone marrow transplantation. *Oncology Nursing Forum, 19*, 31–37.

Boyle, D., Blodgett, L., Gnesdiloff, S., White, J., Bamford, A., Sheridan, M., et al. (2000). Caregiver quality of life after autologous bone marrow transplantation. *Cancer Nursing, 23*, 193–203.

Broers, S., Kaptein, A., Cessie, S., Fibbe, W., & Hengeveld, M. (2000). Psychological functioning and quality of life following bone marrow transplantation: A 3-year follow-up study. *Journal of Psychosomatic Research, 48*, 11–21.

Bush, N., Donaldson, G., Haberman, M., Dacanay, R., & Sullivan, K. (2000). Conditional and unconditional estimation of multidimensional quality of life after hematopoietic stem cell transplantation: A longitudinal follow-up of 415 patients. *Biology of Blood and Marrow Transplantation, 6*, 576–591.

Bush, N., Haberman, M., Donaldson, G., & Sullivan, S. (1995). Quality of life of 125 adults surviving 6–18 years after bone marrow transplantation. *Social Science and Medicine, 40*, 479–490.

Caplan, K.C. (1984). The quality of life in cancer patients: An hypothesis. *Journal of Medical Ethics, 10*, 124–127.

Chiodi, S., Spinelli, S., Ravera, G., Petti, A., van Lint, M., Lamparelli, T., et al. (2000). Quality of life in 244 recipients of allogeneic bone marrow transplantation. *British Journal of Hematology, 110*, 614–619.

Cohen, M., Headley, J., & Sherwood, G. (2000). Spirituality and bone marrow transplantation: When faith is stronger than fear. *International Journal for Human Caring, 20*, 40–46.

Compton, K., McDonald, J., & Stetz, K. (1996). Understanding the caring relationship during marrow transplantation: Family caregivers and health care professionals. *Oncology Nursing Forum, 23*, 1428–1432.

Curbow, B., Legro, M.W., Baker, F., Wingard, J.R., & Somerfield, M.R. (1993). Loss and recovery themes of long-term survivors of bone marrow transplants. *Journal of Psychosocial Oncology, 10*(4), 1–20.

Duell, T., van Lint, M., Ljungman, P., Tichelli, A., Socie, G., Apperley, J., et al. (1997). Health and functional status of long-term survivors of bone marrow transplantation. *Annals of Internal Medicine, 166*, 184–192.

Ersek, M. (1992). The process of maintaining hope in adults undergoing bone marrow transplantation for leukemia. *Oncology Nursing Forum, 19*, 883–889.

Felder-Puig, R., Peters, C., Matthes-Martin, S., Lamche, M., Felsberger, C., Gadner, H., et al. (1999). Psychosocial adjustment of pediatric patients after allogeneic stem cell transplantation. *Bone Marrow Transplantation, 24*, 75–80.

Ferrans, C.E. (1990). Development of a quality of life index for cancer patients. *Oncology Nursing Forum, 17*, 15–21.

Ferrell, B., Grant, M., Schmidt, G., Rhiner, M., Whitehead, C., Fonbuena, P., et al. (1992a). The meaning of quality of life for bone marrow transplant survivors. The impact of bone marrow transplant on quality of life. *Cancer Nursing, 15*, 153–160.

Ferrell, B., Grant, M., Schmidt, G.M., Rhiner, M., Whitehead, C., Fonbuena, P., et al. (1992b). The meaning of quality of life for bone marrow transplant survivors. Part 2. Improving quality of life for bone marrow transplant survivors. *Cancer Nursing, 15*, 247–253.

Ferrell, B.R. (1996). The quality of lives: 1,525 voices of cancer. *Oncology Nursing Forum, 23*, 909–916.

Fromm, K., Andrykowski, M., & Hunt, J. (1996). Positive and negative psychosocial sequelae of bone marrow transplantation: Implications for quality of life assessment. *Journal of Behavioral Medicine, 19*, 221–240.

Foxall, M., & Gaston-Johansson, F. (1996). Burden and health outcomes of family caregivers of hospitalized bone marrow transplant patients. *Journal of Advanced Nursing, 24*, 915–923.

Haberman, M., Bush, N., Young, K., & Sullivan, K. (1993). Quality of life of adult long-term survivors of bone marrow transplantation: A qualitative analysis of narrative data. *Oncology Nursing Forum, 20*, 1545–1553.

Heinomen, H., Volin, L., Uutela, A., Zevon, M., Barrick, C., & Ruutu, T. (2001). Quality of life and factors related to perceived satisfaction with quality of life after allogeneic bone marrow transplantation. *Annals of Hematology, 80*, 137–143.

King, C.R., Haberman, M., Berry, D.L., Bush, N., Butler, L., Dow, K.H., et al. (1997). Quality of life and the cancer experience: The state-of-the knowledge. *Oncology Nursing Forum, 24*, 27–41.

Lee, S.L., Fairclough, D., Parsons, S.K., Soiffer, R.J., Fisher, D.C., Schlossman, R.L., et al. (2001). Recovery after stem-cell transplantation for hematologic diseases. *Journal of Clinical Oncology, 19*, 242–252.

Marks, D., Gale, D., Vedhara, K., & Bird, J. (1999). A quality of life study in 20 adult long-term survivors of unrelated donor bone marrow transplantation. *Bone Marrow Transplantation, 24*, 191–195.

Matthes-Martin, S., Lamche, M., Ladenstein, R., Emminger, W., Felsberger, C., Topf, R., et al. (1999). Organ toxicity and quality of life after allogeneic bone marrow transplantation in pediatric patients: A single center retrospective analysis. *Bone Marrow Transplantation, 23*, 1049–1053.

Molassiotis, A. (1997). Psychosocial transitions in the long-term survivors of bone marrow transplantation. *European Journal of Cancer Care, 6*, 100–107.

Molassiotis, A., Boughton, B.J., Burgoyne, T., & van den Akker, O. (1995). Comparison of the overall quality of life in 50 long-term survivors of autologous and allogeneic bone marrow transplantation. *Journal of Advanced Nursing, 22*, 509–516.

Molassiotis, A., van den Akker, O., & Boughton, B. (1997). Perceived social support, family environment and psychosocial recovery in bone marrow transplant long-term survivors. *Social Science Medicine, 44*, 317–325.

Mumma, G., Mashberg, D., & Lesko, L. (1992). Long-term psychosexual adjustment of acute leukemia survivors: Impact of marrow transplantation versus conventional chemotherapy. *General Hospital Psychiatry, 14*, 43–55.

Neitzert, C., Dancey, J., Murray, C., & Avery, J. (1998). The psychosocial impact of bone marrow transplantation: A review of the literature. *Bone Marrow Transplantation, 22*, 409–422.

Nespoli, L., Verri, A., Lacatelli, F., & Bertuggia, L. (1995). The impact of pediatric bone marrow transplantation on quality of life. *Quality of Life Research, 4*, 233–240.

Phipps, S., & Mulhern, R. (1995). Family cohesion and expressiveness promote resilience to the stress of pediatric bone marrow transplant: a preliminary report. *Journal of Developmental and Behavioral Pediatrics, 16*, 257–263.

Prieto, J., Saez, R., Carreras, E., Atala, J., Sierra, J., Rovira, M., et al. (1996). Physical and psychosocial functioning of 117 survivors of bone marrow transplantation. *Bone Marrow Transplantation, 17*, 1133–1142.

Rivera, L. (1997). Blood cell transplantation: Its impact on one family. *Seminars in Oncology Nursing, 13*, 94–99.

Saunders, J.E., Buckner, C.D., Amos, D., Levy, W., Appelbaum, F.R., Doney, K., et al. (1988). Ovarian function following marrow transplantation for aplastic anemia or leukemia. *Journal of Clinical Oncology, 6*, 813–818.

Somerfield, M., Curbow, B., Wingard, J., Baker, F., & Fogarty, L. (1996). Coping with the physical and psychosocial sequelae of bone marrow transplantation among long-term survivors. *Journal of Behavioral Medicine, 19*, 163–184.

Steeves, R.H. (1992). Patients who have undergone bone marrow transplantation: Their quest for meaning. *Oncology Nursing Forum, 19*, 899–905.

Stetz, K., McDonald, J., & Compton, K. (1996). Needs and experiences of family caregivers during marrow transplantation. *Oncology Nursing Forum, 23*, 1422–1427.

Sutherland, H., Fyles, G., Adams, G., Hao, Y., Lipton, J., Minden, M., et al. (1997). *Bone Marrow Transplantation, 19*, 1129–1136.

Syrjala, K., Roth-Roemer, S., Abrams, J., Scanlan, J., Chopko, M., Visser, S., et al. (1998). Prevalence and predictors of sexual dysfunction in long-term survivors of marrow transplantation. *Journal of Clinical Oncology, 16*, 3148–3157.

Syrjala, K.L., Chapko, M.K., Vitaliano, P.P., Cummings, C., & Sullivan, K.M. (1993). Recovery after allogeneic marrow transplantation: Prospective study of predictors of long-term physical and psychosocial functioning. *Bone Marrow Transplantation, 11*, 319–327.

Vallwrand, A., Breckenridge, D., & Hodgson, N. (1998). Theories and conceptual models to guide quality of life related research. In C. King & P. Hinds (Eds.), *Quality of life* (pp. 37–53). Sudbury, MA: Jones and Bartlett.

Vickberg, S., Duhamel, K., Smith, M., Manne, S., Winkel, G., Papadopoulos, E., et al. (2001). Global meaning and psychological adjustment among survivors of bone marrow transplant. *Psycho-Oncology, 10*, 29–39.

Whedon, M., & Ferrell, B. (1994). Quality of life in adult bone marrow transplant patients: Beyond the first year. *Seminars in Oncology Nursing, 10*, 42–57.

Whedon, M., Stearns, D., & Mills, L.E. (1995). Quality of life of long-term adult survivors of autologous bone marrow transplantation. *Oncology Nursing Forum, 22*, 1527–1535.

Wingard, J.R. (1994). Functional ability and quality of life of patients after allogeneic bone marrow transplantation. *Bone Marrow Transplantation, 14*(Suppl. 4), 529–533.

Wingard, J.R., Curbow, B., Baker, F., Zabora, J., & Piantadosi, S. (1992). Sexual satisfaction in survivors of bone marrow transplantation. *Bone Marrow Transplantation, 7*, 311–316.

Wochna, V. (1997). Anxiety, needs, and coping in family members of the bone marrow transplant patient. *Cancer Nursing, 20*, 244–250.

Wolcott, D., Wellisch, D., Fawzy, F., & Landsverk, J. (1986). Adaptation of adult bone marrow transplant recipient long-term survivors. *Transplantation, 41*, 478–484.

Zittoun, R., Suciu, S., Watson, M., Solbu, G., Muus, P., Mandelli, F., et al. (1997). Quality of life in patients with acute myelogenous leukemia in prolonged first complete remission after bone marrow transplantation (allogeneic or autologous) of chemotherapy: A cross-sectional study of the EORTC-GIMEMA AML, 8A trial. *Bone Marrow Transplantation, 20*, 307–315.

CHAPTER 16

Shelley Burcat, RN, MSN

Current Research and Future Directions in Hematopoietic Stem Cell Transplantation

Introduction

Research studies leading to wide application of hematopoietic stem cell transplant (HSCT) began more than 50 years ago (Thomas, 1999). In 1977, a transplant team in Seattle reported on 100 patients with advanced acute leukemia who were prepared with cyclophosphamide and total body irradiation and then given marrow from a human leukocyte antigen (HLA)-matched sibling. Seventeen of the patients were alive one to three years later (Thomas et al., 1977). The success of HSCT in even a few patients with advanced disease allowed researchers to consider treating patients earlier in the course of their disease (Thomas). Presently, more than 20,000 human transplants of hematopoietic cells from marrow, peripheral blood, or cord blood are performed annually (Thomas). In spite of the advances made by the hundreds of teams performing HSCTs, there remain obstacles to overcome (Bishop, 1999; Dupont, 1997). The major obstacles to HSCT plaguing researchers today include donor availability, graft versus host disease (GVHD), treatment-related complications, and relapse of disease (Bishop).

A limitation of HSCT is the lack of suitable HLA-matched donors and the complications of GVHD associated with HLA disparities. In the absence of a suitable HLA-identical sibling donor, alternative donors such as mismatched related or matched unrelated donors may be used (Gluckman, Rocha, & Chastang, 1998). Research is an integral and ongoing part of HSCT. It is helping to define the role of HSCT in the treatment of many malignant and nonmalignant disease processes, including autoimmune diseases and primary immune deficiency diseases. This chapter will review current research and future directions in HSCT.

Unrelated Donor Transplants

Speaking at a symposium during the American Society of Hematology (ASH) Conference 2000, Dr. D. Confer, medical director of the National Marrow Donor Program (NMDP), discussed unrelated donor transplants. Currently, more than four million donors are registered with the NMDP; 57% of these are fully typed. The number of potential donors from racial and ethnic minorities is increasing.

More than 9,000 transplants have been performed using marrow from unrelated donors, and approximately 300 transplants have been performed from unrelated peripheral stem cell donors. More than 1,400 transplants currently are performed annually using unrelated donors (NMDP, 2000). Through the NMDP, the probability of finding at least one HLA-A, -B, and -DR–matched donor on the initial search has increased from 15% in 1987 to more than 80% (Anasetti, Petersdorf, Martin, Woolfrey, & Hansen, 2001). The increasing number of unrelated transplants being performed has led to the development of many clinical trials.

Davies et al. (2000) analyzed engraftment of matched unrelated donor (MUD) bone marrow (BM). They studied 5,246 patients who received transplants facilitated by the NMDP between August 1991 and June 1999. A 4% primary graft failure was seen in patients surviving at least 28 days. Multivariate logistic regression analysis showed that engraftment was associated with marrow matched at HLA-A, HLA-B, DRBI, high cell dose, younger recipient, male recipient, and recipient from a non–African American ethnic group. A platelet count higher than $50 \times 10^9/l$ was achieved by 47% of patients by day 100. Conditional on survival to day 100, survival at three years was 61% in those with platelet engraftment between day 30 and 100 and 33% in those without engraftment at day 100. This study demonstrated the importance of HLA matching on primary engraftment after MUD bone marrow transplant (BMT) and that platelet recovery is a strong predictor of survival. Remberger et al. (2001) studied BM versus peripheral blood stem cell (PBSC) from unrelated donors and found that the use of PBSC from unrelated donors is a safe and well-tolerated procedure resulting in faster engraftment than BM, a good survival rate, and a good disease-free survival rate. In a recent study, 107 patients receiving PBSCs mobilized by granulocyte–colony-stimulating factor (G-CSF) from HLA-A, HLA-B, and HLA-DR–compatible unrelated donors were compared to 107 matched controls receiving unrelated marrow. Engraftment was achieved in 94% of patients in both groups. The PBSC recipients had a significantly shorter time to neutrophil and platelet engraftment ($p < 0.001$). Probabilities of acute and chronic GVHD were not statistically significant. Three-year transplant-related mortality rates were 42% in the PBSC group and 31% in the BM control ($p = 0.7$). Survival rates were 46% and 51%, respectively. The probability of relapse was 25% and 31% in both groups.

Umbilical Cord Blood Transplants

Another alternative donor source of stem cells under investigation is cord blood. More than 30,000 units of frozen cord blood are available, and more than 1,500 cases of cord blood transplant have been reported (Gluckman, 2000). The numbers of umbilical cord blood transplants (UCBTs) are increasing, and researchers are evaluating their results and comparing the outcomes of UCBT with allogeneic BMTs (Gluckman). The future objectives of Eurocord (2003) are to compare the results of UCBT to BMT in each indication, including unrelated BMT and haploidentical related BMT, to analyze prognostic factors associated with each transplant source, and to publish recommendations for each of these strategies (Gluckman).

Eurocord has analyzed the outcomes of 527 UCBTs from 121 transplant centers. These transplants involved 138 related donors and 399 unrelated donors. The results showed that survival with UCBT was comparable to that with related or unrelated BMTs. Engraftment with cord blood was delayed, resulting in an increased incidence of early transplant complications. The incidence of acute and chronic GVHD was reduced with cord blood grafts even in HLA-mismatched transplants and adults. In patients with leukemia, the rate of relapse was similar to the rate of relapse after BMT. The overall event-free survival with UCBT was not statistically different compared to BMT (Gluckman, 2000).

Rocha et al. (2000) analyzed GVHD in children who had received a cord blood or marrow transplant from an HLA-identical sibling. The records of 113 recipients of cord blood from HLA-identical siblings from the period 1990 through 1997 were studied and compared with the records of 2,052 recipients of BM from HLA-identical siblings during the same period. The study population consisted of children up to the age of 15. The researchers compared rates of GVHD, hematopoietic recovery, and survival using Cox proportional hazards regression to adjust for potentially confounding factors. The results showed recipients of cord blood were younger than recipients of BM (median age five years versus eight years; $p < 0.001$), weighed less (median weight 17 kg versus 26 kg; $p < 0.001$), and were less likely to have received methotrexate (MTX) for prophylaxis against GVHD (28% versus 65%; $p < 0.001$). Multivariate analysis demonstrated a lower risk of acute GVHD (relative risk 0.41; $p = 0.001$) and chronic GVHD (relative risk 0.35; $p = 0.02$) among recipients of cord-blood transplants. As compared with recovery after BMT, the likelihood of recovery of the neutrophil count and the platelet count was significantly lower in the first month after cord-blood transplantation (relative risk 0.40 [$p < 0.001$] and 0.20 [$p < 0.001$], respectively). Mortality was similar in the two groups (relative risk of death in the recipients of cord blood 1.15; $p = 0.43$). The researchers concluded from this study that recipients of cord-blood transplants from HLA-identi-

cal siblings have a lower incidence of acute and chronic GVHD than recipients of marrow transplants from HLA-identical siblings. Laughlin et al. (2001) reported results of a study of hematopoietic engraftment and survival in adult recipients of umbilical cord blood (UCB) from unrelated donors. Sixty-eight adults with life-threatening hematologic disorders received intensive chemotherapy or total-body irradiation and then transplants of HLA-mismatched UCB. They evaluated the outcomes in terms of hematologic reconstitution, the occurrence of acute and chronic GVHD, relapses, and event-free survival. Of the 68 patients, 48 (71%) received grafts of UCB that were mismatched for two or more HLA antigens. Of the 60 patients who survived 28 days or more after transplantation, 55 had neutrophil engraftment at a median of 27 days (range = 13–59). The estimated probability of neutrophil recovery in the 68 patients was 0.90 (95% confidence interval [CI], 0.85–1.0). The presence of a relatively high number of nucleated cells in the UCB before it was frozen was associated with faster recovery of neutrophils. Severe acute GVHD (of grade III or IV) occurred in 11 of 55 patients who could be evaluated within the first 100 days after transplantation. The median follow-up for survivors was 22 months (range = 11–51). Of the 68 patients, 19 were alive and 18 of these (26%) were disease-free 40 months after transplantation. The presence of a high number of CD34+ cells in the graft was associated with improved event-free survival ($p = 0.05$). The researchers concluded that UCB from unrelated donors can restore hematopoiesis in adults who receive myeloablative therapy and is associated with acceptable rates of severe acute and chronic GVHD.

Barker et al. (2001) performed a matched-pair analysis of survival after transplantation of unrelated donor UCB compared to HLA-matched unrelated donor BM. To investigate the relative merits of unrelated donor UCB versus BM, a matched-pair analysis comparing the outcomes of recipients of 0 to 3 HLA-mismatched UCB and HLA-A, -B, -DRB1–matched BM was performed. UCB patients, who received cyclosporine (CSA) and methylprednisolone (MP), were matched for age, diagnosis, and disease stage with BM patients, who received either MTX and CSA (26 pairs) or T cell depletion and CSA/MP (31 pairs). Patients were predominantly children (median age five years) undergoing transplantation for malignancy, storage diseases, BM failure, and immunodeficiency syndromes between 1991 and 1999. Although neutrophil recovery was significantly slower after UCB transplantation, the probability of donor-derived engraftment at day 45 was 88% in UCB versus 96% in BM-MTX recipients ($p = 0.41$) and 85% in UCB versus 90% in BM-T cell–depleted recipients ($p = 0.32$), respectively. Platelet recovery was similar in UCB versus BM pairs. Incidences of acute and chronic GVHD were similar in UCB and BM recipients, with 53% of UBC versus 41% of BM-MTX recipients alive ($p = 0.40$) and 52% of UCB versus 56% of UCBT cell-depleted recipients alive at two years ($p > 0.80$), respectively. These data suggest that, despite increased HLA disparity, probabilities of engraftment, GVHD, and survival after

UCB transplantation are comparable to those observed after HLA-matched BM transplantation.

Rocha et al. (2001) performed a comparison of outcomes of unrelated BMT and UCBT in children with acute leukemia. Five-hundred forty-one children with acute leukemia undergoing UCBT (n = 99), T cell–depleted unrelated BMT (T-UBMT) (n = 180), or nonmanipulated unrelated BMT (UBMT) (n = 262) were analyzed in a retrospective multicenter study. Comparisons were performed after adjustment for patient, disease, and transplant variables. The major difference among the three groups was the higher number of HLA mismatches (defined by serology for class I and molecular typing for DRB1) in the UCBT group. The donor was HLA mismatched in 92% of UCBTs, in 18% of UBMTs, and 43% of T-UBMTs (p < 0.001). Other significant differences were observed in pretransplant disease characteristics, preparative regimens, GVHD prophylaxis, and number of cells infused. Nonadjusted estimates of two-year survival rates were 40% and 43%, respectively, in the UBMT group and 41% and 37% in the UCBT group. After adjustment, differences in outcomes appeared in the first 100 days after the transplantation. Compared with UBMT recipients, UCBT recipients had delayed hematopoietic recovery (hazard ration [HR] = 0.37; 95% CI: 0.27–0.52; p < 0.001), increased 100 day transplant-related mortality (HR = 2.13; 95% CI: 1.20–3.76; p < 0.01), and decreased acute GVHD (HR = 0.50; 95% CI: 0.34–0.73; p < 0.001). T-UBMT recipients had decreased acute GVHD (HR = 0.25; 95% CI: 0.17–0.36; p < 0.0001) and increased risk of relapse (HR = 1.96; 95% CI: 1.11–3.45; p = 0.02). After day 100 post-transplant, the three groups achieved similar results in terms of relapse. Chronic GVHD was decreased after T-UBMT (HR = 0.21; 95% CI: 0.11–0.37; p < 0.0001) and UCBT (HR = 0.24; 95% CI: 0.01–0.66; p = 0.002), and overall mortality was higher in T-UBMT recipients (HR = 1.39; 95% CI: 0.97–1.99; p < 0.07). The researchers concluded the use of UCBT, as a source of hematopoietic stem cells (HSCs), is a reasonable option for children with acute leukemia lacking an acceptably matched unrelated marrow donor.

Clinical trials in UCBT have revealed delayed engraftment. To speed engraftment, several methods can be investigated, including the use of hematopoietic growth factors such as G-CSF, Kit ligand, or thrombopoietin. At this stage, the usefulness of these factors has not been demonstrated and deserves further investigation. Also, protocols for studying cord blood stem cell expansion for improving short-term engraftment could be clinically useful (Gluckman et al., 1998).

Haploidentical Transplants

Genetically haploidentical family members can provide alternative donors for patients in need of HSCT. Haploidentical donors are available in 90% of patients. They have been used for patients with advanced disease who urgently require transplant and cannot wait for a donor search (Rowe & Lazarus, 2001).

Aversa et al. (1998) studied patients with acute leukemia and tried to achieve successful transplantation with the use of HSCs from donors who shared only one HLA haplotype with the recipient (a "full-haplotype mismatch"). To prevent graft failure, large doses of T cell–depleted HSCs were transplanted after a conditioning regimen of enhanced myeloablation and immunosuppression was administered to the recipient. Forty-three patients with high-risk acute leukemia who were scheduled for transplantation received total body irradiation, thiotepa, fludarabine, and antithymocyte globulin (ATG). The graft consisted of peripheral blood progenitor cells that had been mobilized in the donor with recombinant G-CSF and also, in 28 cases, marrow. BM from the donor was depleted of T lymphocytes by processing with soybean agglutinin and E-rosetting. T cell depletion of peripheral blood mononuclear cells was achieved by E-rosetting followed by positive selection of CD34+ cells. No post-transplantation prophylaxis against GVHD was administered. In all of the patients, full donor-type engraftment was achieved. Neither acute nor chronic GVHD developed in the patients who could be evaluated. Regimen-related toxicity was minimal. Eleven of the 23 patients with acute lymphoblastic leukemia had a relapse, as did 2 of the 20 patients with acute myeloid leukemia. Transplantation-related mortality was 40%. After a median follow-up of 18 months (range = 8–30), 12 of the 43 patients were alive and free of disease. All surviving patients had a good quality of life. The researchers concluded the main limitations of transplantation of marrow from donors who are matched with the recipient for only one HLA haplotype, GVHD and graft failure, can be overcome. Because most patients have a relative with one haplotype mismatch, advances in this method will increase the availability of hematopoietic cell transplantation as curative therapy for acute leukemia.

Henslee-Downey et al. (1996) studied 40 patients using an approach combining in vitro and in vivo T cell depletion with T lymphocyte-targeted monoclonal antibodies (mAbs) and intensified conditioning therapy, including fractionated total body irradiation before etoposide, cytosine arabinoside, cyclophosphamide, and MP. Grafts were treated with T10B9.1A-31 mAb, directed against the alpha-beta heterodimer of the T cell receptor, and rabbit complement. In vivo depletion was attempted with an anti-CD5 mAb-Ricin A-chain (H65-RTA) immunotoxin (IT). Study patients were compared with a historical control group of 17 patients not given H65-RTA. Rates of engraftment were not significantly different (93% versus 100%, p = 0.12), although patients receiving IT engrafted more rapidly. The probability of developing > grade I GVHD was significantly lower in the study group when compared with the control group (36% versus 100%, p = 0.0001), as well as for severe grade III–IV GVHD (19% versus 92%, p = 0.0001). Five-year survival tended to be improved in the study group (40% versus 18%, p = 0.21). The researchers concluded that transplant from haploidentical family members is indicated for patients without a matched sibling in whom allogeneic BMT offers the best opportunity to achieve cure.

Bunjes et al. (2000) reported on 10 patients with incurable hematologic malignancies who were treated with haploidentical PBSC transplant. Conditioning consisted of ATG, total body irradiation, thiotepa, cyclophosphamide, and additional radioimmunotherapy in five patients. All patients received G-CSF mobilized PBSC grafts. GVHD prophylaxis consisted of T cell depletion by CD34+ selection; nine patients received no post-transplant immunosuppression. Stable engraftment was achieved in nine patients; one case of acute graft rejection was observed. Seven patients developed grade I acute GVHD, and six patients developed chronic GVHD. Infections were the most significant clinical problem post-transplant. Two patients suffered a relapse of their disease, and two further patients died of transplant-related complications. After a median follow-up of 13 months (range 5–37 months), six patients were surviving in remission. The researchers concluded that haploidentical stem cell transplant is a reasonable alternative to matched unrelated transplant.

Aversa and colleagues at the University of Perugia, Italy, reported the successful use of a relatively nontoxic conditioning regimen using thiotepa, a single dose of 800 cGy of total body irradiation, fludarabine, and ATG. Thirty-day treatment-related mortality is approximately 10% and relies on fundamental work that established the concept that escalation of the stem cell dose directly contributed to the likelihood of the establishment of donor type chimerism (Aversa, Velardi, Tabilio, Reisner, & Martelli, 2001; Rowe & Lazarus, 2001). Aversa and colleagues treated 76 patients with acute leukemia between October 1995 and October 2000 using immunoselected CD34+ cell transplant (2001). Seventy (92%) of the 76 patients achieved primary and sustained engraftment. Immunologic rejection was reversed in five of the remaining six patients by the transplantation of T cell–depleted PBSCs from a different haploidentical family member who did not share the same haplotype as the first after further immunosuppression, which was started medianly 30 days after the first conditioning regimen ended. Thus, sustained engraftment was achieved in 75 of 76 patients. Hematopoietic recovery was rapid, with neutrophil counts reaching $1 \times 10^9/l$ and platelet counts $25 \times 10^9/l$ at a median of 10 days (range = 8–19) and 17 days (range = 12–18), respectively. All patients achieved and sustained a full donor type chimerism in the peripheral blood and the marrow. Three patients developed acute GVHD grade II–IV, which progressed to chronic in two patients. The extra-hematologic toxicity of this conditioning regimen was minimal. Two of the first 16 patients died from toxic acute pulmonary decompensation soon after transplant. The total dose of lung radiation was reduced from 6 to 4 Gy, and no further acute lung toxicity was observed. No significant late effects were observed in the 19 patients surviving more than one year after transplant (range = 12–68 months, with a median of 28 months). Twenty-four of the 34 nonleukemic deaths in the 76 patients transplanted were caused by infection. To date, the event-free survival (EFS) compares favorably with what has been reported in patients at the same stage of disease who received transplants from matched donors (Aversa et al., 2001).

The major focus of performing haploidentical transplantation was aimed at engraftment and GVHD. As these problems have largely been surmounted, the single most important barrier still to be overcome is infection (Rowe & Lazarus, 2001). The major challenge for future years is to achieve engraftment of allogeneic hematopoietic cells following nonmyeloablative conditioning, in the absence of alloreactive T cells. It has been suggested that this goal might be achieved by using megadoses of CD34+ stem cells in conjunction with nonalloreactive anti–third-party cytotoxic T lymphocytes. This hypothesis currently is being tested in primates (Reisner & Martelli, 2000). With less-toxic conditioning regimens, transplantation will be possible for patients who are not eligible for conventional cytoreductive treatments and those for whom the risk of supralethal radiochemotherapy is not justified, such as patients with nonmalignant hematologic disorders (Aversa et al., 2001). The use of prospective, multicenter, controlled clinical trials and companion translational studies will further improve upon this modality (Rowe & Lazarus).

Graft Versus Host Disease

GVHD continues to be a cause of morbidity and mortality for patients undergoing allogeneic HSCT (Arai & Vogelsang, 2000; Basara, Kiehl, & Fauser, 2001; Goker, Hazendaroglu, & Chao, 2001). Approximately 30%–60% of patients receiving histocompatible matched sibling allografts develop acute GVHD (Arai & Vogelsang). Incidence of GVHD is higher for alternative donor transplants (Arai & Vogelsang; Basara et al.). Chronic GVHD develops in 35%–50% of patients after transplant (Arai & Vogelsang). Recent clinical trials have used and compared immunosuppressive agents, changed conditioning regimens, and used mAbs to prevent and treat GVHD (Arai & Vogelsang; Basara et al.; Goker et al.; Murphy & Blazar, 1999). Currently, researchers are attempting to prevent and treat GVHD with emphasis on the variables that affect its induction and severity, the effector mechanisms, and whether GVHD can be suppressed while maintaining graft versus tumor effects (Murphy & Blazar).

Ratanatharathorn et al. (1998) conducted a phase III randomized trial testing the role of tacrolimus/MTX versus CSA/MTX for GVHD prophylaxis after HLA-identical sibling marrow transplantation in patients with hematologic malignancies (Goker et al., 2001; Ratanatharathorn et al.). The incidence of grade II–IV acute GVHD was found to be significantly lower in patients who received tacrolimus compared to patients in the CSA group (31.9% versus 44.4%, $p = 0.01$), although grade III–IV acute GVHD was similar (13.3% versus 17.1%), chronic GVHD between groups was similar (55.9% versus 49.4%, $p = 0.8$), and relapse rates also were not different. The patients who received CSA had significantly better survival rates than patients who received tacrolimus (57.2% versus 46.9%). This study demonstrated that tacrolimus (FK506) appeared to be a better choice for the prophylaxis of acute GVHD, but it did not allow a survival advantage (Goker et al.; Ratanatharathorn et al.).

Chao et al. (1999) conducted a prospective randomized trial comparing the three-drug regimen (CSA/MTX [three doses]/prednisone [PSE]) to the "standard" two-drug regimen (CSA/MTX [four doses]) to investigate the benefit of PSE used up front for the prevention of acute and chronic GVHD (Chao et al., 1999; Goker et al., 2001). In this study, 193 patients were randomized, and 186 patients were included in the analysis (5 were not evaluable because of death before engraftment, and 2 were deemed ineligible). All patients received marrow from a fully histocompatible sibling donor. The preparatory regimen consisted of fractionated total body irradiation and etoposide in all but 13 patients, who received fractionated total body irradiation/cyclophosphamide. The patients were randomized to receive either CSA/MTX/PSE or CSA/MTX. The two groups were well balanced with respect to diagnosis, age, donor-recipient gender match, and parity. In an intent-to-treat analysis, the incidence of acute GVHD was 18% (CI: 12–28 for CSA/MTX/PSE) compared to 20% (CI: 10–26) for CSA/MTX ($p = 0.60$). Overall survival was 65% for those receiving CSA/MTX/PSE and 72% for CSA/MTX ($p = 0.10$), with a relapse rate of 15% for the CSA/MTX/PSE group and 12% for the CSA/MTX group ($p = 0.83$). The incidence of chronic GVHD was similar (46% versus 52%, $p = 0.38$), with a follow-up of 0.7–6 years. Nineteen patients went off study because of GVHD, 4 in the group receiving CSA/MTX/PSE and 15 of those receiving CSA/MTX ($p = 0.20$); and 11 patients went off study because of alveolar hemorrhage, 3 in the CSA/MTX/PSE arm and 8 in the CSA/MTX arm ($p = 0.22$). The addition of PSE did not result in higher incidence of infectious complications: bacterial (66% versus 58%), viral (77% versus 66%), and fungal (20% versus 20%) in those receiving CSA/MTX/PSE or CSA/MTX, respectively. These data suggest that the addition of PSE is associated with a somewhat lower incidence of early post-transplant complications but did not have a positive impact on overall incidence of acute or chronic GVHD or event-free or overall survival (Chao et al., 1999; Goker et al.).

Chao et al. (1996) reported results of a prospective, randomized, double-blind study comparing thalidomide to placebo as prophylaxis against the development of chronic GVHD (Arai & Vogelsang, 2000; Chao et al., 1996). This group randomized 59 patients to receive either placebo or thalidomide (200 mg orally twice a day) starting on day 80 after allogeneic HSCT. Fifty-four patients were evaluable at the time of the first interim analysis, and the study was stopped at that time. Not only was there a higher incidence of GVHD among the patients receiving thalidomide compared to those receiving placebo ($p = 0.60$), but overall survival also was significantly worse among those receiving thalidomide ($p = 0.006$). The authors concluded that the early use of thalidomide shifted the balance between GVHD and induction of tolerance, thus leading to the negative effects of thalidomide, of incidence of chronic GVHD, and overall survival (Arai & Vogelsang; Chao et al., 1996).

Przepiorka et al. (2000) studied daclizumab, a humanized anti-interleukin-2 receptor alpha chain antibody, for treatment of acute GVHD. Forty-three patients with advanced or steroid-refractory GVHD were treated with daclizumab. The first cohort of 24 patients was treated with daclizumab 1 mg/kg on days 1, 8, 15, 22, and 29. On day 43, the complete response (CR) rate was 29% (95% CI, 13%–51%). Survival on day 120 was 29% (95% CI, 13%–51%). A second cohort of 19 patients was treated with daclizumab 1 mg/kg on days 1, 4, 8, 15, and 22. For these patients, the CR rate on day 43 was 47% (95% CI, 24%–71%) and survival on day 120 was 53% (95% CI, 29%–76%). No infusion-related reactions and no serious side effects related to daclizumab were observed. Following treatment, there was a reduction in serum concentrations of soluble IL-2R and peripheral blood CD3+25+ lymphocytes, but these changes were not predictive of response. Daclizumab has substantial activity for the treatment of acute GVHD, and the second regimen evaluated is recommended for a controlled study (Przepiorka et al.).

Krijanovski et al. (1999) studied the administration of human recombinant keratinocyte growth factor (KGF) in a well-characterized murine BMT model for its effects on GVHD. KGF administration from day –3 to +7 significantly reduced GVHD mortality and the severity of GVHD in the gastrointestinal (GI) tract, reducing serum lipopolysaccharide and tumor necrosis factor (TNF)-alpha levels but preserving donor T cell responses (cytotoxic T lymphocyte activity, proliferation, and interleukin [IL]-2 production) to host antigens. When mice received lethal doses of p815 leukemia cells at the time of BMT, KGF treatment significantly decreased acute GVHD compared with control-treated allogeneic mice and resulted in a significantly improved leukemia-free survival (42% versus 4%, $p = < 0.001$). KGF administration thus offers a novel approach to the separation of graft versus leukemia effects from GVHD (Krijanovski et al.).

Anticytokine antibodies are being investigated and include IL-1 receptor antibody, TNF-alpha antibody, and IL-2 receptor antibody and have had encouraging results (Arai & Vogelsang , 2000). Antin et al. (1994) conducted a phase I/II trial to evaluate the effectiveness of an IL-1 receptor antagonist in 16 patients with steroid-resistant GVHD. The infused antibody was given as a 24-hour continuous infusion over seven days, and doses were escalated from 400 to 3,200 mg/day. Improvement was noted in the skin (8/14), GI tract (9/11), and liver (2/11) (Antin et al.; Arai & Vogelsang). Anti-TNF-alpha monoclonal antibody has been used in the treatment of GVHD. In 24 patients with resistant grade III–IV GVHD who were given anti-TNF-alpha, no CRs were seen, but 17 patients had a partial response (Arai & Vogelsang).

Herve et al. (1991) reported the efficacy of IL-2 receptor antibody (IgG1 murine monoclonal antibody) in patients with steroid-resistant GVHD. Twenty-nine of 58 patients (50%) had complete resolution of GVHD (Arai & Vogelsang, 2000; Herve et al.). Anasetti and colleagues reported similar results (Anasetti et al., 1992; Arai & Vogelsang). Humanized anti-TAC (a genetically engineered human IgG1 monoclonal antibody specific for the alpha subunit of the IL-2 receptor) is now available, and it has been used in 20 patients with steroid-refractory GVHD. Improvement in GVHD was noted in eight patients (Anasetti et al., 1992; Arai & Vogelsang). Some progress in therapy for GVHD has been made, but further research is needed to better understand the pathogenesis of GVHD so that new therapeutic approaches may be developed (Arai & Vogelsang).

Nonmyeloablative Transplants

A current focus of research in HSCT is the nonmyeloablative or "mini" transplant. HSCT was thought of as a rescue technique for restoring hematopoiesis after high-dose therapy. It is now known that high-dose therapy alone does not eradicate malignancy in many patients, and the benefit of allogeneic transplant lies in the associated immune-mediated graft versus malignancy (Champlin et al., 1999, 2000). Nonmyeloablative transplants have allowed researchers to effectively treat patients using the principles of graft versus malignancy and adoptive immunotherapy. Nonmyeloablative transplants are responsible for safer allografting procedures that can be better tolerated by older patients as well as patients with comorbid conditions who would be ineligible for conventional allogeneic transplant (Carella, Champlin, Slavin, McSweeney, & Storb, 2000).

Nonmyeloablative transplants use a less-intensive preparative regimen designed not to eradicate the malignancy but to provide sufficient immunosuppression to achieve engraftment of an allogeneic blood stem cell or marrow graft, allowing the development of an immune graft versus malignancy effect (Champlin et al., 2000). Many transplant centers currently are performing trials evaluating nonmyeloablative conditioning regimens (Spitzer, 2000).

Giralt et al. (1997) treated 15 patients with acute myeloid leukemia or myelodysplastic syndrome. Preparative regimens were either fludarabine (30 mg/m^2/d x 4 days) and idarubicin (12 mg/m^2/d x 3 days) with either cytosine arabinoside (2,000 mg/m^2/d x 4 days) or high-dose melphalan (140 mg/m^2/d), or 2-chlorodeoxyadenosine ([2CDA], 12 mg/m^2/d x 5 days) and cytosine arabinoside (1,000 mg/m^2/d x 5 days). Thirteen patients received PBSC transplants from HLA-genotypically identical sibling donors and two from a one-antigen–mismatched sibling donor. Chemotherapy generally was well tolerated, with only one death occurring as a result of multiorgan failure. Thirteen patients had engraftment as evidenced by an absolute neutrophil count of greater than 0.5 x 10^9 per liter. Chimerism was measured by either conventional cytogenetic or restriction fragment length polymorphism (RFLP) analysis. Seven patients achieved greater than 90% donor hematopoiesis 14–30 days post-transplant. Four patients had no evidence of donor hematopoiesis. Five patients experienced early relapse (between 43 and 127 days) post-transplant. Six of 15 patients were alive between 34 and 175 days post-transplant. Acute GVHD occurred in three patients. None of the five evaluable patients had evidence of chronic GVHD (Giralt et al.; Spitzer, 2000).

Khouri et al. (1998) described 15 patients with chronic lymphocytic leukemia (CLL) or low to intermediate-grade non-Hodgkin's lymphoma (NHL) who received fludarabine (30 mg/m^2/d x 3 days) and cyclophosphamide (300 mg/m^2/d x 3 days) or fludarabine (30 mg/m^2/d x 2 days), cisplatin (25 mg/m^2/d x 4 days), and cytosine arabinoside (500 mg/m^2/d x 2 days). Eleven of 15 patients had donor cell engraftment as measured by RFLP analysis of the bone marrow. The percentage of donor cells ranged from 50% to 100% at one month post-transplant. Seven patients had greater than or equal to 90% donor cells. Four patients had exclusively recipient marrow cells and recovered autologous hematopoiesis promptly. Only four patients received delayed donor lymphocyte infusion (DLI) from 55 to 100 days post-transplant. One of the patients converted from 75% donor cells at six weeks post-transplant to 100% donor cells following DLI. Five patients developed acute GVHD following the initial transplant. Two patients developed extensive chronic GVHD, which was fatal in one patient. Three patients developed GVHD following DLI; one of these patients had grade IV GVHD, which was fatal. Eight patients achieved a CR. At an initial median follow-up of 180 days, five of six patients (83.3%) with chemosensitive disease were alive compared to only two of nine patients (22.3%) who had chemo-refractory or untested disease (Khouri et al.; Spitzer, 2000).

Slavin et al. (1998) treated 22 patients with hematologic malignancies and 4 patients with genetic diseases using a busulfan-based regimen. Preparative therapy consisted of busulfan (8 mg/kg), fludarabine (180 mg/m^2) and anti–T lymphocyte globulin. Fourteen of the 22 patients with hematologic malignancy had low-risk disease (acute myeloid leukemia in first remission or chronic myeloid leukemia [CML] in chronic phase). G-CSF–mobilized PBSCs were used as the source of stem cell support. GVHD prophylaxis consisted of CSA. Twenty-five patients received HLA-genotypically identical sibling donor transplants. One patient received stem cells from a donor with a single antigen mismatch at the A and C locus. Chimerism was evaluated by standard cytogenetic analysis, by analysis of residual Ph+ cells in patients with CML, or by polymerase chain reaction (PCR)-based variable number of tandem repeat sequence analysis in sex matched donor recipient combinations. Treatment generally was well tolerated. All patients had evidence of donor engraftment. In 9 of 26 evaluable patients, transient mixed chimerism was observed. Acute GVHD occurred in 12 of 26 patients. Six patients developed grade III–IV GVHD that was the sole cause of mortality in 4 patients. Limited chronic GVHD developed in 9 of 25 evaluable patients. At a median of eight months post-transplant, 22 of 26 patients (85%) were alive, 21 of whom (81%) were clinically disease free (Slavin et al.; Spitzer, 2000).

McSweeney et al. (1999) used low-dose total body irradiation (200 cGy) and post-transplant immunosuppression (mycophenolate mofetil [MMF] and CSA) to treat 44 patients with hematologic malignancies who were ineligible for conventional allografting because of age, prior therapy, or organ dysfunction. Of 42 evaluable patients, all had persistent donor chimerism at two months post-transplant. The regimen was well tolerated with no significant myelosuppression, GI toxicities, or alopecia and the achievement of major disease responses in 70% of the patients (McSweeney et al.; Spitzer, 2000).

Childs et al. (1999) described the engraftment kinetics after nonmyeloablative therapy with cyclophosphamide (60 mg/kg/d x 2 days) and fludarabine (25 mg/m²/d x 5 days) and HLA-matched or one antigen-mismatched donor PBSC transplantation for hematologic malignancy (n = 8) or solid tumors (melanoma, n = 4; renal cell cancer [RCC], n = 3). Patients who achieved mixed chimerism were eligible for monthly escalating doses of DLI. Full donor T cell engraftment was more rapid than donor myeloid engraftment and was a prerequisite for acute GVHD and disease regression. Ten patients had a response (three patients with metastatic RCC; two with CML in chronic phase; one with chronic myelomonocytic leukemia; one with myelodysplastic syndrome; one with diffuse large-cell NHL; one with melanoma; and one with extramedullary plasmacytoma), five of whom were in a sustained CR (one metastatic RCC, three with CML, and one with NHL). Eight were alive between 121 and 409 days post-transplant (Childs et al., 1999; Spitzer, 2000).

Spitzer (2000) and colleagues reliably induced mixed lymphohematopoietic chimerism in patients with chemoradiotherapy refractory hematologic malignancies. Preparative therapy consisted of cyclophosphamide (150–200 mg/kg), ATG (15–30 mg/kg/d on days –2, –1 and +1 or –1, +1, +3, and +5), and thymic irradiation in patients who had not previously received mediastinal radiation therapy. Post-transplant CSA was given as GVHD prophylaxis. Twenty-eight patients received an HLA-matched (HLA genotypically matched in 27 and phenotypically matched in 1) donor transplant, while 16 received an HLA-mismatched donor transplant (1 HLA 3-antigen, 11 HLA 2-antigen, and 4 HLA 1-antigen mismatch). Therapy was well tolerated. Cyclophosphamide-induced cardiac toxicity has been observed in six patients and has been reversible in five. Severe ATG toxicities at a dose of 30 mg/kg in two patients necessitated a dose reduction to 15 mg/kg. Of 23 evaluable patients of HLA-matched donor transplantation, 20 have achieved stable mixed lymphohematopoietic chimerism. Ten patients with stable mixed chimerism, who had no evidence of GVHD, received DLI beginning on day +35 post-transplant. Conversion of mixed chimerism to fully donor hematopoiesis has occurred in 6 of the 10 patients. Seven of 10 evaluable recipients of HLA-mismatched donor marrow transplants have achieved stable mixed chimerism. Antitumor responses have been seen in the majority of these patients with refractory hematologic malignancies. Of 23 evaluable patients with chemorefractory Hodgkin's disease or NHL, seven (29%) achieved a partial remission and eight (33%) a complete response. Twenty-two patients are presently alive. Thirteen of these 22 patients are evaluable for response, and 8 are clinically progression free. Of the 10 patients who received delayed DLIs beginning at day +35 post-transplant for conversion of their chimerism, six patients have achieved a complete remission and seven remain progression free (Spitzer).

What effect, if any, the immune-mediated graft versus tumor effect will have in solid tumors remains to be seen (McCarthy & Bishop, 2000). A number of transplant programs are performing studies to evaluate the effect of an allogeneic graft on solid tumors.

Childs et al. (2000) reported on the regression of metastatic RCC after nonmyeloablative allogeneic PBSC transplant. Nineteen patients with refractory metastatic RCC who had suitable donors received a preparative regimen of cyclophosphamide (60 mg/kg/d x 2 days) and fludarabine (25 mg/m² x 5 days). Two patients who received a transplant from a donor with a single HLA locus mismatch also received ATG (40 mg/kg/d x 4 days). Patients received an infusion of PBSC allograft from an HLA-identical sibling or a sibling with a mismatch of a single HLA antigen. CSA, used to prevent GVHD, was withdrawn early in patients with mixed T cell chimerism or disease progression. Patients with no response received up to three infusions of donor lymphocytes. At the time of last follow-up, 9 of the 19 patients were alive 287 to 831 days after transplantation (median follow-up 402 days). Two had died of transplant-related causes and eight from progressive disease. In 10 patients (53%), metastatic disease regressed; 3 had a CR, and 7 had a partial response. The patients who had a CR remained in remission 27, 25, and 16 months after transplant. Regression of metastases was delayed, occurring a median of 129 days after transplantation and often followed the withdrawal of CSA and the establishment of complete donor T cell chimerism. These results are consistent with a graft versus tumor effect. The researchers concluded that nonmyeloablative allogeneic stem cell transplantation could induce sustained regression of metastatic RCC in patients who have had no response to conventional immunotherapy (Childs et al., 2000).

A number of questions remain for researchers to answer related to nonmyeloablative transplants. Nonmyeloablative HSCT primarily has been used to treat patients with hematologic disorders. The absolute numbers of individuals that have been treated are small, with the largest reported single series consisting of 50 patients. This approach has been applied to older patients who would have been excluded from allogeneic transplant on the basis of age, poor performance status, or comorbid disease.

The primary goal of achieving donor engraftment has been achieved, but the optimal regimen to achieve this goal has yet to be determined (McCarthy & Bishop, 2000). Further studies are needed to clearly outline definitions and management of mixed chimerism. Questions still to be answered about DLI include optimal timing of delivery, most effective and least toxic dose, and durability of tumor response in the nonmyeloablative setting (McCarthy & Bishop).

The Nonmyeloablative Transplant Trials Group was developed to encourage multi-institutional studies and decrease the number of single institution studies. Composed of approximately 20 centers, this trials group is based out of the Medical College of Wisconsin (MCW) and the International Bone Marrow Transplant Registry (IBMTR)/Autologous Blood and Marrow Transplant Registry (ABMTR); it is led by Christopher Bredeson (MCW and IBMTR/ABMTR) and Robert Collins (University of Texas-Southwestern). Currently, the group has two trials available: one in CLL and one for hematologic malignancies in general (personal communication, J. Filicko, May, 27, 2001).

Clinical Trials

Currently, the numbers of ongoing clinical trials related to HSCT are too numerous to list. In spite of the importance of clinical trials in setting a standard for care, only about 4% of adult patients with cancer are entered in clinical trials (Lara et al., 2001). Dr. Mary Horowitz, scientific director of the IBMTR, spoke at a symposium titled "Technologies that Make Transplant Safer" during the annual meeting of ASH in December 2000. The discussion focused on difficulties of enrolling patients in clinical trials for HSCT. Dr. Horowitz cited the lack of a cohesive network of transplant and referral centers for multicenter trials, which resulted in most transplant-related technologies never being evaluated in randomized trials (NMDP, 2000). Other problems identified by Dr. Horowitz that have slowed advances in HSCT include a lack of standardized objectives and validation of criteria for diagnosing and grading transplant complications (NMDP).

The general consensus of transplant researchers is that current systems to foster rapid translation of advances in transplantation biology are inadequate (O'Reilly, 2000). There also is concern that the existing infrastructure for the conduct of phase II trials evaluating new strategies for transplantation, transplantation-associated tumor-targeted therapies, and the treatment of transplant-associated complications is inadequate to exploit, in a timely manner, the many opportunities suggested by current research (O'Reilly). Currently, transplant researchers are working with the National Cancer Institute (NCI) and National Heart, Lung, and Blood Institute to develop new organizational structures that will support ongoing research in HSCT (O'Reilly). Researchers are attempting to develop a system that will encourage participation by most of the transplant centers in the country, exploit transplant biology in its development, include prioritization of clinical trials, and allow for rapid accrual of patients into the clinical trials (O'Reilly). Recognizing the need to develop new strategies for HSCT, the National Institutes of Health (2001) awarded a five-year grant to IBMTR/ABMTR in collaboration with the NMDP and EMMES Corporation for the development of a Blood and Marrow Transplant Clinical Trials Network (BMT CTN). The National Heart, Lung, and Blood Institute and NCI are providing funding for this network. This consortium is establishing a Data Coordinating Center for a national network of centers performing clinical trials focused on HSCT. Additional goals of the consortium include the development of consensus guidelines for diagnosing, monitoring, and grading important transplant-related endpoints and the development and use of novel study designs to increase the efficiency and scientific validity of clinical trials in blood and marrow transplantation. Additional information about the BMT CTN is available by calling 414-456-8325, sending an e-mail message to ibmtr@mcw.edu, or visiting the IBMTR Web site at www.ibmtr.org.

Changing existing systems for conducting clinical trials will partially help to expedite clinical trials. Low accrual rates clearly have a negative impact on clinical trials, often prolonging the duration of the trial, delaying the analysis of important results, or leading to early closure of important studies (Lara et al., 2001). Survey results indicated that patients as well as physicians have many misperceptions about the clinical trial process that must be overcome (Finn, 2000). An effort currently is under way to disseminate information about clinical trials to the public in an effort to increase participation in clinical trials. Figure 16-1 provides a list of Web sites that contain information on clinical trials.

Nurses are in an excellent position to educate patients about the existence and role of clinical trials. Nurses working with transplant recipients should be familiar with clinical trials, as many patients undergoing HSCT are involved in research studies. See Figure 16-2 for a listing of clinical trials in HSCT available through NCI-sponsored groups. Nurses responsible for providing care for patients undergoing transplant usually administer study medications and record patient responses. Many nurses also are employed as study coordinators and data managers for clinical trials. Nurses usually are the member of the healthcare team that spends the most time with patients and their families and frequently are the ones patients and families turn to for interpretation of a doctor's explanation and information and support about treatment decisions.

Nurses can provide counsel, education, and emotional support for families who are making difficult treatment decisions based on their knowledge and experience in working with patients undergoing clinical trials. Many resources are available for patients that explain and list available clinical trials. Some resources for a starting point are included in Figure 16-1.

Gene Transfer Therapy

Gene therapy is a technique used to correct or replace abnormal, nonfunctioning, or missing genes. Clinical trials in gene therapy have been disappointing (Beutler, 1999). Efficiency and accuracy of gene therapy remain the most significant barriers to date (Vile, Russell, & Lemoine, 2000). In spite of this, researchers are optimistic that gene therapy will become an effective treatment for a wide range of diseases. The spectrum ranges from the treatment of inherited or acquired genetic disorders to cancer, AIDS, cardiopathies, and neurologic diseases (Romano, Pacilio, & Giordano, 1999).

The goals of gene transfer are destruction of tumor cells, protection of marrow cells from the effects of chemotherapy, and marking of cells to determine the source of relapse (Bank, 2000; Wheeler, 1995). The requirements necessary for successful gene transfer to take place include an ability to insert

Figure 16-1. Clinical Trial Resource List

American Bone Marrow Donor Registry is a nonprofit organization that coordinates donor searches among participating donor centers in the United States and throughout the world.
American Bone Marrow Donor Registry
PO Box 8841
Mandeville, LA 70470-8841
800-745-2452
www.charityadvantage.com/abmdr/Home.asp

American Society for Blood and Marrow Transplantation is a national professional association that promotes advancement of the field of blood and bone marrow transplantation. ASBMT members are both in clinical practice and in research.
American Society for Blood and Marrow Transplantation
85 W. Algonquin Road, Suite 550
Arlington Heights, IL 60005
847-427-0224
www.asbmt.org

Astis Trial is a multicenter, prospective randomized phase III study to compare efficacy and safety of high-dose immunoablation and autologous hematopoietic stem cell transplantation with IV pulse therapy cyclophosphamide for the treatment of patients with severe systemic sclerosis.
www.astistrial.com

BMT*net* is a new portal to blood and marrow transplantation resources on the World Wide Web. The portal, or doorway, with links to multiple Web sites is a joint project of seven blood and marrow transplantation organizations, supported by an unrestricted educational grant from Pfizer, Inc.
At a single Web address, www.bmtnet.org, healthcare professionals, patients, and the general public can find blood and marrow transplantation information and easily move back and forth among the Web sites of the seven participating organizations:
• American Society for Blood and Marrow Transplantation (ASBMT)
• Canadian Blood and Marrow Transplant Group (CBMTG)
• European Group for Blood and Marrow Transplantation (EBMT)
• Foundation for Accreditation of Hematopoietic Cell Therapy (FAHCT)
• International Bone Marrow Transplant Registry (IBMTR) and Autologous Blood and Marrow Transplant Registry (ABMTR)
• International Society for Hematotherapy and Graft Engineering (ISHAGE)
• National Marrow Donor Program (NMDP)
www.bmtnet.org

Bone Marrow Donors Worldwide is the continuing effort to collect the HLA phenotypes of volunteer bone marrow donors and cord blood units and for the coordination of their worldwide distribution. Participants are 53 bone marrow donor registries from 39 countries, and 33 cord blood registries from 21 countries. The current number of donors and cord blood units is 8,698,428 (as of September 2003).
www.bmdw.org

Canadian Blood and Marrow Transplant Group (CBMTG) is a national, voluntary, multidisciplinary organization providing leadership and promoting excellence in patient care, research, and education in the field of blood and marrow transplantation.
CBMTG Head Office
777 West Broadway, Suite 401
Vancouver, BC, Canada V5Z 4J7
604-874-4944
www.cbmtg.org

Cancer.gov: A service of the National Cancer Institute (NCI). Has accurate information on cancer from NCI, including site-specific information, clinical trials, statistics, and research funding.
www.cancer.gov

Coalition of National Cancer Cooperative Groups offers Trial Check, an easy-to-search database of more than 300 cooperative group cancer clinical trials.
www.trialcheck.org

EORTC, the European Organization for Research and Treatment of Cancer has a Web site that features a list of clinical trials available in Europe.
www.eortc.be

European Group for Blood and Marrow Transplantation (EBMT) is a nonprofit organization based in Nijmegen, The Netherlands, that was established in 1974 to allow scientists and physicians involved in clinical bone marrow transplantation to share their experience and develop cooperative studies. EBMT aims to promote all aspects associated with the transplantation of hematopoietic stem cells from all donor sources and donor types, including basic and clinical research, education, standardization, quality control, and accreditation for transplant procedures.
EBMT Central Office
Dept. of Haematology
Macdonald Buchanan Building
Middlesex Hospital
London W1N 8AA, United Kingdom
44-207-380-9772
www.ebmt.org

International Bone Marrow Transplant Registry/Autologous Blood and Marrow Transplant Registry are voluntary organizations of basic and clinical scientists collaborating in an effort to address important issues in blood and marrow transplantation. (They do not make donor matches.) Staff are available to answer questions about transplantation.
IBMTR/ABMTR Statistical Center
Health Policy Institute
Medical College of Wisconsin
8701 Watertown Plank Road
PO Box 26509
Milwaukee, WI 53226
414-456-8325
www.ibmtr.org

Journal of Gene Medicine clinical trial site allows users to search for trials by clinical phase and also by status (e.g., open, closed, under review), in addition to searching by country, investigator, disease, vector, and gene.
www.wiley.co.uk/genetherapy/clinical

National Marrow Donor Program is funded by a federal contract with the American Red Cross, the American Association of Blood Banks, and the Council of Community Blood Centers. It was created to improve the efficiency and effectiveness of the donor search so that a larger number of unrelated bone marrow transplantations can be carried out. Their Web site contains an information page on clinical trials with links for sources of clinical trials.
National Marrow Donor Program
Suite 400 3433 Broadway St. NE
Minneapolis, MN 55413
Donor information: 800-654-1247
Patient search information: 800-526-7809
www.marrow.org/MEDICAL/clinical_trials.html

(Continued on next page)

the correct gene into the correct cell type, and the cell must adequately express the inserted gene (Hwu & Rosenberg, 1997). Currently, HSCs, most commonly autologous, are the favorite target for implementation of human trials of gene therapy because stem cells carrying a therapeutic gene could be a lifelong source of the gene (Kirby, 1999). Transfer of genes into the cell is performed using either viral vectors or nonviral vectors (Abernathy & Wilson, 2000; Bank; Beutler, 1999; Havenga, Hoogerbrugge, Valerio, & van Es, 1997; Wheeler).

HSCs are desirable targets for gene therapy for several reasons; for example, they are easily accessible, and they are able to replicate into all the cell lineages (Fraser & Hoffman, 1995; Kirby, 1999). HSCs have been used successfully as a source of long-term repopulation of cells, so these cells should provide a lifelong source of amplified progeny expressing the introduced gene (Cavazzana-Calvo, Bagnis, Mannoni, & Fischer, 1999; Civin, 2000; Schmitz et al., 1996). Progenitors of the HSC are involved in many human disorders (Havenga et al., 1997). Natural and laboratory viruses can gain entry to and integrate into the DNA of early hematopoietic progenitor cells (Civin).

Stem cell transduction, or the ability to transfer the gene of interest to the stem cell, has remained a challenging problem for researchers (Cuaron & Gallucci, 1997; Kirby, 1999). HSCs constitute not more than one cell in 10,000 and perhaps as few as one in 100,000 (Kirby). The number of harvested HSCs represents only a small percentage of the HSCs in the body, making it impossible to transduce a majority of the cells with the intended gene (Beutler, 1999). Stem cells resist transduction because they have trace receptors on the cell surface for the vectors to interact with (Kirby). HSCs spend most of their time in a resting stage, making transduc-

tion efficiency low because they are not dividing. Attempts to induce the HSC to enter a dividing state with 5-fluorouracil and/or colony-stimulating factor has led to the loss of some of the properties of the stem cell. HSCs were abnormally incapable of engrafting when forced to cycle (Kirby; Romano, Michelli, Pacilio, & Giordano, 2000). Humans have evolved mechanisms for inactivating externally introduced fragments of DNA, and these must be overcome for gene therapy to be successful (Beutler).

The purification of HSCs for gene therapy relies mainly on mobilizing the stem cells from the marrow into the peripheral circulation, using an agent such as colony-stimulating factor or chemotherapy; cells are then selected. Using a positive-enrichment method requires the existence of cell-surface markers that are potentially specific for stem cells. The search for new stem cell–specific markers is an extremely active area of research at present (Fry & Wood, 1999). Gene therapy with HSCT consists of the replication of incompetent retroviral vectors that are modified to carry the gene of interest into pluripotent stem cells of the body. A commonly used strategy involves harvesting the progenitor cells, incubating a portion of these cells with the transducing vector, and then reinfusing these cells back in the patient after a regimen of conditioning therapy designed to reduce the number of cancerous cells (Cuaron & Gallucci, 1997; Giles, Hanania, Fu, & Deisseroth, 1995).

Nonmalignant Diseases Treated With Hematopoietic Stem Cell Transplant

The use of HSCT has expanded to include many nonmalignant diseases, including genetic disorders, errors in metabolism, and autoimmune diseases. The first successful allogeneic HSCTs reported were for patients with primary immunodeficiencies (Sullivan, Parkman, & Walters, 2000). Transplant-related morbidity and mortality remain serious concerns when considering HSCT for the treatment of nonmalignant diseases. These include regimen-related toxicities, fertility issues, GVHD, nonengraftment, and infection (Steward, 2000; Sullivan et al., 1998). Advances in supportive care for patients with many genetic disorders, autoimmune diseases, and errors in metabolism can allow patients to experience good quality of life for many years after diagnosis (Steward). However, HSCT is the only curative therapy for patients with many primary immunodeficiencies and metabolic diseases (Sullivan et al., 1998). The risk versus benefit of HSCT for these patients is sometimes difficult to determine with current transplant techniques.

Primary Immunodeficiency Diseases

HSCT is an established therapy for patients with immunodeficiency diseases and is the treatment of choice for patients with severe combined immunodeficiency disease (SCID) (Sullivan et al., 2000). The majority of these patients are treated with T cell–depleted haploidentical stem cells (Sullivan et al., 2000). Overall survival is reported at 80%

Figure 16-2. Clinical Trials in HSCT Available Through NCI-Sponsored Cooperative Groups

Eastern Cooperative Oncology Group (www.ecog.org)

- Phase I Study of Amifostine and High-Dose Melphalan in Patients with Primary Systemic Amyloidosis Undergoing Autologous Peripheral Blood Stem Cell Transplantation. (Date last modified: 09/16/2003)

- Phase II Study of a Nonmyeloablative Conditioning Regimen Followed by Allogeneic Bone Marrow Transplantation in Patients with Relapsed Non-Hodgkin's or Hodgkin's Lymphoma. (Date first published: 03/24/2003)

- Phase II Study of a Reduced-Intensity Preparative Regimen with Allogeneic Bone Marrow Transplantation in Patients with Myelodysplastic Syndromes. (Date last modified: 06/03/2003)

- Phase II Study of Alemtuzumab (Monoclonal Antibody CD52; Campath-1H) and Peripheral Blood Stem Cell Transplantation in Patients with Chronic Lymphocytic Leukemia. (Date last modified: 01/05/2003)

- Phase III Randomized Study of Allogeneic Bone Marrow Transplantation (BMT) or Conventional Consolidation and Maintenance Chemotherapy Versus Autologous BMT in Patients with Acute Lymphoblastic Leukemia in First Remission. (Date last modified: 04/01/2003)

- Phase III Randomized Study of Autologous Stem Cell Transplantation with or without Rituximab in Patients with Relapsed or Progressive B-Cell Diffuse Large Cell Lymphoma. (Date last modified: 04/03/2003)

- Phase III Randomized Study of Daunorubicin and Cytarabine with or without Gemtuzumab Ozogamicin Followed by Autologous Hematopoietic Stem Cell Transplantation in Patients with Acute Myeloid Leukemia. (Date last modified: 03/21/2003)

Southwestern Oncology Group (www.swog.org)

- Phase II Study of Allogeneic Peripheral Blood Stem Cell Transplantation with Pre-Conditioning Low-Dose Total Body Irradiation and Fludarabine Followed by Mycophenolate Mofetil and Cyclosporine in Elderly Patients with Acute Myeloid Leukemia in First Complete Remission. (Date last modified: 04/01/2003)

- Phase II Study of Fludarabine and Cyclophosphamide Followed by Allogeneic Peripheral Blood Stem Cell Transplantation in Patients with Metastatic or Unresectable Renal Cell Cancer. (Date last modified: 02/25/2003)

- Phase II Study of High-Dose Melphalan and Autologous Peripheral Blood Stem Cell Transplantation in Patients with High-Risk Multiple Myeloma or Primary Systemic Amyloidosis. (Date last modified: 08/12/2003)

- Phase II Study of Thalidomide and Dexamethasone Induction Followed by Tandem Melphalan and Peripheral Blood Stem Cell Transplantation Followed by Prednisone and Thalidomide Maintenance in Patients with Multiple Myeloma. (Date last modified: 08/18/2003)

- Phase III Randomized Study of Interleukin-2 Versus Observation Only After Total Body Irradiation, High-Dose Etoposide, Cyclophosphamide, and Autologous Peripheral Blood Stem Cell Transplantation in Patients with Adult Non-Hodgkin's Lymphoma. (Date last modified: 09/15/2003)

- Phase III Study of Early High-Dose Chemoradiotherapy and Autologous Peripheral Blood Stem Cell Transplantation Versus Conventional Dose Cyclophosphamide, Doxorubicin, Vincristine, and Prednisone (CHOP) in Patients with Intermediate or High-Grade Non-Hodgkin's Lymphoma. (Date last modified: 09/15/2003)

Children's Oncology Group (www.nccf.org/nccf/cancer/protocol/prot_dir.htm)

- Phase I Pilot Study of Induction Chemotherapy Including Cyclophosphamide and Topotecan in Patients with Newly Diagnosed or Progressive High-Risk Neuroblastoma Undergoing Autologous Peripheral Blood Stem Cell Transplantation. (Date last modified: 09/24/2003)

- Phase I Study of Rituximab Followed by Yttrium Y 90 Ibritumomab Tiuxetan with or without Autologous Peripheral Blood Stem Cell Transplantation in Children with Recurrent or Refractory CD20-Posititve Lymphoma. (Date last modified: 11/02/2003)

- Phase II Pilot Study of Dexamethasone-Based Induction Chemotherapy Followed by Augmented Berlin-Frankfurt-Munster (BFM) Consolidation Chemotherapy with or without Allogeneic Bone Marrow Transplantation in Infants with Previously Untreated Acute Lymphoblastic Leukemia. (Date last modified: 12/09/2003)

- Phase II Pilot Study of Gemtuzumab Ozogamicin in Children with Newly Diagnosed Acute Myeloid Leukemia Undergoing Intensive Remission Induction and Intensification Therapy. (Date first published: 09/24/2003)

- Phase II Pilot Study of Intensification Comprising High-Dose Thiotepa and Cyclophosphamide with Autologous Peripheral Blood Stem Cell Transplantation (PBSCT) and Sargramostim (GM-CSF) Followed by High-Dose Carboplatin, Etoposide, and Melphalan with Second PBSCT, GM-CSF, and Isotretinoin After Induction Therapy in Children with Newly Diagnosed High-Risk Neuroblastoma. (Date last modified: 09/30/2003)

- Phase II Pilot Study of Intensified Chemotherapy with or without Allogeneic Hematopoietic Stem Cell Transplantation in Children with Very High-Risk Acute Lymphoblastic Leukemia. (Date last modified: 07/15/2003)

- Phase II Study of Neoadjuvant Chemotherapy with or without Second-Look Surgery Followed by Radiotherapy with or without Peripheral Blood Stem Cell Rescue in Patients with Intracranial Non-Germinomatous Germ Cell Tumors. (Date last modified: 10/01/2003)

- Phase II Study of R11577, Isotretinoin, Cytarabine, and Fludarabine Followed by Allogeneic Bone Marrow or Umbilical Cord Blood Transplantation in Children with Newly Diagnosed Juvenile Myelomonocytic Leukemia. (Date last modified: 03/01/2003)

- Phase II/III Randomized Study of Immunotherapy Comprising Cyclosporine, Interferon Gamma, and Interleukin-2 After High-Dose Myeloablative Chemotherapy with Autologous Stem Cell Transplantation in Patients with Refractory or Relapsed Hodgkin's Lymphoma. (Date first published: 09/24/2003)

- Phase III Randomized Study of Purged Versus Unpurged Peripheral Blood Stem Cell Transplantation After Dose-Intensive Induction Chemotherapy in Patients with Newly Diagnosed High Risk Neuroblastoma. (Date last modified: 09/22/2003)

(Continued on next page)

Cancer and Leukemia Group B (www.calgb.org)

- Phase II Study of a Nonmyeloablative Preparative Regimen Comprising Fludarabine and Busulfan Followed by Allogeneic Stem Cell Transplantation in Older Patients with Acute Myeloid Leukemia in First Complete Remission. (Date first published: 09/24/2003)

- Phase II Study of Autologous Peripheral Blood Stem Cell (PBSC) Transplantation Followed by Non-Myeloablative Allogeneic PBSC Transplantation in Patients with Multiple Myeloma. (Date last modified: 02/06/2003)

- Phase II Study of Fludarabine and Cyclophosphamide Followed by Allogeneic Peripheral Blood Stem Cell Transplantation in Patients with Chronic Lymphocytic Leukemia, Prolymphocytic Leukemia, Low-Grade Non-Hodgkin's Lymphoma or Mantle Cell Lymphoma. (Date last modified: 01/24/2003)

- Phase II Study of Non-Myeloablative Allogeneic Hematopoietic Stem Cell Transplantation in Patients with Relapsed Hematologic Malignancies After Prior High-Dose Chemotherapy and Autologous Stem Cell Transplantation. (Date first published: 12/21/2002)

- Phase II Study of Sequential Chemotherapy, Imatinib Mesylate, and Peripheral Blood Stem Cell Transplantation in Patients with Newly Diagnosed Philadelphia Chromosome-Positive Acute Lymphoblastic Leukemia. (Date last modified: 07/02/2003)

- Phase III Randomized Study of Induction Chemotherapy with or without PSC 833 Followed by Cytogenetic Risk Adapted Intensification Therapy Followed by Interleukin-2 Versus No Further Therapy in Patients with Previously Untreated Acute Myeloid Leukemia. (Date last modified: 05/01/2003)

for patients receiving histocompatible HSCT and 60%–70% in those receiving haploidentical transplants (Sullivan et al., 2000).

An area of controversy for HSCT in SCID remains whether there is a need for pretransplant chemotherapy (Sullivan et al., 2000). The absence of conditioning therapy has been associated with graft failure in patients with T-B-NK+ SCID and adenosine deaminase (ADA) deficiency (Amrolia et al., 2000; Porta & Friedrich, 1998). Many patients have poor B cell reconstitution requiring continued IV immune globulin (IVIGG) administration (Amrolia et al.; Buckley et al., 1999; Sullivan et al., 2000). In patients receiving T cell-depleted transplants, the time course of T cell reconstitution may be prolonged, which may necessitate a subsequent stem cell boost to improve stem cell recovery (Amrolia et al.). Use of conditioning prior to HLA-haploidentical HSCT appears to be a prerequisite for reliable engraftment and complete immune reconstitution. The beneficial effect of cytoreductive conditioning, however, is counterbalanced by increased short- and long-term toxicity. Toxicity includes infection and end organ decompensation, which leads to the high treatment-related mortality rates seen with conventionally conditioned HSCT in older children who have acquired organ dysfunction. Other late effects, such as growth retardation, infertility, and secondary malignancy, are difficult to justify in children with nonmalignant disorders (Amrolia et al.).

Buckley and colleagues (1999) prospectively studied immunologic function in 89 consecutive infants with SCID who received HSCT at Duke Medical Center between May 1982 and September 1998. Seventy-seven of the infants received T cell-depleted, HLA-haploidentical parental marrow, and 12 received HLA-identical marrow from a related donor; 3 of the recipients of haploidentical marrow also received placental blood transplants from unrelated donors. Except for two patients who received placental blood, none of the recipients received chemotherapy before transplantation or prophylaxis against GVHD. Of the 89 infants, 72 (81%) were alive 3 months to 16.5 years after transplantation, including all of the 12 who received HLA-identical marrow, 60 of the 77 (78%) who were given haploidentical marrow, and 2 of the 3 (67%) who received both haploidentical marrow and placental blood. T cell function became normal within two weeks after transplantation in the patients who received unfractionated HLA-identical marrow but usually not until three to four months after transplantation in those who received T cell-depleted marrow. At the time of the most recent evaluation, all but 4 of the 72 survivors had normal T cell function, and all the T cells in their blood were of donor origin. B cell function remained abnormal in many of the recipients of haploidentical marrow. In 26 children (5 recipients of HLA-identical marrow and 21 recipients of haploidentical marrow), between 2% and 100% of B cells were of donor origin. Forty-five of the 72 children were receiving IV immune globulin. The results of this study showed transplantation of marrow from a related donor is a life-saving and life-sustaining treatment for patients with any type of SCID, even when there is no HLA-identical donor (Buckley et al.).

Kane et al. (2001) evaluated the outcome following neonatal BMT for SCID. They performed a retrospective review of cases referred and transplanted between 1987 and 1999, focusing on infectious and GVHD complications as well as T and B lymphocyte function. Thirteen patients received 18 HSCTs: 4 whole marrow, 1 cord blood, 10 parental T cell–depleted haploidentical, and 3 T cell–depleted unrelated donor BMT. Nine were conditioned with busulfan and cyclophosphamide. All patients are alive and well (6 months to 11.5 years after HSCT). Six had grade I–II acute GVHD and two chronic GVHD (now resolved). Three had a top up BMT for poor T cell function, one had a third BMT for graft failure, and one had a third BMT for graft failure and chronic GVHD. At the time of the study, 12 had good in vitro proliferation to T cell mitogens, and all had normal serum IgA levels. Three were receiving IV immunoglobulin; for one of these, it was less than one year since BMT. Nine were above the second centile, and 10 of 12 who were old enough to be assessed had normal neurological development. The researchers found that early postnatal BMT should be the preferred option in neonatal SCID (Kane et al.).

Amrolia et al. (2000) reported the use of nonmyeloablative stem cell transplant for congenital immunodeficiencies. Eight patients with severe immunodeficiency states underwent T cell-replete BMT from an HLA antigen–matched unrelated (n = 6) or sibling (n = 2) donor with nonmyeloablative conditioning using a fludarabine-melphalan-anti-lymphocyte globulin-based regimen. All patients had severe organ dysfunction that precluded transplantation with conventional conditioning. All patients were engrafted with predominantly donor hematopoiesis, and the duration of neutropenia was brief. Significant acute GVHD did not develop, but one patient had limited chronic GVHD. One patient died of disease recurrence, and three had stable, mixed chimerism. At a median follow-up of one year, all patients had had good recovery of CD34+ T cell numbers, and six of seven evaluable patients had normal phyto-hemagglutinin stimulation indices. The rate of immune reconstitution is comparable with that of historical controls undergoing standard myeloablative protocols. The researchers concluded that nonmyeloablative HSCT permits rapid engraftment from both sibling and unrelated donors with minimal toxicity even in patients with severe organ dysfunction. If long-term immune reconstitution of patients treated with this protocol is demonstrated, it is believed this approach might offer significant advantages compared with standard protocols by combining adequate immune reconstitution with reduced short- and long-term toxicity (Amrolia et al.).

Wiscott-Aldrich syndrome (WAS) is a disease also treated with HSCT, and patients require pretransplant immunosuppression and ablation of host HSCs (Sullivan et al., 2000). Initially, the combination of cyclophosphamide and total body irradiation were utilized; however, total-body irradiation has been replaced by busulfan and cyclophosphamide to permit adequate immunosuppression and ablation of the abnormal recipient HSC without the long-term toxicity of irradiation (Sullivan et al., 2000). At this time, 145 transplants for WAS have been reported to the IBMTR (Sullivan et al., 2000). Overall survival for patients transplanted from a histocompatible donor was 86%; mismatched related donor was 51%. Survival of unrelated donor recipients younger than five years of age was 83%, and for recipients of unrelated donor stem cells who were older than five years, survival was 26% (Sullivan et al., 2000). Histocompatible or unrelated donor transplant in patients under five years is the treatment of choice for patients with WAS (Sullivan et al., 2000).

ß-Thalassemia Major

ß-thalassemia major is the nonmalignant disease for which transplants most commonly are performed. More than 1,500 patients have received matched sibling stem cell transplants worldwide (Hoppe & Walters, 2001; Steward, 2000). The largest number of transplants at a single center for thalassemia has been reported in Pesaro, Italy, where more than 800 transplants were performed (Rund & Rachmilewitz, 2000; Steward). Lucarelli et al. (1998) performed analyses of results of transplantation in patients under age 17 who

had thalassemia and developed three classes of risk using criteria of degree of hepatomegaly, degree of portal fibrosis, and quality of chelation treatment given before transplant. Patients for whom all three criteria were adverse constituted Class 3, patients with none of the adverse criteria constituted Class 1, and patients with one or various associations of two of the adverse criteria formed Class 2. Most patients older than age 16 have disease characteristics that place them in Class 3, with very few in Class 2. All of the patients with an HLA-identical donor are assigned to two protocols based on the class the patient belongs to at the time of transplant and independent of age. One hundred-four patients in Class 1 and 262 in Class 2 received conditioning with busulfan 14 mg/kg, cyclophosphamide 200 mg/kg, and CSA; the probabilities of survival and of event-free survival are 95% and 90% for Class 1 and 87% and 84% for Class 2. For 33 Class 3 patients who received conditioning for transplant with busulfan 14 mg/kg, cyclophosphamide 160 mg/kg, CSA, and "short" MTX, the probabilities of survival and event-free survival are 89% and 64%. Fifty-seven adult patients (17–35 years) underwent transplant after preparation with the same protocol used for Class 3; the probabilities of survival and event-free survival are 70% and 60%, respectively (Lucarelli et al.). Use of HLA-identical cord blood transplant has been reported in 12 thalassemia patients aged one to eight years. Eight patients were Class 1–2 and four were Class 2 based on the Pesaro risk scoring system. Preparative regimen consisted of busulfan (14–16 mg/kg) and cyclophosphamide (100–200 mg/kg). Median nucleated cell number infused was 3.3×10^7/kg. All patients are alive with an event-free survival of 49%. Incidence of GVHD was low (one case had grade II GVHD), and five of the patients have had autologous reconstitution. The researchers recommend use of cord blood for younger children to increase the dosing of stem cells infused (Gluckman et al., 1997; Miniero et al., 1998; Rund & Rachmilewicz). Based on studies conducted, the best time to transplant is in very young patients with HLA-identical siblings; however, current supportive therapy can provide good quality of life for these patients (Sullivan et al., 2000). Patients who are at high risk of dying from complications of iron overload would seem to be ideal candidates for transplant, but these patients do not have good transplant outcomes (Sullivan et al., 2000). Poor-risk patients have organ damage caused by inadequate iron chelation, hepatic fibrosis, and hepatomegaly (Olivieri, 1999; Rund & Rachmilewitz; Sullivan et al., 2000). Currently, studies are ongoing to evaluate transplant in high-risk and older patients with thalassemia (Steward). Nonmyeloablative transplantation may be an option considered for older patients who have been heavily transfused (Sullivan et al., 2000).

Sickle Cell Disease

Clinical trials using HSCT to treat sickle cell disease began in 1984, and approximately 175 children have been transplanted from matched siblings (Hoppe & Walters, 2001). All patients treated for the indication of sickle cell anemia received pretransplant preparation with myeloablative doses of busulfan and cyclophosphamide. Most patients received an anti-T lymphocyte antibody before HSCT, and a smaller number received total lymphoid irradiation for pretransplant immunosuppression. Most common GVHD prophylaxis consisted of a combination of MTX and CSA (Hoppe & Walters). Results of these trials have shown that sickle cell disease can be cured and organ damage stabilized (Vermylen, Cornu, Ferster, Ninane, & Sariban, 1993). Patients selected for transplant had preexisting complications of sickle cell disease, such as stroke, recurrent episodes of acute chest syndrome, or vaso-occlusive crises (Hoppe & Walters).

Walters et al. (2000) reviewed the impact of transplantation for symptomatic sickle cell disease. Fifty children who had symptomatic sickle cell disease received matched sibling marrow allografts between September 1991 and March 1999, with Kaplan-Meier probabilities of survival and event-free survival of 94% and 84%, respectively. Twenty-six patients (16 male, 10 female) had at least two years of follow-up and were evaluated for the impact of transplant on sickle cell-related central nervous system and pulmonary disease. Patients ranged from 3.3 to 14.0 years of age (median = 9.4 years) and had a median follow-up of 57.9 months after transplantation (range = 38–95 months). Among 22 of 26 patients who had stable donor engraftment, complications related to sickle cell disease resolved, and none experienced further episodes of pain, stroke, or acute chest syndrome. All 10 engrafted patients with a prior history of stroke had stable or improved cerebral magnetic resonance imaging results. Pulmonary function tests were stable in 22 of 26 patients, worse in 2, and not studied in 2. Seven of eight patients transplanted for recurrent acute chest syndrome had stable pulmonary function (Walters et al.). Age at transplant appears to be a factor in survival, indicating that patients younger than 16 years of age tolerate transplant better (Hoppe & Walters, 2001).

In spite of the success seen with the use of stem cell transplant in SCID, the national collaborative group study found that 315 (6.5%) of 4,848 sickle cell patients younger than age 16 met eligibility for the study. Two-hundred thirty-nine of these patients had siblings, of whom 46% were not HLA typed because of parental refusal, physician concerns, lack of financial support, or other reasons. Eight percent of eligible patients were transplanted (Vichinsky, Brugnara, Styles, & Wagner, 1998).

As with all allogeneic transplants, only one-third of patients eligible for transplant will have an HLA-matched sibling, so alternate sources of stem cells are being evaluated (Vichinsky et al., 1998). Several studies have demonstrated that UCB is an acceptable source of stem cells for transplant (Gluckman et al., 1997; Wagner, Kernan, Steinbuch, Broxmeyer, & Gluckman, 1995). There have been no reported controlled trials examining matched unrelated or mismatched related transplants for SCID (Hoppe & Walters, 2001).

Nonmyeloablative regimens have been used for adult SCID patients. In one reported study using total body irradiation alone or with fludarabine followed by MMF and CSA post-transplant, 68% of patients were alive, with 42% in complete remission (Sandmaier, McSweeney, Yu, & Storb, 2000). Researchers are in the process of developing optimum conditioning regimens including nonmyeloablative regimens that are sufficient for donor engraftment and decrease transplant-related toxicity (Hoppe & Walters, 2001).

Autoimmune Diseases

HSCT has been proposed for the treatment of autoimmune diseases including rheumatoid arthritis (RA), systemic lupus erythematosus (SLE), multiple sclerosis (MS), and systemic sclerosis (SSc). The rationales for the use of HSCT in autoimmune diseases are twofold. First, trials in animal models have demonstrated cures of autoimmune diseases with HSCT (Brodsky & Smith, 1999; Snowden, Brooks, & Biggs, 1997; van Bekkum, 1999). Second, researchers have found that some patients treated with allogeneic HSCT that have an autoimmune disease experienced prolonged remissions of their autoimmune disease (Snowden et al.). Snowden et al. reported on three patients with RA transplanted for aplastic anemia. Two of the three patients remained in complete remission 11 and 13 years following BMT. The third patient relapsed two years post-BMT; however, the disease ran an attenuated course, and the patient was in treatment-free remission for more than 11 years (Brodsky & Smith; Snowden, 1998). Patients undergoing autologous transplant have experienced transient remissions in their autoimmune disease (Snowden et al.; Sullivan et al., 1998) especially when receiving unmanipulated stem cells (Sullivan et al., 2000). Jantunen, Myllykangas-Luosujarvi, Kaipiainen-Seppanen, and Nousiainen (2000) reported on a patient with advanced ankylosing spondylitis (AS) receiving treatment with three antirheumatic drugs who was diagnosed with large B cell lymphoma with poor prognostic features. The patient received eight cycles of CHOP (cyclophosphamide [750 mg/m^2] day 1, doxorubicin [50 mg/m^2] day 1, vincristine [2 mg] day 1, and prednisolone [100 mg] on days 1–5); all antirheumatic drugs were stopped, and the patient attained a complete remission. PBSC mobilization was performed with high-dose cyclophosphamide (4 g/m^2) and filgrastim (5 mg/kg/day). The patient was consolidated with BEAM (carmustine [300 mg/m^2] day –7, etoposide [200 mg/m^2] days –6 to –3, cytosine arabinoside [200 mg/m^2] days –6 to –3, and melphalan [140 mg/m^2] day –3) followed by infusion of unselected graft (2.6 x 10^6/kg CD34+ cells). Post-transplant course was uneventful. The patient has been in remission for lymphoma and without signs of peripheral arthritis or other signs of active AS. At most recent follow-up, the patient was well without any medication 27 months after transplant (Jantunen et al.).

Meloni, Capria, Vignetti, Mandelli, and Modena (1997) described a 23-year-old female with long-lasting SLE and subsequent CML. At the time of diagnosis, the patient fulfilled six criteria of the revised classification for the diagnosis of SLE. Treatment consisted of 1 mg/kg prednisone for two months, followed by gradual taper without the possibility of complete discontinuation because of persistent positivity of serum autoantibodies. Approximately nine years later, this patient was diagnosed with Ph+ CML and was treated with subcutaneous interferon at 9 x 10^6 IU/d. Marrow harvested after 24 months of treatment with interferon showed a major cytogenetic response. The patient went on to develop blast crisis and was treated with vincristine, idarubicin, prednisone, and intrathecal MTX, achieving a second chronic phase. The patient then received an autologous BMT because she lacked an HLA-identical sibling. The patient was conditioned with BAVC (800 mg/m^2 BCNU on day +1; 300 mg/m^2 ARA-c; 150 mg/m^2 AMSA; + 150 mg/m^2 VP16 on days +2, +3, and +4) followed by unmanipulated autologous BMT. Transplant toxicity was mild, and on day +21, the patient was discharged in good clinical general condition. After 30 months of follow-up, the patient remained in complete hematologic remission of CML (Ph+ 80%) without clinical and serological evidence of autoimmune disease (Meloni et al.).

Consensus conferences have been held in the United States and Europe to define the role of HSCT in autoimmune diseases as well as strategies for conducting trials. The decision of the consensus conferences were to initially treat patients with autoimmune diseases using autologous transplant because of lower morbidity and mortality associated with this type of transplant (Sullivan et al., 1998; van Bekkum, 1999). Using allografting of stem cells from a matched sibling donor may have theoretical appeal; however, if environmental triggers are no longer operative or if resetting immunoregulatory control after lymphoablative conditioning is successful, then safety concerns favor initial trials of autologous transplantation (Sullivan et al., 2000).

The European League Against Rheumatism (EULAR) and the European Group for Bone Marrow Transplantation (EBMT) have set forth transplant recommendations for autoimmune diseases. HSCT should not be considered a standard treatment for patients with autoimmune disease. Transplantation initially should be used as a treatment for patients with severe life-threatening or organ-threatening autoimmunity for which conventional treatment has failed (Sullivan et al., 1998). Identification of patients who will have a bad outcome is becoming possible in RA, which will allow some of these patients to be transplanted earlier in the course of their disease (Brooks, 1997). The optimum patients for this approach as well as the ideal preparative regimens will evolve over the next several years (Brodsky & Smith, 1999).

Approximately 480 patients have been treated for autoimmune diseases using autologous HSCT (Tyndall, 2002). Most of the patients treated had either a progressive form of MS (n = 102) or SSc (n = 60). Other diseases transplanted include RA (n = 63), juvenile idiopathic arthritis (n = 43), SLE (n = 33), and idiopathic thrombocytopenia purpura (n = 9) (Tyndall). Overall actuarially adjusted transplant-related mortality was 7%. A large difference in mortality has been observed between diseases, with a 12.5% transplant-related mortality in SSc and only one death in 63 RA patients (Tyndall).

Burt et al. (1998) reported on 10 patients with autoimmune diseases (MS, SLE, and RA) treated with autologous transplant. Autologous HSCs were collected from BM or mobilized from peripheral blood with either G-CSF or cyclophosphamide and G-CSF. Stem cells were enriched ex vivo using CD34+ selection and reinfused after either myelosuppressive conditioning with cyclophosphamide (200 mg/kg), methylprednisone (4 g), and ATG (90 mg/kg) or myeloablative conditioning with total body irradiation (1,200 cGy), methylprednisone (4 g) and cyclophosphamide (120 mg/kg). Six patients with MS, two with SLE, and two with RA have undergone HSCT. Mean time to engraftment of an absolute neutrophil count greater than 500/ml (0.5 x 10^9/l) and a nontransfused platelet count greater than 20,000/ml (20 x 10^9/l) occurred on day 10 and 14, respectively. Regimen-related nonhematopoietic toxicity was minimal. All patients improved and/or had stabilization of disease with a follow-up of 5 to 17 months (median = 11 months). The researchers concluded that intense immunosuppressive conditioning and autologous T cell–depleted hematopoietic transplantation was safely used to treat these 10 patients; however, the durability of response remains unknown (Burt et al.).

Fassas et al. (1997) conducted a phase I/II pilot study, treating 15 progressive MS patients with BEAM followed by autologous blood HSCT and ATG. Cyclophosphamide (4 g/m^2) and G/GM-CSF (5 mcg/kg/d) were used for stem cell mobilization, which caused no neurotoxicity. On day +1 and +2, ATG (2.5–5 mg/kg) was given for in vivo T cell depletion. Allergy (93%) and infections (87%) were the principal toxic complications. Mild, transient neurotoxicity was observed in six patients in the immediate post-transplant period. The median follow-up time was six months (range = 6–18). Durable neurologic improvements were detected. One patient worsened at three months, and two have relapsed. The researchers concluded that autologous HSCT appears to be feasible in MS; however, these observations need confirmation, and long-term outcomes will show if benefits counterbalance toxicity and cost (Fassas et al.).

Based on results of early phase I/II trials, several randomized, prospective controlled trials have been sponsored by EBMT and EULAR.

The ASTIS (Autologous Stem-Cell Transplantation International Scleroderma) Trial: Diffuse skin SSc patients are selected who have less than four years of diffuse skin involvement and evidence of progressive organ- or life-threatening disease. The primary endpoint for the trial is event-free survival at two years, with events being arbitrarily but precisely defined to capture irreversible and severe organ failure or death (see Figure 16-3) (Tyndall, 2002).

Figure 16-3. Study Flow Chart

A multicenter, prospective randomized phase III study to compare efficacy and safety of high-dose immunoablation and autologous hematopoietic stem cell transplantation with intravenous pulse therapy cyclophosphamide for the treatment of patients with severe systemic sclerosis

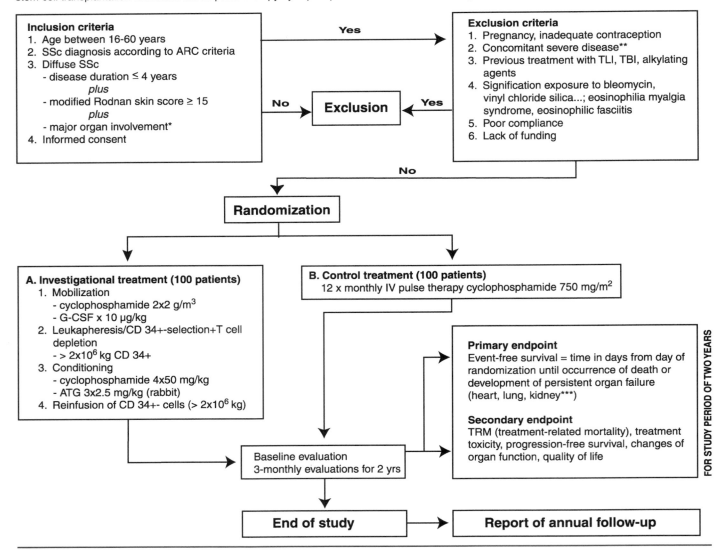

* Respiratory: DLCO and/or (F)VC < 70% plus interstitial lung disease
Renal: Hypertension (> 160/110 mm Hg), persistent urinalysis abnormalities, microangiopathic hemolytic anemia or new renal insufficiency
Cardiac: Congestive heart failure (reversible), rhythm disturbances or pericardial effusion

** Respiratory: PAP > 50 mm Hg, DLCO < 40%, respiratory failure
Renal: Creatinin clearance < 40 ml/min.
Cardiac: Refractory congestive heart failure, LVEF < 45%, uncontrolled atrial or ventricular arrythmia; pericardial effusion with hemodynamic consequences
Liver failure, uncontrolled infections, neoplasms, myelodysplasia, bone marrow insufficiency, uncontrolled hypertension, psychiatric disorders

*** Heart: LVEF < 30%
Lungs: Respiratory failure (PaO$_2$ < 8 kPa/60 mm Hg +/or PCO$_2$ > 6.7 kPa/50 mm Hg)
Kidney: Need for renal replacement therapy

ASTIMS (Autologous Stem-Cell Transplantation International Multiple Sclerosis) Trial: Secondary progressive MS patients with an Expanded Disability Status Scale score between 3.5 and 6.0 will be randomized to either HSCT (BEAM and ATG) followed by an unmanipulated graft or mitoxantrone. The primary endpoint is progression-free survival at three years. Each arm will recruit 80 patients (Tyndall, 2002).

ASTIRA (Autologous Stem-cell Transplantation International Rheumatoid Arthritis) Trial: Active RA patients with disease duration between 2 and 15 years who have failed to respond to at least four disease modifying antirheumatic drugs (including MTX and anti-TNF-alpha programs) will all receive stem cell mobilization with cyclophosphamide (4 g/m^2) and G-CSF. Randomization then will occur to either continued conventional therapy using either MTX or leflunamide or conditioning with cyclophosphamide (200 mg/kg) and ATG. The graft will not be manipulated, and maintenance with MTX or leflunamide will be given. The primary endpoint is the number of patients reaching a good or moderate EULAR response and/or ACR 20 (the standard assessment of disease activity) at six months. Each arm requires 16 patients, calculated on a > 50% difference in the two groups (Tyndall, 2002).

Phase I/II trials are continuing in an effort to determine which autoimmune diseases respond to transplant as well as the ideal timing of transplantation with autoimmune diseases. To eliminate the problem of reinfusing autoreactive lymphocytes with the autograft, many investigators are studying the effects of T cell depletion on autologous transplant for autoimmune diseases (Brodsky & Smith, 1999; Fassas et al., 1997). If donor chimerism is successful in allowing durable engraftment of stem cells without excess toxicity in hematologic malignancies, then the application of nonmyeloablative allogeneic transplant for autoimmune diseases can proceed to clinical trials (Sullivan et al., 2000). Systematic long-term follow up of current patients is essential to trace the durability of remission and any associated late complications of the transplant procedure (Sullivan et al., 2000). Single institutions cannot accrue enough patients to provide meaningful data. International multicenter trials should be undertaken to avoid duplication of effort and to ensure that a minimum amount of time is devoted to determining the role of this potentially life-saving procedure (Tyndall & Gratwohl, 2000).

AIDS

HSCT has been reported for the treatment of 32 patients with the diagnosis of AIDS (Huzicka, 1999). Two of the 32 patients reported demonstrated negative polymerase chain reaction (PCR) for HIV after transplant, but one died of relapsed disease and the other died of transplant complications within four months of transplant (Contu et al., 1993; Huzicka; Saral & Holland, 1994). Saral et al. reported on seven patients who were HIV positive. All were treated with marrow from an HLA-matched sibling. Pretransplant conditioning consisted of cyclophosphamide and total body irradiation for six and busulfan and cyclosphophamide for one. Patients also were given zidovudine. One patient was PCR negative from 40–120 days post-transplant and died of GVHD. The other patients in the study had a 1- to 2-log decrease in virus titer (Huzicka; Saral & Holland). Contu et al. reported on one patient with AIDS treated with allogeneic transplant. The patient received conditioning with busulfan, cyclophosphamide, antilymphocyte globulin, zidovudine, and sargramostim. The patient died on day 301 from adult respiratory distress syndrome but was PCR negative from day 30 for HIV and had anti-HIV antibodies negative from four

months (Contu et al.; Huzicka). Some researchers feel there is still an indication for continued clinical trials of HSCT for the treatment of AIDS. Issues related to AIDS and HSCT that need further investigation through clinical trials include the optimum conditioning regimen and graft versus virus effect on AIDS (Huzicka).

Nursing Research

HSCT is a rapidly growing field. Nurses caring for transplant recipients work in many varied settings, including but not limited to inpatient and outpatient transplant units, physician offices, and home care. Nurses working with HSCT recipients are expected to have the knowledge to provide care for patients experiencing a wide range of transplant-related side effects, symptoms, and problems. These may be physical or psychosocial in nature and involve the patient directly or a family member. As with most specialties in nursing, HSCT nurses strive to base nursing interventions on research-based solutions. However, the conceptual foundation that currently guides HSCT nursing practice is stronger than the existing empirical or research base for practice (Haberman, 1997).

In a review from 1997, Molassiotis reported that HSCT nursing research and empirical knowledge are limited and that only about 14% of the publications in the nursing literature were research-based. The majority of nursing interventions used in HSCT are based on research from other disciplines such as medicine, nutrition, psychology, and dentistry (Winters, Miller, Maracich, Compton, & Haberman, 1994).

The body of nursing research in HSCT currently is increasing, and the majority of studies published relate to psychosocial issues (see Table 16-1). A search of the Cumulative Index of Nursing and Allied Health Literature database (CINAHL) lists quality-of-life studies in transplant patients as well as studies examining isolation and isolation techniques (i.e., gowning), mucositis and oral care, coping abilities, hope, stress, adaptation after transplant, sexual functioning, pain, and massage. Despite large numbers of studies, there is a lack of valid and reliable research suitable for clinical implementation (Hunt, 2001). There clearly remains a need for continued nursing research in the field of HSCT.

Several studies have been done examining utilization of nursing research and barriers to utilization of research in cancer practice (Rutledge, Greene, Mooney, Nail, & Ropka, 1996; Rutledge, Ropka, Greene, Nail, & Mooney, 1998). The studies reported that dissemination of the findings through reading literature, attending educational offerings, and observing the practice of others were important. Barriers to utilization included a lack of time to read research and implement new ideas as well as a lack of authority to change patient care. Other reasons cited were the research is not generalizable to every practice setting, lack of support from physicians and other staff, as well as difficulty understanding research language and statistics.

When valid research findings are identified, implementing them into practice should be a priority. Policies, procedures, and standards should be revised to incorporate

Authors	Title	Study Design	Sample	Comments
Brandt, DePalma, Irwin, Shogan, & Lucke, 1996	Comparison of Central Venous Catheter Dressings in Bone Marrow Transplant Recipients	Quantitative: Experimental randomized two-group clinical trial	101 adult patients undergoing autologous hematopoietic stem cell transplant (HSCT)	For adults undergoing autologous bone marrow transplant (BMT), either dry sterile gauze dressing or transparent moisture vapor–permeable dressing can be used safely based on patient preference and skin tolerance to the dressing material.
Campos de Carvalho, Goncalves, Bontempo, & Soler, 2000	Interpersonal Needs Expressed by Patients During Bone Marrow Transplantation	Qualitative: Semi-structured interviews during three phases of BMT	23 patients undergoing BMT	Nursing staff should seek strategies to stimulate expression of feelings and actions regarding needs, to preserve desired control whenever possible and to be sensitive to affection and inclusion manifestations.
Duquette-Petersen, Francis, Dohnalek, Skinner, & Dudas, 1999	The Role of Protective Clothing in Infection Prevention in Patients Undergoing Autologous Bone Marrow Transplantation	Quantitative: Randomized two-group controlled clinical trial	40 patients undergoing autologous BMT for hematologic and solid tumor malignancy	Use of cover gowns and shoe covers did not have an impact on time to first antibiotic or length of antibiotic treatment. Elimination of cover gowns and shoe covers will save nursing time and hospital resources as well as eliminate one isolation barrier experienced by patients.
Ezzone, Baker, Rosselet, & Terepka, 1998	Music as an Adjunct to Antiemetic Therapy	Qualitative: Randomized two-group clinical trial	39 patients undergoing BMT	Using music as a diversional adjunct intervention to antiemetic therapy is helpful in decreasing nausea and vomiting.
Ezzone, Jolly, Replogle, Kapoor, & Tutschka, 1993	Survey of Oral Hygiene Regimens Among Bone Marrow Transplant Centers	Quantitative: Descriptive survey	92 BMT centers	Few similarities existed in the assessment and management of oral care.
Gaskill, Henderson, & Fraser, 1997	Exploring the Everyday World of the Patient in Isolation	Qualitative: Interpretive, phenomenologic	7 BMT recipients	Elements of caring for the patient appeared to dominate the comments associated with staff contact. Other forms of care emphasized the importance of nurses understanding and connecting with people's meanings and experiences of their illness and treatment.
McGuire et al., 1998	Acute Oral Pain and Mucositis in Bone Marrow Transplant and Leukemia Patients: Data From a Pilot Study	Quantitative, qualitative Prospective, repeated measures Descriptive	18 patients undergoing BMT or induction for leukemia	Nurses should continue to assess oral pain and mucositis vigorously and assist patients in selecting multiple management strategies.
Molassiotis, Boughton, Burgoyne, & van den Akker, 1995	Comparison of the Overall Quality of Life in 50 Long-Term Survivors of Autologous and Allogeneic Bone Marrow Transplantation	Quantitative: use of three standardized questionnaires	50 BMT survivors: 24 autologous and 26 allogeneic	Patients post-autologous transplant had mainly psychological difficulties in their post–transplant adaptation, whereas patients post–allogeneic transplant developed more physical problems.
Molassiotis & Morris, 1999	Quality of Life in Patients With Chronic Myeloid Leukemia After Unrelated Donor Bone Marrow Transplantation	Qualitative: descriptive study	28 BMT survivors	Unrelated-donor BMT long-term survivors have an acceptable degree of quality of life, but rehabilitative services still need to be used for those who exhibit difficulties with their daily life.

(Continued on next page)

Table 16-1. Nursing Research Studies in Hematopoietic Stem Cell Transplant (Continued)

Authors	Title	Study Design	Sample	Comments
Molassiotis, van den Akker, Milligan, & Boughton, 1995	Gonadal Function and Psychosexual Adjustment in Male Long-Term Survivors of Bone Marrow Transplantation	Quantitative: Descriptive Comparative	29 male survivors of BMT	BMT survivors and patients with cancer had significantly higher psychosexual dysfunction compared with healthy subjects. Type of chemotherapy, total body irradiation, type of transplant, and post-BMT time did not correlate with either gonadal or psychosexual functioning.
Pederson & Parran, 1999	Pain and Distress in Adults and Children Undergoing Peripheral Blood Stem Cell or Bone Marrow Transplant	Quantitative: Descriptive, longitudinal design	40 patients undergoing HSCT 20 adults and 20 children	Administering opioid therapy by continuous infusion with titration or bolus doses as needed was effective in managing pain in transplant recipients.
Pederson & Parran, 2000	Opioid Tapering in Hematopoietic Progenitor Cell Transplant Recipients	Quantitative and qualitative: Descriptive, exploratory, prospective	45 HSCT recipients	Use of an opioid-taper guideline may promote consistency of tapering while not increasing levels of pain or withdrawal symptoms.
Stetz, McDonald, & Compton, 1996	Needs and Experiences of Family Caregivers During Marrow Transplantation	Qualitative: Descriptive, cross-sectional	19 adult family members of people who underwent BMT	Healthcare professionals need to acknowledge the caregiving role and actively involve and support the family caregiver throughout the transplant experience.
Whedon, Stearns, & Mills, 1995	Quality of Life of Long-Term Adult Survivors of Autologous Bone Marrow Transplantation	Qualitative, quantitative: Cross-sectional, descriptive, replication study	29 survivors of autologous BMT	Most survivors of autologous BMT can expect above-average quality of life.

new findings into practice. Communication of changes in practice should be made to all healthcare workers involved in the patients' care, including physicians. Changes in practice can be piloted on selected units to work out the identified institutional problems, and then thorough educational in-servicing is recommended to implement the practice change throughout the hospital.

Nursing management should encourage staff to join specialty organizations and attend conferences to maintain up-to-date knowledge of transplantation and to network with other healthcare workers involved in the care of HSCT recipients. Managers should support introduction of new nursing interventions based on valid research findings and should encourage staff endeavors to implement new research findings when possible. Clinical staff should be encouraged to review current journals for new, relevant research findings. Staff also should be encouraged to question current nursing practice and look for gaps where there is a lack of research-based practice (Haberman, 1997). Nurses at the bedside are in the best position to identify problems for research. Nurses working at the bedside and nurses conducting research must work together so that areas of interest can be identified for research and studied. Managers and advanced practice nurses are in a position to act as a bridge between nurses at the bedside and nurse researchers. Currently, staff interested in conducting research can consult with a nurse researcher via the Oncology Nursing Society (ONS) Research Consultation Program. Information is available online at www.ons.org/xp6/ONS/Research.xml/

Consultation.xml. The only requirement for use of the program is membership in ONS. ONS also has a survey program to assist nurses with development of surveys; information is available at www.ons.org/xp6/ONS/Research.xml/Survey.xml.

Strategies to develop nursing infrastructures to complete valid and viable nursing research mirror those of the medical transplant community. Currently, most of the nursing studies performed involve single institutions with small patient samples. To develop meaningful research-based practice, nurses need to form cooperative groups consisting of researchers and clinicians representing the different areas of HSCT. These groups could develop research priorities that would be translated into studies conducted in multi-institutional trials. Performing multi-institutional trials increases the number of patient accruals and allows studies to be generalizable for more patients (Haberman, 1997). Recruitment of physicians and other healthcare team members in developing and conducting interdisciplinary research is another way for nurses to become involved in the research process. Because no single discipline is wholly responsible for the care of patients undergoing HSCT, it makes sense to perform research as a team. Including members from a number of disciplines will allow studies to address the different interests identified by each of these disciplines in conducting the study. A small number of interdisciplinary research studies have been published (see Table 16-2), and it is hoped that this trend will continue in the future.

Table 16-2. Interdisciplinary Research in Hematopoietic Stem Cell Transplant

Authors	Title	Study Design	Sample	Comments
Ahles et al., 1999	Massage Therapy for Patients Undergoing Autologous Bone Marrow Transplantation	Quantitative: Randomized	35 patients undergoing autologous bone marrow transplant (BMT)	Initial results suggest that massage is a useful technique for enhancing the quality of life of patients undergoing BMT. However, further research is necessary.
Baker, Zabora, Polland, & Wingard, 1999	Reintegration After Bone Marrow Transplantation	Qualitative: Descriptive	84 patients post-BMT	Three areas of psychosocial morbidity were identified: physical problems, psychological problems, and community reintegration problems.
Bush, Donaldson, Haberman, Dacanay, & Sullivan, 2000	Conditional and Unconditional Estimation of Multidimensional Quality of Life After Hematopoietic Stem Cell Transplantation: A Longitudinal Follow-Up of 415 Patients	Quantitative	415 adult patients post-BMT	Although some problems can be anticipated, typical patients can look forward to a quality of life after transplantation that is broadly comparable to that of the normal population.
Bush, Haberman, Donaldson, & Sullivan, 1995	Quality of Life of 125 Adults Surviving 6–18 Years After Bone Marrow Transplantation	Quantitative: Descriptive	125 adult survivors of BMT	Almost all long-term survivors were leading full and meaningful lives. Persistent complications were, on the whole, dismissed as relatively trivial, and the overwhelming majority viewed themselves as cured and well.
Sonis et al., 2001	Oral Mucositis and the Clinical and Economic Outcomes of Hematopoietic Stem-Cell Transplantation	Quantitative	92 transplant patients	Oral mucositis is associated with significantly worse clinical and economic outcomes in blood and marrow transplantation.

Conclusion

Research in HSCT is progressing at a rapid pace with hundreds of transplant centers worldwide. As the toxicities of transplant decrease with the use of nonmyeloablative transplants and researchers gain a better understanding of the graft versus malignancy phenomena, the potential applications for HSCT are increasing. Researchers currently are developing systems that will enable rapid translation of biological science to clinical trials to make transplants a more available and safer procedure. Clinical trials also are ongoing to evaluate psychosocial and physical aspects of HSCT, ensuring that patients will have optimal experiences before, during, and after transplant.

References

Abernathy, E., & Wilson, H. (2000). Gene therapy: An overview and implications for peripheral stem cell transplantation. In P.C. Buchsel & P. Kapustay (Eds.), *Stem cell transplantation: A clinical textbook* (pp. 11.3–11.19). Pittsburgh, PA: Oncology Nursing Society.

Ahles, T.A., Tope, D.M., Pinkson, B., Walch, S., Hann, D., Whedon, M., et al. (1999). Massage therapy for patients undergoing autologous bone marrow transplantation. *Journal of Pain and Symptom Management, 18,* 157–163.

Amrolia, P., Gaspar, H.B., Hassan, A., Webb, D., Jones, A., Sturt, N., et al. (2000). Nonmyeloablative stem cell transplantation for congenital immunodeficiencies. *Blood, 96,* 1239–1246.

Anasetti, C., Hansen, J., Waldmann, T., Binger, M.H., Mould, D., Satoh, H., et al. (1992). Treatment of graft-versus-host disease with a humanized monoclonal antibody specific for the interleukin 2 receptor [Abstract 1484]. *Blood, 80*(Suppl. 1), 373a.

Anasetti, C., Petersdorf, E., Martin, P., Woolfrey, A., & Hansen, J. (2001). Trends in transplantation of stem cells from unrelated donors. *Current Opinion in Hematology, 8,* 337–341.

Antin, J.H., Weinstein, H.J., Guinan, E.C., McCarthy, P., Bierer, B.E., Gilliland, D.G., et al. (1994). Recombinant human interleukin-1 receptor antagonist in the treatment of steroid-resistant graft-versus-host disease. *Blood, 84,* 1342–1348.

Arai, S., & Vogelsang, G.B. (2000). Management of graft-versus-host disease. *Blood Reviews, 14*(4), 190–204.

Aversa, F., Tabilio, A., Velardi, A., Cunningham, I., Terenzi, A., Falzetti, F., et al. (1998). Treatment of high-risk acute leukemia with T-cell-depleted stem cells from related donors with one fully mismatched HLA haplotype. *New England Journal of Medicine, 339,* 1186–1193.

Aversa, F., Velardi, A., Tabilio, A., Reisner, Y., & Martelli, M.F. (2001). Haploidentical stem cell transplantation in leukemia. *Blood Reviews, 15*(3), 111–119.

Baker, F., Zabora, J., Polland, A., & Wingard, J. (1999). Reintegration after bone marrow transplantation. *Cancer Practice, 7,* 190–197.

Bank, A. (2000). Gene therapy. In J. Armitage & K. Antman (Eds.), *High-dose cancer therapy: Pharmacology, hematopoietins, stem cells* (3rd ed., pp. 167–181). Philadelphia: Lippincott Williams and Wilkins.

Barker, J., Davies, S., DeFor, T., Ramsay, N., Weisdorf, D., & Wagner, J. (2001). survival after transplantation of unrelated donor umbilical cord blood is comparable to that of human leukocyte antigen-matched unrelated donor bone marrow: results of a matched-pair analysis. *Blood, 97,* 2957–2961.

Basara, N., Kiehl, M.G., & Fauser, A.A. (2001). New therapeutic modalities in the treatment of graft-versus-host disease. *Critical Reviews in Oncology-Hematology, 38*(2), 129–138.

Beutler, E. (1999). Gene therapy. *Biology of Blood and Marrow Transplantation, 5,* 273–276.

Bishop, M. (1999). The Champlin et al. article reviewed. *Oncology, 13,* 631, 635.

Brandt, B., DePalma, J., Irwin, M., Shogan, J., & Lucke, J.F. (1996). Comparison of central venous catheter dressings in bone marrow transplant recipients. *Oncology Nursing Forum, 23,* 829–836.

Brooks, P. (1997). Hematopoietic stem cell transplantation for autoimmune diseases. *Journal of Rheumatology, 24*(Suppl. 48), 19–22.

Brodsky, R.A., & Smith, B.D. (1999). Bone marrow transplantation for autoimmune diseases. *Current Opinion in Oncology, 11*(2), 83–86.

Buckley, R.H., Schiff, S.E., Schiff, R.I., Markert, L., Williams, L.W., Roberts, J.L, et al. (1999). Hematopoietic stem-cell transplantation for the treatment of severe combined immunodeficiency. *New England Journal of Medicine, 340,* 508–516.

Bunjes, D., Duncker, C., Wiesneth, M., Stefanic, M., Dohr, D., Harsdorf, S., et al. (2000). CD34+ selected cells in mismatched stem cell transplantation: a single center experience of haploidentical peripheral blood stem cell transplantation. *Bone Marrow Transplantation, 25*(Suppl. 2), S9–S11.

Burt, R.K., Traynor, A.E., Pope, R., Schroeder, J., Cohen, B., Karlin, K.H., et al. (1998). Treatment of autoimmune disease by intense immunosuppressive conditioning and autologous hematopoietic stem cell transplantation. *Blood, 92,* 3505–3514.

Bush, N.E., Donaldson, G.W., Haberman, M.H., Dacanay, R., & Sullivan, K.M. (2000). Conditional and unconditional estimation of multidimensional quality of life after hematopoietic stem cell transplantation: a longitudinal follow-up of 415 patients. *Biology of Blood and Marrow Transplantation, 6,* 576–591.

Bush, N.E., Haberman, M., Donaldson, G., & Sullivan, K.M. (1995). Quality of life of 125 adults surviving 6-18 years after bone marrow transplantation. *Social Science and Medicine, 40,* 479–490.

Campos de Carvalho, E., Goncalves, P.G., Bontempo, A.P.M., & Soler, V.M. (2000). Interpersonal needs expressed by patients during bone marrow transplantation. *Cancer Nursing, 23,* 462–467.

Carella, A.M., Champlin, R., Slavin, S., McSweeney, P., & Storb, R. (2000). Mini-allografts: Ongoing trials in humans. *Bone Marrow Transplantation, 25,* 345–350.

Cavazzana-Calvo, M., Bagnis, C., Mannoni, P., & Fischer, A. (1999). Peripheral blood stem cell and gene therapy. *Baillieres Clinical Hematology, 12*(1/2), 129–138.

Champlin, R., Khouri, I., Komblau, S., Molidrem, J., & Giralt, S. (1999). Reinventing bone marrow transplantation nonmyeloablative preparative regimens and induction of graft-vs.-malignancy effect. *Oncology, 13,* 621–628.

Champlin, R., Khouri, I., Shimoni, A., Gajewski, J., Kornblau, S., Molldrem, J., et al. (2000). Harnessing graft-versus-malignancy: Non-myeloablative preparative regimens for allogeneic haematopoietic transplantation, an evolving strategy for adoptive immunotherapy. *British Journal of Haematology, 111,* 18–29.

Chao, N.J., Parker, P.M., Niland, J.C., Wong, R.M., Dagis, A., Long, G.D., et al. (1996). Paradoxical effect of thalidomide prophylaxis on chronic graft-vs.-host disease. *Biology of Blood and Marrow Transplantation, 2*(2), 86–92.

Chao, N., Snyder, D., Jain, M., Wong, R., Niland, J., Negrin, R., et al. (1999). Equivalence of two effective GVHD prophylaxis regimes: results of a prospective blinded randomized trial [Abstract 2957a]. *Blood, 94*(Suppl.1), 666a.

Childs, R., Chernoff, A., Contentin, N., Bahceci, E., Schrump, D., Leitman, S., et al. (2000). Regression of metastatic renal-cell carcinoma after nonmyeloablative allogeneic peripheral-blood stem-cell transplantation. *New England Journal of Medicine, 343,* 750–758.

Childs, R., Clave, E., Contentin, N., Jayasekera, D., Hensel, N., Leitman, S., et al. (1999). Engraftment kinetics after nonmyeloablative allogeneic peripheral blood stem cell transplantation: Full donor T-cell chimerism precedes alloimmune responses. *Blood, 94,* 3234–3241.

Civin, C. (2000). Gene therapy in clinical application. *Stem Cells, 18,* 150–156.

Contu, L., La Nasa, G., Arras, M., Pizzati, A., Vacca, A., Carcassi, C., et al. (1993). Allogeneic bone marrow transplantation combined with multiple anti-HIV-1 treatment in a case of AIDS. *Bone Marrow Transplantation, 12,* 669–671.

Cuaron, L.J., & Gallucci, B. (1997). Gene therapy and blood cell transplantation. *Seminars in Oncology Nursing, 13,* 200–207.

Davies, S.M., Kollman, C., Anasetti, C., Antin, J.H., Gajewski, J., Casper, J.T., et al. (2000). Engraftment and survival after unrelated-donor bone marrow transplantation: A report from the National Marrow Donor Program. *Blood, 96,* 4096–4102.

Dupont, B. (1997). Immunology of hematopoietic stem cell transplantation: A brief review of its history. *Immunological Reviews, 157,* 5–12.

Duquette-Petersen, L., Francis, M.E., Dohnalek, L., Skinner, R., & Dudas, P. (1999). The role of protective clothing in infection prevention in patients undergoing autologous bone marrow transplantation. *Oncology Nursing Forum, 26,* 1319–1324.

Eurocord. (2003). *European research on cord blood banking and use for transplantation.* Retrieved October 14, 2003, from http://www.aramis-research.ch/e/6137.html#basicinformation

Ezzone, S., Baker, C., Rosselet, R., & Terepka, E. (1998). Music as an adjunct to antiemetic therapy. *Oncology Nursing Forum, 25,* 1551–1556.

Ezzone, S., Jolly, D., Replogle, K., Kapoor, N., & Tutschka, P.J. (1993). Survey of oral hygiene regimens among bone marrow transplant centers. *Oncology Nursing Forum, 20,* 1375–1381.

Fassas, A., Anagnostopoulos, A., Kazis, A., Kapinas, K., Sakellari, I., Kimiskidis, V., et al. (1997). Peripheral blood stem transplantation in the treatment of progressive multiple sclerosis: First results of a pilot study. *Bone Marrow Transplantation, 20,* 631–638.

Finn, R. (2000). Oncologist's role critical to clinical trial enrollment. *Journal of the National Cancer Institute, 92,* 1632–1634.

Fraser, C.C., & Hoffman, R. (1995). Hematopoietic stem cell behavior: Potential implications for gene therapy. *Journal of Laboratory Clinical Medicine, 125,* 692–702.

Fry, J.W., & Wood, K.J. (1999, June). Gene therapy: Potential applications in clinical transplantation. *Expert Reviews in Molecular Medicine.* Retrieved October 1, 2003, from http://www-ermm.cbcu. cam.ac.uk/99000691a.pdf

Gaskill, D., Henderson, A., & Fraser, M. (1997). Exploring the everyday world of the patient in isolation. *Oncology Nursing Forum, 24,* 695–700.

Giles, R.E., Hanania, E.G., Fu, S., & Deisseroth, A. (1995). Genetic therapy using bone marrow transplantation. *Cancer Treatment and Research, 76,* 271–280.

Giralt, S., Estey, E., Albitar, M., van Besien, K., Rondon, G., Anderlini, P., et al. (1997). Engraftment of allogeneic hematopoietic progenitor cells with purine analog-containing chemotherapy: Harnessing graft-versus-leukemia without myeloablative therapy. *Blood, 89,* 4531–4536.

Gluckman, E. (2000). Current status of umbilical cord blood hematopoietic stem cell transplantation. *Experimental Hematology, 28,* 1197–1120.

Gluckman, E., Rocha, V., Boyer-Chammard, A., Locatelli, F., Arcese, W., Pasquini, R., et al. (1997). Outcome of cord-blood-transplantation from related and unrelated donors. Eurocord Transplant Group and the European Blood and Marrow Transplantation Group. *New England Journal of Medicine, 337,* 373–381.

Gluckman, E., Rocha, V., & Chastang, C.I., on behalf of Eurocord-Cord Blood Transplant Group. (1998). Cord blood hematopoietic stem cells biology and transplantation. *American Society of Hematology education book,* pp. 1–14. Retrieved October 1, 2003, from http://www.hematology.org/education/hema98/gluckman.pdf

Goker, H., Hazendaroglu, I.C., & Chao, N. (2001). Acute graft-vs-host disease: Pathobiology and management. *Experimental Hematology, 29*, 259–277.

Haberman, M.R. (1997). Nursing research in blood cell and marrow transplantation. In M.B. Whedon & D. Wujcik (Eds.), *Blood and marrow stem cell transplantation: Principles, practice and nursing insights* (2nd ed., pp. 497–505). Sudbury, MA: Jones and Bartlett.

Havenga, M., Hoogerbrugge, P., Valerio, D., & van Es, H. (1997). Retroviral stem cell gene therapy. *Stem Cells, 15*(3), 162–179.

Henslee-Downey, P.J., Parrish, R.S., MacDonald, J.S., Romond, E.H., Marciniak, E., Coffey, C., et al. (1996). Combined in vitro and in vivo T lymphocyte depletion for the control of graft-versus-host disease following haploidentical marrow transplant. *Transplantation, 61*, 738–745.

Herve, P., Racadot, E., Wijdenes, J., Flesch, M., Tiberghien, P., Bordigoni, P., et al. (1991). Monoclonal anti TNF alpha antibody in the treatment of acute GvHD refractory both to corticosteroids and anti IL-2 R antibody. *Bone Marrow Transplantation, 7*(Suppl. 2), 149.

Hoppe, C., & Walters, M. (2001). Bone marrow transplantation in sickle cell anemia. *Current Opinion in Oncology, 13*(2), 85–90.

Hunt, J. (2001). Research into practice: The foundation for evidence-based care. *Cancer Nursing, 24*(2), 78–87.

Huzicka, I. (1999). Could bone marrow transplantation cure AIDS? Review. *Medical Hypothesis, 52*, 247–257.

Hwu, P., & Rosenberg, S. (1997). Gene therapy of cancer In V.T. DeVita, S. Hellman, & S.A. Rosenberg (Eds.), *Cancer: Principles and practice of oncology* (5th ed., pp. 3005–3022). Philadelphia: Lippincott-Raven.

Jantunen, E., Myllykangas-Luosujarvi, R., Kaipiainen-Seppanen, O., & Nousiainen, T. (2000). Autologous stem cell transplantation in a lymphoma patient with a long history of ankylosing spondylitis. *Rheumatology, 39*, 563–564.

Kane, L., Gennery, A.R., Crooks, B.N., Flood, T.J., Abinun, M., & Cant, A.J. (2001). Neonatal bone marrow transplantation for severe combined immunodeficiency. *Archives of Disease in Childhood: Fetal and Neonatal Edition, 85*(2), F110–F113.

Khouri, I.F., Keating, M., Korbling, M., Przepiorka, D., Anderlini, P., O'Brien, S., et al. (1998). Transplant-lite: Induction of graft-versus-malignancy using fludarabine-based non ablative chemotherapy and allogeneic blood progenitor-cell transplantation as treatment for lymphoid malignancies. *Journal of Clinical Oncology, 16*, 2817–2824.

Kirby, S. (1999). Bone marrow: Target for gene transfer. *Hospital Practice, 34*(13), 59–63, 69–70, 73–74.

Krijanovski, O., Hill, G., Cooke, K., Teshima, T., Crawford, J., Brinson, Y., et al. (1999). Keratinocyte growth factor separates graft-versus-leukemia effects from graft-versus-host disease. *Blood, 94*, 825–831.

Lara, P., Higdon, R., Lim, N., Kwan, K., Tanaka, M., Lau, D., et al. (2001). Prospective evaluation of cancer clinical trial accrual patterns: Identifying potential barriers to enrollment. *Journal of Clinical Oncology, 19*, 1728–1733.

Laughlin, M., Barker, J., Bambach, B., Koc, O., Rizzieri, D., Wagner, J., et al. (2001). Hematopoietic engraftment and survival in adult recipients of umbilical-cord blood from unrelated donors. *New England Journal of Medicine, 344*, 1815–1822.

Lucarelli, G., Galimberti, M., Giardini, C., Polchi, P., Angelucci, E., Baronciani, D., et al. (1998). Bone marrow transplantation in thalassemia: The experience of Pesaro. *Annals of New York Academy of Science, 850*, 270–275.

McCarthy, N., & Bishop, M. (2000). Nonmyeloablative allogeneic stem cell transplantation: Early promise and limitations. *Oncologist, 5*, 487–496.

McGuire, D.B., Yeager, K.A., Dudley, W.N., Peterson, D.E., Owen, D.C., Lin, L.S., et al. (1998). Acute oral pain and mucositis in bone marrow transplant and leukemia patients: Data from a pilot study. *Cancer Nursing, 21*, 385–393.

McSweeney, P., Niederwieser, D., Shizuru, J., Molina, A., Wagner, J., Minor, S., et al. (1999). Outpatient allografting with minimally myelosuppressive, immunosuppressive conditioning of low-dose TBI and postgrafting cyclosporine (CSP) and mycophenolate mofetil (MMF) [Abstract 1742]. *Blood, 94*(Suppl. 1), 393a.

Meloni, G., Capria, S., Vignetti, M., Mandelli, F., & Modena, V. (1997). Blast crisis of chronic myelogenous leukemia in long-lasting systemic lupus erythematosus: Regression of both diseases after autologous bone marrow transplantation. *Blood, 89*, 4659.

Miniero, R., Rocha, V., Saracco, P., Locatelli, F., Brichard, B., Nagler, A., et al. (1998). Cord blood transplantation (CBT) in hemoglobinopathies. Eurocord. *Bone Marrow Transplantation, 22*(Suppl. 1), S78–S79.

Molassiotis, A. (1997). Nursing research within bone marrow transplantation in Europe: An evaluation. *European Journal of Cancer Care, 6*, 257–261.

Molassiotis, A., Boughton, B.J., Burgoyne, T., & van den Akker, O.B. (1995). Comparison of the overall quality of life in 50 long-term survivors of autologous and allogeneic bone marrow transplantation. *Journal of Advanced Nursing, 22*, 509–516.

Molassiotis, A., & Morris, P.J. (1999). Quality of life in patients with chronic myeloid leukemia after unrelated donor bone marrow transplantation. *Cancer Nursing, 22*, 340–349.

Molassiotis, A., van den Akker, O.B., Milligan, D.W., & Boughton, B.J. (1995). Gonadal function and psychosexual adjustment in male long-term survivors of bone marrow transplantation. *Bone Marrow Transplantation, 16*, 253–259.

Murphy, W.J., & Blazar, B.R. (1999). New strategies for preventing graft-versus-host disease. *Current Opinion in Immunology, 11*, 509–515.

National Institutes of Health. (2001). *NIH grant awarded to develop a blood and marrow transplant clinical trials network*. Retrieved November 25, 2001, from http://www.ibmtr.org/news.asp?id=37

National Marrow Donor Program. (2000). *NMDP hosts symposium on advances in transplantation*. (2000). Retrieved November 25, 2001, from http://www.marrow.org/NEWS/ARTICLES/ashfollowup 12272000.html

Olivieri, N.F. (1999). The beta-thalassemias. *New England Journal of Medicine, 341*, 99–109.

O'Reilly, R. (2000). Clinical trials of hematopoietic cell transplantations: Current needs and future strategies. *Biology of Blood and Marrow Transplant, 6*, 79–89.

Pederson, C., & Parran, L. (1999). Pain and distress in adults and children undergoing peripheral blood stem cell or bone marrow transplant. *Oncology Nursing Forum, 26*, 575–582.

Pederson, C., & Parran, L. (2000). Opioid tapering in hematopoietic progenitor cell transplant recipients. *Oncology Nursing Forum, 27*, 1371–1380.

Porta, F., & Friedrich, W. (1998). Bone marrow transplantation in congenital immunodeficiency diseases. *Bone Marrow Transplantation, 21*(Suppl. 2), S21–S23.

Przepiorka, D., Kernan, N., Ippoliti, C., Papadoupoulos, B., Giralt, S., Khouri, I., et al. (2000). Daclizumab, a humanized anti-interleukin-2 receptor alpha chain antibody, for treatment of acute graft-versus-host disease. *Blood, 95*, 83–89.

Ratanatharathorn, V., Nash, R.A., Przepiorka, D., Devine, S.M., Klein, J.L., Weisdorf, D., et al. (1998). Phase III study comparing methotrexate and tacrolimus (prograf, FK506) with methotrexate and cyclosporine for graft-versus-host disease prophylaxis after HLA-identical sibling bone marrow transplantation. *Blood, 92*, 2303–2314.

Reisner, Y., & Martelli, M.F. (2000). Tolerance introduction by "Magadose" transplants of CD34+ stem cells: A new option for leukemia patients without an HLA-matched donor. *Current Opinion in Immunology, 12*, 536–541.

Remberger, M., Ringden, O., Blau, I.W., Ottinger, H., Kremens, B., Kiehl, M.G., et al. (2001). No difference in graft-versus-host disease, relapse, and survival comparing peripheral stem cells to bone marrow using unrelated donors. *Blood, 98,* 1739–1745.

Rocha, V., Cornish, J., Sievers, E., Filipovich, A., Locatelli, F., Peters, C., et al. (2001). Comparison of outcomes of unrelated bone marrow and umbilical cord blood transplants in children with acute leukemia. *Blood, 97,* 2962–2970.

Rocha, V., Wagner, J., Sobocinski, K., Klein, J., Zhang, M., Horowitz, M., et al. (2000). Graft-versus-host disease in children who have received a cord-blood or bone marrow transplant from an HLA-identical sibling. *New England Journal of Medicine, 342,* 1846–1854.

Romano, G., Michelli, P., Pacilio, C., & Giordano, A. (2000). Latest developments in gene transfer technology: achievements, perspectives and controversies over therapeutic applications. *Stem Cells, 18,* 19–39.

Romano, G., Pacilio, C., & Giordano, A. (1999). Gene transfer technology in therapy: Current applications and future goals. *Stem Cells, 17,* 191–202.

Rowe, J.M., & Lazarus, H.M. (2001). Genetically haploidentical stem cell transplantation for acute leukemia. *Bone Marrow Transplantation, 27,* 669–676.

Rund, D., & Rachmilewitz, E. (2000). New trends in the treatment of ß-thalassemia. *Critical Reviews in Oncology/Hematology, 33,* 105–118.

Rutledge, D., Greene, P., Mooney, K., Nail, L., & Ropka, M. (1996). Use of research-based practices by oncology staff nurses. *Oncology Nursing Forum, 23,* 1235–1244.

Rutledge, D., Ropka, M., Greene, P., Nail, L., & Mooney, K. (1998). Barriers to research utilization for oncology staff nurses and nurse managers/clinical nurse specialists. *Oncology Nursing Forum, 25,* 497–505.

Sandmaier, B., McSweeney P., Yu, C., & Storb, R. (2000). Nonmyeloablative transplants: Preclinical and clinical results. *Seminars in Oncology, 27*(2 Suppl. 5), 78–81.

Saral, R., & Holland, H.K. (1994). Bone marrow transplantation for the acquired immune deficiency syndrome. In S.J. Forman, K.G. Blume, & E.D. Thomas (Eds.), *Bone marrow transplantation* (pp. 654–664). Boston: Blackwell Scientific.

Schmitz, N., Linch, D.C., Dreger, P., Goldstone, A.H., Boogaeerts, M.A., Ferrant, A., et al. (1996). Randomized trial of filgrastim-mobilized peripheral blood progenitor cell transplantation in lymphoma patients. *Lancet, 347,* 353–357.

Slavin, S., Nagler, A., Naparstek, E., Kapelushnik, Y., Aker, M., Cividalli, G., et al. (1998). Nonmyeloablative stem cell transplantation and cell therapy as an alternative to conventional bone marrow transplantation with lethal cytoreduction for the treatment of malignant and nonmalignant hematologic diseases. *Blood, 91,* 756–763.

Snowden, J. (1998). Long-term outcome of autoimmune disease following allogeneic bone marrow transplantation. *Arthritis and Rheumatism, 41,* 453–459.

Snowden, J., Brooks, P., & Biggs, J. (1997). Haemopoietic stem cell transplantation for autoimmune diseases. *British Journal of Haematology, 99,* 9–22.

Sonis, S.T., Oster, G., Fuchs, H., Bellm, L., Bradford, W.Z., Edelsberg, J., et al. (2001). Oral mucositis and the clinical and economic outcomes of hematopoietic stem-cell transplantation. *Journal of Clinical Oncology, 19,* 2201–2205.

Spitzer, T. (2000). Nonmyeloablative allogeneic stem cell transplant strategies and the role of mixed chimerism. *Oncologist, 5,* 215–223.

Stetz, K.M., McDonald, J.C., & Compton, K. (1996). Needs and experiences of family caregivers during marrow transplantation. *Oncology Nursing Forum, 23,* 1422–1477.

Steward, C. (2000). Stem cell transplant for non-malignant disorders. *Baillieres Clinical Hematology, 13,* 343–363.

Sullivan, K., Nelson, J.L., Arnason, B., Good, R., Burt, R., & Gratwohl, A. (1998). Evolving role of hematopoietic stem cell transplantation in autoimmune disease. In *American Society of Hematology education book,* pp. 198–214. Retrieved October 2, 2003, from www.hematology.org/education/hema98/sullivan.pdf

Sullivan, K., Parkman, R., & Walters, M. (2000). Bone marrow transplantation for non-malignant disease. *American Society of Hematology education book,* pp. 319–338. Retrieved October 2, 2003, from http://www.asheducationbook.org/cgi/reprint/2000/1/319.pdf

Thomas, E.D. (1999). A history of haemopoietic cell transplantation. *British Journal of Haematology, 105,* 330–339.

Thomas, E.D., Buckner, C.D., Banaji, M., Clift, R.A., Fefer, A., Flournoy, N., et al. (1977). One hundred patients with acute leukemia treated by chemotherapy, total body irradiation, and allogeneic marrow transplantation. *Blood, 49,* 511–533.

Tyndall, A. (2002). Restoring control the use of hematopoietic stem-cell support therapy in severe autoimmune diseases. *Helix, Amgen's Magazine of Biotechnology, 1,* 16–22.

Tyndall, A., & Gratwohl, A. (2000). Immune ablation and stem cell therapy in autoimmune disease. Clinical experience. *Arthritis Research, 2,* 276–280.

van Bekkum, D.W. (1999). Autologous stem cell transplantation for treatment of autoimmune diseases. *Stem Cells, 17,* 172–178.

Vermylen, C., Cornu, G., Ferster, G., Ninane, A., & Sariban, E. (1993). Bone marrow transplantation for sickle cell disease: The Belgian experience. *Bone Marrow Transplantation, 12*(Suppl. 1), 1167.

Vichinsky, E., Brugnara, C., Styles, L., & Wagner, J. (1998). Future therapy for sickle cell disease. *American Society of Hematology education book,* pp. 1129–1135. Retrieved October 2, 2003, from http://www.hematology.org/education/hema98/vichinsky.pdf

Vile, R.G., Russell, S.J., & Lemoine, N.R. (2000). Cancer gene therapy: Hard lessons and new courses. *Gene Therapy, 7*(1), 2–8.

Wagner, J.E., Kernan, N.A., Steinbuch, M., Broxmeyer, H.E., & Gluckman, E. (1995). Allogeneic sibling umbilical-cord-blood transplantation in children with malignant and non-malignant disease. *Lancet, 346,* 214–219.

Walters, M.C., Storb, R., Patience, M., Leisenring, W., Taylor, T., Sanders, J.E., et al. (2000). Impact of bone marrow transplantation for symptomatic sickle cell disease: an interim report. Multicenter investigation of bone marrow transplantation for sickle cell disease. *Blood, 95,* 1918–1924.

Whedon, M., Stearns, D., & Mills, L.E. (1995). Quality of life of long-term adult survivors of autologous bone marrow transplantation. *Oncology Nursing Forum, 22,* 1527–1535.

Wheeler, V. (1995). Gene therapy: Current strategies and future applications. *Oncology Nursing Forum, 22*(Suppl. 2), 20–26.

Winters, G., Miller, C., Maracich, L., Compton, K., & Haberman, M.R. (1994). Provisional practice: The nature of psychosocial bone marrow transplant nursing. *Oncology Nursing Forum, 21,* 1147–1165.

Index

The letter *f* after the page number indicates that relevant content is in a figure; the letter *t*, in a table.

A

ABO-incompatible BMT, complications of, 141–142, 142*t*
accreditation, of HSCT programs, 18, 19*f*, 61, 66–67, 74–77, 76*f*–77*f*
acetazolamide, 49
acrolein, 173
Actigall® (ursodeoxycholic acid), 98, 111
Activase® (alteplase, recombinant), 33
acute GVHD (aGVHD), 85. *See also* graft versus host disease
  in allogeneic transplants, 33
  associated with GVT effect, 11
  biology/pathogenesis of, 85–87, 86*f*
  clinical/histopathologic features of, 88–91, 90*f*
  grading/staging systems for, 91, 92*t*, 93*f*, 110
  hepatic, 169–170*t*
  HLA mismatch and, 10
  onset/incidence of, 91
  in PBSCT vs. BMT, 10
  predictive factors for, 88–91, 89*t*
  prevention/treatment for, 97–109, 99*f*, 100*t*–105*t*, 109–110, 110*t*, 112*t*
  tumor necrosis factor and, 10
acute lymphoid/lymphocytic/ lymphoblastic leukemia (ALL)
  allogeneic HSCT for, 15*t*
  autologous HSCT for, 14
  and leukoencephalopathy, 196
  preparative regimens for, 17*t*
  sanctuary sites in, 202
acute myeloid/myelogenous/ myeloblastic leukemia (AML)
  allogeneic HSCT for, 15*t*
  autologous HSCT for, 14

donor lymphocyte infusion in, 202
graft versus tumor effect in, 121
and intercranial hemorrhages, 196
preparative regimens for, 17*t*
as secondary malignancy, 203
acute promyelocytic leukemia, DIC associated with, 50
acute respiratory distress syndrome (ARDS), 178*f*, 182
acute tumor lysis syndrome (ATLS), 48–49
acyclovir, 135, 171, 194, 214*t*
adenoids, 5
adenovirus, 53, 149, 171, 173
adhesion cascade, 54
adhesion molecules, 2–3, 54
adrenoleukodystrophy, allogeneic HSCT for, 15*t*
advance directives, 233
advanced practice nurses, 66, 70, 73
adverse effects. *See* side effects
Aeromonas, 149
AIDS, 265. *See also* HIV
air filtration systems, 135, 137
alemtuzumab (Campath-1®), 18, 103*t*, 107, 110, 201
alkalization, of urine, 49
allergic reaction, 45*t*–46*t*
allogeneic HSCT, 14, 14*t*, 26, 27*f*, 55, 61, 133–134. *See also* hematopoietic stem cell transplantation
  anemia in, 141
  BLPD and, 203
  and cognitive effects of TBI, 193
  collection for, 33–35
  dietary recommendations for, 162–163
  diseases treated with, 14, 15*t*
  first successful, 13, 33
  graft failure in, 143
  HLA mismatch in, 9–10, 38
  immune system recovery after, 8–9, 54, 133–134
  infections after, 133, 135–138

mortality from, 14
neurologic complications in, 195, 197
pulmonary complications in, 177–178
relapse following, 202, 215
risks/benefits of, 14, 33
TBI use in, 44
total parenteral nutrition in, 163
travel restrictions following, 210–211
alloimmunization, 140, 143
allopurinol, 49
alopecia, 45*t*
American Red Cross UCB banks, 37*f*
American Society for Histocompatibility and Immunogenetics, 9*t*
American Society of Clinical Oncology (ASCO), 74
American Society of Hematology (ASH), 74
American Society of Histocompatibility and Immunogenetics, 75
amikacin, 135
aminoglycosides, 135, 172, 172*f*, 194
amitriptyline, 51
amphotericin, 135, 170–172, 177*f*, 184–186
amsacrine, 49
anaphylaxis, 45*t*–46*t*
anemia, 140–142, 141*t*–142*t*
  allogeneic HSCT for, 15*t*
  grading of, 141, 142*t*
  from GVHD, 90
  preparative regimen for, 17*t*
  as side effect of preparative regimen, 45*t*
anorexia, as side effect of preparative regimen, 45*t*
Anthony Nolan Trust, 9*t*
antibiotics/antimicrobials/ antivirals, 53–54, 135, 151, 186, 194–195. *See also specific medications*
antibodies, 5, 5*t*
antibody-dependent cell-mediated cytotoxicity, 5

anticoagulants
  causing cardiac tamponade, 186
  for pulmonary embolism, 180
  for VOD, 168
anticytokine antibodies, 253
antidiuretic hormone (ADH), excessive release of, 51–52
antiemetic agents, 156, 157*t*, 192. *See also* nausea/ vomiting
antigens, 4
antithrombin III levels, in DIC, 51
antithymocyte globulin (ATG), 18, 44*t*–45*t*, 103*t*, 107, 109–110, 110*t*
antitoxin, 5
anxiety, of patient/family, 20. *See also* psychosocial stress; quality of life
Anzemet® (granisetron), 157*t*
apheresis, 16, 30–33, 31*t*, 32*f*, 34*t*. *See also* collection; mobilization
  in children, 35
  education regarding, 72
  large-volume, 32, 37
  machines/devices for, 30–32, 32*f*, 35
  for phototherapy, 108
  side effects of, 31*t*, 33, 34*t*, 35
  timing of, 30
  transient thrombocytopenia from, 140
aplastic anemia
  allogeneic HSCT for, 15*t*
  preparative regimen for, 17*t*
apoptosis, 3
appendix, 5
arginine vasopressin, 51
arrhythmias, 185
ascitic fluid, 50–51
Ashley Ross Cord Blood Program, 37*f*
Aspergillus/aspergillosis, 110, 135, 136*t*, 139, 170, 178*f*, 184–185, 195–196
ASTIMS Trial, 264

cephalosporin, 54, 135, 194
cerebral ischemia, 193, 196
cerebral vasospasm, 193
certified nursing assistants, 64
Chagas' disease, 53
chaplaincy program, 67
Chédiak-Higashi syndrome, allogeneic HSCT for, 15t
chemoreceptor trigger zone (CTZ), 156
chemotherapy, 17–18. See also specific agents
  cardiotoxicity of, 187t–188t
  combined with TBI, 43–44, 44t
  with growth factor use, 30
  high-dose, 17, 38–39, 43, 44t–45t, 167, 201
  neurologic complications from, 191–192
  post-transplant, 214
  pulmonary toxicity from, 178f, 178–179, 179t
  risks/benefits of, 27–28
  side effects of, 45t, 156–157, 159, 172, 172f, 202–203. See also side effects; specific agents
  stem cells mobilized by, 27–28
chest tubes, 180
children
  BSC collections in, 35
  clinical trials involving, 259f
  dental evaluation/management in, 152
  education of, 19
  IQ reduction in, after radiation therapy, 192
  leukoencephalopathy in, 196
  nausea in, behavioral interventions for, 157
  neuropsychological testing, prior to HSCT, 18
  pain management in, 152
  perineal/rectal skin alterations in, 159–160, 161t
  quality-of-life issues for, 246
  RBC transfusion in, 142
  relapse in, 215
  seizures in, 191
  TBI for, 46
Children's Hospital of Orange County Cord Blood Bank, 37f
chimeric state, 11, 55
chlorhexidine mouthwash, 151
chloroacetaldehyde, 191
cholestasis
  drug-induced, 170
  TPN-induced, 170
cholestyramine (Questran®), 98t

chromosomal analysis, engraftment confirmed by, 55
chronic granulomatous disease, allogeneic HSCT for, 15t
chronic GVHD (cGVHD), 85, 91–96. See also graft versus host disease
  in allogeneic transplants, 33
  classification/grading of, 96–97, 97t–99t
  clinical/histopathological features of, 93f, 93–96, 94f–96f
  hepatic, 169–170, 170t
  HLA mismatch and, 10
  and immune recovery, 96
  incidence of, 92, 169
  and increased IL-6, 10
  pathogenesis of, 91–92
  in PBSCT vs. BMT, 10, 16
  prevention/treatment for, 97–109, 99f, 100t–105t, 110–112, 112t
  risk factors for, 92–93
  timing of onset, 97
chronic lymphocytic leukemia
  graft versus tumor effect in, 121
  NST for, 15
chronic myelogenous leukemia (CML)
  allogeneic HSCT for, 15t
  donor lymphocyte infusion in, 202
  graft versus tumor effect in, 121
  preparative regimens for, 17t
cidofovir, 173
cisplatin, 17t, 52, 139, 155, 157, 185, 186f, 187t, 192, 194
City of Hope National Medical Center, 69
cladribine, 49
clindamycin, 195
clinical evaluation
  of donors, 18, 19f, 23, 24f–26f
  prior to HSCT, 18, 19f
clinical nurse specialist, 66
clinical trials, 256, 257f–260f, 263–265
clofazimine, 111
clonal succession, 3
Clostridium, 89–90, 149–151, 185
clotrimazole, 135
clots
  in acute DIC, 51
  and catheter occlusion, 33
cluster of differentiation. See CD proteins
coagulation, overstimulation of, 50–51

COBE® Spectra™ apheresis machine, 30
Coccidiomycosis, 136t
cognitive effects, of radiation therapy, 192–193
"cold hypodynamic" clinical presentation, 52
collection, 33, 34t, 35. See also apheresis; mobilization
  of allogeneic BSCs, 33–35
  of BMSCs vs. PBSCs, 16
  facilities for, 75–77
  future directions in, 38–39
  of PBSCs, 16, 26–27, 27f, 32–33
  in pediatric patients, 35
  side effects of, 33, 34t, 35
colony assay, 32
colony-forming units (CFUs), 3. See also hematopoietic progenitor cells
colony-stimulating factors (CSFs), 2, 4, 16, 28, 33–35, 53, 133–134
  guidelines for using, 134
Common Toxicity Criteria (NCI), 34, 133, 134t, 138, 158
communication, during patient follow-up, 207f, 207–208
community cancer centers, 69–70
complement, 5, 7
complications. See side effects
comprehensive model, of outpatient care, 69
conditioning regimens, 17t, 17–18, 43–46, 44t–45t. See also specific immunosuppressants
  and acute GVHD development, 86
  anemia caused by, 141
  nursing management of, 46t, 46–47
congenital neutropenia, allogeneic HSCT for, 15t
congestive heart failure, 181
conjunctivitis, 45t, 94
constipation, as side effect of preparative regimen, 45t
continuing education, for HSCT center staff, 65–66
COPE model of education, 71
corneal testing, 94
corticosteroids
  ATLS associated with, 49
  for BOOP treatment, 181
  for BO treatment, 182
  for chemotherapy-associated pulmonary toxicity, 179, 179t

  for DAH treatment, 139, 178
  for GVHD control, 87, 92–93, 99, 101t, 105, 109–110, 110t, 111, 112t, 169
  ineffective for IPS, 178
  for nausea/vomiting, 157t
  neurological effects of, 193–194, 194f
  for radiation-induced pulmonary toxicity, 179
costs, housing, for outpatient care, 69
cryopreservation, of stem cells, 37–38, 47, 77, 77t
cryoprotectant, in stem cell product, 37–38, 47, 193
Cryptococcus neoformans, 136t
Cryptosporidium, 163, 210
cutaneous effects. See skin
cyclin-dependent kinases (CDKs), 3
cyclins, 3
cyclophosphamide, 17t, 18, 27, 43, 44t–45t, 46, 51–52, 139, 155, 157, 173t, 177f, 185, 186f, 187t, 193, 203
cyclosporine, 87, 96, 100t, 105–106, 106t, 109–110, 110t, 111, 112t, 139, 142, 170, 172–173, 182, 193, 202, 214t, 252–253
cystitis, 45t
cytarabine, 44t–45t, 139, 177f, 178, 186f, 187t–188t, 191–192
cytogenetic relapse, 202
cytokine cascade, 86f, 86–87, 91–92
cytokine receptors, 2
cytokines, 2–3, 86–87, 202. See also colony-stimulating factors; erythropoietin; interleukins; stem cell factor; tumor necrosis factor
cytokine shields, 118
cytomegalovirus, 53
  associated with BOOP, 181
  associated with GVHD, 87–88, 90, 94, 110, 171, 173
  causing thrombocytopenia, 139
  gastrointestinal, 149–151
  with HHV-6 infection, 195
  lower risk in UCB, 36
  and oral mucositis, 148
  pneumonia from, 178f, 182–183, 183t

hepatocytes, 167
hepatorenal syndrome, 173–174
Herceptin® (trastuzumab), 202
herpes simplex virus (HSV), 53
    associated with GVHD, 87–88, 90, 111, 171
    and oral mucositis, 148
    post-transplant, 135, 136t, 137–138
high-dose chemotherapy, 17, 38–39, 43, 44t–45t, 167, 201
HIV, 53, 139, 142, 265
HLA genes, 7–8, 8t–9t
    naming of, 8
HLA haplotypes, 8, 9f
HLA matching, 9–10, 35–36, 38, 91
HLA typing, 7, 9t, 14
    engraftment confirmed by, 55
Hodgkin's disease
    autologous HSCT for, 15t
    HST for, 15
    preparative regimens for, 17t, 43
home care, of HSCT patient, 70, 137–138, 211–214, 215f
homing, of transplanted cells, 54
Hope Village, 69
Hospital Infection Control Practice Advisory Committee (HICPAC), 52
household pets, 210
HSCT networks, 78–81, 81t, 81f
HSCT programs
    accreditation of, 18, 19f, 61, 66–67, 74–77, 76f–77f
    budget/startup costs for, 78, 79f–80f
    development of, 61–63, 62t, 63f
        by for-profit corporations, 80–81
    feasibility evaluation of, 61, 63f
    highest areas of expense in, 78
    multidisciplinary team approach in, 66–67, 115
    networking of, 78–81, 81t, 81f
    policy/procedure development, 73–74
    reimbursement methodologies for, 78, 81t
    staff development/education in, 63–66, 65f–66f, 75

standards of care developed for, 73t, 73–74, 74f
Human Genome Project, 7
human herpes virus 6 (HHV-6), 195
human leukocyte antigens (HLAs), 7, 13. *See also under* HLA
human T cell leukemia virus-1, 142
humoral hypercalcemia, 50
humoral immune response, 5, 7
Hunter's disease, allogeneic HSCT for, 15t
Hurler's syndrome, allogeneic HSCT for, 15t
hydration, 46, 48, 50, 159t
hydrogen peroxide, for mouth rinses, 151
hydroxychloroquine, 111
hydroxyethyl starch (HES) (cryoprotectant), 38
hyperacute GVHD, 91
hyperbilirubinemia, 106, 107t
hypercalcemia, 49–50
hyperkalemia, 49
hypernephroma, hypercalcemia with, 17t
hyperosmotic supplements, 159
hyperphosphatemia, 49
hyperpigmentation, 45t, 93, 95f
hypertension, 45t
hyperuricemia, 49
hypoalbuminemia, 89
hypocalcemia, 49
    during stem cell collection, 34t, 35
hypogammaglobulinemia, 90
hypogeusia, 155. *See also* taste changes
hyponatremia, 52
hypopigmentation, 93
hypotension, 45t, 142, 193
hypovolemia, 52
    during stem cell collection, 34t

I

IBMTR Severity Index, for staging GVHD, 91, 92t
ICU, 67–68, 185–186
idiopathic pneumonia syndrome, 44, 177–178, 178f
ifosfamide, 172f, 172–173, 185, 186f, 187t, 191
imipenem-cisplatin, 194
immune hemolytic anemia, 141
immune-mediated neurologic toxicities, 197
immune system, 4–11, 5t–6t
    activity/responses of, 6–7

cells of, 5t, 5–6, 6t
    effect of GVHD on, 90–91, 96, 99t, 112, 169
    genetic basis of, 7–8, 8t–9t, 9f
    and HSCT, 8–10
    manipulation of, post-transplant, 214–215
    organs of, 5
    recovery after HSCT, 8–9, 54, 108, 133, 214–215
    sepsis and, 52
immunodeficiency diseases
    allogeneic HSCT for, 15t, 258–261
    high-dose chemotherapy for, 17, 38–39
immunoglobulin allele typing, engraftment confirmed by, 55
immunoglobulin C (IgC), 53
immunoglobulins, 5, 5t, 54, 183
immunologic effects, of HSC infusion, 46t
Imuran® (azathioprine), 102t
inappropriate medical care, discontinuation of (futility), 234
infections. *See also* neutropenia; *specific infections*
    associated with SIADH, 51
    bacterial
        associated with GVHD, 89–90, 112–113
        associated with MMF, 106
        cardiac, 185–186
        gastrointestinal, 149
        neurologic, 195
        oral, 148
        post-transplant, 135–138, 136t
        pulmonary, 184
        transmitted through blood products, 53
    of central nervous system, 96
    costs associated with, 133
    during follow-up, 208–211, 210t
    fungal
        associated with GVHD, 89–90, 111–113
        hepatic, 170–171, 172t
        neurologic, 195–196
        oral, 148
        post-transplant, 135, 136t, 138, 147
        pulmonary, 184
    lower risk in UCBT, 36
    nursing management of, 117f
    periodontal, 152
    prevention of, 53, 112–113, 208–211, 210t

sepsis from, 52–54
    transmitted through blood products, 53, 142–143
    during transplant process, 135–138, 136t–137t
    viral
        associated with GVHD, 87, 90, 94, 111–113
        associated with MMF, 106
        causing thrombocytopenia, 139
        gastrointestinal, 149
        hepatic, 171, 172t, 173
        lower risk in UCBT, 36, 90
        neurologic, 195
        oral, 148
        post-transplant, 135–138, 136t
        pulmonary, 181–184, 183t
        from transfusions, 53, 142–143
infertility, 45t
inflammatory demyelinating polyneuropathy, 197
infliximab (Remicade®), 87, 103t, 107, 110
influenza, 53, 113, 136t–137t, 138, 181, 183
influenza vaccination, 208–210
informed consent, 18, 23, 75, 222–228
    in UCB transplant, 36–37
infusion
    fresh, 48
    of HSCs, 46t, 47–48
inpatient care, 67
Institutes of Quality, 78–81, 81t, 81f
insurance, for outpatient costs, 69
integrins, 3, 54
integumentary effects, of preparative regimens, 45t
intelligence, affected by TBI, 192
intensive care, 67–68, 185–186
intercranial hemorrhage, 196
interferon, 6t, 49, 86–87, 171, 215
interleukin-1 (IL-1), 4, 6t, 86–87, 107, 148
interleukin-2 (IL-2), 4, 6t, 86–87, 106, 202, 215
interleukin-3 (IL-3), 2, 4, 6t, 28
interleukin-4 (IL-4), 4, 6t
interleukin-5 (IL-5), 4, 6t
interleukin-6 (IL-6), 4, 6t, 10, 148
interleukin-7 (IL-7), 6t
interleukin-8 (IL-8), 6t
interleukin-9 (IL-9), 6t

nursing management of, 117f
oral, 94, 152, 153f–154f
pancreatic insufficiency, with chronic GVHD, 94
parainfluenza, 138, 178f, 183
parathyroid hormone, 50
parotitis, 45t
parvovirus B19, 142
pastoral care, 67
patient acuity tools, 64, 65f, 75
patient-controlled analgesia (PCA), 152
patient education, 18–19, 46–48, 54, 71, 72t, 113, 137–138, 149, 179, 181, 183–184, 223f–226f, 228, 229f–232f
payor mix, of HSCT program, 78
PBSCT. See peripheral blood stem cell transplant
Pedialyte®, 159
pediatric patients
  BSC collections in, 35
  clinical trials involving, 259f
  dental evaluation/management in, 152
  education of, 19
  IQ reduction in, after radiation therapy, 192
  leukoencephalopathy in, 196
  nausea in, behavioral interventions for, 157
  neuropsychological testing, prior to HSCT, 18
  pain management in, 152
  perineal/rectal skin alterations in, 159–160, 161t
  quality-of-life issues for, 246
  RBC transfusion in, 142
  relapse in, 215
  seizures in, 191
  TBI for, 46
penicillin, 54, 139, 194, 214t
pentamidine, 137, 184
pentoxifylline, 110
Pen-Vee K®, 135
performance standards, in HSCT programs, 73t, 73–74, 74f
pericardial effusion, 96
pericardial window, 186
pericardiocentesis, 186
perineal skin alterations, 159–160, 161t
periodontal infections, 152
peripheral blood stem cells (PBSCs)
  added to BM harvest, 29
  collection of, 16, 26–27, 27f, 32–35
  mobilization of, 16, 27–30

peripheral blood stem cell transplant (PBSCT), 13
  vs. BMT, 10, 16, 23, 26, 27f, 55, 78, 88, 92, 133, 135, 249–250
  immune system recovery after, 8–9, 54. See also immune system
  from unrelated donor, 35
Peripheral Blood Stem Cell Transplantation: Recommendations for Nursing Education and Practice (ONS), 73
peripheral nervous system effects, of chemotherapy, 191–192
peripheral neuropathy, 45t, 95
peripheral venous access, vs. central venous catheters, 30
pets, in patient household, 210
Peyers patches, 5
phagocytes, 5–6
pharmacists, 66
phenytoin, 139
photophobia, 90
phototherapy, for GVHD, 108–109, 111
physical therapy
  for GVHD patients, 115
  post-transplant, 211
physician assistant, 66
PIXY321 (growth factor), 28, 53
placental blood stem cells, 36. See also UCB stem cells
plasma cell, 5
plasma volume exchange, 140
plasmin, 51
platelet refractoriness, 196
platelets, 1, 4, 54
  average number in circulation, 4
  decrease in, 138–140, 139t
  effect of GVHD on, 90
  increased in DIC, 51
  replenishment/transfusion of, 33–34, 55, 138, 140
  complications of, 142–143
  sources for transfusion, 140
pleural effusion, 178f, 180
pleurodesis, 180
pluripotent hematopoietic stem cells (PHSCs), 1–4, 86
Pneumococcus, 113, 195
Pneumocystis carinii, 53, 112–113, 136t–137t, 137–138, 178f, 184
pneumonia, 44, 53, 90, 112, 138–139, 183–184
pneumonitis, 45t, 181

pneumothorax, from mobilization, 34
poikiloderma, 93
polyclonal antibodies, for GVHD therapy, 106–107
polymorphisms, 7
polymyositis, 197
polyserositis, 96
positive cell selection, 38, 109
practice standards, in HSCT programs, 73t, 73–74, 74f, 75
prednisone, 182, 253
premedications, before HSC infusion, 47
preparative regimens, 17t, 17–18, 43–46, 44t–45t. See also specific immunosuppressants
  and acute GVHD development, 86
  anemia caused by, 141
  nursing management of, 46t, 46–47
primary graft failure, 143. See also graft failure
Primaxin®, 135
processing, of stem cells, 37–38, 48, 67, 77, 77t, 201
prochlorperazine, 157t, 192
Prograf®, 98, 100t–101t, 142. See also tacrolimus
programmed cell death. See apoptosis
progressive chronic GVHD, 96–97, 97t
protein tyrosine kinase (PTK), 2
proteoglycans, 54
prothrombin time, in DIC, 51
Prudential Insurance Company of America, 78–80
Pseudomonas, 135, 148–151, 185, 195
psoralen and UVA irradiation (PUVA), 108–109, 111
psychological assessment
  in HSCT programs, 67
  prior to HSCT, 18
psychosocial stress
  of bone marrow harvest, 24–26
  experienced by patient/family, 20, 72–73, 245–246
  nursing management of, 117f–118f
  of rehospitalization, 216–217
Puget Sound Blood Center, 37f
pulmonary complications, 177–185, 178f
  from chemotherapy, 178f, 178–179, 179t
  of chronic GVHD, 95, 98t, 111

of HSC infusion, 46t
of preparative regimens, 44, 45t
from radiation, 179
pulmonary edema, 178f, 180–181
pulmonary embolism, 179–180
pulmonary fibrosis, 95
pulmonary function tests, 179
pulmonary veno-occlusive disease (PVOD), 178f, 181
pulsus paradoxus, 186
PUVA. See psoralen and UVA irradiation
pyrimethamine, 195

Q

quality assurance/improvement, in HSCT programs, 74, 74f, 75
quality of life, 115, 193
  conceptual model of, 237, 238f
  definitions of, 237
  family/caregiver, 246
  literature review concerning, 238–246, 239t–245t
  pediatric, 246
quantal mitosis, 3
Questran® (cholestyramine), 98t
quiescent onset GVHD, 96–97, 97t
quinidine, 139
quinine, 139
quinolones, 135

R

radiation fibrosis, 179
radiation-induced myelitis, 192
radiation pneumonitis, 179
radiation therapy. See also total body irradiation
  post-transplant, 214
random donor platelets, 140
Rapamune®, 169
rapamycin, 104t, 110, 118
Ras-dependent signaling pathway, 2
recruitment/retention, of transplant center staff, 64
rectal skin alterations, 159–160, 161t
recurrence anxiety, 20
red blood cells (RBCs), 1, 4, 54
  average number in circulation, 4
  breakdown of, 47
  decrease in, 140–142. See also anemia